Peripheral nerve disorders: pathology and genetics

Peripheral nerve disorders: pathology and genetics

EDITED BY

Jean-Michel Vallat

Neurology Laboratory
National Referral Center for Rare Peripheral Neuropathies
University Hospital
Limoges
France

Joachim Weis

Director, Institute of Neuropathology
RWTH Aachen University Hospital
JARA Brain Translational Medicine
Aachen
Germany

SERIES EDITORS

Francoise Gray

Department of Pathology
Lariboisière Hospital (AP-HP)
University Denis Diderot-Paris 7
France

Katy Keohane

Consultant Neuropathologist
Cork University Hospital
Ireland

FOREWORD BY

Peter J. Dyck

Department of Neurology, Mayo Clinic
Rochester, Minnesota
USA

WILEY Blackwell

Registered Office
John Wiley & Sons, Ltd, The Atrium, Southern Gate, Chichester, West Sussex, PO19 8SQ, UK

Editorial Offices
9600 Garsington Road, Oxford, OX4 2DQ, UK
111 River Street, Hoboken, NJ 07030-5774, USA

For details of our global editorial offices, for customer services and for information about how to apply for permission to reuse the copyright material in this book please see our website at www.wiley.com/wiley-blackwell

Library of Congress Cataloging-in-Publication Data

Peripheral nerve disorders (Vallat)
Peripheral nerve disorders : pathology and genetics / edited by Jean-Michel Vallat, Joachim Weis.
p. ; cm.
Includes bibliographical references and index.
ISBN 978-1-118-61843-1 (cloth)
I. Vallat, Jean-Michel, editor. II. Weis, Joachim, 1960– editor. III. International Society of Neuropathology, issuing body. IV. Title.
[DNLM: 1. Peripheral Nervous System Diseases–physiopathology. 2. Peripheral Nervous System Diseases–genetics. WL 520]
RC409
616.85′6–dc23

2014013299

A catalogue record for this book is available from the British Library.

Wiley also publishes its books in a variety of electronic formats. Some content that appears in print may not be available in electronic books.

hardback: 978-111-86184-3-1
ePDF: 978-111-86184-0-0 oBook: 978-111-86184-2-4
epub: 978-111-86184-1-7 mobi: 978-111-86183-9-4

Set in 8.5/12pts Meridien by SPi Publisher Services, Pondicherry, India
Printed and bound in Malaysia by Vivar Printing Sdn Bhd

1 2014

Contents

Contributor list

Douglas C. Anthony
Professor of Pathology and Laboratory Medicine
Department of Pathology and Laboratory Medicine
Alpert Medical School of Brown University
Pathologist-in-chief, Lifespan Academic Medical Center
Rhode Island, USA

Jean-Christophe Antoine MD
Service de Neurologie, Hôpital Nord
CHU de Saint-Etienne
France

Juan M. Bilbao MD, FRCP
Professor (Emeritus) of Laboratory Medicine
Department of Laboratory Medicine
University of Toronto
Ontario, Canada

Pierre Bouche MD
Department of Clinical Neurophysiology
APHP, Groupe Hospitalier Pitié-Salpêtrière
Paris, France

Sebastian Brandner MD, FRCPath
Professor of Neuropathology
Division of Neuropathology and Department of Neurodegenerative Disease
National Hospital for Neurology and Neurosurgery and UCL Institute of Neurology
London, UK

Leila Chimelli MD
Professor of Neuropathology
Department of Pathology, University Hospital
Federal University of Rio de Janeiro
Rio de Janeiro, Brazil

Kristl G. Claeys MD, PhD
Institute of Neuropathology and Department of Neurology
RWTH Aachen University Hospital and JARA Brain Translational Medicine
Aachen, Germany

Michael P. Collins MD
Associate Professor of Neurology
Department of Neurology
Medical College of Wisconsin
Wisconsin, USA

Umberto De Girolami MD
Professor of Pathology
Department of Pathology
Harvard Medical School and
Neuropathologist, Brigham and Women's Hospital
Boston, USA

P. James B. Dyck MD
Professor of Neurology
Department of Neurology
Mayo Clinic
Rochester, USA

Benjamin Ellezam MD, PhD
Assistant Clinical Professor
Department of Pathology and Cell Biology
Université de Montréal
CHU Sainte-Justine
Montreal, Canada

Benoît Funalot MD, PhD
Departments of Biochemistry, Genetics, and Neurology
National Referral Center for Rare Peripheral Neuropathies, CHU Limoges and EA6309 "Myelin Maintenance and Peripheral Neuropathies"
Limoges University Medicine School
Limoges, France

António Guimarães, MD
Department of Neuropathology
Hospital de Santo António, Centro Hospitalar do Porto
Instituto de Ciências Biomédicas Abel Salazar
Universidade do Porto
Porto, Portugal

Richard A.C. Hughes MD, FRCP, FMedSci
Emeritus Professor of Neurology
Department of Neurology
King's College London and Cochrane Neuromuscular Disease Group
MRC Centre for Neuromuscular Disease
National Hospital for Neurology and Neurosurgery
London, UK

Or Kakhlon PhD
Department of Neurology
Hadassah-Hebrew University Medical Centre
Jerusalem, Israel

Istvan Katona
Institute of Neuropathology
RWTH Aachen University Hospital and
JARA Brain Translational Medicine
Aachen, Germany

Yuichi Kawagashira MD, PhD
Department of Neurology
Nagoya University Graduate School of Medicine
Nagoya, Japan

Rosalind King
Honorary Principal Research Fellow
Department of Clinical Neurosciences, Institute of Neurology
University College London
London, UK

Haruki Koike MD, PhD
Lecturer, Department of Neurology
Nagoya University Graduate School of Medicine
Nagoya, Japan

David Lacomis MD
Professor, Department of Neurology and Pathology
University of Pittsburgh School of Medicine
Pittsburgh, USA

Martin Lammens MD, PhD
Head, Department of Pathology
Antwerp University Hospital
Edegem, and University of Antwerp
Antwerp, Belgium

Alexander Lossos MD
Department of Neurology
Hadassah-Hebrew University Medical Centre
Jerusalem, Israel

Laurent Magy MD, PhD
Neurology Laboratory
National Referral Center for Rare Peripheral Neuropathies
University Hospital
Limoges
France

Stéphane Mathis
Neurologist, Department of Neurology
La Milétrie University Hospital
Poitiers, France

Manoj Menezes FRACP
Department of Neurology
The Children's Hospital at Westmead
Sydney, Australia

Maria Nolano MD, PhD
Department of Neurology
"Salvatore Maugeri" Foundation
Telese, Italy

Carlos Ortiz-Hidalgo MD
Professor of Histology
Department of Tissue and Cell Biology
Universidad Panamericana
Chairman, Department of Surgical and Molecular Pathology
The American British Cowdray (ABC) Medical Centre
Mexico

Robert Ouvrier MD, FRACP
Emeritus Professor, The University of Sydney
Department of Neurology
The Children's Hospital at Westmead
Sydney, Australia

Manuel Melo Pires MD, PhD
Department of Neuropathology
Hospital de Santo António, Centro Hospitalar do Porto
Instituto de Ciências Biomédicas Abel Salazar
Universidade do Porto
Porto, Portugal

Andreas Roos
Institute of Neuropathology
RWTH Aachen University Hospital and
JARA Brain Translational Medicine
Aachen, Germany

Robert E. Schmidt MD, PhD
Department of Pathology and Immunology
Division of Neuropathology
Washington University School of Medicine
St. Louis, USA

J. Michael Schröder MD
Institute of Neuropathology
RWTH Aachen University Hospital and
JARA Brain Translational Medicine
Aachen, Germany

Jan Senderek
Friedrich Baur Institute
Department of Neurology
Ludwig-Maximilians University
Munich, Germany

Gen Sobue MD
Department of Neurology
Nagoya University Graduate School of Medicine
Nagoya, Japan

Dov Soffer MD
Department of Pathology
Hadassah-Hebrew University Medical Centre
Israel

Claudia Sommer MD
Professor of Neurology
Department of Neurology
University of Würzburg
Würzburg, Germany

Ricardo Taipa MD, FEBN
Department of Neuropathology
Hospital de Santo António, Centro Hospitalar do Porto
Instituto de Ciências Biomédicas Abel Salazar,
Universidade do Porto
Porto, Portugal

Meriem Tazir MD
Professor of Neurology
Laboratoire de Recherche de Neurosciences,
Service de Neurologie
Mustapha Bacha University Hospital
Algiers, Algeria

Anne Vital MD, PhD
Professor, Department of Pathology-Neuropathology
Service de Pathologie
Hôpital Pellegrin
Bordeaux, France

Roy O. Weller MD, PhD, FRCPath
Emeritus Professor of Neuropathology
Department of Neuropathology
Clinical and Experimental Sciences
Faculty of Medicine
University of Southampton
Southampton, UK

Foreword

It is exciting to welcome *Peripheral Nerve Disorders: Pathology and Genetics*. Like most future readers, I was not involved in the choice of authors and topics so it will be fun to explore the contents of this textbook. With you, I will enjoy seeing what topics are covered, new insights and mechanisms revealed, and adequacy of the illustrations. I hope and expect to be pleasantly surprised by the quality of the book, because I am familiar with many of the authors who are known for their contributions to the peripheral neuropathy field.

A quick look at the chapter headings indicates that the book will emphasize pathologic alterations and molecular genetics. To give these subjects context there will also be extensive descriptions of clinical disorders. This restricted approach probably makes sense because as we found (I and P. K. Thomas) it is increasingly difficult to review the whole subject of the neurobiology and diseases of the peripheral nervous system in a two-volume set of books as we attempted to do in our four editions of *Peripheral Neuropathy* (W. B. Saunders and Elsevier, Inc. 1975, 1984, 1993, and 2005). In confronting the issue of the breadth and complexity of knowledge about the peripheral nervous system, Co-editors of *Companion to Peripheral Neuropathy* (Elsevier, Inc., 2010) focused on new topics of interest to neuromuscular physicians (e.g., MRI targeted fascicular nerve biopsy, pathologic alterations, especially of focal nerve lesions and genetic topics). The present textbook edited by Vallat, Weis, Gray, and Keohane made the sensible decision to focus on pathology and genetics on the background of clinical disorders.

Europeans have contributed in a major way to the contents of this text. This is entirely reasonable considering the historic role Europeans have played in the history of peripheral nerve discovery (e.g., Remak; Virchow; Waller; Ranvier; Gombault and Mallet; Charcot, Marie, and Tooth; Friedreich; Aran and Duchenne; Cajal and Krücke – to name only a few).

From reading the Contents list, I judge that molecular genetic abnormalities are described by known clinical patterns of involvement. For the clinician it is helpful to classify neuropathies by which classes of neurons (fibers) are affected, by clinical and physiologic characterization of the pathologic abnormalities, and by the temporal pattern of involvement. With increasingly detailed information about molecular genetic abnormalities, it will be necessary to relate these genetic derangements to known clinical patterns of involvement. It is likely that, in a short period of time, chips with diverse multiple probes representing different genetic disorders will be available to decrease confusion.

Finally, I thank the authors and John Wiley & Sons, Ltd for their willingness to produce a textbook at this time, knowing that the writing of medical textbooks no longer provides high financial rewards. Hopefully, many readers will express their thanks by buying the book in print or online.

Peter J. Dyck, M.D.
Roy E. and Merle Meyer Professor of Neuroscience
Professor of Neurology, Mayo Medical School
Head of the Peripheral Neuropathy Research Laboratory, Mayo Clinic
Consultant in Neurology, Mayo Clinic, Rochester, MN

Preface

With this book, the International Society of Neuropathology is devoting a volume of the established series of "Pathology and Genetics" textbooks to the pathology of peripheral nerve diseases. It is regrettable but true that nerve biopsy has become less frequent in recent years, so neuropathologists have less experience than before in this technique. The knowledge accrued is diminishing, with long term implications for its sustainability. This also applies to electron microscopic (EM) examination. EM requires a dedicated team and elaborate instrumentation, and is thus nowadays often regarded as too expensive.

These views are held even though nerve biopsy (with electron microscopy) can provide a diagnosis, can point to a disease mechanism that will guide treatment, and can redirect investigation toward a hereditary neuropathy with implications for genetic counseling. For example, when neuropathy develops in patients undergoing chemotherapy for a hematological disorder, the differential diagnosis includes a neurotoxic effect of treatment or spread of the underlying process such as immunoglobulin or amyloid deposition or infiltration of malignant cells to directly involve nerves. Defining the exact pathological process leads to specific therapeutic intervention such as reduction of toxic therapy, or conversely, modification of immune therapy, a requirement for bone marrow transplant. As another example, even though clinical and electrophysiological criteria are useful for the diagnosis of Chronic Inflammatory Demyelinating Polyneuropathy (CIDP) or peripheral nerve vasculitis, in practice these criteria are often not sufficient; nerve biopsy will lead to diagnosis and treatment of patients with atypical clinical and neurophysiological features.

Regarding the hereditary neuropathies, correlation of histological and genetic findings is essential for a number of reasons. It is accepted that mutations of more than 60 genes are likely to be responsible for hereditary neuropathies. Nowadays the diagnosis is achieved in many cases by molecular genetic analysis; however, nerve biopsy can be helpful in identifying the decisive pathomechanisms especially in the growing number of cases where next generation sequencing techniques are employed and often reveal several candidate gene defects. Nerve biopsy will also uncover concomitant (e.g., inflammatory) pathology. Moreover, it is expected to provide clues for eventual therapeutic interventions, for example, by defining subgroups of patients. Finally, nerve biopsy analysis has contributed greatly to the understanding of the pathophysiology of neuropathies including hereditary neuropathies. Nerve biopsy studies will even increase in importance with the ever growing number of animal models that need to be correlated with and adjusted to the human pathology. Thus, contrary to earlier oversimplified views, at this point in time, it is not true that molecular biology will replace pathology. For a certain number of patients, all these techniques are very useful and complement each other, it being understood that nerve biopsy is an invasive process, so the decision to undertake it must be discussed on a case-by-case basis.

For the purpose of this volume, we felt it was important to devote a special chapter to skin biopsy in the investigation of small fiber or painful sensory neuropathies, given that this technique essentially studies unmyelinated intra-epidermal nerve fibers and that skin biopsies for this purpose are rapidly increasing in number.

We also included some clinical, electrophysiological, and other ancillary investigative data, depending on the context of the entities discussed. In practice integrating these combined variables together with the nerve biopsy results is key to a correct diagnosis. In fact this monograph is hoped to be of interest to all those involved in the study of peripheral nerve disorders: clinicians, neurophysiologists, neuropathologists, and molecular biologists.

Of course we have been able to benefit from the efforts of numerous international authors who wrote about their own area of expertise in human peripheral neuropathies, often also summarizing studies in animal models. Each chapter is accompanied by quality illustrations of the lesions described in the text. The interactions with the authors have been most productive, interesting, and constructive, and we sincerely thank them all.

We must also express our huge gratitude to Professors Francoise Gray and Katy Keohane for their editorial skills and patience and for their input into every chapter, to improve the overall style and English, and for ensuring that a quality volume was produced.

Jean-Michel Vallat and Joachim Weis
Limoges and Aachen

Abbreviations

(genes are written in italics)

α-Gal Alpha-Galactosidase
α -NAGA α -N-Acetylgalactosaminidase
AARS Alanyl-tRNA-synthetase
AAV ANCA-Associated Vasculitides
ABCA1 ATP-Binding Cassette Transporter A1
ACA Acrodermatitis chronica atrophicans
ACE Angiotensin-Converting Enzyme
ACR American College of Rheumatology
AD Autosomal Dominant
ADCA Autosomal dominant spinocerebellar atrophies
AFB Acid Fast Bacilli
AFLP Amplified Fragment Length Polymorphism
AIDP Acute Inflammatory Demyelinating Polyneuropathy
ALN Alcohol Related Neuropathy
ALS Amyotrophic Lateral Sclerosis
ALS11 Amyotrophic Lateral Sclerosis of Type 11
AMAN Acute Motor Axonal Neuropathy
AMP Adenosine Monophosphate
AMSAN Acute Motor and Sensory Axonal Neuropathy
ANA Antinuclear Antibody
ANCA Anti-Neutrophil Cytoplasmic Antibody
ANS Ataxia Neuropathy Spectrum
APBD Adult Polyglucosan Body Disease
APC antigen-Presenting Cell
Apo Apolipoproteins
ApoA-I Apolipoprotein A-I
ApoB Apolipoprotein B
AR Autosomal Recessive
AR CMT Autosomal Recessive Charcot–Marie–Tooth Neuropathy
AR CMT1 Autosomal Recessive Charcot–Marie–Tooth Neuropathy, of Demyelinating Type
AR CMT2 Autosomal Recessive Charcot–Marie–Tooth Neuropathy, of Axonal Type
ARHGEF10 Rho Guanine-Nucleotide Exchange [GEF] Factor 10
ARSA Arylsulfatase A
ATL1 Atlastin 1
B.b Borrelia burgdorferi
BBW rats Biobreeding Wor rats
BDNF Brain Derived Neurotrophic Factor
BEAR Brain Stem Evoked Auditory Responses
CAN Congenital Amyelinating Neuropathy
CANOMAD Chronic Ataxic Neuropathy, Ophthalmoplegia, IgM paraprotein, cold Agglutinins and Disialosyl antibodies
CCT Cytosolic Chaparonin-Containing T-complex peptide
CD4 Cluster of Differentiation 4
CES Cholesterol Emboli Syndrome
CETP Cholesteryl Ester Transfer Protein
CG Cryoglobulinemia
CHCC Chapel Hill Consensus Conference
CHIKV Chikungunya Virus
CHN Congenital Hypomyelination Neuropathy
CHS Chediak–Higashi Syndrome
CIDP Chronic Inflammatory Demyelinating Polyneuropathy/Polyradiculoneuropathy
CIM Critical Illness Myopathy
CIP Critical Illness Polyneuropathy
CIPA Congenital Insensitivity to Pain with Anhydrosis
CIPN Chemotherapy-Induced Toxic Peripheral Neuropathies
CMAP Compound Muscle Action Potential(s)
CMT Charcot–Marie–Tooth
CMT DI Charcot–Marie–Tooth Neuropathy, Autosomal Dominant, of Intermediate type
CMT RIA Charcot–Marie–Tooth Neuropathy, Autosomal Recessive, of Intermediate type A
CMT X X-linked Charcot–Marie–Tooth Neuropathy
CMT Charcot–Marie–Tooth disease/neuropathy
CMT1 Charcot–Marie–Tooth neuropathy, autosomal dominant, of demyelinating type
CMT2 Charcot–Marie–Tooth neuropathy, autosomal dominant, of axonal type/type 2
CMT4 Charcot–Marie–Tooth neuropathy, autosomal recessive, of demyelinating type
CMTID Intermediate Charcot–Marie–Tooth
CMTX X-linked Charcot–Marie–Tooth
CMV Cytomegalovirus
CNM Centronuclear Myopathy
CNS Central Nervous System
CNTF Ciliary Neuron Trophic Factor
COPD Chronic Obstructive Pulmonary Disease
COX Cytochrome c OXidase
CRMP5 Collapsin Response Mediator Protein 5
CSAP Compound Sensory Action Potential
CSF Cerebrospinal Fluid

CSNAP Compound Sensory Nerve Action Potential
CTD Connective Tissue Disease
CTL Cytotoxic T Lymphocyte
CTX Cerebrotendinous Xanthomatosis
Cx31 Connexin 31 (=GJB3)
Cx32 Connexin 32
DANP Diabetic Autonomic Neuropathy
DCBU Dorsal Cutaneous Branch of the Ulnar nerve
DCCT Diabetes Control and Complications Trial
DCRPN Diabetic Cervical Radiculoplexus Neuropathy
DDT Dichloro-Diphenyl-Trichloroethane
DHH Desert Hedgehog Homolog (*Drosophila*)
dHMN Distal Hereditary Motor Neuropathy
DIC Disseminated Intravascular Coagulation
DILS Diffuse Infiltrative Lymphocytic Syndrome
DLRPN Diabetic Lumbosacral Radiculoplexus Neuropathy
DNA DeoxyRiboNucleic Acid
DNM Dynamin
DNM2 Dynamin 2
DNMT DNA Methyl Transferase
DNP Diabetic Neuropathy
DRG Dorsal Root Ganglia
DSD Déjérine–Sottas Disease
DSS Déjérine–Sottas Syndrome
dSMA Distal SMA
DSP Distal Sensory Polyneuropathy
DβH Dopamine β-hydroxylase
EAN Experimental Allergic Neuritis
EBV Epstein–Barr virus
EEG Electroencephalogram
EGPA Eosinophilic Granulomatosis with PolyAngiitis
EGR Early Growth Response Gene
EGR2 Early Growth Response 2 encoding gene
ELISA Enzyme-Linked Immunosorbent Assay
EM Electron Microscopy
EMA Epithelial Membrane Antigen
EMG Electromyography
ENF Epidermal Nerve Fibres
ENMG ElectroNeuroMyoGraphy
ER Endoplasmic Reticulum
ERK/MAPK Extracellular Signal-Regulated Kinases/ Mitogen-Activated Protein Kinases
ERT Enzyme Replacement Therapy
ESR Erythrocyte Sedimentation Rate
FAM134B FAMily with sequence similarity 134, member B
FAP Familial Amyloid Neuropathy
FBLN5 Fibulin 5
FFM Focally Folded Myelin
FGD4 FYVE, RhoGEF and PH Domain-containing protein 4 encoding gene
FIG4 Polyphosphoinositide phosphatase encoding gene
FLAIR Fluid-Attenuated Inversion-Recovery
FLC Fibrous Long-spacing Collagen
Frabin FGD1-related F-actin binding protein
FSGS Focal Segmental GlomeruloSclerosis
GAN Giant Axonal Neuropathy (*GAN1*)
GAP-43 Growth Associated Protein-43
GARS Glycyl-tRNA Synthetase
Gb3 GloBotriaosylceramide
GBA GlucocereBrosidase
GBE Glycogen Branching Enzyme
GBE1 Glycogen Branching Enzyme gene 1
GBS Guillain–Barré Syndrome
GCA Giant Cell Arteritis
GDAP1 Ganglioside-Induced Differentiation-Associated PROTEIN 1 encoding gene
GJB1 Gap Junction Protein Beta 1
GLA Galactosidase A
GLB1 β-Galactosidase
GLUT-1 Glucose Transporter 1
GM1 Monosialoganglioside
GM2 Disialoganglioside
GPA Granulomatosis with Polyangiitis
GPCR G-Protein-Coupled-Receptor
GSD IV Glycogen Storage Disease type IV
GTPase Guanosine Triphosphate Hydrolase
Gβ_4 Guanine-nucleotide-binding protein subunit beta-4
H&E Hematoxylin and Eosin
HAART High Activity Antiretroviral Treatment
HB Hansen's Bacilli
HBV Hepatitis B Virus
HCV Hepatitis C Virus
HDL High-Density Lipoprotein
HEXA Hexosaminidase A
HHV Human Herpes Viruses
HINT1 Histidine triad Nucleotide binding protein 1 encoding gene
HIV Human Immunodeficiency Virus
HK1 Hexokinase 1 encoding gene
HMG-Co-A Hydroxymethylglutaryl coenzyme-A
HMN Hereditary Motor Neuropathy
HMSN Hereditary Motor and Sensory Neuropathy
HMSN II Hereditary Motor and Sensory Neuropathy, autosomal dominant, of axonal type
HMSN III Hereditary Motor and Sensory Neuropathy of type 3 (same as DSS)
HMSNL Hereditary Motor and Sensory Neuropathy, of type Lom
HMSNR Hereditary Motor and Sensory Neuropathy, of type Russe
HNPP Hereditary Neuropathy with Liability to Pressure Palsy
HSAN Hereditary Sensory and Autonomic Neuropathies
HSF1 Heat Shock Transcription Factor 1
HSN Hereditary Sensory (and autonomic) Neuropathies

HSP	Hereditary Spastic Paraplegia
HSP	Heat Shock Protein
HSPB1	Heat Shock 27kD protein 1 encoding gene (same as *HSP27*)
HSV	Herpes Simplex Virus
HTLV1	Human T Lymphocytic Virus 1
HUV	Hyopcomplementemic Urticarial Vasculitis
ICOS	Inducible Costimulator/T cell Stimulator
ICU	Intensive Care Unit
ID CMT	Intermediate Dominant CMT
IDPN	Iminodipropionitrile
IENF	Intra-Epidermal Nerve Fibers
IENFD	Intra-Epidermal Nerve Fiber Density
IF	Immunofluorescence
Ig	Immunoglobulin
IgA	Immunoglobulin A
IGT	Impaired Glucose Tolerance
INAD	Infantile Neuroaxonal Dystrophy
INF2	Inverted Formin2
IOSCA	Infantile-Onset Spinocerebellar Ataxia
IRIS	Immune Reconstitution Inflammatory Syndrome
ISEL	*In Situ* End-Labeling
IVIg	Intravenous Immunoglobulin
KARS	lysyl-tRNA synthetase gene
kDa	Kilodalton
KSS	Kearns–Sayre Syndrome
LCB1	Long Chain Base one
LD	Lyme Disease
LDL	Low Density Lipoproteins
LHN	Localized Hypertrophic Neuropathy
LHON	Leber's Hereditary Optic Neuropathy
LITAF	Lipopolysaccharide-Induced TNF Factor
LLON	Leprosy Late-Onset Neuropathy
LMNA	Lamin A/C Encoding Gene
LOTS	Late-Onset Tay–Sachs disease
LRSAM1	Leucine Rich repeat and Sterile Alpha Motif containing 1 gene
LS	Leigh Syndrome
LS	Lumbosacral
LTX	Liver Transplant
LWR	London White Resin
MADSAM	Multifocal Acquired Demyelinating Sensory And Motor (neuropathy)
MAG	Myelin-Associated Glycoprotein
MAL	Myelin and Lymphocyte Protein
MBP	Myelin Basic Protein
MCHS	Myo-Cerebro-Hepatopathy Spectrum
MED25	Mediator complex subunit 25 encoding gene
MELAS	Mitochondrial Encephalopathy, Lactic Acidosis, and Stroke-like episodes
MEMSA	Myoclonic Epilepsy, Myopathy, and Sensory Ataxia
Merlin	Moesin-Ezrin-Radixin-Like protein
MERRF	Myoclonic Epilepsy with Ragged Red Fibers
MFN2	Mitofusin 2 encoding gene
MFNP	Minifascicular neuropathy
MFS	Miller–Fisher Syndrome
MG	Monoclonal Gammopathy
MGUS	Monoclonal Gammopathy of Undetermined Significance
MHC	Major Histocompatibility Complex
MIRAS	Mitochondrial Recessive Ataxia Syndrome
MM	Multiple Mononeuropathy
MN	Morton's Neuroma
MNCV	Motor Nerve Conduction Velocity
MNGIE	Mitochondrial Neuro-Gastro-Intestinal Encephalomyopathy
MPA	Microscopic Polyangiitis
MPNST	Malignant Peripheral Nerve Sheath Tumor
MPO	Myeloperoxidase
MPZ	Myelin Protein Zero
MRC	Medical Research Council
MRC scale	Medical Research Council scale
MRI	Magnetic Resonance Imaging
mRNA	Messenger Ribonucleic Acid
MRS	Magnetic Resonance Spectroscopy
mtDNA	mitochondrial DNA
MTM1	Myotubularin 1 protein
MTMR13	Myotubularin-Related protein 13 encoding gene
MTMR2	Myotubularin-Related protein-2 encoding gene
MTMR5	Myotubularin-Related protein 5
MTP	Microsomal Triglyceride Transfer Protein
MUP	Motor-Unit action Potential
NANA	N-Acetylneuraminic (sialic) Acid
NARP	Neuropathy, Ataxia, and Retinitis Pigmentosa
NB	Nerve Biopsy
NBIA	Neurodegeneration with Brain Iron Accumulation
NCS	Nerve Conduction Study
NCV	Nerve Conduction Velocity
NDRG1	N-myc Downstream-Regulated Gene 1
NEFL	Neurofilament Light encoding gene/ polypeptide
NF1	Neurofibromatosis 1
NF2	Neurofibromatosis 2
NF-L	Neurofilament Light chains
NGF	Nerve Growth Factor
NGFB	Nerve Growth Factor β
NOS	Nitric Oxide Synthase
NRG-1	Axonal Neuregulin-1
NSVN	Nonsystemic Vasculitic Neuropathy
NT-1	Neurotrophin-3
NT-4/5	Neurotrophin 4/5
NT-6	Neurotrophin-6
NTRK	Neurotrophic Tyrosine Kinase
P0	Myelin Protein zero
P100	P100 wave (P for positive, and 100 for 100 milliseconds)

PAN	Polyarteritis Nodosa
PAS	Periodic Acid-Schiff stain
PBM	Peroneus Brevis Muscle
PCR	Polymerase Chain Reaction
PCWH	Peripheral demyelinating neuropathy, Central dysmyelinating leukodystrophy, Waardenburg syndrome, and Hirschsprung disease
PE	Plasma Exchange
PEO	Progressive External Ophtalmoplegia
PGB	Polyglucosan Body
PGP 9.5	Protein-Gene-Product 9.5
PGP	Protein Gene Product
PH	Pleckstrin Homology
PHYH	Phytanoyl-CoA Hydroxylase
$PI(3,5)P_2$	Phosphatidylinositol 3,5-bisphosphate
PI3K	Phosphatidylinositol 3-kinase
PIG-7	P53 inductible gene-7
PKAN	Pantothenate Kinase-Associated Neurodegeneration
PLEKHG5	Pleckstrin Homology domain-containing, family G, member 5
PLP	Proteolipid Protein
PMP22	Peripheral Myelin Protein 22
PN	Painful Neuropathy
PN	Polyneuropathies
PNP	Peripheral Neuropathy
PNS	Paraneoplastic Neurological Syndromes
PNS	Peripheral Nervous System
POEMS	Polyneuropathy, Organomegaly, Endocrine features, M (Monoclonal) protein, Skin lesions
PP	Progressive Polyneuropathy
PR3	Proteinase 3
PRKWNL	Protein Kinase-With-No-Lysine
PRPSI	Phosphoribosylpyrophosphate Synthetase I
PRX	Periaxin encoding gene
PS2	type 2 peroxisomal targeting signal
PSW	Positive Sharp Waves
QST	Quantitative Sensory Testing
RAB7	RAS-related protein 7 gene/oncogene
RAPD	Ribosomal gene probes, random Amplification of Polymorphic DNA
RF	Rheumatoid Factor
RhoGTPases	Rho family of small Guanosine Triphosphatase (GTP)-binding proteins
RLS	Roussy–Levy syndrome
RPH	Reactive Perineurial Hyperplasia
RPN	Radiculoplexus Neuropathy
SAC3	SAC domain containing inositol phosphatase 3 encoding gene
SANDO	Sensory Ataxic Neuropathy with Dysarthria and Ophthalmoplegia
SAP 1	Saposin
SBF1	SET Binding Factor 1 encoding gene
SBF2	SET Binding Factor 2 encoding gene
SC	Schwann Cell
SCA	Spinocerebellar Ataxia
SCAE	Spino-Cerebellar Ataxia with Epilepsy
SCAN1	Spinocerebellar Ataxia with axonal neuropathy
SCLC	Small Cell Lung Cancer
SCN	Solitary Circumscribed Neuroma
SCN9A	Sodium Channel voltage gated type IX alpha subunit
SD	Standard Deviation
SDH	Succinate Dehydrogenase
SEPs	Somatosensory Evoked Potentials
SH3	Src-Homology-3
SH3TC2	SH3 domain and Tetratricopeptide repeat domain 2 encoding gene
SIMPLE	Small Integral Membrane Protein of Lysosomal/Late Endosome
SMA	Spinal Muscular Atrophy
SMARCB1	SWI/SNF-related, Matrix-associated, Actin-dependent Regulator of Chromatin, subfamily B, member 1
SNAP	Sensory Nerve Action Potential
SPG	Spastic Paraplegia
SPN	superficial Peroneal Nerve
SPOAN	Spastic Paraplegia, Optic Atrophy, and Neuropathy
SPSMA	Scapuloperoneal SMA
SPTLC1	Serine Palmitoyltranferase long chain base subunit 1
SSEPs	Somatosensory Evoked Action Potentials
SSN	Subacute Sensory Neuronopathy (SSN)
SVN	Systemic Vasculitic Neuropathy
TAN	Tropical Ataxic Neuropathy
TLI	Terminal Latency Index
TN	Traumatic Neuroma
TNF	Tumor Necrosis Factor
TRPA-1	Transient Receptor Potential Ankyrin 1
TRPV1	Transient Receptor Potential Vanilloid type 1
TRPV4	Transient Receptor Potential cation channel, subfamily V, member 4 gene
TSP	Tropical Spastic Paraparesis
TTR	Transthyretin
TyrRS	Tyrosyl-tRNA synthetase
UML	Uncompacted Myelin Lamellae
VEGF	Vascular Endothelial Growth Factor
VIP	Vasoactive Intestinal Polypeptide
VLDL	Very Low Density Lipoproteins
VZV	Varicella Zoster Virus
WHO	World Health Organization
WldS	Slow Wallerian Degeneration
WNK1	WNK lysine deficient protein kinase 1
WSM	Widely Spaced Myelin
ZDF rats	Zucker Diabetic Fatty rats

CHAPTER 1

Clinical assessment and classification of peripheral nerve diseases

Pierre Bouche

Department of Clinical Neurophysiology, APHP, Groupe Hospitalier Pitié-Salpêtrière, Paris, France

Pathophysiology

The major processes underlying peripheral nerve lesions will be detailed in Chapter 7 entitled "Basic pathologic reactions."

- *Wallerian degeneration* occurs following a physical interruption of healthy axons in a nerve trunk. The changes occur distal to the transection site. There is complete paralysis and loss of sensation in the territory of the nerve trunk immediately following the nerve lesion. Axons and myelin sheaths degenerate distal to the site of transection. Nerve conduction disappears in a few days in myelinated fibers (usually between 5 and 8 days) but takes longer to vanish in unmyelinated fibers.
- *Segmental demyelination* is due to damage to the myelin sheath, sparing the axons. Depending on the extent of demyelination, nerve conduction is slowed or blocked. Slowing of nerve conduction without block does not lead to a motor deficit. Conduction block may be transient and remyelination may be rapid with complete recovery in few days but may take up to 3 months. Pure segmental demyelination is not common and there is usually a variable degree of associated axonal degeneration. In chronic polyneuropathies, demyelination and remyelination proceed, leading to hypertrophic nerve fibers (onion bulb formations).
- *Axonal degeneration* causes a distal breakdown of axons. Paralysis is roughly proportional to axonal loss. The clinical features are usually a symmetric distal sensorimotor deficit in the lower limbs. It is frequently due to metabolic disorders or toxins. Recovery takes much longer than in demyelinating neuropathies; axonal regeneration may take more than a year.
- *Neuronopathy* corresponds to a lesion of the nerve cell body and can be a motor neuronopathy (anterior horn cell) or a sensory ganglionopathy (sensory ganglion).

Clinical examination

Pattern of distribution of nerve involvement

The pattern of distribution of peripheral nerve involvement is very helpful and important for initial diagnostic workup.

The main patterns are:

- *Mononeuropathy*, which comprises focal lesions of peripheral nerves. The usual causes are trauma, focal compression by external pressure or entrapment. It may also be an isolated feature of a more widespread process such as a vasculitis or a hereditary neuropathy with liability to pressure palsies (HNPP).
- *Multiple mononeuropathy (or multiplex mononeuropathy, mononeuritis multiplex)* is the involvement of multiple separate peripheral nerves, which may appear simultaneously or serially. The main causes are vasculitis, diabetes, and leprosy but it may also be due to a focal variant of chronic inflammatory demyelinating polyneuropathy (CIDP, or a multifocal motor neuropathy. HNPP may also present as a multiple mononeuropathy.
- *Polyneuropathy* is a generalized neuropathy and is symmetrical or slightly asymmetrical. It may be distal or distal and proximal if roots are also involved as in

Peripheral Nerve Disorders: Pathology and Genetics, First Edition. Edited by Jean-Michel Vallat, Joachim Weis, Francoise Gray, and Katy Keohane.

polyradiculoneuropathy. In distal symmetrical polyneuropathy, nerve fibers appear affected in a length-dependent way: toes and feet are affected first. This type of polyneuropathy is mainly due to metabolic diseases (diabetes). In polyradiculoneuropathy, both roots and nerves are affected and an inflammatory/immune cause is generally found.
- Other presentations are *plexopathy* and *radiculopathy*.

Medical history

Clinical assessment of neuropathies should include a careful past medical history, current and past medications, exposure to heavy metals and solvents, social and family history, and review of systemic diseases.

Social history review includes patient's occupation, hobbies, and behavior (smoking, alcohol, sexual preference, recreational or intravenous drug use).

Family history is important, especially in chronic, long-standing neuropathies. General inquiries are frequently not helpful; examination of family members is better.

Course of the disease: The course may be acute, over days to four weeks, subacute, weeks to months, chronic, or long standing (onset during childhood). The course may be monophasic, progressive, or relapsing.

Clinical presentation

Peripheral nerve diseases may present with motor and/or sensory and autonomic symptoms (see Table 1.1).

Table 1.1 Causes of neuropathy according to the clinical presentation.

Predominantly motor neuropathies	
Inflammatory/immune neuropathies	Acute (Guillain–Barré syndrome)
	Subacute
	Chronic (CIDP) progressive or relapsing
Acute intermittent porphyria	
Diphteritic neuropathy	
Lead neuropathy	Frequently upper limb onset
Diabetic neuropathy	Lumbosacral plexopathy
	Lower limb proximal neuropathy (diabetic amyotrophy)
Inherited motor-sensory neuropathies	Charcot–Marie–Tooth diseases (I, II, III)
Predominantly sensory neuropathies	
Global sensory loss	Carcinomatous sensory neuropathy
	Diabetic sensory neuropathy
	Most of the metabolic/endocrine neuropathies
	Most of the toxic neuropathies
	Hereditary sensory neuropathies
Loss of large-fiber modalities: ataxic form	Idiopathic sensory neuropathy
	Ganglionopathies
	Neuropathy associated with Sjögren syndrome
	Cisplatin neuropathy
Loss of small-fiber modalities	Hereditary sensory neuropathies
	Lepromatous neuropathy
	Diabetic small fiber neuropathy
	Amyloid neuropathies
	Fabry disease
	Tangier disease
	Painful small fiber neuropathy
Predominant autonomic dysfunction	
	Diabetic neuropathies
	Amyloid neuropathies
	Pandysautonomia
	Hereditary dysautonomia (Riley–Day syndrome)
	Rare alcoholic neuropathies

The main presenting complaints for most neuropathies are some combination of weakness, sensory disturbance, and walking difficulties.

Patients variably describe their sensory symptoms as tingling, swelling, stabbing, bunched-up socks, prickling, icy, hot, and clumsy. Frequently all these abnormal feelings are referred to as *paresthesia*. Neuropathic painful symptoms may be described as throbbing, burning, or like an electric shock.

Motor symptoms are frequently distal at the onset: patients often complain of tripping over kerbs, or difficulty walking. They may notice a stepping gait due to foot drop. Limb ataxia is the major complaint in large-fiber neuropathies (ganglionopathies). Whether the onset is proximal or distal, in upper or lower limbs, is diagnostically important.

Other positive motor symptoms include tremor, fasciculation, myotonia, cramps, neuromyotonia, and the syndrome of continuous motor unit activity, moving toes (in the painful legs and moving toes syndrome), and restless legs syndrome.

Examination

Neurological examination needs to be complete. A general physical examination may provide clues to the diagnosis.

Neurological examination

Motor examination

It is a good practice to begin by watching the patient stand and walk, then do the Romberg's test, asking the patient to rise onto their heels and toes. Thereafter, look for wasting of distal upper and lower limb muscles, especially in the peroneal muscles in the lower limbs and the intrinsic muscles of the hand.

Strength is usually graded using the Medical Research Council (MRC) grading scale (see Table 1.2).

Mild or early weakness is best assessed in muscles such as the toe flexors and extensors. The interosseous and thenar intrinsic muscles of the hands must be examined as well as the proximal muscles in the upper and lower limbs.

The distribution of weakness is crucial for diagnosis. Does the weakness involve distal extremities, or is it both proximal and distal? Does the weakness have a symmetric distribution? Does the weakness involve neck or facial muscles?

Table 1.2 Expanded MRC scale for manual muscle testing [1].

Grade	Degree of strength
5	Normal strength
5–	Equivocal, barely detectable weakness
4+	Definite but slight weakness
4	Able to move the joint against combination of gravity and some resistance
4–	Capable of minimal resistance
3+	Capable of transient resistance but collapses abruptly
3	Able to move through full range against gravity without resistance to the movement
3–	Able to move against gravity but not through full range
2	Able to move with gravity eliminated
1	Flicker of movement
0	No movement

Source: Bromberg & Smith, 2002. Reproduced with permission of Lippincott Williams & Wilkins.

Sensory examination

Sensory examination is difficult since it is mainly subjective and dependent on the patient's cooperation. Examination should involve testing for light touch, pain, vibration, and proprioception.

The inability to distinguish between touch and pin suggests a loss of nociceptive fibers.

The joint position sense that assesses large diameter fibers is usually tested in the big toe.

Temperature must be tested using cold and hot tubes over the skin. It assesses unmyelinated and small fibers.

Deep tendon reflexes

Sensory fibers of the reflex arc are more vulnerable than motor fibers.

Loss of tendon reflex is usually an indication of loss or lesions of large-diameter fibers and is common in peripheral neuropathy, but may not develop until late stage in small-fiber neuropathy.

Autonomic signs

Few neuropathies have subjective and severe autonomic disturbances (orthostatic hypotension, bowel or bladder dysfunction, impotence in men).

Evaluation of autonomic and small nerve fiber involvement requires specialized tests, including *quantitative sensory testing* (QST) and skin biopsy (cf. Chapter 3).

Neuropathies associated with autonomic disturbances are very similar to those associated with small fiber involvement (diabetes, amyloidosis). Rare purely autonomic disturbances include pandysautonomia (usually acute), hereditary dysautonomia (Riley–Day syndrome), and idiopathic dysautonomia (usually cholinergic or adrenergic).

General examination

- *Skeletal deformities* are usually associated with inherited neuropathies with an onset in infancy. They frequently involve the foot (pes cavus) and spine (scoliosis). Joint deformities are associated with disorders in which there is a marked loss of sensory fibers. Neuropathic joint deformities are called Charcot or pseudotabetic joints, resulting from repeated trauma in the absence of pain sensation. Bone resorption, pathologic fractures, and osteomyelitis are features of inherited sensory neuropathy.
- *Changes in skin, hair, and nails.* Mutilating acropathy is characterized by plantar painless ulcerations and is observed in diabetes, amyloidosis, lepromatous, alcoholic, hereditary sensory, and autonomic neuropathies. Hyperpigmentation (melanodermia) may be present in the POEMS syndrome (polyneuropathy, organomegaly, endocrine features, M protein, skin lesions). Purpura, livedo reticularis can be seen in vasculitic neuropathies with or without cryoglobulinemia. Angiokeratomas are especially associated with the Fabry disease. Curly hair is the main sign of giant axonal neuropathy. Mee's lines are observed in arsenic and thallium neuropathies.
- *Xerostomia, xerosis or cutaneous sicca (dry mouth, eyes, and skin), and salivary gland swelling* are features of Sjögren's syndrome. Enlarged orange tonsils are the main mucosal sign in Tangier disease.
- *Ocular manifestations.* Uveitis may be observed in sarcoid and rheumatoid arthritis neuropathies. Scleritis is mainly found in connective tissue disease and vasculitic neuropathies. Corneal opacities are seen in Fabry disease and are the main characteristic feature of gelsolin amyloid neuropathy. Vitreous opacities are found in transthyretin amyloid neuropathies. In Refsum's disease, lens subluxation, optic atrophy, and retinitis pigmentosa are the main ocular signs.

Electrophysiological examination

Electrophysiological examination must be considered as an extension of the clinical evaluation.

Electrodiagnostic studies are the most useful laboratory test in the assessment of a patient with peripheral neuropathy. They can validate peripheral nerve involvement and eliminate other causes (central nervous system diseases, myopathic disorders, non-organic symptoms). They provide crucial information as to the type of fibers involved (motor, sensory, or both), the pathophysiology (axonal or demyelinating neuropathy), the pattern of involvement (symmetric or multifocal), the severity and time course (mild, severe, acute, or chronic). Electrodiagnostic testing for neuropathies includes needle electromyography (EMG) and nerve conduction studies.

Electromyography

EMG is important to differentiate neurogenic from myopathic disorders.

Spontaneous activity

In normal subjects, needle insertion in muscles is normal at rest, outside the end-plate zone. In the end-plate zone spontaneous activity may be observed (end-plate noise). Elsewhere there is no spontaneous activity.

In acute ongoing denervation of muscle, *fibrillation potentials* and/or *positive sharp waves* (PSW) are observed. They appear within 1–3 weeks after loss of axonal continuity, depending on the length of the distal nerve stump. Therefore, fibrillation potentials can persist for many years after denervation. They also are observed in some myopathies, mainly in the inflammatory myopathies (myositis) and some muscular dystrophies.

Fibrillation potentials and PSW have the same significance. In acute nerve lesions, fibrillation potentials do not appear before 7 days in short nerve segments. In chronic neuropathies, it indicates the amount of axonal damage.

Other abnormal spontaneous activities may occur in pathological muscles:

- *Fasciculation potentials:* these are similar to motor unit action potentials in dimensions and have been attributed to spontaneous activation of muscle fibers of individual motor units. They are found in pathological processes involving the anterior horn cell, especially amyotrophic lateral sclerosis.
- *Myotonic discharges:* these consist of high-frequency trains of action potentials. Their frequency waxes and wanes (they sound like a dive bomber on

loudspeaker). They are found in patients with various forms of myotonia.

Involuntary muscle contraction

In normal subjects, with minimal muscle contraction, single motor-unit action potentials (MUPs) are elicited and the shape, voltage (amplitude), duration, and frequency of firing must be noted. Amplitude and duration depend on the number of muscle fibers within the motor unit.

In patients with disorders due to peripheral nerve disease, functional motor units are reduced. The density of electrical activity recorded from affected muscles is diminished when the voluntary contraction is maximal (loss of MUPs). To respond to the maximal contraction, there is an increase in the rate of firing of motor units. The morphology of MUPs is modified: there is an increase in amplitude due to augmentation of the motor unit territory as a consequence of "collateral sprouting," sometimes giving rise to giant MUPs. This feature is best observed in anterior horn cell diseases. In peripheral nerve lesions, MUPs do not increase significantly, except sometimes in very chronic polyneuropathies such as some CIDP and CMT cases.

Nerve conduction studies

Motor conduction studies

These studies involve stimulation of a nerve and recording an evoked response from the corresponding muscle. For example, the ulnar nerve is stimulated at the wrist, below and above the elbow and at the axilla, the evoked response is taken from the abductor digiti minimi in the hand (see Fig. 1.1). If possible, the nerve should be stimulated all along its length. Generally, muscular evoked responses (compound muscle action potential, CMAP) are expressed in millivolts (mV). Duration, area, and amplitude of the CMAP are measured.

Distal latency (i.e., the time between the stimulation and the onset of the negative wave of the CMAP) is measured. Nerve conduction velocity is expressed in meters per second (m/s) and is calculated by dividing the distance between two points of stimulation by the time delay between these two points (conduction velocity in m/s = distance in mm/(proximal latency minus distal latency in m/s). The conduction velocity cannot be measured accurately in the distal segment as the latency is partly due to conduction along the neuromuscular junction and within the muscle.

Reduction of the CMAP amplitude reflects the amount of fiber loss and is mainly observed in rapidly progressive neuropathies. In more chronic disorders, the CMAP amplitude does not correlate well with fiber loss, because motor units remodel during collateral sprouting. Motor nerve conduction velocity is determined by the largest fibers of the nerve. The nerve conduction velocity value may therefore be normal if the large fibers are spared, although the CMAP amplitude may be markedly reduced. This is found in axonal disorders (see Table 1.3 here).

In demyelinating neuropathy, motor nerve conduction velocity is markedly reduced if the study incorporates

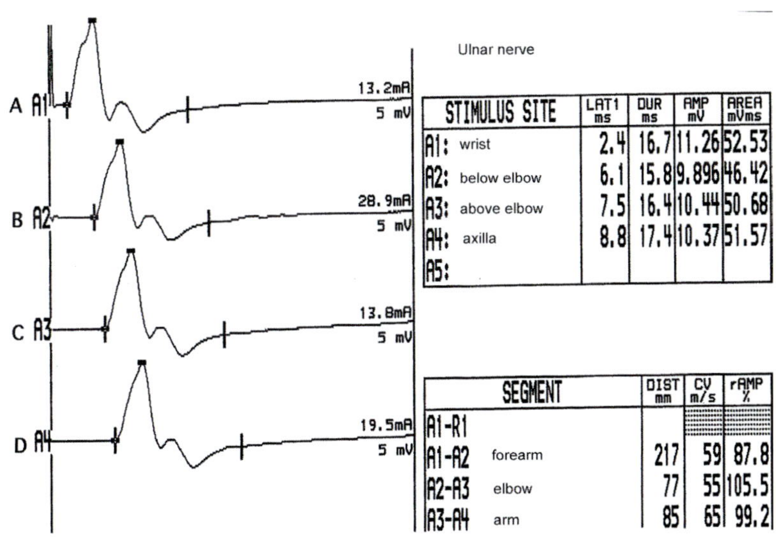

Figure 1.1 Motor nerve conduction study of the ulnar nerve in a normal subject.

Table 1.3 Electrodiagnostic criteria to distinguish primary demyelinating neuropathy from primary axonal neuropathy.

Primary demyelinating neuropathy	
Distal CMAP amplitude	Mild to moderate reduction, depending on the amount of axonal damage and temporal dispersion
Conduction block	May be present (in acquired polyneuropathy)
Temporal dispersion	Present mainly in inflammatory neuropathy
Distal latency	Moderately to markedly prolonged
Conduction velocity	Moderately to markedly slowed
F-wave latency	Moderately to markedly prolonged
Needle EMG	Mild to moderate denervation, depending on the degree of associated fiber loss
Primary axonal neuropathy	
Distal CMAP amplitude	Slightly to markedly reduced, depending on the degree of fiber loss
Conduction block	Absent
Temporal dispersion	Absent
Distal latency	Normal to mildly prolonged
Conduction velocity	Normal to mildly slowed
F-wave latency	Normal to mildly prolonged
Needle EMG	Mild to severe denervation

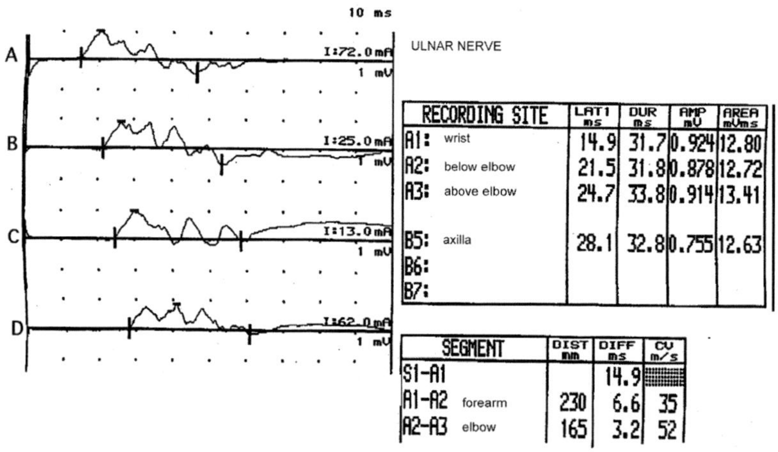

Figure 1.2 Temporal dispersion in a patient with a chronic inflammatory demyelinating polyneuropathy.

the demyelinating zone. Conduction block and temporal dispersion may also be observed. Focal conduction block is due to the inability of the stimulated nerve fibers to normally conduct action potentials. It may be complete or partial. The clinical effect of conduction block is a motor deficit which correlates with the number of nerve fibers that are blocked. Conduction block may be located at every part of the nerve. In focal neuropathies (compressive or entrapment) it is located at the site of entrapment or compression due to focal paranodal or segmental demyelination. When located outside the usual sites of compression, conduction block usually occurs in acquired demyelinating neuropathies. Detection of conduction blocks is important to distinguish between acquired and hereditary demyelinating neuropathies; it may be a transient phenomenon with a rapid recovery, which is mainly due to ischemia.

Temporal dispersion results from the spectrum of arrival times of nerve impulses into the muscle. It is due to slow conduction velocities of individual nerve fibers caused by demyelination. Temporal dispersion may be observed with distal stimulation (see Fig. 1.2) and is

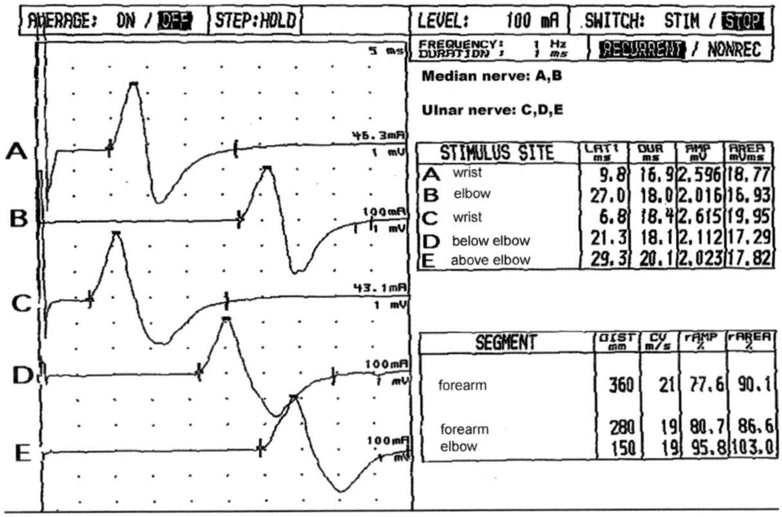

Figure 1.3 Motor conduction velocity in a patient with CMT 1A.

characteristic of chronic demyelinating polyneuropathy. In multifocal motor neuropathy conduction block occurs alone, usually without temporal dispersion. It is observed in acute inflammatory polyneuropathy (Guillain–Barré syndrome), especially during the early stages. They may be difficult to elicit because of their very proximal localization. In chronic demyelinating polyneuropathy, conduction blocks and temporal dispersion usually occur in the inflammatory forms. Conduction blocks are not observed in demyelinating polyneuropathy associated with paraproteinemia, including IgM monoclonal gammopathy. In CMT, there is neither conduction block nor temporal dispersion as the demyelination is uniform all along the nerve length (see Fig. 1.3).

The terminal latency index (TLI) is the ratio between proximal and distal conduction velocities. For example, the median nerve TLI is the ratio between motor conduction velocity at the forearm and distal conduction from distal stimulation at the wrist over a 6-cm distance. In normal subjects, the TLI is 0.34. In patients with distal demyelination (in some CIDP and IgM polyneuropathies) the TLI is low, usually under 0.25. In CMT type 1A, the TLI is the same as in normal subjects, because the demyelination is uniform, identical in proximal and distal segments of the nerve.

Sensory nerve conduction study

The nerve is stimulated, usually using surface electrodes; the evoked potential is recorded over the same nerve using either needle or surface electrodes. The sensory nerve action potential (SNAP) amplitude is much lower than the motor evoked potential and is usually expressed in microvolts (μv). The nerve may be stimulated using orthodromic or antidromic techniques. Sensory conduction velocity is measured in the most rapidly conducting fibers from the site of stimulation to the onset of the negative peak of the *compound sensory action potential* (CSAP). Small fibers cannot be tested and the *compound sensory nerve action potential* (CSNAP) amplitude depends on the number of large myelinated fibers (8–9 μm or more).

A normal SNAP implies that large diameter dorsal root ganglion cells and large distal myelinated axons are normally functioning.

Other techniques

F-wave study. This measures the latency over the complete length of the motor nerve pathway in both antidromic and orthodromic directions, that is, towards and as far as the anterior horn cell and back to the muscle. It is easily obtained by stimulating the distal part of the nerve (peroneal, tibial, median, and ulnar). The results are expressed in milliseconds. F-wave study is useful in investigating patients with suspected more proximal peripheral nerve lesions, such as in polyradiculoneuropathies, especially in very early Guillain–Barré syndrome.

H-reflex study is not very useful in studying patients with polyneuropathy.

Somatosensory evoked potentials (SEPs) are elicited by stimulation of peripheral nerves and recorded at various sites along the sensory pathway. Electrical transcutaneous stimulation is applied at a peripheral nerve and the corresponding area of sensory cortex or dorsal column recorded (e.g., for the median nerve, stimulate at the wrist, and record over the neck and the contralateral central area of the scalp). The investigation should be limited to centers with expertise in the techniques but it is useful in patients with suspected radicular lesions, especially in CIDP when the classical electrophysiological criteria are lacking or unconvincing [2].

Laboratory investigations in peripheral neuropathies

Peripheral neuropathies especially generalized ones, are often the expression of an underlying disease (diabetes, toxins, etc. . .). The cause of most polyneuropathies is evident from the medical history, neurologic examination, and electrodiagnostic studies combined with simple screening laboratory tests as recommended by the American Academy of Neurology [3].

Routine and specialized tests will be guided by the clinical and electrophysiological features of the neuropathy (See subsequent chapters).

Clinical classification of peripheral neuropathies

According to the clinical presentation, time course and electrophysiological results, peripheral neuropathies can be classified into different types; they have varying underlying causes and therefore require different investigations:

- *Focal neuropathies* are mainly entrapment or compressive neuropathies
- *Multifocal neuropathies* may have an acute onset, a subacute or chronic course (see Table 1.4). Among *generalized neuropathies* one may separate:
  - ◦ Acute forms corresponding to Guillain–Barré syndrome which may present either as acute demyelinating polyneuropathies or acute axonal neuropathies
  - ◦ Chronic demyelinating polyneuropathies (see Table 1.5)
  - ◦ Subacute/chronic axonal polyneuropathies (see Tables 1.6)

Table 1.4 Multifocal neuropathies.

Acute onset	
	Vasculitic neuropathy (painful)
	HNPP (painless)
Subacute course	
	MADSAM or Lewis–Sumner syndrome
	Lymphomatous neuropathy
	Diabetes [4]
	Primary amyloidosis [5]
	Transthyretin amyloidosis [6]
Chronic course	
	Multifocal motor neuropathy with persistent conduction block [7]

Table 1.5 Chronic demyelinating polyneuropathies.

Uniform slowing	
	CMT type 1A
	CMT type 4
	Some CMT type 1B
	CMT type 3
	Leucodystrophies
	• adrenomyeloneuropathy
	• metachromatic
	• Krabbe's disease
	• Cockaynes disease
	Refsum's disease
	Tangier disease
	Cerebrotendinous xanthomatosis
	Congenital hypomyelinating neuropathy
Non-uniform slowing	
	CIDP with conduction block and temporal dispersion. Different forms:
	• distal
	• multifocal (Lewis–Sumner syndrome)
	Paraproteinemia neuropathy:
	• IgM with anti-MAG antibody
	• Osteosclerotic myeloma
	• POEMS syndrome
	Usually without conduction block and mainly distal demyelination

Table 1.6 Causes of subacute/chronic axonal polyneuropathies.

Amyloidosis	Primary or hereditary [8]
Nutritional diseases	Vitamin B12 deficiency
	Folate deficiency
	Thiamine deficiency
	Bariatric neuropathy
Alcoholism	With or without thiamine deficiency
Sarcoidosis	
Connective tissue diseases	Rheumatoid arthritis
	Periarteritis nodosa
	Systemic lupus erythematosus
	Churg–Strauss vasculitis
	Cryoglobulinemia [9, 10]
	Sjögren's syndrome
Carcinomatous	Sensorimotor neuropathy
Hypothyroidism	
Lyme disease	
AIDS	
Multiple myeloma	
Drug neuropathy	Amiodarone
	Bortezomib
	Chloroquine
	Dapsone
	Disulfiram
	Isoniazid
	Metronidazole
	Nitrous oxide
	Nucleosides (ddC, ddI, d4T)
	Platinum salts
	Pyridoxine (vitamin B6) with high doses
	Taxanes
	Thalidomide
	Vincristine
Chemical neuropathy	Acrylamide
	Carbon disulfide
	Ethylene oxide
	Hexacarbons
	Carbon monoxide
	Glue sniffing
Metal neuropathy	Arsenic
	Thallium
	Gold
Diabetes mellitus [11]	

- Small fiber neuropathies (see Table 1.7)
- Ataxic neuropathies (large fiber neuropathies) (see Table 1.8)
- Neuronopathies (ganglionopathies) (see Table 1.9)

Table 1.7 Causes of small fiber neuropathy.

Inherited	Familial amyloidosis
	Autosomal recessive hereditary neuropathy
	Hereditary sensory and autonomic neuropathy
	Fabry disease
	Tangier disease
Acquired	Diabetes mellitus
	Impaired glucose tolerance, metabolic syndrome
	Alcoholism
	Systemic amyloidosis
	Vasculitis
	CryoglobulinemiaSarcoidosis
	Sjögren's syndrome
	Systemic lupus erythematosus
	HIV neuropathy
	Paraneoplastic syndrome
Idiopathic	

Table 1.8 Causes of ataxic neuropathy.

Inherited diseases	
	Mitochondrial neuropathies associated with POLG mutations, SANDO, NARP
	Inherited disorders of fat absorption (vitamin E deficiency)
Acquired diseases	
	Demyelinating neuropathies: IgM anti-MAG neuropathy
	CANOMAD
	Acute: Miller–Fisher syndrome and ataxic sensory Guillain–Barré syndrome
	Chronic immune sensory polyradiculopathy

Indications for nerve biopsy

Nerve biopsy has been widely used to investigate patients with peripheral neuropathy (see Table 1.10) and is often the final step in the diagnostic work-up of a neuropathy of unknown origin.

It should be reserved for selected cases when looking for a specific diagnosis, but may be performed to clarify the mechanism of the neuropathy. Patients for whom a nerve biopsy appears necessary should be referred to a specialized center with expertise in performance and interpretation of nerve and muscle biopsy samples.

The choice of nerve to biopsy and techniques employed are described in Chapters 2, 3, and 4.

Table 1.9 Causes of neuronopathy (ganglionopathy).

	Onset	Disease association
Paraneoplastic	Subacute	Small cell lung cancer, bronchial carcinoma, breast cancer, ovarian cancer, lymphoma, neuroendocrine tumors
Inflammatory, immune	Acute/subacute/chronic	Sjögren's syndrome, systemic lupus, autoimmune hepatitis, gluten sensitivity
Infectious-related	Subacute	HIV (also EBV, VZV, measles, HTLV1)
Drugs	Subacute/chronic	Platinum chemotherapy (cisplatin, oxaliplatin, carboplatin)
Vitamin associated	Subacute/chronic	Vitamin B6 toxicity
Idiopathic	Acute/subacute/chronic	

Table 1.10 Conditions for which a nerve biopsy may be indicated.

Neuropathies with specific diagnostic abnormalities	
Abnormal stroma /diagnostic histological features within the stroma	
	Vasculitis (systemic or localized to nerves)
	Sarcoidosis (specific granuloma)
	Amyloidosis, acquired or familial (amyloid deposits)
	Tumor infiltrates (mainly lymphoma)
	Fabry disease
	Leprosy (Hansen's bacilli)
Abnormal axons	
	Giant axonal neuropathy
	Adult polyglucosan body disease
Abnormal myelin sheaths or Schwann cells	
	HNPP
	IgM monoclonal with anti-MAG neuropathy
	Drug neuropathy: amiodarone
Storage diseases	
	Globoid cell leucodystrophy
	Niemann–Pick disease
	Metachromatic leucodystrophy
	Farber disease
Other diseases	Mitochondrial neuropathies (ragged red fibers in muscle)
Neuropathies with non-specific abnormalities supporting a diagnosis	
	CMT type 1A and 3 (onion bulb formations)
	CMT type 4B
	Some forms of X-linked CMT
	Inflammatory neuropathy (CIDP)

Nerve selection

Nerve biopsy involves sensory nerves usually the sural or the superficial peroneal nerves. The latter procedure allows access to the adjacent muscle within the same incision.

In some specific diseases, such as vasculitis or sarcoidosis, it can be important to examine combined muscle and nerve samples (see Chapters 2, 24, and 26).

The nerve to be sampled depends on the clinical and electrophysiological findings. It is preferable to take an affected nerve. In polyneuropathy, the sural or the superficial peroneal nerve should be taken. In multiple mononeuropathy in which the upper limbs are preferentially involved, the superficial sensory branch of the radial nerve may be taken. In rare cases of lower limb proximal diabetic amyotrophy (lumbosacral radiculoplexus neuropathy), a sensory branch of the femoral nerve may be biopsied [12].

Skin biopsy is performed for the investigation of small fiber neuropathies (cf. Chapter 3).

Indications for and information from nerve biopsy

The indications for peripheral nerve biopsy vary according to the clinical context and results of a case by case discussion. It is still a useful diagnostic tool and is strongly indicated in many conditions such as:

1. Acute or subacute multiple mononeuropathies. They are usually painful. The electrophysiological studies show an axonal pattern.
2. Subacute/chronic axonal sensorimotor polyneuropathies with a rapid evolution, with clinical and electrophysiological deterioration from about 6 weeks to 6 months and negative investigations, clinical and electrophysiological asymmetry, general symptoms: cutaneous signs of vasculitis such as livedo or purpura, renal or digestive tract involvement, recent weight loss, context of systemic disease, B or C virus hepatitis, HIV infection, or cryoglobulinemia, and biological inflammatory syndromes. The same underlying causes as those for multiple mononeuropathies should be investigated: vasculitis, lymphoma, sarcoidosis, acquired, or familial amyloidosis, leprosy. Nerve biopsy may also be useful in chronic axonal polyneuropathies in which the clinical and electrophysiological studies show atypical features or where no cause is found, even after a complete check-up.
3. In CIDP patients when the clinical and electrophysiological features are compatible with the diagnosis, but general symptoms (weight loss), biological or immunological abnormalities, rapid axonal loss, or resistance to treatment may be present. Lymphoma, sarcoidosis, POEMS syndrome or amyloid neuropathy may be responsible.
4. In CIDP patients where the clinical features are compatible with the diagnosis but are not confirmed by the electrophysiological results.
5. As the final step in the diagnostic work-up of a neuropathy of unknown origin.

References

1 Bromberg MB, Smith AG (2002) Toward an efficient method to evaluate peripheral neuropathies. *J Clin Neuromusc Dis* 3, 172–182.

2 Yannikas C, Vusic S (2008) Utility of somatosensory evoked potentials in chronic acquired demyelinating neuropathy. *Muscle Nerve* 38, 1447–1454.

3 England JD, Gronseth GS, Franklin G, Carter G, Kinsella LJ, Cohen JA, *et al.* (2009) Evaluation of distal symmetric polyneuropathy: the role of laboratory and genetic testing (an evidence-based review). *Muscle Nerve* 39, 116–125.

4 Dyck PJ, Albers JW, Andersen H, Arezzo JC, Biessels GJ, Bril V, *et al.* (2011) Diabetic polyneuropathies: update on research definition, diagnostic criteria and estimation of severity. *Diabetes Metab Res Rev* 27, 620–628.

5 Tracy JA, Dyck PJ, Dyck PJB (2010) Primary amyloidosis presenting as upper limb multiple mononeuropathies. *Muscle Nerve* 41, 710–715.

6 Briemberg HR, Amato AA (2004) Transthyretin amyloidosis presenting with multifocal demyelinating mononeuropathies. *Muscle Nerve* 29, 318–322.

7 Bouche P, Moulonguet A, Younes-Chennoufi AB, Adams D, Baumann N, Meininger V, *et al.* (1995) Multifocal motor neuropathy with conduction block: a study of 24 patients. *J Neurol Neurosurg Psychiatry* 59, 38–44.

8 Said G, Planté-Bordeneuve V (2009) Familial amyloid polyneuropathy. A clinico-pathologic study. *J Neurol Sci* 284, 149–154.

9 Ammendola A, Sampaolo S, Ambrosone L, Ammendola E, Ciccone G, Migliaresi S, *et al.* (2005) Peripheral neuropathy in hepatitis-related cryoglobulinemia: electrophysiological follow-up study. *Muscle Nerve* 31, 382–385.

10 Yoon M-S, Obermann M, Dockweiler C, Assert R, Canbay A, Haag S, *et al.* (2011) Sensory neuropathy in patients with cryoglobulin negative hepatitis-C infection. *J Neurol* 258, 80–88.

11 Tesfaye S (2011) Recent advances in the management of diabetic distal symmetrical polyneuropathy. *J Diabetes Invest* 2, 33–42.

12 Dyck PJ, Norell JE, Dyck PJ (1999) Microvasculitis and ischemia in diabetic lumbosacral radiculoplexus neuropathy. *Neurology* 53, 2113–2121.

CHAPTER 2

Combined muscle and nerve biopsy

Anne Vital

Department of Pathology-Neuropathology, Hôpital Pellegrin, Bordeaux, France

Introduction

Simultaneous combined superficial peroneal nerve and peroneous brevis muscle biopsy allows examination of several tissue specimens and significantly improves the diagnosis of systemic diseases with peripheral nerve involvement, particularly in vasculitis, intra-vascular lymphoma, sarcoidosis, amyloidosis, mitochondrial disorders, and storage diseases.

Technique

Combined nerve and muscle biopsy requires an appropriate surgical area, competent staff, and aseptic conditions. The aim is to biopsy the superficial peroneal nerve and the peroneous brevis muscle via a single skin incision on the antero-lateral surface of the leg. Under local anesthesia, a 5-cm incision is performed on the lower third of the leg, 1 cm anterior to a line joining the fibular apex to the lateral malleolus at the ankle. Having proximally sectioned the superficial peroneal nerve, a 3-cm specimen is gently lifted without stretching or crushing, and then removed by distal section. This specimen is divided into three pieces; one is immersed in buffered formalin for light microscopy, another in buffered glutaraldehyde for electron microscopy, and the third is frozen mainly for immunofluorescence. The peroneous brevis muscle biopsy is fixed for routine light microscopy, for electron microscopy, and frozen for histochemistry, biochemistry, and genetic studies if necessary. To avoid post-operative hematoma, the sutured wound is compressed by a bandage for 2 h, and the patient avoids standing for 2 days.

Results

Combined nerve and muscle biopsy allows examination of several tissue specimens, which significantly improves the diagnosis of systemic diseases with peripheral nerve involvement.

Vasculitis

Detection of a characteristic histological lesion is mandatory to confirm the diagnosis of *vasculitis*, and muscle biopsy in addition to nerve biopsy increases the number of medium-sized arterioles and/or small vessels available for examination [1–4] (cf. Chapter 24). Vessel walls are infiltrated by inflammatory cells, and mural fibrinoid necrosis is the most significant lesion. Vasculitic lesions correspond mainly to four necrotizing vasculitides: panarteritis nodosa (PAN), microscopic polyangiitis (MPA), Churg–Strauss syndrome, and Wegener's granulomatosis. Microvasculitis corresponds to small vessel wall infiltration by inflammatory cells, as observed in PAN and MPA, but without any necrosis. Microvasculitis has to be differentiated from non-specific inflammatory cell infiltrates surrounding small vessels. However, such perivascular inflammatory cell infiltrates enable a diagnosis of probable vasculitis when associated with cicatricial vessel wall fibrosis, clusters of newly formed vessels, hemosiderin deposits, or focal damage of nerve fibers. In a series of 100

Peripheral Nerve Disorders: Pathology and Genetics, First Edition. Edited by Jean-Michel Vallat, Joachim Weis, Francoise Gray, and Katy Keohane.

patients with necrotizing vasculitis, muscle biopsy was more frequently positive for vasculitis (80%) than was nerve biopsy (55%) [1]. In a larger series of 202 cases, available muscle specimens improved the yield of definite vasculitis by 31.6% in necrotizing vasculitis and by 27% in *microvasculitis* [4].

Intra-vascular lymphoma

An unsuspected diagnosis of *intra-vascular lymphoma* may be established when numerous malignant B lymphocytes are visible within the lumen of several small vessels in nerve and muscle specimens [5]. Other lymphomas may infiltrate peripheral nerve [6], but infiltration of muscle is uncommon [7]. Meningeal or radicular involvement by lymphoma generally does not involve peripheral nerve or muscle [8].

Sarcoidosis

Sarcoid neuropathy is diagnosed histologically by identifying at least one non-caseating granuloma composed of epithelioid cells with a few multinucleated giant cells and lymphocytes (cf. Chapter 26). In a review of 38 sarcoid neuropathy cases, characteristic sarcoid granulomas were present in nerve in 11 cases, in muscle alone in 5, in both muscle and nerve in 10, in nerve and another tissue in 4, and in another tissue in 8 [9]. Non-caseating granulomas are well developed between muscle fibers, whereas they are frequently smaller within epineurium or endoneurium. In addition, evidence of granulomas in muscle is diagnostic in differentiating sarcoidosis from tuberculoid leprosy, in which muscle is always spared [10].

Amyloid polyneuropathies

At the present time, most cases of familial amyloid polyneuropathy are diagnosed by molecular genetic analysis of the transthyretin gene on blood specimens [11] (cf. Chapter 16). Nevertheless, it is still not rare to establish the diagnosis on combined nerve and muscle biopsy. When present, endoneurial amyloid deposits are easily visible on hematoxylin-eosin stains as patchy acellular eosinophilic areas. It is important to note that on muscle specimens stained with hematoxylin-eosin, amyloid deposits are easily overlooked, but Congo-red staining gives these deposits an "amber" color and characteristic "apple-green" birefringence under polarized light. Transthyretin immunohistochemistry may also reveal small amyloid deposits encasing an isolated muscle fiber or surrounding adjacent fat cells [12]. Other amyloid deposits are isolated, derived from a light chain, or associated with an IgA, IgG, or IgM monoclonal gammopathy. The light chain amyloid component is better identified by immunofluorescence on frozen nerve and/or muscle biopsy specimens. Ultrastructural examination may be very helpful if bundles of straight fibrils are seen, sometimes close to a macrophage and corresponding to very small amyloid deposits not even visible on semithin sections [12]. Electron microscopy also differentiates granular non-amyloid light chain deposits from fibrillar amyloid deposits [13].

Mitochondrial cytopathies

Additional muscle specimens can be important in the diagnosis of *neuropathies related to mitochondrial cytopathies* [14–16] (cf. Chapter 17). Typical changes are seen on muscle frozen sections after Gomori trichrome staining, with ragged red fibers corresponding to sub-sarcolemmal accumulation of abnormal mitochondria. This is confirmed by histochemical reactions for the mitochondrial enzymes succinate dehydrogenase (SDH) and cytochrome c oxidase (COX). However, these characteristic appearances are often absent in children as well as in some adult cases. On ultrastructural examination of muscle specimens, abnormal mitochondria are seen as rectangular crystalloid inclusions with a geometric lattice appearance, most often located beneath the sarcolemma. In addition, mitochondrial DNA (mtDNA) is better analyzed on frozen muscle specimens than on lymphocytes from circulating blood. A few cases of mitochondrial neuropathies, due to a mtDNA point mutation, are responsible for MELAS or MERRF phenotypes, but most cases are secondary to nuclear mutations with ensuing mitochondrial dysfunction, and usually associated with multiple small deletions of mtDNA. Most of these cases are adults with an autosomal dominant or autosomal recessive inheritance, but a few cases are sporadic. Progressive external ophtalmoplegia (PEO) is present is some cases, and may be associated with a sensory ataxic polyneuropathy. Ultrastructural examination of nerve specimens can show intra-axonal mitochondria with distorted cristae, but enlarged mitochondria with abnormal cristae within the Schwann cell cytoplasm of a few myelinated fibers are more characteristic [15, 16].

Storage diseases

Storage diseases have mainly been studied on isolated nerve biopsies [17–19] with characteristic features of storage materials on ultrastructural examination, but concomitant study of muscle specimens proved to be very useful in some cases [20, 21] (cf. Chapter 20).

Cholesterol emboli

In cholesterol emboli syndrome, peripheral neuropathy may be the initial manifestation (cf. Chapter 35). Biopsy of peripheral nerve may reveal cholesterol clefts in the lumina of small epineurial arteries. However, this is a very rare occurrence and emboli are more frequently observed in muscle biopsy.

References

1 Said G, Lacroix-Ciaudo C, Fujimura H, *et al.* (1988) The peripheral neuropathy of necrotizing arteritis: a clinicopathological study. *Ann Neurol* 23, 461–465.

2 Collins MP, Mendell JR, Periquet MI, *et al.* (2000) Superficial peroneal nerve/peroneus brevis muscle biopsy in vasculitic neuropathy. *Neurology* 55, 636–643.

3 Griffin JW (2001) Vasculitic neuropathies. *Rheum Dis Clin North Am* 27, 751–760.

4 Vital C, Vital A, Canron MH, *et al.* (2006) Combined nerve and muscle biopsy in the diagnosis of vasculitic neuropathy. A 16-year retrospective study of 202 cases. *J Periph Nerv Syst* 11, 20–29.

5 Vital C, Heraud A, Vital A, *et al.* (1989) Acute mononeuropathy with angiotropic lymphoma. *Acta Neuropathol* 78, 105–107.

6 Vital C, Vital A, Julien J, *et al.* (1990) Peripheral neuropathies and lymphomas without monoclonal gammopathy: a new classification. *J Neurol* 237, 177–185.

7 Odabasi Z, Parrott JH, Reddy VVB, *et al.* (2001) Neurolymphomatosis associated with muscle and cerebral involvement caused by natural killer cell lymphoma: a case report and review of literature. *J Periph Nerv Syst* 6, 197–203.

8 Grisold W, Klimpfinger M, Maehr B, *et al.* (2007) Peripheral nerve involvement in lymphoma: the meninges as the crucial barrier between meningoradicular spread and neurolymphomatosis. *J Periph Nerv Syst* 12, 58–60.

9 Vital A, Lagueny A, Ferrer X, *et al.* (2008) Sarcoid neuropathy: clinico-pathological study of 4 new cases and review of the literature. *Clin Neuropathol* 27, 96–105.

10 Said G, Lacroix C, Plante-Bordeneuve V, *et al.* (2002) Nerve granulomas and vasculitis in sarcoid peripheral neuropathy. A clinicopathological study of 11 patients. *Brain* 125, 264–275.

11 Benson MD, Kincaid JC. (2007) The molecular biology and clinical features of amyloid neuropathy. *Muscle Nerve* 36, 411–423.

12 Vital C, Lagueny A, Mercie P, *et al.* (2010) Usefulness of combined nerve and muscle biopsy in the diagnosis of amyloid neuropathy – a study of 6 new cases. *Clin Neuropathol* 29, 59–64.

13 Vital A. (2001) Paraproteinemic neuropathies. *Brain Pathol* 11, 399–407.

14 Vogel H. (2001) Mitochondrial myopathies and the role of the pathologist in the molecular era. *J Neuropathol Exp Neurol* 60, 217–227.

15 Bouillot S, Martin-Negrier ML, Vital A, *et al.* (2002) Peripheral neuropathy associated with mitochondrial disorders: 8 cases and review of the literature. *J Periph Nerv Syst* 7, 213–220.

16 Vital A, Vital C. (2012) Mitochondria and peripheral neuropathies. *J Neuropathol Exp Neurol* 71, 1036–1046.

17 Midroni G, Bilbao JM. (1995) Biopsy diagnosis of peripheral neuropathy. Butterworth-Heinemann, Boston.

18 King RHM. (1999) *Atlas of Peripheral Nerve Pathology*. Arnold, London.

19 Schroeder JM. (2001) *Pathology of Peripheral Nerves. An Atlas of Structural and Molecular Pathological Changes*. Springer, Philadelphia.

20 Vital C, Vallat JM. (1987) *Ultrastructural Study of the Human Diseased Peripheral Nerve*. Elsevier, New York.

21 Vital A, Vital C, Maleville J. (1984) Fabry's disease: an ultrastructural study of muscle and peripheral nerve. *Clin Neuropathol* 3, 168–172.

CHAPTER 3

Cutaneous nerve biopsy

Claudia Sommer[1] and Maria Nolano[2]

[1] Department of Neurology, University of Würzburg, Würzburg, Germany

[2] Department of Neurology, "Salvatore Maugeri" Foundation, Telese, Italy

Introduction

Skin biopsy is increasingly used to study the nervous system. Using appropriate immunohistochemistry, a number of different nerve fiber types can be investigated in skin. Standards and normal values are available for intra-epidermal innervation (Fig. 3.1A), and the technique has been used extensively in the work-up of small fiber neuropathy [1, 2]. Skin biopsy also enables the investigation of nerve fibers innervating cutaneous mechanoreceptors such as Meissner corpuscles (Fig. 3.1B,D), Merkel complexes (Fig. 3.1E), Pacinian corpuscles (Fig. 3.1F) and hair bulbs (Fig. 3.1C). The autonomic innervation of sweat glands (Fig. 3.2A,B), arrector pili muscle (Fig. 3.2C,D), and blood vessels (Fig. 3.2E, F) can also be studied, and subepidermal myelinated fibers can be identified and quantified [3].

The most common indication for nerve fiber analysis in skin is the suspicion of small fiber neuropathy, that is, patients presenting with distal neuropathic pain without abnormalities in routine electrophysiological tests. Before undertaking skin biopsies for neuropathic diagnosis, training in a center experienced in cutaneous nerve analysis is highly recommended. Here, we summarize data on the best methods for studying nerve fibers in skin biopsies.

Technique

Skin biopsy and location

Biopsy is most commonly performed with small disposable circular punches under sterile conditions following local cutaneous anesthesia. Adhesive strips (*SteriStrip* ®) can be used to close the wound; sutures are usually not required. In most instances healing occurs within 7–10 days.

Punches with diameters from 2–5 mm are used, depending on the location. The biopsy should contain the epidermis and dermis, including sweat glands. For diagnostic purposes in peripheral neuropathies, one biopsy is taken from the distal leg (10 cm above the lateral malleolus) and a second from the proximal thigh (20 cm below the iliac spine) to gain information on whether the disease is length-dependent. If the patient also has a sural nerve biopsy, the distal skin biopsy can be taken from the incision site. If touch organelles or myelinated fibers need to be studied, a 2-mm skin biopsy from the fingertip or the lateral proximal phalanx may be needed.

Tissue preparation

The biopsy is fixed in cold fixative for up to 24 h at 4 °C. Suitable fixatives are 4% paraformaldehyde, 2% para formaldehyde-lysine periodate, or Zamboni's fixative (2% paraformaldehyde and picric acid). The fixative is washed off with 0.1 M phosphate buffer, the specimen is kept in a cryoprotective solution, usually sucrose 10 or 20%, overnight at 4 °C. Serial 50-µm sections are cut using a cryostat and immunostained using antibodies labeling the different skin structures (e.g., nerve fibers, basement membranes, vessels, resident, or infiltrating cells). The most commonly used markers for nerve fibers are antibodies against the protein-gene-product 9.5 (PGP 9.5), a predominantly neuronal form of ubiquitin carboxyl-terminal hydrolase. [4]. Immunohistochemistry with brightfield microscopy and immunofluorescence with or without confocal microscopy are used. The

Peripheral Nerve Disorders: Pathology and Genetics, First Edition. Edited by Jean-Michel Vallat, Joachim Weis, Francoise Gray, and Katy Keohane.

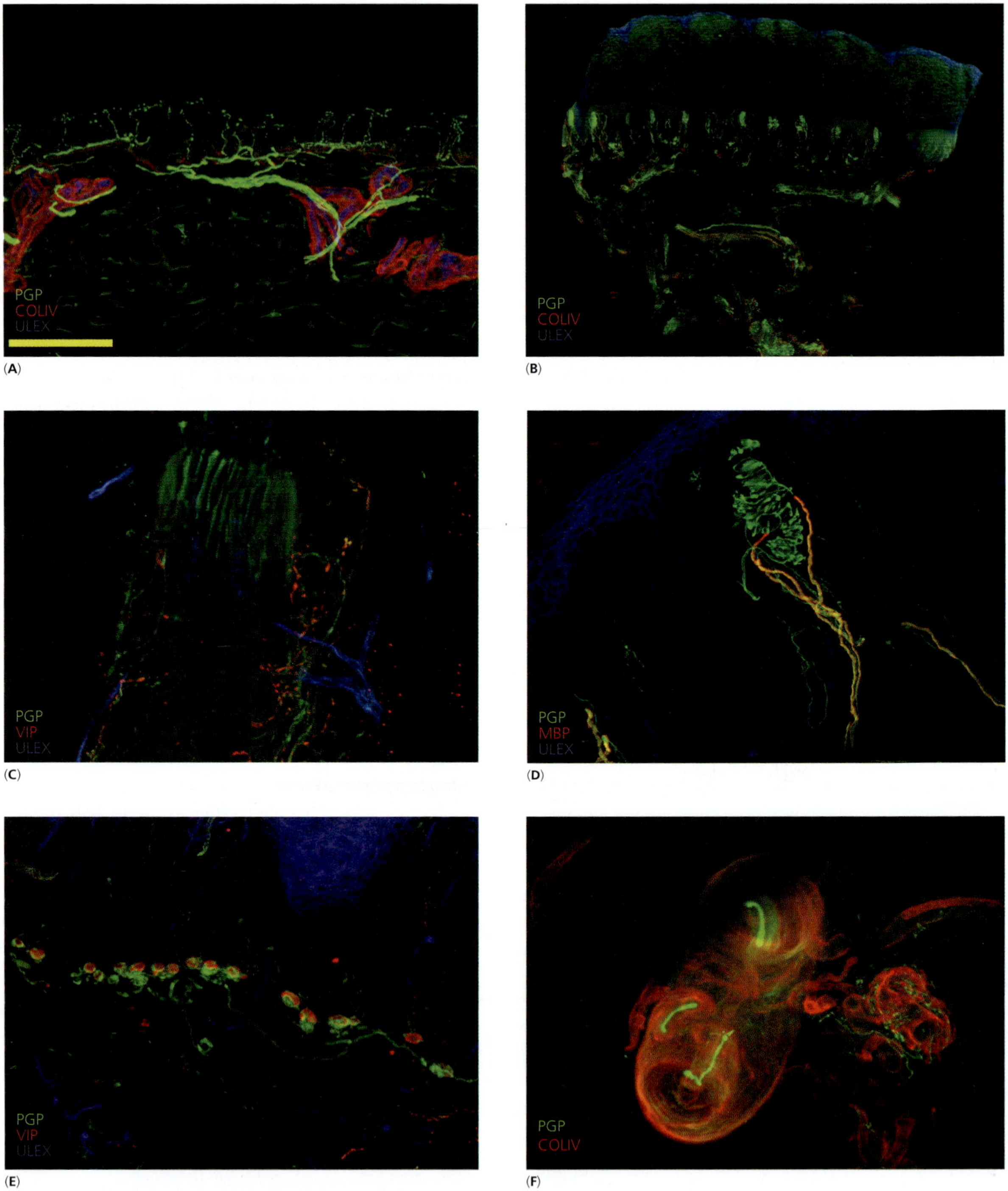

Figure 3.1 Confocal digital images of cutaneous innervation from fingertip smooth skin (**B**, **D**, **E**, and **F**) and thigh hairy skin (A and C) of a normal subject. (**A**) Regular distribution of epidermal nerve fibers with a rich subepidermal neural plexus. (**B**) Regular distribution of Meissner corpuscles at the apex of dermal papillae. (**C**) Hair follicle showing both the typical palisade-like innervation (originating from myelinated fibers) and the unmyelinated component. (**D**) Meissner corpuscle innervated by myelinated endings. (**E**) Merkel complex at the base of a dermal papilla. Both the neural expansions (green) and the cellular counterpart (red) of the receptor are visible. (**F**) Pacinian corpuscle with the typical onion bulb aspect and its Aβ afferents. Scale bar = 100 μm in **A**, **D**, and **F**, 800 μm in **B**, 50 μm in **C**, and 400 μm in **F**.

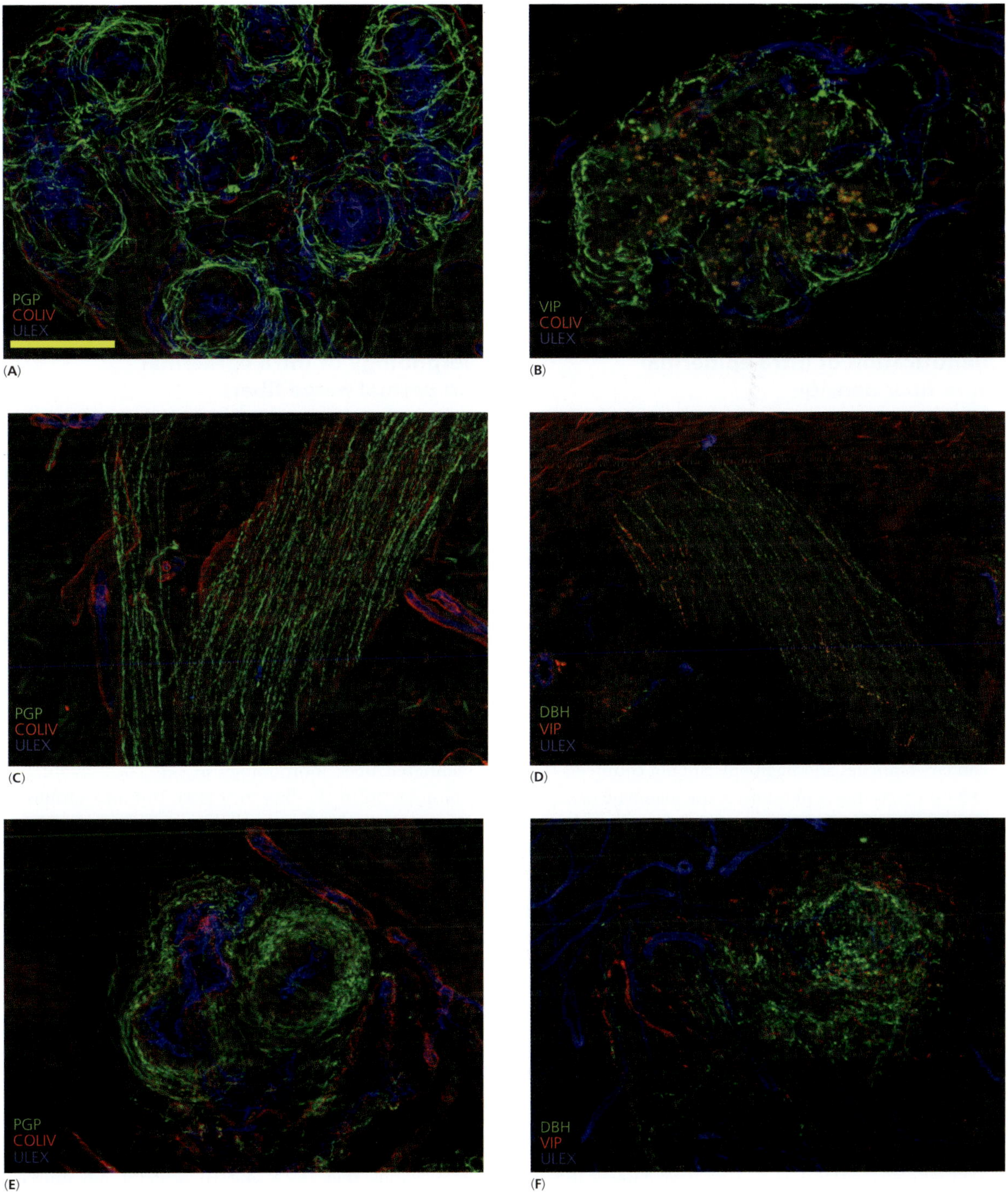

Figure 3.2 Confocal digital images of cutaneous autonomic innervation of sweat gland (**A** and **B**), arrector pili muscle (**C** and **D**), and arteriovenous anastomoses (**E** and **F**) in a normal subject. The figures show the different patterns of innervation of the cutaneous adnexae. The complexity increases from the quite regular pilomotor innervation to the irregular plexus of the arteriovenous anastomosis. Sudomotor innervation is predominantly cholinergic while within pilomotor and vasomotor plexuses cholinergic and noradrenergic components are both expressed.

staining procedure requires experience with both techniques. Preparation of specimens for brightfield microscopy takes 3 days of tissue processing and requires handling of free-floating sections. Immunofluorescence allows multiple antigens to be studied in the same nerve (e.g., axon and myelin sheath) or in different structures (e.g., mechanoreceptor and nerve fiber, dermal-epidermal junction and nerve fibers). With brightfield microscopy, stains are generally stable when stored at room temperature, while with immunofluorescence there is a risk of stains fading. The newer fluorescent stains are more stable so this risk is now negligible.

Quantification of intra-epidermal nerve fiber density

To determine intra-epidermal nerve fiber density (IENFD) individual PGP 9.5 positive intra-epidermal nerve fibers crossing the dermal–epidermal junction (epidermal basement membrane) are counted in at least three non-consecutive sections using the 40× objective (Fig. 3.1A). Branches separating within the epidermis are not counted. Some investigators use a slightly different counting method also including isolated nerve fragments in the epidermis as this yields a higher number of intra-epidermal nerve fibers [5, 6]. Most groups, however, apply the previously described rule that those intra-epidermal nerve fibers, which are counted have to cross or originate at the dermal-epidermal junction and that secondary branches and fragments are not counted [7].

IENFD (nerve fibers per mm) is calculated by measuring the length of epidermis using morphometry software (e.g., ImageJ) or an intraocular lens ruler. Both approaches give similar results [8]. IENFD can also be derived simply by dividing the number of counted fibers by three in a 3-mm disposable circular punch; this correlates well with nerve fiber density measured by image analysis [9]. With strict counting rules and proper training, a high degree of intra- and inter-observer reliability is achieved [10].

Normal reference values for IENFD exist for both brightfield immunohistochemistry and indirect immunofluorescence at several sites, including lower and upper leg, forearm, finger, and trunk [11]. Gender, age, and height influence distal IENFD. Men have a lower IENFD than women and IENFD decreases with age [10, 12].

Several statistical methods (Z scores, fifth percentile, and ROC analysis) are used to define an abnormal IENFD. Comparing all three methods, Z scores and fifth percentile have a high specificity (98 and 95%, respectively), but a low sensitivity (31 and 35%), whereas ROC analysis has a specificity of 64% and a sensitivity of 78% [13]. In a study using fluorescence imaging, a cut-off value of 8.8 had a specificity of 80% and sensitivity of 77% [3]. Recently it has been recommended to use a minimum of two sections for values well in the normal or abnormal range and 10 sections in borderline cases, using fifth percentiles [14].

Results

Morphology of intra-epidermal and dermal nerve fibers

Distinguishing normal from pathological morphology of skin nerve fibers is tricky, since some features previously regarded as pathological can be found in normal subjects [15]. Swellings and varicosities as well as branching and sprouting may be present in the distal leg skin biopsy of healthy individuals. Large (>1.5 μm) axonal swellings are considered as evidence of a pathological process. They can occur early in the course of HIV and diabetic neuropathy and are regarded as pre-degenerative changes [16]. Prominent swellings have also been shown during axonal regeneration subsequent to capsaicin denervation [17].

As methods improve, there is increased interest in myelinated fiber morphology in skin, best evaluated in biopsies from the fingertip [18], but also visible in skin from the thigh [19]. In patients with Charcot–Marie–Tooth disease (CMT) -1A, internodal length shortening was demonstrated using double immunofluorescence for PGP 9.5 and myelin basic protein, (MBP) [20]. Another study demonstrated elongated nodes of Ranvier in skin biopsies of patients with demyelinating peripheral neuropathy and myelinated dermal nerve fibers were reduced in peripheral neuropathy in general [19].

Autonomic innervation

Skin is a rich reservoir of postganglionic sympathetic autonomic fibers which innervate skin adnexae, such as sweat glands (Fig. 3.2A and B) arrector pili muscles (Fig. 3.2C and D) arteriovenous anastomoses (Fig. 3.2E and F) with a complex network of noradrenergic and cholinergic fibers [21]. Accurate quantification of these complex neural networks is challenging.

Several approaches to quantify sudomotor innervation have been tried, for example, semi-quantitative evaluation [22], quantification of nerve-related fluorescence [23], and manual nerve tracing of total nerve length [24]. More reliable methods based on manual morphometry [25] or on area-based morphometric analysis [26] in brightfield microscopy, validated by comparison with stereological methods are recently described.

Innervation of arrector pili muscle is less complex. Pilomotor fibers are regularly orientated along the major axis of the muscle (Fig. 3.2C and D). A novel method to quantify pilomotor innervation uses immunofluorescence and PGP, VIP, and DβH markers [27]. It was reliable and suitable for rapid quantification of cholinergic and noradrenergic nerve fibers in diabetic and healthy subjects.

Examples of the diagnostic value of cutaneous nerve biopsy in peripheral nerve disease

Small fiber neuropathy

A suspected small fiber neuropathy is the most frequent indication for cutaneous nerve biopsy. Patients often present with burning feet and few other symptoms or signs. The diagnostic criteria are (1) clinical signs of small fiber impairment, (2) abnormal small fiber function shown by quantitative sensory testing or specialized neurophysiology, and (3) reduced IENFD in the distal leg [28, 29]. Small fiber neuropathy is accepted as definite if all three criteria are present, and probable if two of the three criteria are fulfilled: Exclusion criteria are any signs or symptoms of large fiber neuropathy, such as pareses or abnormal nerve conduction studies.

Small fiber neuropathy is frequently length-dependent, that is, patients have reduced IENFD at the calf with normal or less severely reduced proximal IENFD. In non-length dependent small fiber neuropathy, both proximal and distal IENFDs are reduced [30], possibly indicating a ganglionopathy. In contrast, length-dependent small fiber neuropathy is more likely to have a peripheral inflammatory component [30].

Small fiber neuropathy is frequent in early diabetes (see next), hypothyroidism [31, 32], and alcohol abuse [33]. Other causes are sarcoidosis [34], drug-induced and inflammatory neuropathies that may start as a small fiber neuropathy, for review see [35]. Recently, mutations in voltage-gated sodium channels are recognized as causing painful small fiber neuropathy [36, 37].

Diabetic neuropathy

Length-dependent distal axon loss in type I and type II diabetes can easily be shown by IENFD in skin biopsies [38–46]. Impaired glucose tolerance was associated with a reduced IENFD [40, 46], but not reproduced by all groups [47].

Hereditary neuropathies

Some hereditary neuropathies predominantly affect small fibers, so skin biopsy is important to verify the diagnosis and stage of disease. Examples are Fabry's disease [48–50], familial dysautonomia [51] and congenital insensitivity to pain [52]. In patients with Friedreich's ataxia, with degeneration of large sensory afferents, skin biopsy revealed small fiber involvement [53].

In CMT caused by mutations in myelin proteins, myelinated dermal nerve fibers can show abnormal axolemmal molecular architecture [54, 55]. Shortened internodal length has been described in dermal myelinated fibers of CMT 1A [20]. Mutations in voltage-gated sodium channels are increasingly recognized as causes of otherwise "idiopathic" small fiber neuropathies (see previously).

Demyelinating and vasculitic neuropathies

Longitudinal sections of myelinated fibers, in thick sections of the dermis, allow analysis of nodes of Ranvier in order to demonstrate segmental demyelination (Fig. 3.3) [19, 20]. Ranvier node length and size of internodes can be measured and nodal and paranodal proteins such as ion channels, contactin associated protein (caspr) (Fig. 3.3C, D), and neurofascin can be analyzed. Further research is needed, but this method is a promising tool for distinguishing hereditary and inflammatory demyelinating neuropathies.

Traditionally, peripheral nerve vasculitis is the domain of nerve and muscle biopsy. A recent pilot study showed a good correlation between the detection of vasculitic infiltrates in skin and in sural nerve in non-systemic vasculitic neuropathy [56].

Nerve regeneration

Skin biopsy, being minimally invasive, lends itself to serial investigation, so that nerve regeneration in skin has been studied. The rate of regeneration was lower

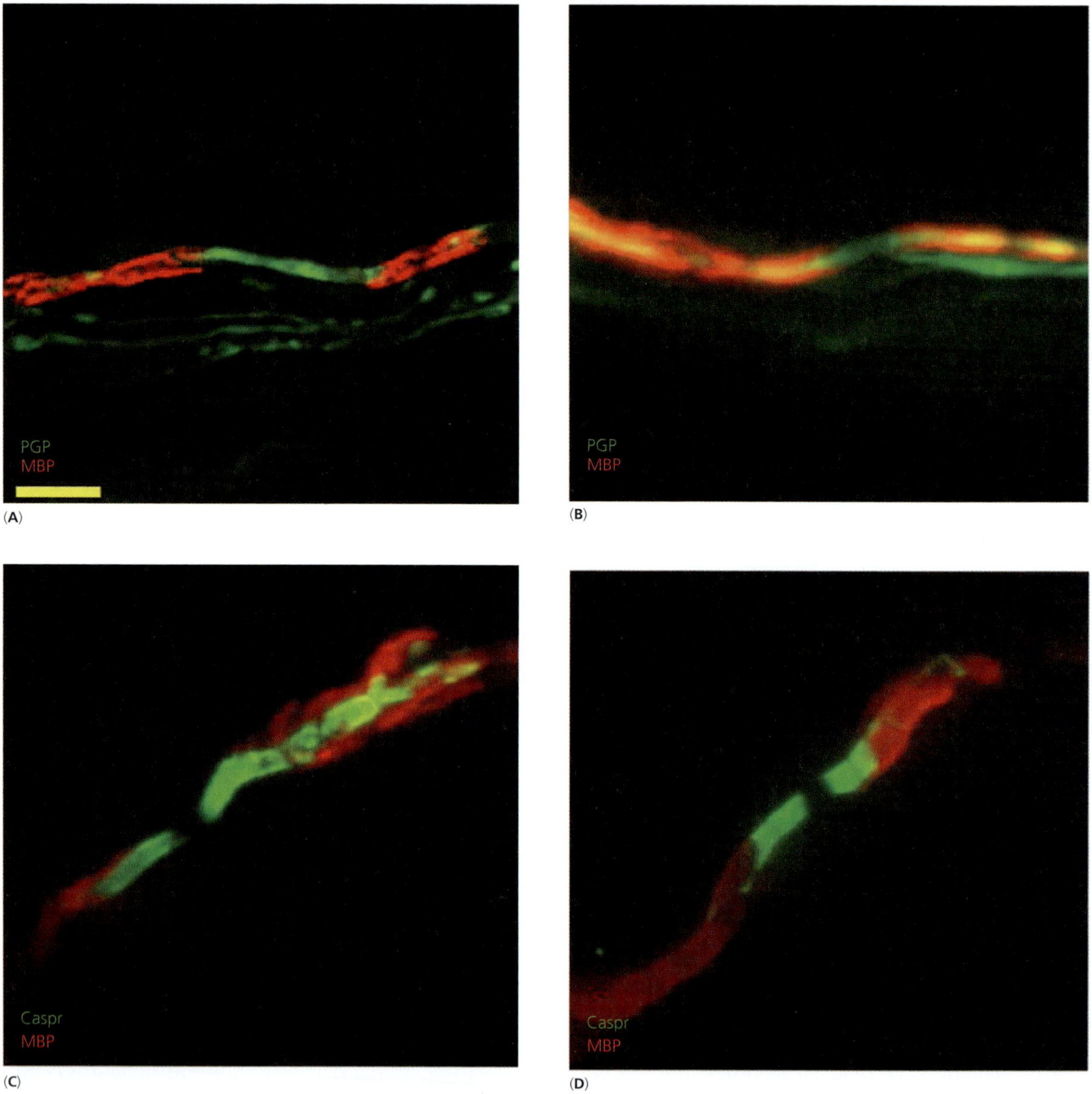

Figure 3.3 Node of Ranvier in a patient with chronic inflammatory demyelinating neuropathy (CIDP). Double immunofluorescence with antibodies to myelin basic protein and PGP 9.5 shows an elongated node of Ranvier in a patient with CIDP (**A**) compared to control (**B**). The paranodal protein contactin associated protein (caspr) is present in a short paranodal band in a normal control (**D**); this band is elongated in a patient with CIDP (**C**). Scale bar = 5 μm. (Courtesy of Dr Kathrin Doppler).

in diabetics, even preceding signs or symptoms of neuropathy [57]. Intra-epidermal nerve fiber regeneration was also shown in individual diabetic patients with changed lifestyle [42], or following pancreatic transplant [45], in HIV neuropathy treated with nerve growth factor [58], and in Fabry's disease following enzyme replacement therapy [50]. Another approach to study regenerating cutaneous nerve fibers is immunostaining for growth associated protein-43 (GAP-43) [59, 60].

Conclusions and recommendations for practical application

Skin biopsy analysis of nerve fibers has improved our understanding of cutaneous innervation in health and disease. PGP9.5 immunostaining demonstrates small unmyelinated fibers allowing objective assessment of small nerve fiber neuropathy. In 2005, the European Federation of Neurological Societies task force published guidelines for quantification of IENFD and summarized its uses [11], and an update was presented by a joint task force of the European Federation of Neurological Societies and the Peripheral Nerve Society in 2010 [61]. Normal age and gender matched control data from healthy subjects, and quality control measures should be used to interpret neuropathy in skin biopsies. Artifacts and errors may occur at any stage of the process. Intra- and inter-observer ratings and quality control between laboratories should be regularly assessed. With these caveats, skin biopsy with quantification of IENFD is a reliable technique to diagnose small fiber neuropathy. Myelinated fibers, subepidermal nerve plexus densities, subepidermal nerve bundles, touch receptor innervation, and nodes of Ranvier can also be studied. Given the autonomic system involvement in many neurodegenerative diseases, study of cutaneous autonomic innervation is likely to become more important in the future.

References

1 Sommer C, Lauria G. (2007) Skin biopsy in the management of peripheral neuropathy. *Lancet Neurol* 6, 632–642.

2 Lauria G, Lombardi R. (2012) Skin biopsy in painful and immune-mediated neuropathies. *J Peripher Nerv Syst* 17 Suppl 3, 38–45.

3 Vlckova-Moravcova E, Bednarik J, Dusek L, Toyka KV, Sommer C. (2008) Diagnostic validity of epidermal nerve fiber densities in painful sensory neuropathies. *Muscle Nerve* 37, 50–60.

4 Wilkinson KD, Lee KM, Deshpande S, Duerksen-Hughes P, Boss JM, Pohl J. (1989) The neuron-specific protein PGP 9.5 is a ubiquitin carboxyl-terminal hydrolase. *Science* 246, 670–673.

5 Ebenezer GJ, Hauer P, Gibbons C, McArthur JC, Polydefkis M. (2007) Assessment of epidermal nerve fibers: a new diagnostic and predictive tool for peripheral neuropathies. *J Neuropathol Exp Neurol* 66, 1059–1073.

6 Weis J, Katona I, Muller-Newen G, Sommer C, Necula G, Hendrich C, *et al.* (2011) Small-fiber neuropathy in patients with ALS. *Neurology* 76, 2024–2029.

7 Kennedy WR, McArthur JC, Polydefkis M, Wendelschafer-Crabb G. (2005) Pathology and quantitation of cutaneous innervation. In: Dyck PJ, Thomas PK (eds). *Peripheral Neuropathy*. 4th edn, pp. 869–895. Philadelphia: Elsevier Saunders.

8 Wilder-Smith EP, Chow A. (2006) Comparison of a simple method for quantitation of intraepidermal nerve fibres with a standard image analysis method using hypothenar skin. *J Neurol* 253, 1011–1015.

9 Chien HF, Tseng TJ, Lin WM, Yang CC, Chang YC, Chen RC, *et al.* (2001) Quantitative pathology of cutaneous nerve terminal degeneration in the human skin. *Acta Neuropathol* 102, 455–461.

10 Lauria G, Bakkers M, Schmitz C, Lombardi R, Penza P, Devigili G, *et al.* (2010) Intraepidermal nerve fiber density at the distal leg: a worldwide normative reference study. *J Peripher Nerv Syst* 15, 202–207.

11 Lauria G, Cornblath DR, Johansson O, McArthur JC, Mellgren SI, Nolano M, *et al.* (2005) EFNS guidelines on the use of skin biopsy in the diagnosis of peripheral neuropathy. *Eur J Neurol* 12, 747–758.

12 Bakkers M, Merkies IS, Lauria G, Devigili G, Penza P, Lombardi R, *et al.* (2009) Intraepidermal nerve fiber density and its application in sarcoidosis. *Neurology* 73, 1142–1148.

13 Nebuchennykh M, Loseth S, Lindal S, Mellgren SI. (2009) The value of skin biopsy with recording of intraepidermal nerve fiber density and quantitative sensory testing in the assessment of small fiber involvement in patients with different causes of polyneuropathy. *J Neurol* 256, 1067–1075.

14 Engelstad JK, Taylor SW, Witt LV, Hoebing BJ, Herrmann DN, Dyck PJ, *et al.* (2012) Epidermal nerve fibers: confidence intervals and continuous measures with nerve conduction. *Neurology* 79, 2187–2193.

15 Wendelschafer-Crabb G, Kennedy WR, Walk D. (2006) Morphological features of nerves in skin biopsies. *J Neurol Sci* 242, 15–21.

16 Hsieh ST, Chiang HY, Lin WM. (2000) Pathology of nerve terminal degeneration in the skin. *J Neuropathol Exp Neurol* 59, 297–307.

17 Nolano M, Simone DA, Wendelschafer-Crabb G, Johnson T, Hazen E, Kennedy WR. (1999) Topical capsaicin in humans: parallel loss of epidermal nerve fibers and pain sensation. *Pain* 81, 135–145.

18 Nolano M, Provitera V, Crisci C, Stancanelli A, Wendelschafer-Crabb G, Kennedy WR, *et al.* (2003) Quantification of myelinated endings and mechanoreceptors in human digital skin. *Ann Neurol* 54, 197–205.

19 Doppler K, Werner C, Henneges C, Sommer C. (2012) Analysis of myelinated fibers in human skin biopsies of patients with neuropathies. *J Neurol* 259, 1879–1887.

20 Saporta MA, Katona I, Lewis RA, Masse S, Shy ME, Li J. (2009) Shortened internodal length of dermal myelinated nerve fibres in Charcot–Marie–Tooth disease type 1A. *Brain* 132, 3263–3273.

21 Donadio V, Nolano M, Provitera V, Stancanelli A, Lullo F, Liguori R, *et al.* (2006) Skin sympathetic adrenergic innervation: an immunofluorescence confocal study. *Ann Neurol* 59, 376–381.

22 Donadio V, Cortelli P, Elam M, Di Stasi V, Montagna P, Holmberg B, *et al.* (2010) Autonomic innervation in multiple system atrophy and pure autonomic failure. *J Neurol Neurosurg Psychiatry* 81, 1327–1335.

23 Sommer C, Lindenlaub T, Zillikens D, Toyka KV, Naumann M. (2002) Selective loss of cholinergic sudomotor fibers causes anhidrosis in Ross syndrome. *Ann Neurol* 52, 247–250.

24 Hirai A, Yasuda H, Joko M, Maeda T, Kikkawa R. (2000) Evaluation of diabetic neuropathy through the quantitation of cutaneous nerves. *J Neurol Sci* 172, 55–62.

25 Gibbons CH, Illigens BM, Wang N, Freeman R. (2009) Quantification of sweat gland innervation: a clinical-pathologic correlation. *Neurology* 72, 1479–1486.

26 Luo KR, Chao CC, Chen YT, Huang CM, Yang NC, Kan HW, *et al.* (2011) Quantitation of sudomotor innervation in skin biopsies of patients with diabetic neuropathy. *J Neuropathol Exp Neurol* 70, 930–938.

27 Nolano M, Provitera V, Caporaso G, Stancanelli A, Vitale DF, Santoro L. (2010) Quantification of pilomotor nerves: a new tool to evaluate autonomic involvement in diabetes. *Neurology* 75, 1089–1097.

28 Lacomis D. (2002) Small-fiber neuropathy. *Muscle Nerve* 26, 173–188.

29 Devigili G, Tugnoli V, Penza P, Camozzi F, Lombardi R, Melli G, *et al.* (2008) The diagnostic criteria for small fibre neuropathy: from symptoms to neuropathology. *Brain* 131, 1912–1925.

30 Uçeyler N, Kafke W, Riediger N, He L, Necula G, Toyka KV, *et al.* (2010) Elevated proinflammatory cytokine expression in affected skin in small fiber neuropathy. *Neurology* 74, 1806–1813.

31 Orstavik K, Norheim I, Jorum E. (2006) Pain and small-fiber neuropathy in patients with hypothyroidism. *Neurology* 67, 786–791.

32 Penza P, Lombardi R, Camozzi F, Ciano C, Lauria G. (2009) Painful neuropathy in subclinical hypothyroidism: clinical and neuropathological recovery after hormone replacement therapy. *Neurol Sci* 30, 149–151.

33 Bednarik J, Vlckova-Moravcova E, Bursova S, Belobradkova J, Dusek L, Sommer C. (2009) Etiology of small-fiber neuropathy. *J Peripher Nerv Syst* 14, 177–183.

34 Hoitsma E, Marziniak M, Faber CG, Reulen JP, Sommer C, De Baets M, *et al.* (2002) Small fibre neuropathy in sarcoidosis. *The Lancet* 359, 2085–2086.

35 Lauria G, Merkies IS, Faber CG. (2012) Small fibre neuropathy. *Curr Opin Neurol* 25, 542–549.

36 Faber CG, Hoeijmakers JG, Ahn HS, Cheng X, Han C, Choi JS, *et al.* (2012) Gain of function Nanu1.7 mutations in idiopathic small fiber neuropathy. *Ann Neurol* 71, 26–39.

37 Hoeijmakers JG, Merkies IS, Gerrits MM, Waxman SG, Faber CG. (2012) Genetic aspects of sodium channelopathy in small fiber neuropathy. *Clin Genet* 82, 351–358.

38 Levy DM, Karanth SS, Springall DR, Polak JM. (1989) Depletion of cutaneous nerves and neuropeptides in diabetes mellitus: an immunocytochemical study. *Diabetologia* 32, 427–433.

39 Kennedy WR, Wendelschafer-Crabb G, Johnson T. (1996) Quantitation of epidermal nerves in diabetic neuropathy. *Neurology* 47, 1042–1048.

40 Smith AG, Ramachandran P, Tripp S, Singleton JR. (2001) Epidermal nerve innervation in impaired glucose tolerance and diabetes-associated neuropathy. *Neurology* 57, 1701–1704.

41 Sumner CJ, Sheth S, Griffin JW, Cornblath DR, Polydefkis M. (2003) The spectrum of neuropathy in diabetes and impaired glucose tolerance. *Neurology* 60, 108–111.

42 Smith AG, Russell J, Feldman EL, Goldstein J, Peltier A, Smith S, *et al.* (2006) Lifestyle intervention for pre-diabetic neuropathy. *Diabetes Care* 29, 1294–1299.

43 Quattrini C, Tavakoli M, Jeziorska M, Kallinikos P, Tesfaye S, Finnigan J, *et al.* (2007) Surrogate markers of small fiber damage in human diabetic neuropathy. *Diabetes* 56, 2148–2154.

44 Loseth S, Stalberg E, Jorde R, Mellgren SI. (2008) Early diabetic neuropathy: thermal thresholds and intraepidermal nerve fibre density in patients with normal nerve conduction studies. *J Neurol* 255, 1197–1202.

45 Boucek P, Havrdova T, Voska L, Lodererova A, He L, Saudek F, *et al.* (2008) Epidermal innervation in type 1 diabetic patients: a 2.5-year prospective study after simultaneous pancreas/kidney transplantation. *Diabetes Care* 31, 1611–1612.

46 Vlckova-Moravcova E, Bednarik J, Belobradkova J, Sommer C. (2008) Small-fibre involvement in diabetic patients with neuropathic foot pain. *Diabet Med* 25, 692–699.

47 Nebuchennykh M, Loseth S, Jorde R, Mellgren SI. (2008) Idiopathic polyneuropathy and impaired glucose metabolism in a Norwegian patient series. *Eur J Neurol* 15, 810–816.

48 Scott LJ, Griffin JW, Luciano C, Barton NW, Banerjee T, Crawford T, *et al.* (1999) Quantitative analysis of epidermal innervation in Fabry disease. *Neurology* 52, 1249–1254.

49 Torvin Moller A, Winther Bach F, Feldt-Rasmussen U, Rasmussen A, Hasholt L, Lan H, *et al.* (2009) Functional and structural nerve fiber findings in heterozygote patients with Fabry disease. *Pain* 145, 237–245.

50 Üçeyler N, He L, Schonfeld D, Kahn AK, Reiners K, Hilz MJ, *et al.* (2011) Small fibers in Fabry disease: baseline and follow-up data under enzyme replacement therapy. *J Peripher Nerv Syst* 16, 304–314.

51 Hilz MJ, Axelrod FB, Bickel A, Stemper B, Brys M, Wendelschafer-Crabb G, *et al.* (2004) Assessing function and pathology in familial dysautonomia: assessment of temperature perception, sweating and cutaneous innervation. *Brain* 127, 2090–2098.

52 Nolano M, Crisci C, Santoro L, Barbieri F, Casale R, Kennedy WR, *et al.* (2000) Absent innervation of skin and sweat glands in congenital insensitivity to pain with anhidrosis. *Clin Neurophysiol* 111, 1596–1601.

53 Nolano M, Provitera V, Crisci C, Saltalamacchia AM, Wendelschafer-Crabb G, Kennedy WR, *et al.* (2001) Small fibers involvement in Friedreich's ataxia. *Ann Neurol* 50, 17–25.

54 Li J, Bai Y, Ghandour K, Qin P, Grandis M, Trostinskaia A, *et al.* (2005) Skin biopsies in myelin-related neuropathies: bringing molecular pathology to the bedside. *Brain* 128, 1168–1177.

55 Sabet A, Li J, Ghandour K, Pu Q, Wu X, Kamholz J, *et al.* (2006) Skin biopsies demonstrate MPZ splicing abnormalities in Charcot–Marie–Tooth neuropathy 1B. *Neurology* 67, 1141–1146.

56 Üçeyler N, Devigili G, Toyka KV, Sommer C. (2010) Skin biopsy as an additional diagnostic tool in non-systemic vasculitic neuropathy. *Acta Neuropathol* 120, 109–116.

57 Polydefkis M, Hauer P, Sheth S, Sirdofsky M, Griffin JW, McArthur JC. (2004) The time course of epidermal nerve fibre regeneration: studies in normal controls and in people with diabetes, with and without neuropathy. *Brain* 127, 1606–1615.

58 Schifitto G, Yiannoutsos C, Simpson DM, Adornato BT, Singer EJ, Hollander H, *et al.* (2001) Long-term treatment with recombinant nerve growth factor for HIV-associated sensory neuropathy. *Neurology* 57, 1313–1316.

59 Bursova S, Dubovy P, Vlckova-Moravcova E, Nemec M, Klusakova I, Belobradkova J, *et al.* (2012) Expression of growth-associated protein 43 in the skin nerve fibers of patients with type 2 diabetes mellitus. *J Neurol Sci* 315, 60–63.

60 Narayanaswamy H, Facer P, Misra VP, Timmers M, Byttebier G, Meert T, *et al.* (2012) A longitudinal study of sensory biomarkers of progression in patients with diabetic peripheral neuropathy using skin biopsies. *J Clin Neurosci* 19, 1490–1496.

61 (2010) European Federation of Neurological Societies/Peripheral Nerve Society Guideline on management of paraproteinemic demyelinating neuropathies. *Report of a Joint Task Force of the European Federation of Neurological Societies and the Peripheral Nerve Society* – first revision. *J Peripher Nerv Syst* 15, 185–195.

CHAPTER 4

Methods for examination of peripheral nerve

Juan M. Bilbao,[1] Douglas C. Anthony,[2] and Umberto De Girolami[3]

[1] *Department of Laboratory Medicine, University of Toronto, Ontario, Canada*

[2] *Department of Pathology and Laboratory Medicine, Alpert Medical School of Brown University, and Lifespan Academic Medical Center, Rhode Island, USA*

[3] *Department of Pathology, Harvard Medical School and Neuropathologist, Brigham and Women's Hospital, Boston, USA*

General considerations

Nerve biopsy

Indications

There are fewer indications for nerve biopsies today due to improved electrophysiological methods and new molecular tests; however, certain clinical diagnostic issues continue to require a nerve biopsy [1–3]. The highest diagnostic yield is in the patient population with focal (or asymmetric) neuropathies, demyelinating neuropathies, or small-fiber neuropathies. The lowest yield is in biopsies from patients with chronic slowly-progressive diffuse symmetric axonal peripheral neuropathies. When a nerve biopsy is undertaken, the biopsy of a sensory peripheral nerve, such as the sural nerve, is preferred. The biopsy procedure is accompanied by the risk of potential adverse side effects that include wound infection, neuroma formation, post-operative pain, and persistent numbness [4]. Biopsy of a motor nerve, when necessary, is accompanied by loss of motor function, and is considered only when the function of the selected nerve is of limited distribution and has already been compromised. Even then, a fascicular biopsy, as opposed to whole nerve biopsy, is recommended in order to reduce the postoperative motor deficit.

Many nerve biopsy specimens do not demonstrate the histologic findings to resolve the differential diagnosis, a problem that is complicated whenever the sample is not optimally processed. Nevertheless, nerve biopsy continues to have a useful role in some clinical settings, and careful handling assures optimal information will be obtained [1–3, 5].

Site of biopsy

In practice, since many neuropathies are length-dependent, two nerves in the lower limb are ideal and are the most commonly obtained: the sural nerve (a branch of the common fibular nerve) or the superficial peroneal nerve (a branch of the lateral popliteal nerve). There is extensive and detailed information on the normal fiber composition of both these nerves, especially the sural nerve [6–13]. The superficial peroneal nerve is sometimes chosen, especially in the absence of sensory involvement, because the underlying peroneus brevis muscle may also be sampled with a single surgical incision when both a nerve and a muscle biopsy are needed (cf. Chapter 2). If symptoms predominantly affect the upper limbs, the superficial radial sensory nerve may be the preferred site for biopsy.

Biopsy procedure

The surgeon performing the biopsy should take care that a 2–4-cm segment of the nerve is gently exposed, without undue manipulation [14, 15]. The most common mistake is putting pressure on the nerve fascicles, such as clasping the nerve with forceps, which distorts the axons and myelin sheaths, and complicates further analysis of fine structure or quantitation. Care must also be taken not to cause damage by infiltration with local anesthetic or other undue manipulations during surgery. Once exposed, the nerve is cut with a sharp blade, first at the proximal end. It is removed by gentle traction on the epineurium, without direct pressure applied across the fascicles. The nerve must be rapidly transported to the laboratory and apportioned as needed,

Peripheral Nerve Disorders: Pathology and Genetics, First Edition. Edited by Jean-Michel Vallat, Joachim Weis, Francoise Gray, and Katy Keohane.

according to the clinical differential diagnosis. At many institutions, this is achieved by intra-operative consultation with the pathologist, using the same operative procedure as for the frozen section. The pathologist or technologist may then assist with the type of fixation, embedding media and the method of preparing the specimen as described in more detail next. If intraoperative consultation is not possible, the nerve segment should be placed on saline-soaked gauze (without excess medium, and not floating in fluid), and transported immediately to the laboratory. Selected references are offered for the reader who wishes detailed information [14–21].

Postmortem examination

Postmortem examination offers an opportunity to study the pathology of the peripheral nervous system in detail. Inadequate autopsy sampling often results in insufficient material for study of the pathology of diseases of the peripheral nervous system. Since the "organ" cannot simply be removed for examination, the customary autopsy samples are biopsies of the brachial or lumbosacral plexus or one or two proximal limb nerves. This sampling is inadequate for a full evaluation of the peripheral nervous system.

Having detailed clinical neurologic data and suspected diagnosis at the time of autopsy is ideal for planning the autopsy strategy; however, in its absence, sampling the peripheral nervous system is performed by selective biopsies. The best approach is to obtain multiple nerves for examination that reflect the topography of the patient's symptoms; in the absence of detailed neurologic information at the time of autopsy, a distribution of sampling that reflects the sensory system, motor system, and autonomic system (including both proximal and distal nerves and ganglia) is critical to fully study diseases of the peripheral nervous system.

In a sensorimotor polyneuropathy, the main objective is to study proximal and distal samples of the peripheral nervous system, combined with the routine examination of the spinal cord and brainstem. Segments of distal nerves, plexuses, and spinal and proximal nerves must be removed and identified as to their location. Several dorsal root spinal ganglia, anterior and posterior roots, and corresponding segments of the spinal cord should be excised after formalin fixation. The vagus nerve, sympathetic ganglia, and plexuses should be sampled, especially when autonomic symptoms were present. Cranial nerves and ganglia should also be carefully studied. Muscle biopsies should also be obtained, preferably from several sites, and skin biopsies may be analyzed for extent of innervation. After fixation, blocks of tissue are prepared for appropriate stains, using frozen section methods and embedding materials as detailed next.

Methods for evaluating nerve biopsies

The optimal examination of nerve biopsies requires routine paraffin histology, frozen samples for histology and molecular testing, plastic embedding for the preparation of semithin sections and electron microscopy, and nerve teasing. Since a broad range of specialized techniques are used to evaluate peripheral nerve biopsies, the clinical team should inform the pathologist about the indications for the biopsy and the specific clinical questions that need to be addressed.

In order to protect the nerve from air-drying, it is wrapped in a saline-moistened gauze (with all excess saline decanted), and transferred to the laboratory immediately after biopsy. One of the most critical aspects of handling a nerve biopsy is maintaining it as a straight segment, because its natural elasticity will allow the nerve to recoil when immersed in fixative. Before fixation or freezing, the fresh specimen may be gently stretched and the two ends of the nerve secured as a linear segment. There are multiple options in use, depending on the individual laboratory: securing between the clasps of a muscle biopsy clamp; suspending with light weights in fixative; or attaching to a fixed support, such as dental wax or cork board, with pins. Nerve biopsies are best analyzed by the combination of both cross sections and longitudinal sections.

The longitudinal 2–4 cm segment of biopsied nerve is apportioned, with a very sharp blade and very gentle handling of the tissue, into four or five segments with the following objectives: (1) routine paraffin histology, ideally with both longitudinal and cross sections; (2) plastic embedding for semithin sections and electron microscopy in cross section; (3) nerve teasing, requiring at least 1 cm of tissue for longitudinal evaluation; (4) frozen sections in cross section; and (5) snap freezing for biochemical studies.

Routine histology (paraffin embedding)

Fixation in 10% buffered formaldehyde and paraffin embedding is readily available in surgical pathology laboratories; the nerve biopsy should be oriented to obtain both cross and longitudinal sections. This enables the study of abnormalities of epineurial connective tissue and endoneurial structures, including blood vessels. Infiltration of tissue by inflammatory cells or tumor cells, and the presence of deposits of substances such as amyloid are best detected in these routine histologic samples. The stains most commonly employed for paraffin sections include H&E (Figure 4.1), elastic tissue stains, Masson trichrome, silver impregnation for reticulin, myelin stains, silver impregnations for axons, and stains for amyloid deposits (e.g., Congo red). Routine paraffin-embedded tissue is also optimal for additional aniline dye methods, when needed, and immunohistochemistry.

Immunohistochemistry

Immunohistochemistry has been optimized in paraffin-embedded tissue, and a wide range of antibodies are available for evaluation of biopsies. Most surgical pathology laboratories have validated a whole range of immunohistochemical markers in paraffin blocks. Markers allow identification of inflammatory cells, separate identification of T cells and B cells, and their subtypes (CD4, CD8, CD20, etc.). In addition, cell surface markers allow identification of both epithelial and lymphoid tumor cells. Axons may be highlighted with immunohistochemical detection of neurofilaments, or the protein gene product (PGP 9.5). The latter has been used for quantitative assessment of axonal density.

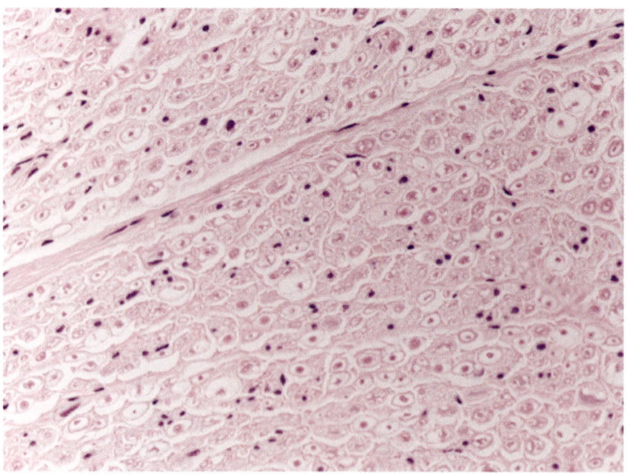

Figure 4.1 Routine histology of peripheral nerve, embedded in paraffin and stained with H&E, in cross section allows identification of large caliber axons (eosinophilic axon with clear halo due to extraction of myelin lipids). In this normal biopsy, axons are abundant and easily identified.

Plastic-resin embedding

Embedding specimens in plastic or resin media allows thinner sections to be obtained. Specimens are immediately fixed in 2.5%-buffered glutaraldehyde, post-fixed with osmium tetroxide, and embedded in a resin (Epon is a common example). This method provides excellent fixation of proteins through the glutaraldehyde, and fixation of lipids (via osmium tetroxide), providing high-resolution microscopy. The resin allows for semithin (1-µm thick) transverse and longitudinal sections to be prepared; this is the method of choice to examine the fine details of both myelinated and unmyelinated fibers (Figure 4.2). Plastic-embedded semithin sections provide higher resolution than paraffin-embedded sections, due to better fixation and thinner sections. Resin embedding also permits quantitative assessment of axonal density, myelin thickness, and subcellular structures that are poorly visualized with routine histology. In addition, this medium is compatible with electron microscopy, should it be required.

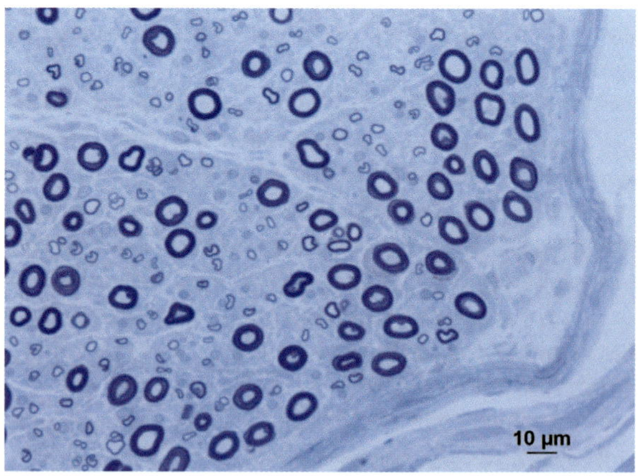

Figure 4.2 Epon-embedded normal nerve biopsy in cross section shows the normal complement of axons. The large caliber axons have thick myelin sheaths and stand out. In reality, the axons show a bimodal distribution, with both large and small caliber axons, with the thickness of the myelin sheath proportional to the axonal diameter. Unmyelinated axons are not well resolved, even with epon-embedded samples, but the cytoplasm of their ensheathing Remak cells stands out from the adjacent paler collagen.

Frozen sections for immunofluorescence

Direct immunofluorescence studies can be carried out using specific antibodies to identify abnormal deposits of immunoglobulins in endoneurium or adjacent to myelinated fibers. Various markers can be employed to identify different proteins (IgG, IgM, complement) as well as different types of inflammatory cells, as recognized by their surface cell markers (B-lymphocytes, T-lymphocytes and subtypes, and macrophages). Some classifications of immune-mediated neuropathies include immunofluorescence criteria. Immunofluorescence requires freezing one short segment of nerve (ideally in cross section) without any aldehyde fixation. Frozen sections can also be used to detect lipid-rich substances that are extracted during routine histologic preparations.

Dissociation of fibers (nerve teasing)

This technique consists of the separation of individual myelinated fibers (around 1 cm long), after aldehyde fixation and osmication. After fixation, following the same protocol as for resin embedding, the nerve is separated into individual fascicles, stripped of perineurium, and individual fibers are teased apart with fine needles under a dissecting microscope. Light microscopic examination of the longitudinally-oriented teased fibers shows osmicated internodes, separated at regular intervals by gaps in the osmication that represent the nodes of Ranvier. The length of each internodal segment and the relative thickness of the myelin from one internode to the next can be assessed, and this is very helpful in discriminating between lesions characteristic of demyelination versus axonal degeneration. The method is also sensitive in the detection of axonal degeneration; however, while degeneration may be seen on resin-embedded sections, the segmental demyelination along the length of a fiber is only visible on teased fiber preparations.

Frozen specimens for molecular analysis

Frozen tissue is also useful when testing for metabolic disorders, both because direct chemical analysis of tissue can be performed, and because storage materials, which may be removed during routine histologic processing, are retained. Many laboratories retain a frozen portion for molecular testing; this portion does not need to be oriented and can simply be snap frozen, such as with liquid nitrogen. This frozen tissue is ideal for direct chemical analysis of tissue for storage materials or deposits.

Deoxyribonucleic acid (DNA) testing for a wide range of conditions is now available on whole blood samples, and it is not necessary to use nerve biopsy tissue to identify most forms of hereditary peripheral neuropathy. However, DNA can be extracted from either paraffin-embedded or frozen tissue, allowing molecular classification of archival material.

Electron microscopy

The resin-embedded sample is the best tissue sample for electron microscopy. Review of the light microscopy of the resin-embedded nerve allows the pathologist to select areas for electron microscopy; most laboratories require a cross-sectional area that is less than the full cross-sectional area of the sural nerve. Those areas of highest interest can then be processed for ultrathin sections; typically the adjacent tissue is trimmed away, the area is sectioned with an ultramicrotome, and sections are placed on copper grids and stained for electron microscopic examination. Electron microscopy is the best method to detect alterations in the myelin layers, and to evaluate unmyelinated fibers (Figure 4.3).

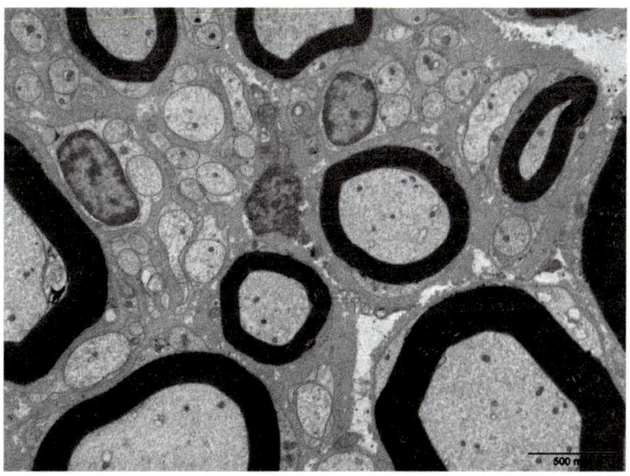

Figure 4.3 An electron micrograph demonstrates larger caliber myelinated axons, smaller caliber myelinated axons, and the unmyelinated axons. Myelin is wrapped concentrically around each myelinated axon, while the unmyelinated axons are grouped together as clusters within a darker cytoplasm of the Remak cell. Each of the Schwann cell types (myelinating and Remak cell) has a basal lamina, while the endoneurial fibroblasts lack a basal lamina.

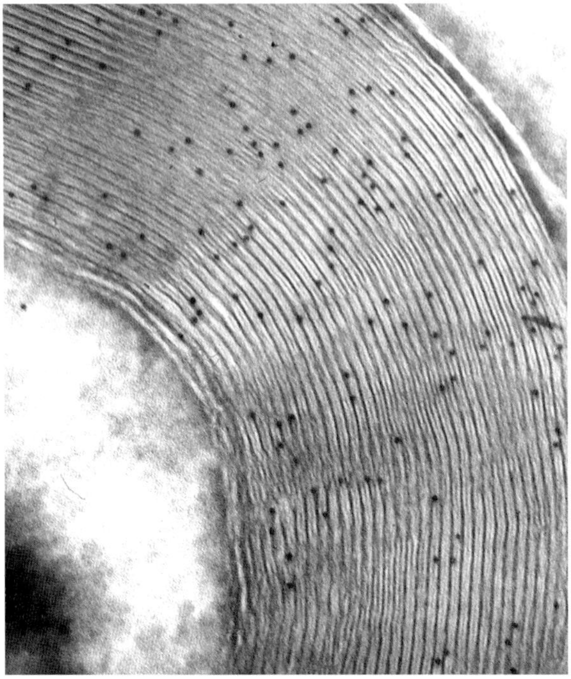

Figure 4.4 Immunoelectron microscopy. Transverse section of a normal nerve. Immunolabeling of P0 by a specific antibody located in this normal myelin sheath, revealed by gold particles. Source: Jean-Michel Vallat, CHU de Limoges, France. Reproduced with permission of Jean-Michel Vallat.

Immuno-electron microscopy may be performed in order to identify specific proteins at ultrastructural level; however, this technique is available in only a few academic medical centers. It is a powerful technique that combines the specificity and flexibility of immunohistochemistry with the resolution of electron microscopy (Figure 4.4). A variety of methods are available, but most require a special embedding resin (such as London white resin; LWR) in order to allow antigen recognition.

Quantitative and morphometric analyses

Morphometric studies of nerve are time-consuming and costly, and are best reserved for research or in the approach to specific differential diagnosis. Instead, an experienced observer can often give a reliable opinion as to the density of myelinated fibers, an estimate of the degree of loss of large or small fibers, and the presence and severity of demyelinating and/or axonal lesions, without the expense and delay that is added by quantitative assessment.

Electron microscopy is probably the best method for quantitative assessments of cross sections, and allows quantification of myelinated and unmyelinated axons. However, resin-embedded cross sections may also be used, and allow assessment of axonal density (fibers per square micrometer), and g ratio (ratio of the inner axonal diameter to the total nerve fiber diameter including the myelin sheath). In addition, PGP 9.5 immunohistochemistry has been used to assess axonal density from paraffin-embedded tissue.

Morphometric analysis of cross-sections may be carried out either after photography or directly by image analysis. In young adults, the average axonal density is between 7000 and 10,000 fibers/mm^2 of endoneurial area. There are marked age-dependent differences, and the number of fibers decreases progressively with age. The diameter of myelinated fibers ranges from 2–12 μm in a bimodal distribution with peaks at 3–6 μm and 9–12 μm; there are more small myelinated fibers than large myelinated fibers.

The relationships between size of the axon and number of myelin lamellae (or thickness of myelin) can only be established with electron microscopic examination, and is a nearly linear relationship. The g ratio is defined as the ratio of axonal diameter to fiber diameter, and is relatively constant over a large range of axonal diameters. It is commonly used to evaluate the severity of demyelination and may be measured on semi-thin sections of high quality.

Unmyelinated fibers may also be quantified, but it requires special expertise to reliably identify them. The diameter of these axons ranges from 0.2–2.5 μm in a unimodal distribution with a peak at 1.4–1.6 μm, and they are located in clusters within Remak cells with 7–10 fibers per cell. The density of unmyelinated fibers ranges from 20,000 to 35,000/mm^2. The ratio of unmyelinated fibers to myelinated fibers is about 4: 1. Other parameters may also be quantified; such as the thickness of the perineurium and the extent of proliferation of endoneurial connective tissue.

In the longitudinal plane, morphometric analysis is best performed on teased fiber preparations. It allows quantification of the internodal lengths on single nerve fibers, and the frequency of fibers involved. Unlike cross sections for which some automated morphometric analyses are possible, the quantitative assessment of teased fibers is an entirely manual process.

References

1 Lacomis D. (2005) Clinical utility of peripheral nerve biopsy. *Curr Neurol Neurosci Rep* 5: 41–47.

2 Schweikert K, Fuhr P, Probst A *et al.* (2007) Contribution of nerve biopsy to unclassified neuropathy. *Eur Neurol* 57: 86–90.

3 Hilton DA, Jacob J, Househam L, Tengah C. (2007) Complications following sural and peroneal nerve biopsies. *J Neurol Neurosurg Psychiatry* 78: 271–1272.

4 Mikell CB, Chan AK, Stein GE *et al.* (2013) Muscle and nerve biopsies: techniques for the neurologist and neurosurgeon. *Clin Neurol Neurosurg* 115: 1206–1214.

5 Gabriel CM, Howard R, Kinsella N, *et al.* (2000) Prospective study of the usefulness of sural nerve biopsy. *J Neurol Neurosurg Psychiatry* 69: 442–446.

6 Midroni G, Bilbao JM. (1995) *Biopsy Diagnosis of Peripheral Neuropathy.* Butterworth-Heinemann, Boston.

7 De Girolami U, Frosch M, Amato AA. (2003) Biopsy of nerve and muscle. In Samuels M, Feske S (eds). *Office Practice of Neurology,* pp. 217–225. Harcourt Health Sciences, Philadelphia.

8 O'Sullivan. (1968) The fiber size and content of the radial and sural nerves. *J Neurol Neurosur Psychiatr* 31: 464–470.

9 Ferreire G, Denef J-F, Rodriguez J, Guzzetta F (1985) Morphometric studies of normal sural nerves in children. *Muscle Nerve* 8: 697–704.

10 Jacobs JM, Love S (1985) Qualitative and quantitative morphology of human sural nerve at different ages. *Brain* 108: 897–924.

11 Ouvrier RA, McLeod JC, Conchin T (1987) Morphometric studies of sural nerve in childhood. *Muscle Nerve* 10: 47–53.

12 Gibbels E (1989) Morphometry of unmyelinated nerve fibers. *Clin Neuropathol* 8: 179–187.

13 Behse F (1990). Morphometric studies on the human sural nerved. *Acta Neuropatholol Scan* 82 (Supp) 132: 1–38.

14 Anthony DC, Crain BJ (1996) Peripheral nerve biopsies. *Arch Pathol Lab Med* 120: 26–34.

15 Weis J, Brander s, Lammens M, Sommer C, Vallat J-M (2012) Processing of nerve biopsies: a practical guide. *Clin Neuropathol* 31: 7–23.

16 Bouche P, Vallat J-M (1992) *Neuropathies Périphériques.* Doin, Paris.

17 Richardson EP, Jr., De Girolami U (1995) Pathology of the Peripheral Nerve. WB Saunders, Philadelphia.

18 Schröder JM (2001) *Pathology of Peripheral Nerves. An Atlas of Structural and Molecular Pathological Changes.* Springer, Berlin

19 Dyck PJ, Dyck PJB, Engelstad J (2005) Pathologic alterations of nerves. In: Dyck PJ, Thomas PK (eds). *Peripheral Neuropathy,* pp. 733–829. W-B Saunders, Philadelphia.

20 DeGirolami UL, Anthony DC (2001) Nerve and muscle biopsy. In: Katirja B, Kaminski HJ, Preston DC, Ruff RL, Shapiro BE, (eds). *Neuromuscular Disorders in Clinical Practice,* pp. 223–46. Butterworth-Heinemann Publishers, Woburn, MA.

21 Amato AA, Russell JA (2008) *Neuromuscular Disorders,* pp. 83–94. McGraw-Hill, New York.

CHAPTER 5

Complications from nerve biopsy

Richard A.C. Hughes

Department of Neurology, King's College London and Cochrane Neuromuscular Disease Group, MRC Centre for Neuromuscular Disease, National Hospital for Neurology and Neurosurgery, London, UK

Introduction: My nerve biopsy

As I write this, I am unaware of any symptoms following a fascicular biopsy of my right sural nerve 20 years ago. Immediately after, I had loss of feeling along the lateral border of the foot from the heel to the base of the little toe associated with a warm tingling feeling [5]. This was replaced by a more or less continuous burning feeling in the numb area and up the back of the calf proximal to the scar, never severe enough to require analgesia. This discomfort persisted for several months and slightly for a couple of years, becoming more apparent when I was tired or stressed; a genuine Achilles' heel. Now, if I rub the scar I can just feel a very faint tingling.

Frequency of complications

All studies addressing complications of nerve biopsy have identified a small percentage of patients who have experienced complications, sometimes severe. Dyck *et al.* [3] surveyed 134 patients by postal questionnaire; 97 replied and 10% reported considerable persistent pain or dysesthesiae. Poburski *et al.* [9] invited 82 patients who had sural nerve biopsies during the previous 4 years at the Medizinischer Hochschule, Hanover, to attend for review. Only 24 (29%) attended. The extent of sensory loss varied from none to 100 cm^2, mean 46 cm^2. Fourteen of the 24 (58%) had discomfort and five (21%) considerable discomfort. Electricity-like sensations prevented one woman from wearing shoes and caused constant aching pain in another. The frequency of side-effects may have been overrepresented because those with problems had greater motivation to attend for review. Solders [12] sent a postal questionnaire to 60 patients, who had a sural nerve biopsy between 6 years and 6 months earlier at the Karolinska Institute, Sweden. Fifty-four replied and six had persistent discomfort, which was severe in three. Oh [7] reported delayed wound healing in 1% and post-traumatic neuralgia in 0.5% of 385 biopsies.

Gabriel *et al.* [4] performed the only prospective study. It included 50 consecutive sural nerve biopsies performed at Guy's Hospital, London, to investigate the cause of peripheral neuropathy. The study design invited patients to return a questionnaire about their experience of nerve biopsy to an independent audit officer. Thirty nine patients completed the questionnaire after 6 weeks and 30 after 6 months. Six (15% of responders) reported "infection" and 21 (67%) increased pain at 6 weeks. Seven (18%) reported having had infection and 10 (33%) increased pain at 6 months. There was no significant difference in the incidence of side effects between different types of neuropathy. The questionnaire also sought answers to how satisfied patients were by the biopsy. Thirty one (79%) of the 39 patients who responded after 6 weeks and 19 (63%) of 30 who responded after 6 months were very or fairly pleased they had the biopsy. Almost all of those who were "slightly" or "very unhappy" had idiopathic axonal neuropathy and were dissatisfied because the biopsy had not disclosed the diagnosis.

The number of patients with severe discomfort after nerve biopsy in the reported series is disconcerting. It should dissuade us from performing biopsies unless absolutely necessary and require us to warn patients of the possibility of severe pain when obtaining consent for the procedure.

Peripheral Nerve Disorders: Pathology and Genetics, First Edition. Edited by Jean-Michel Vallat, Joachim Weis, Francoise Gray, and Katy Keohane.

When to perform a nerve biopsy

Because of the risk of complications, nerve biopsy should not be performed as a diagnostic procedure unless the neuropathy is or is becoming a significant problem to the patient, the diagnosis cannot be reached in some other way and there is a chance of a treatable pathology being revealed [11]. A diagnostically useful biopsy is more likely if the neuropathy is asymmetrical and painful, and possibly if nerve conduction is slowed. However, even in the absence of these features a nerve biopsy may be diagnostically helpful, especially when it shows an unexpected diagnosis. A sural nerve biopsy showed vasculitis in 11% of 53 cases with clinical and electrophysiological features of symmetrical axonal neuropathy [1]. Biopsy revealed chronic inflammatory demyelinating polyradiculoneuropathy in eight patients who had insufficient evidence of demyelination on electrophysiological examination to make the diagnosis [13].

Predicting complications

There is no reliable means of predicting which patients will or will not suffer complications. Common sense dictates that patients who already have dense sensory loss and pain in the territory of the nerve to be biopsied are less likely to have increased sensory loss or pain afterwards. Complications are not commoner in the elderly: in reviewing the nerve biopsies of 100 consecutive patients aged 65 years or more, Said *et al.* (reported in [2]) at the Centre Hospitalier de Bicêtre, Paris, France, did not find any more problems with wound healing, subcutaneous hematomas or infection than in younger patients, although they do not state how common such complications were. Perry and Bril [8] found that mild persistent pain occurred in 18.9% of patients and was no more common in 41 diabetics than 40 non-diabetics with neuropathy; none had severe pain. Delayed healing or infection of the wound is probably more likely in patients who are on corticosteroids.

Reducing complications

It is likely that technique affects the incidence of complications. Counterintuitively, Pollock *et al.* [10] found in a personal series of 16 patients that symptoms and sensory loss were no greater 5–6 years after a full thickness than a fascicular sural nerve biopsy. There is wide variation in the extent of immobilization after the procedure. Said *et al.* [2] immobilized the biopsied limb for 5–7 days in a plastic cast, longer for patients on corticosteroids. There is a need for a randomized controlled trial to compare the effect of longer and shorter periods of immobilization on wound healing and long-term complications. There is also a need to investigate whether and when skin biopsy with examination of the dermal nerve fibers [6] can replace nerve biopsy for diagnostic purposes.

References

1 Bennett DL, Groves M, Blake J *et al.* The use of nerve and muscle biopsy in the diagnosis of vasculitis: a 5 year retrospective study. *J Neurol Neurosurg Psychiatry* 2008; 79: 1376–1381.
2 Chia L, Fernandez A, Lacroix C *et al.* Contribution of nerve biopsy findings to the diagnosis of disabling neuropathy in the elderly: A retrospective review of 100 consecutive patients. *Brain* 1996; 119: 1091–1098.
3 Dyck PJ, Karnes J, Lais AC, Stevens JC. Pathological alterations of the peripheral nervous system. In: Dyck PJ, Thomas PK, Lambert EH, (eds). *Peripheral Neuropathy*. Philadelphia: Saunders WB; 1984.
4 Gabriel CM, Howard R, Kinsella N *et al.* Prospective study of the usefulness of sural nerve biopsy. *J Neurol Neurosurg Psychiatry* 2000; 69: 442–446.
5 Hughes RAC. Me and my nerve biopsy. *Practical Neurology* 2003; 3: 313–314.
6 Lauria G, Cazzato D, Porretta-Serapiglia C *et al.* Morphometry of dermal nerve fibers in human skin. *Neurology* 2011; 77: 242–249.
7 Oh SJ. Diagnostic usefulness and limitations of the sural nerve biopsy. *Yonsei Medical Journal* 1990; 31: 1–26.
8 Perry JR, Bril V. Complications of sural nerve biopsy in diabetic versus non-diabetic patients. *Can J Neurol Sci* 1994; 21: 34–37.
9 Poburski R, Malin JP, Stark E. Sequelae of sural nerve biopsies. *Clin Neurol Neurosurg* 1985; 87: 193–198.
10 Pollock M, Nukada H, Taylor P *et al.* Comparison between fascicular and whole sural nerve biopsy. *Ann Neurol* 1983; 13: 65–68.
11 Said G. Indications and usefulness of nerve biopsy. *Arch Neurol* 2002; 59: 1532–1535.
12 Solders G. Discomfort after fascicular sural nerve biopsy. *Acta Neurol Scand* 1988; 77: 503–504.
13 Vallat J-M, Tabaraud F, Magy L *et al.* Diagnostic value of nerve biopsy for atypical chronic inflammatory demyelinating polyneuropathy: evaluation of eight cases. *Muscle Nerve* 2003; 27: 478–485.

CHAPTER 6
Anatomy of the peripheral nerve

Rosalind King
Department of Clinical Neurosciences, Institute of Neurology, University College London, London, UK

Introduction

Axons are extensions of neurons that enable communication between neurons and the peripheral end organs. In the peripheral nervous system (PNS), they are collected in fascicles defined by perineurial cells and embedded in a collagenous epineurial sheath. All PNS axons are surrounded by and given metabolic support by Schwann cells. Some axons have an insulating myelin sheath, produced during development from Schwann cell processes and consisting of alternating lipid and protein layers in consecutive segments that contact each other at nodes of Ranvier. The function of the myelin sheath is to increase the conduction velocity as the nervous impulse jumps from one node to the next. Smaller axons are not myelinated and conduct much more slowly (Fig. 6.1). Nerve structure is not mature until about 12 years of age. In later life there may be spontaneous breakdown of the myelin sheath and failure of neurons to support the more distal parts of the axon.

Normal anatomy of peripheral nerves

The nerve trunk

This consists of cylindrical fascicles containing nerve fibers originating in the central nervous system or the dorsal root ganglion and autonomic ganglion neurons. The sural nerve at the ankle is the most frequently examined in man and contains between 8 and 13 fascicles. Each fascicle is defined by a cellular sheath or perineurium consisting of several layers of modified fibroblasts separated by layers of fibrillar collagen and connected together by tight and gap junctions [1]. The perineurium forms a diffusion barrier across which access to the interior of the fascicle is provided by active transport. The epineurium surrounds the perineurium. The epineurium provides metabolic and mechanical support (Fig. 6.2) for the fascicles and contains fibroblasts, fibrillar collagen, blood vessels, lymph ducts, and fat cells. Small branches of the blood vessels penetrate the perineurium. Adjacent to the cytoplasmic surface of the perineurial cell are fibrillar patches resembling the actin of smooth muscle; it has been suggested that these are analogous to similar structures on seminiferous tubules and hence that the perineurium has contractile properties [2]. Perineurial cells are ensheathed by a basal lamina, consisting of collagens V and VI, laminin, and glycosaminoglycans. This may be extensively thickened in later life and also in patients with diabetes.

The tube of perineurial cells is continuous from the meninges to terminal encapsulated sensory end organs. In motor nerves and probably also in unencapsulated sensory endings, the perineurium terminates as an open-ended sheath. There are patches of oxytalan fibrils within and underlying the perineurium. True elastic fibers composed of elaunin and oxytalan are only found in the epineurium.

There are two distinct layers of collagen (mostly type I collagen fibrils) in the epineurium. The outer layers may contain considerable numbers of adipocytes in addition to collagen fibrils. Although the collagen fibrils are inextensible, they are arranged in a zig-zag pattern. This changes when placed under tension and this arrangement probably allows extension of the limb without damage to the nerve [3].

Peripheral Nerve Disorders: Pathology and Genetics, First Edition. Edited by Jean-Michel Vallat, Joachim Weis, Francoise Gray, and Katy Keohane.

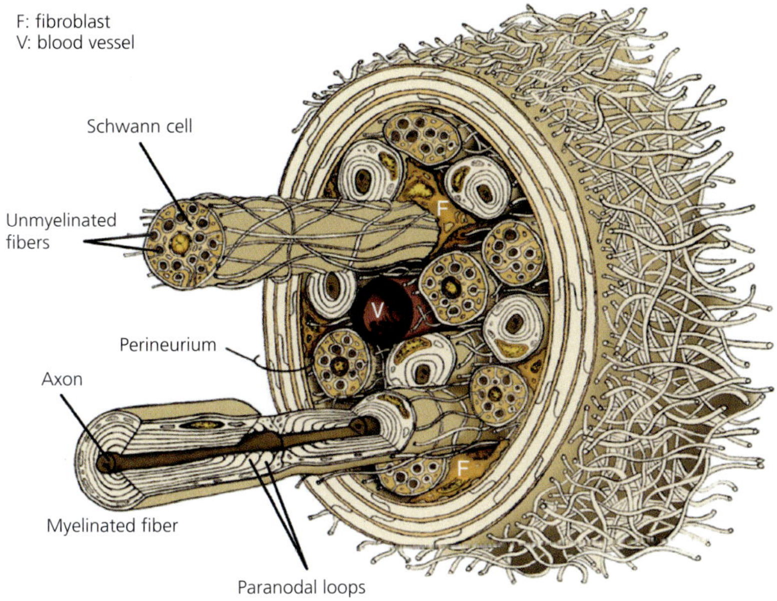

Figure 6.1 Cellular constituents of the endoneurial microenvironment in peripheral nerve. A small nerve fascicle ensheathed by perineurium surrounded by epineurial collagen fibrils is shown with myelinated and unmyelinated fibers, a single endoneurial vessel (V) and scattered fibroblasts (F) embedded in the loose connective tissue of the endoneurium. Not shown are pericytes, resident macrophages, and masts cells. Source: Mizisin & and Weerasuriya, *Acta Neuropathol* 2011; 121:291–312. Reproduced with permission of Springer.

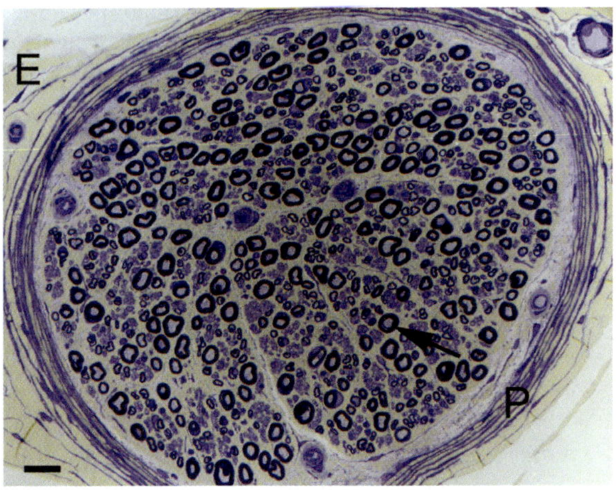

Figure 6.2 Light micrograph, resin section, normal nerve fascicle showing epineurium (E) and perineurium (P). The endoneurium contains large and small myelinated fibers (arrow) embedded in yellow stained fibrillar collagen. Unmyelinated axons are not resolvable at this magnification. Bar = 20 µm.

The nerve fibers themselves are composite structures consisting of axons surrounded and supported by specialized glial cells (Schwann cells). Fibroblasts in the endoneurium produce striated collagen fibrils (mainly type III collagen) that give mechanical strength and support the fragile nerve fibers. In some fascicles there may also be ovoid structures called Renaut bodies, composed of thin fibroblast processes and bundles of collagen. It has been suggested that these act as shock absorbers.

The blood supply to nerve trunks consists of small arteries and veins in the epineurium that divide into smaller vessels and penetrate into the endoneurium. Mast cells and small numbers of resident monocytes/macrophages may also be found in the endoneurium.

Axons

The axons within fascicles vary in size from 0.2–15 µm in diameter. They are all surrounded by Schwann cells but the arrangement differs depending on the diameter of the axon. PNS axons are very long, thin cylindrical extensions originating in neuronal cell bodies lying in the brain, spinal cord or dorsal root, and autonomic ganglia; they connect the central nervous system to peripheral sensory end organs and muscles. Unlike neuronal dendrites, axons do not contain rough endoplasmic reticulum so protein synthesis is in the perikaryon and proteins are transported along the axon. Axons leave the cell body at the axon hillock and there is little or no branching before reaching their terminus where they may divide into many smaller branches.

The axonal cytoskeleton consists of specialized intermediate neurofilaments composed of three types of subunit that polymerize to form 10-nm unbranched filaments with side arms at regular intervals [4]. Microtubules are slightly larger in cross-section being approximately 25 nm in diameter. They are composed of dimers of alpha and beta tubulin that polymerize to form a helical tube with 13 protofilaments. These provide the mechanism for transporting organelles such as mitochondria along the considerable distances from cell body to end organ and back; in the long nerves of the leg, axons may be as much as a meter in length. Anterograde transport from the cell body to the periphery is by means of kinesin molecules acting as motors to move organelles along the tubules. The reverse mechanism is retrograde transport, which is similar but mediated by dynein [5]. Axons are electrically active and carry nerve impulses produced by neurons. They end in synapses where the electrical signal is transduced into a chemical signal that activates the receptor cell.

Myelinated nerve fibers

Where axon diameter is larger than 2–3 μm, it is encased by a chain of Schwann cells whose length is related to the axon diameter, being approximately 100 times as long as the axon diameter. This results in an internode of 300 μmon the smallest axons and 1.5 mm on the largest. Each myelinating Schwann cell produces an insulating myelin sheath around the length of axon that it covers (Fig. 6.3). Myelin is a lipoprotein material with a lamellar structure with a periodicity of 17 nm in fresh material that is reduced to about 14 nm after fixation [6]. At high magnification the structure is resolvable into Major dense lines separated by a less dense intraperiod line (Fig. 6.3 insert). Myelin has the function of increasing the conduction speed of the fiber. In this situation each Schwann cell surrounds only one axon. Adjacent Schwann cells and their myelin segments join at specialized structures called nodes of Ranvier. Adjacent to the node is the paranode where the myelin lamellae terminate on the axon. In small fibers with a diameter of less than 5 μm the lamellae terminate consecutively in a simple arrangement; this has been called a type I node [7]. Where the axon diameter is larger, the paranodal arrangement is more complex with many lamellae terminating on one another before they reach

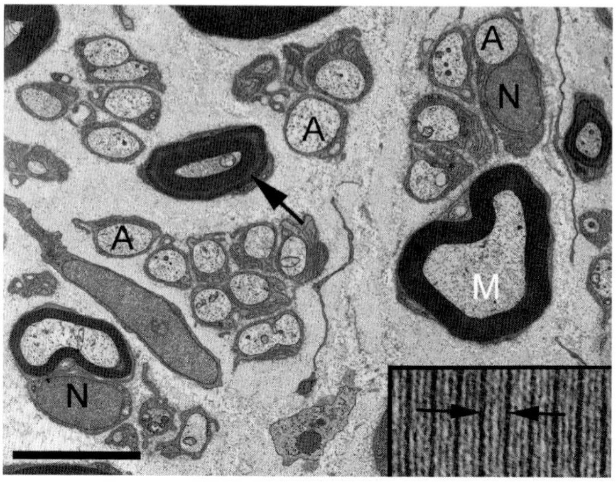

Figure 6.3 Electron micrograph showing unmyelinated axons (A) and myelinated fibers (M), one containing a Schmidt–Lanterman incisure (arrow). N indicates Schwann cell nuclei. *Insert*: detail of myelin structure showing major dense lines (arrows) and intermediate lines between them. Bar = 2 μm.

the axon. This structure has been likened to ears of barley and occupies a much shorter length of axolemma than would be the case if each myelin layer terminated consecutively; this has been called a type 2 node [7].

The nodal gap is the bare length of axon between two myelin segments; sodium channels are located in this region. Schwann cells terminate in villus-like nodal processes that interdigitate and closely approach the axolemma. The Schwann cell basal lamina is continuous across this region, forming a continuous unbroken tube from the origin of the axon to its termination.

The Schwann cell nucleus is located midway along the cell on the exterior surface of the myelin sheath. Most of the Schwann cell cytoplasm is adjacent to the paranode, juxtaparanode, and the perinuclear region. The myelin sheath is circular for most of its length, but in larger fibers near the node it forms deep folds, having a crenated cross appearance with three or four arms enclosing pockets of Schwann cell cytoplasm on cross section. Most of the mitochondria of the cell are located at the paranode [8]. Between the nuclear region and the juxtaparanode, the Schwann cell cytoplasm divides into narrow ribbons on the surface of the myelin sheath. Away from these ribbons, the myelin is separated from the extracellular space only by the Schwann cell basal lamina.

In addition to complete breaks in continuity of the myelin sheath at nodes of Ranvier, there are internodal regions of non-compaction, the Schmidt–Lanterman incisures (Fig. 6.3). Here the lamellae open up to enclose pockets of Schwann cell cytoplasm forming a helical pathway connecting the Schwann cell immediately adjacent to the axon to the cytoplasm on the outer surface of the myelin sheath. The principal function of the axon is to transmit an electrical impulse between the cell body and the end organ. In myelinated nerve fibers the impulse jumps from one node of Ranvier to the next in a process known as saltatory conduction [9]. This increases conductions speeds from about 2 m/s in unmyelinated axons to 60 m/s or more in large myelinated axons [9]. When sodium channels on the axolemma at the nodes of Ranvier open, sodium ions leave the axon and the voltage across the axolemma changes; the result is that the nervous impulse jumps from one node to the next. To reset the resting conditions, potassium ions move into the axon at the juxtaparanode.

The largest myelinated fibers are the sensory afferents to muscle spindles. Slightly smaller ones are motor fibers that terminate on the muscle fibers. Smaller myelinated and unmyelinated axons are sensory and autonomic fibers. In the sural nerve, fiber size distribution is bimodal with a smaller peak of large fibers about 10 μm in diameter, internodal minimum at about 7 μm, and a larger peak of small fibers with a mean diameter of about 5 μm. The thickness of the myelin sheath varies with axon diameter and is often expressed as the ratio of axon diameter to total fiber diameter (g ratio). This ratio is approximately 0.7 in the normal sural nerve but smaller myelinated axons have a relatively thinner myelin sheath and larger fibers are more nearly circular in cross section than smaller ones [10, 11].

Unmyelinated axons

Smaller axons (less than about 2–3 μm) do not have a myelin sheath or individual Schwann cell ensheathment. They are difficult to see by light microscopy; electron microscopy shows them as one or more axons lying partly or completely surrounded by Schwann cell cytoplasm (a Remak fiber) (Fig. 6.3). As they run from one Schwann cell to the next, the association between individual axons and Schwann cells changes frequently [12]. This has implications for regeneration as the Schwann cells form individual disconnected rounded cells when the axons connecting them degenerate. This contrasts with the situation when a myelinated axon degenerates leaving an intact tube of Schwann cell basal lamina to act as a guide for regenerating axon sprouts. In the sural nerve there are approximately four times as many axons without a myelin sheath as myelinated ones.

End organs

Motor nerves contact muscles at motor end plates. Close to the muscle, the myelinated fiber loses its myelin sheath and divides into several smaller branches, each with its own Schwann cell. These closely approach the target muscle. In this region the sarcolemma is highly convoluted and electron dense. The axon terminus contains numerous small vesicles containing acetylcholine. When a nerve impulse arrives these are emitted and travel the short distance to the muscle sarcolemma where they lock onto specialized receptors and trigger muscle contraction.

Sensory endings

These may be encapsulated or free. Specialized types of encapsulated endings include Pacinian corpuscles, Ruffini corpuscles, Golgi tendon organs, and muscle spindles. These all possess a perineurial-like capsule surrounding a single fiber that is unmyelinated at its end. They detect pressure or movement, magnified by the multiple layers surrounding the central fiber. Each type has a specific function and is found in a particular tissue. Free nerve endings are naked endings of unmyelinated axons and are sensory detectors for heat, cold, or pain [13].

Variations according to age

Development

In the embryo, axon sprouts growing out from the CNS into the periphery initially form large groups of small, naked axons surrounded by thin Schwann cell processes. These are difficult to distinguish from adjacent muscle fiber bundles but, as the embryo grows, a loose arrangement of fibroblast-like cells encircles the developing nerve to produce a defined nerve trunk. As this develops, the Schwann cells divide and some extend processes that wrap around individual axons and remove them from the embryonic bundle [14]. Once a one-to-one relationship between one axon and one Schwann cell is established, cytoplasmic processes wrap around the central axon (Fig. 6.4). The layers of cell membrane then compress together and cytoplasm is extruded. At the same time additional proteins are incorporated, mainly myelin basic protein (MBP), myelin protein zero (MPZ), and a small proportion (10%) of peripheral myelin protein MW22 (PMP22). Despite its low percentage, PMP22 is implicated in the most important of the inherited myelin diseases, Charcot–Marie–Tooth disease type 1. The resultant myelin sheath thus consists of alternating lipid and protein layers. The myelin sheath continues to grow in thickness for several years and remains permanently connected to the inner and outer surfaces of the Schwann cell by extensions of the plasma membrane known as inner and outer mesaxons [14, 15]. During development, fibroblasts multiply and segregate bundles of Schwann cells and axons into protofascicles. The fibroblasts then connect together by means of tight and gap junctions to form a continuous multilamellated tube, the *perineurium*. The mature perineurium has a continuous basal laminal ensheathment and layers of fibrous collagen between the cellular laminae. Maturation of the perineurium lags behind myelination possibly rendering the developing nerve more susceptible to deleterious substances than the adult nerve.

The function of an axon is to communicate between the cell bodies in the central nervous system and sensory or motor end organs in the periphery. Unfortunately myelinated fibers have the disadvantage of being more fragile and sensitive to mechanical and chemical insults than unmyelinated axons. Hence where speed of reaction is important such as in motor fibers these are myelinated but when robustness is more important and speed less so, such as pain and temperature sensation, the axons are small and unmyelinated.

Age changes

With age, defects appear more prominent in larger myelinated fibers. The myelin sheath becomes more irregular with prominent infoldings and outfoldings. Intramyelinic edema produces "bubbles" between lamellae or adjacent to the axon (Fig. 6.5). In experimental studies these were more obvious in spinal roots than in peripheral nerve. These changes may be a precursor of demyelination. Metabolic changes in Schwann cells produce spontaneous breakdown of the myelin sheath leading to segmental demyelination and remyelination. Similarly, aging of the neuronal cell body may produce a dying-back type axonal damage, seen as axonal atrophy, and formation of extensive infoldings and outfoldings of the myelin sheath [16, 17].

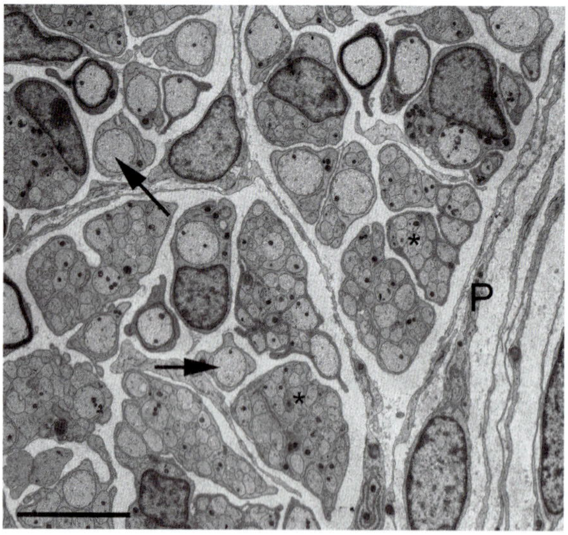

Figure 6.4 EM of developing nerve showing small, thinly myelinated fibers, promyelinated fibers (arrows) and fetal bundles of small axons (asterisk *) surrounded by the developing perineurium, which is still a loose collections of fibroblasts without basal laminae (P). Bar = 5 μm.

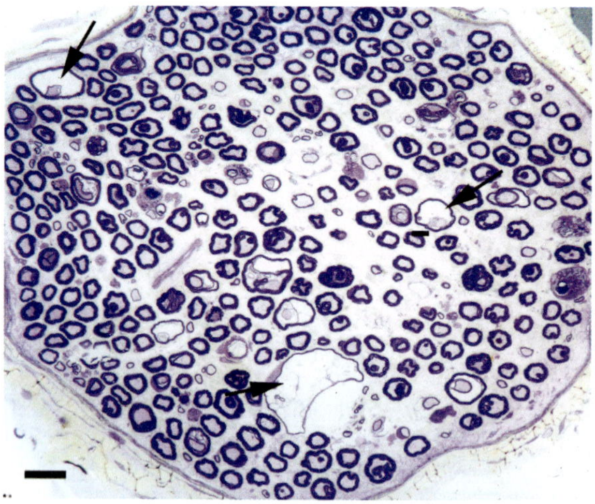

Figure 6.5 Nerve showing age changes; the most prominent of which are spaces due to intramyelinic edema (arrows). There is an increase in extracellular space in the center of the nerve, several axons are dense and shrunken and others have abnormally thin myelin sheaths. 30 month old rat, phrenic nerve. Bar = 20 μm.

References

1 Shantha TR, Bourne GH (1968) The perineurial epithelium – A new concept, In: *The Structure and Function of Nervous Tissue*, Bourne GH (ed.), pp. 379–459. Academic Press, New York.

2 Ross MH, Reith EJ (1969) Perineurium: evidence for contractile elements, *Science* 165, 604–606.

3 Stolinski C (1995) Structure and composition of the outer connective tissue sheaths of peripheral nerve, *Journal of Anatomy* 186, 123–130.

4 Fuchs E, Cleveland DW (1998) A structural scaffolding of intermediate filaments in health and disease, *Science* 279, 514–519.

5 Skoufias DA, Scholey JM (1993) Cytoplasmic microtubule-based motor proteins, *Current Opinion in Cell Biology* 5, 95–104.

6 Robertson JD (1957) New observations on the ultrastructure of the membranes of frog peripheral nerve fibers, *Journal of Biophysical and Biochemical Cytology* 3, 1043–1048.

7 Raine CS (1982) Differences between the nodes of Ranvier of large and small diameter fibres in the P.N.S, *Journal of Neurocytology* 11, 935–947.

8 Williams PL, Landon DN (1963) Paranodal apparatus of peripheral nerve fibres of mammals, *Nature* (London) 198, 670–673.

9 Huxley AF, Stämpfli R (1949) Evidence for saltatory conduction in peripheral myelinated nerve fibres, *Journal of Physiology* 108, 315–339.

10 Coppin CML (1973) *A study of the properties of mammalian peripheral nerve fibres*, D Phil Thesis, University of Oxford.

11 Jack JJB (1976) Electrophysiological properties of peripheral nerve, In: *The Peripheral Nerve*, Landon DN (ed.), pp. 740–818. Chapman and Hall, London.

12 Aguayo AJ, Bray GM, Terry LC, Peyronnard JM. (1973) Analysis of single normal unmyelinated nerve fibers and their reactions to injury, *Transactions of the American Neurological Association* 98, 70–72.

13 Zelena J (1994) *Nerves and Mechanoreceptors. The Role of Innervation in the Development and Maintenance of Mammalian Mechanoreceptors*. Chapman & Hall, London.

14 Friede RL, Samorajski T (1968) Myelin formation in the sciatic nerve of the rat. A quantitative electron microscopic, histochemical and radioautographic study, *Journal of Neuropathology and Experimental Neurology* 27, 546–570.

15 Low PA (1976) Hereditary hypertrophic neuropathy in the Trembler mouse. Part 2. Histopathological studies: electron microscopy, *Journal of the Neurological Sciences* 30, 343–368.

16 Kazui H, Fujisawa K (1988) Radiculoneuropathy of ageing rats: a quantitative study. *Neuropathology and Applied Neurobiology* 14, 137–156.

17 Krinke G, Froehlich E, Herrmann M, *et al.* (1988) Adjustment of the myelin sheath to axonal atrophy in the rat spinal root by the formation of infolded myelin loops. *Acta Anatomica* 131, 182–187.

CHAPTER 7

Basic pathology of the peripheral nervous system

J. Michael Schröder and Joachim Weis

Institute of Neuropathology, RWTH Aachen University Hospital and JARA Brain Translational Medicine, Aachen, Germany

Introduction

The human peripheral nervous system (PNS) with all its branches and connections is a highly complex structure. A large and growing number of hereditary and non-hereditary conditions can cause peripheral neuropathy. Nevertheless, in certain diseases a biopsy of a segment of a single nerve can provide an accurate diagnosis. Structural changes of the PNS may affect any of its various components. These include peripheral motor, sensory, and autonomic neurons and their axons, as well as Schwann cells and myelin sheaths in the radicular and peripheral nerves. The connective tissue components of endoneurium, perineurium, and epineurium, including blood and lymphatic vessels, are also frequently affected either primarily or secondarily.

The main basic alterations in the PNS comprise:

- Maldevelopment of axons and/or Schwann cells (Fig. 7.1, 7.2),
- Segmental demyelination and remyelination (Fig. 7.3, 7.4),
- Axonal degeneration and regeneration (Fig. 7.5–7.10),
- Loss of entire nerve fibers (axons and Schwann cells) with eventual loss of the whole neuron.

Distally accentuated degeneration of axons and anterograde Wallerian degeneration is often an initial event, resulting in the "dying back" of the nerve fibers (dying back neuropathy). Such alterations will be visible early in a biopsy of a distal peripheral nerve, for example, the sural nerve.

Neuropathology traditionally distinguishes neuropathies as:

- Primarily "axonal" (affecting primarily the axon),
- Neuronal (affecting the whole neuron, axon and cell body: including the soma (= perikaryon)),
- Primarily "demyelinating" (primarily affecting the Schwann cell),
- and combined axonal and demyelinating neuropathies ("mixed" or "intermediate," primarily affecting both axons and Schwann cells).

The disorders of the peripheral nervous system can be further subdivided according to:

1 The type of neuron affected (motor, sensory, and/or autonomic),
2 The location of the initial pathological alterations within the neuron
   (a) axonal or dendritic terminals or synapses contacting pre- or postsynaptic elements,
   (b) distal peripheral axons,
   (c) proximal peripheral, central peripheral, or central proximal axons,
   (d) perikaryon (cell body with its nucleus), and
3 The involvement of the myelin sheath with its internode, Schmidt–Lanterman incisures, and paranodes, including the axon-Schwann cell network and the complex attachment zone of myelin loops to the axolemma at the node of Ranvier.

Pathological alterations also vary depending on which organelle is primarily affected: nucleus, mitochondria, endoplasmic reticulum of the perikaryon and axon, Golgi complex, pinocytotic or coated vesicles, lysosomes,

Peripheral Nerve Disorders: Pathology and Genetics, First Edition. Edited by Jean-Michel Vallat, Joachim Weis, Francoise Gray, and Katy Keohane.

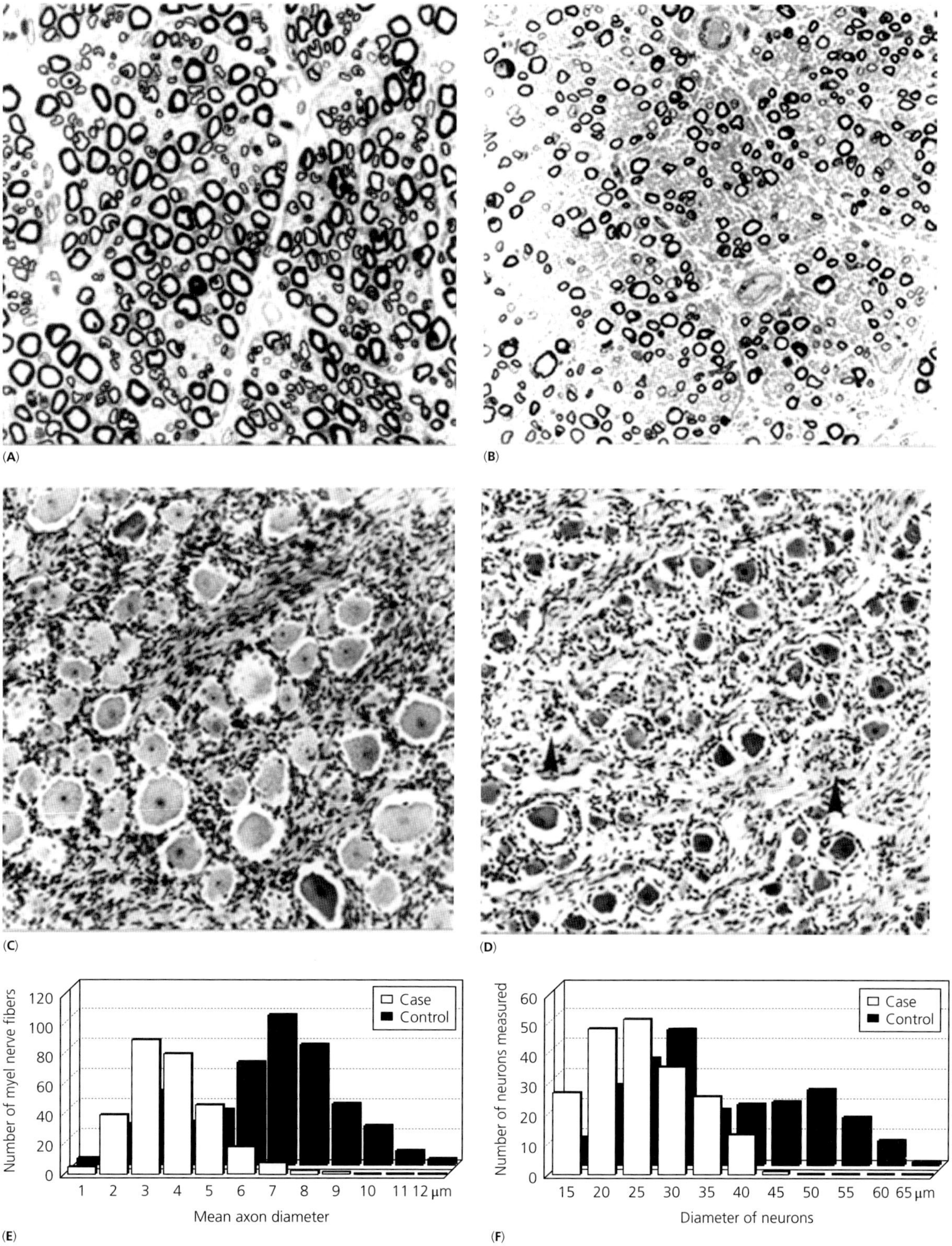

Figure 7.1 Aplasia of large myelinated nerve fibers in the sural nerve (**B**) and of corresponding neurons in a dorsal root ganglion (**D**) of a 30-month-old girl with HMSN, deafness, and mental retardation in comparison to an age-matched control (**A**, **C**). Occasional nodules of Nageotte (arrowheads in **D**) indicate some degree of progression. Total absence of large nerve fibers and neurons was morphometrically confirmed (**E**, **F**) Source: Schröder, 1999. Reproduced with permission of Springer.

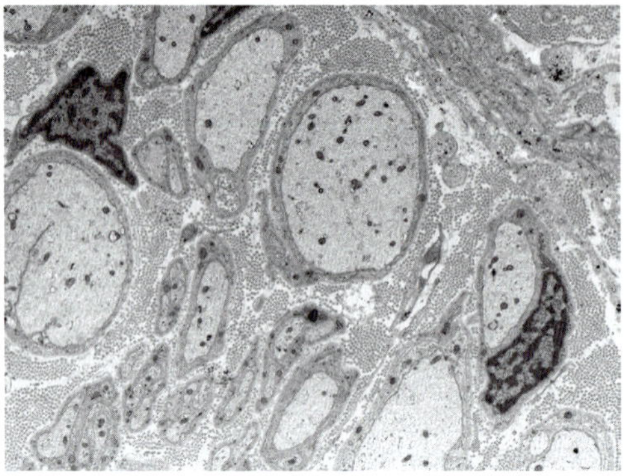

Figure 7.2 Peripheral amyelination. Schwann cells are present, but myelin sheaths are absent in this segment of the sural nerve of a term infant with SOX10 mutation. Axolemmal indentations are apparent in a large axon on the left. EM.

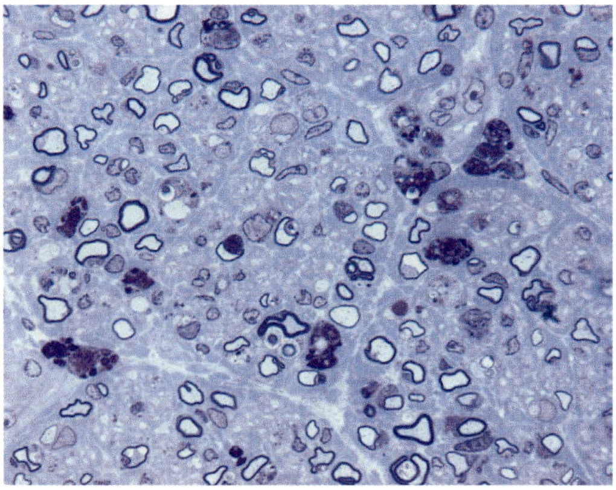

Figure 7.3 Metachromatic leukodystrophy. Most axons show disproportionately thin or absent myelin sheaths and many macrophages contain metachromatic (reddish) granular material. Semithin section, Toluidine blue.

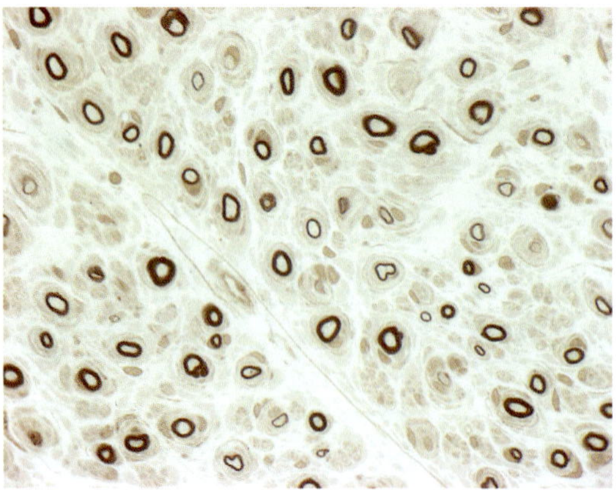

Figure 7.4 Frequent onion bulb formations around more or less thinly myelinated or demyelinated nerve fibers in CMT1A. Semithin section, paraphenylenediamine.

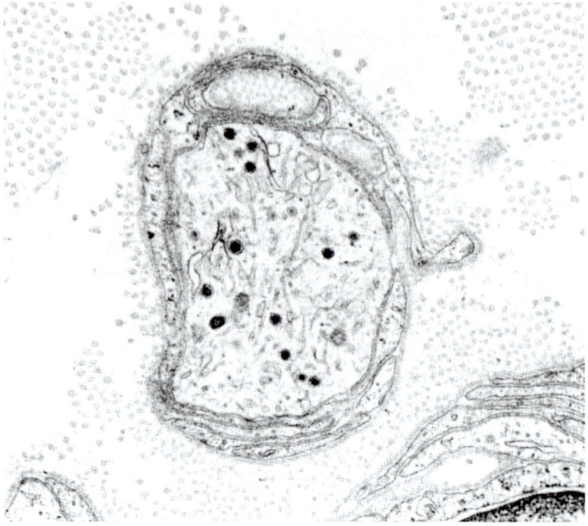

(A)

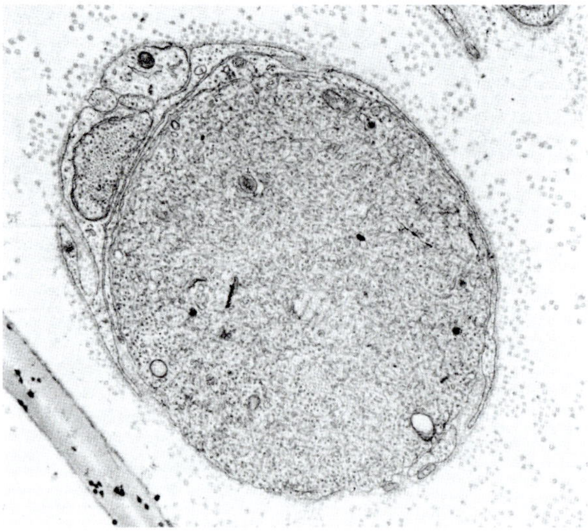

(B)

Figure 7.5 (**A**) Vesicular, tubular and membranous material accumulating in an unmyelinated axon. EM. (**B**) Intra-axonal filamentous aggregate in an unmyelinated nerve fiber. EM.

peroxisomes, microtubules, intermediate filaments ("neurofilaments"), microfilaments (actin), and others. Furthermore, the metabolism of lipids, carbohydrates, iron, copper, sodium, potassium, and calcium ions may be affected within neurons, Schwann cells, endoneurial fibroblasts and perineurial cells as well as endoneurial and epineurial blood vessels including endothelial and smooth muscle cells, and rarely, lymph vessels. Each of these elements may be primarily or secondarily affected.

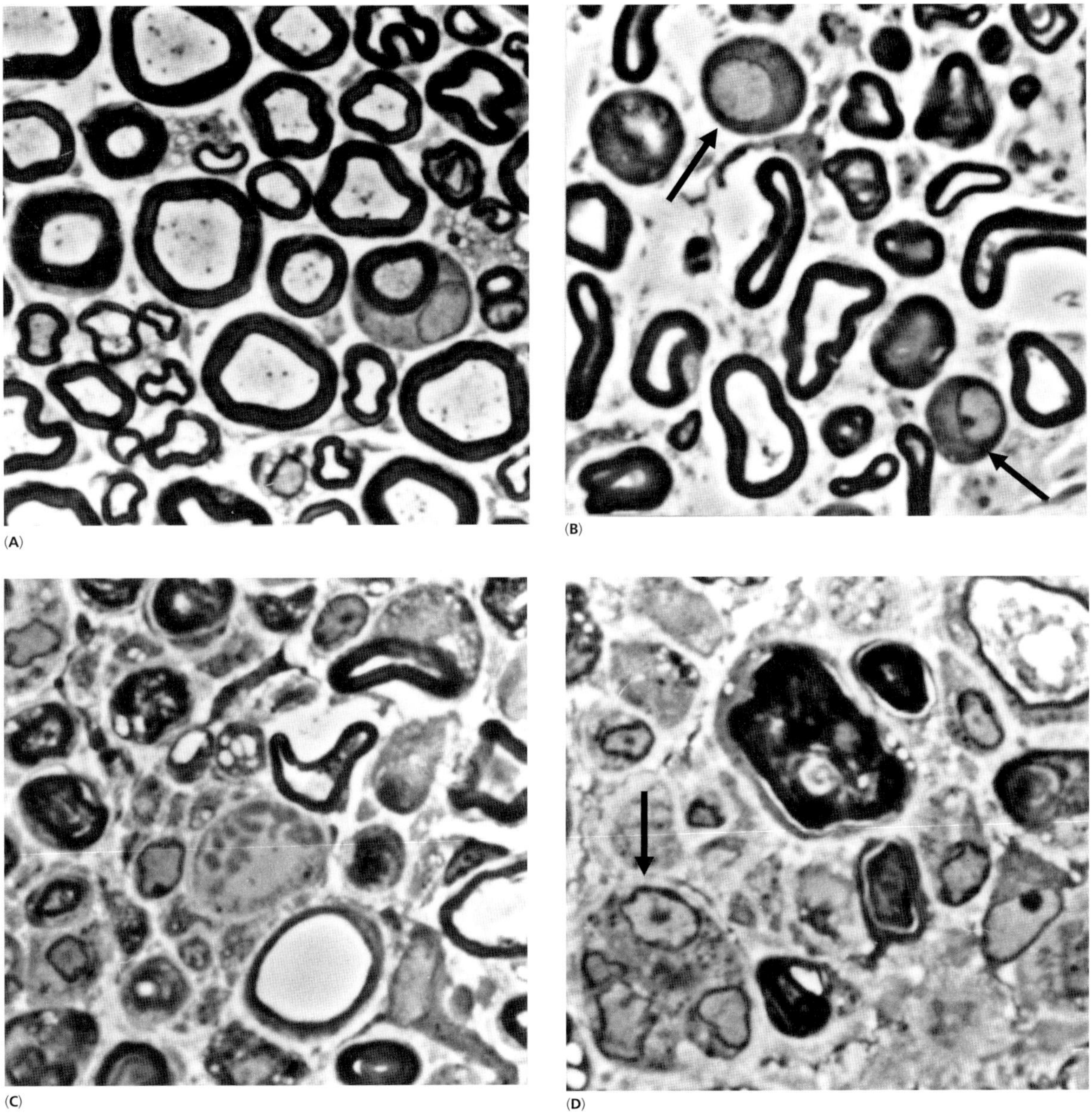

Figure 7.6 Wallerian degeneration at 1 day (**A**), 2 days (**B**), 10 days (**C**), and 20 days (**D**) after transection of the sciatic nerve in rats. At 1 day (**A**), the axons of large fibers appear moderately swollen. At 2 days (**B**), several myelin sheaths are collapsed. Other degenerating fibers are cut at the level of the Schwann cell nucleus where the myelin sheath is already disconnected leaving space for the enlarged nucleus (arrows). Myelin ovoids are also seen as well as a moderate degree of endoneurial edema. At 10 days (**C**), myelin degradation within bands of Büngner is progressing. A mitotic cell (arrow) is seen adjacent to a capillary as is a fibroblast or macrophage extending its processes. At 2 weeks (**D**), the number of nuclei is increased by a factor of 8. There are four nuclei in a single band of Büngner (arrow) at some distance from a giant myelin degradation product. The number of other nuclei is also increased. Semithin section, paraphenylenediamine. Source: Schröder, 1987 [130]. Reproduced with permission of VCH Publishers.

Selective changes in each of these structures may give rise to both inherited and sporadic (acquired) peripheral nerve disorders. Some of these disorders are restricted to the PNS; other, "complex" diseases affect the PNS and other systems.

Few morphological alterations detectable by light and electron microscopy in a nerve biopsy are specific for a certain disease. The vast majority of changes encountered in a nerve biopsy are non-specific and not pathognomonic [1–5]. However, many changes are characteristic for a particular disease or a distinct group of disorders. They can also help to assess the severity and time course of the disease.

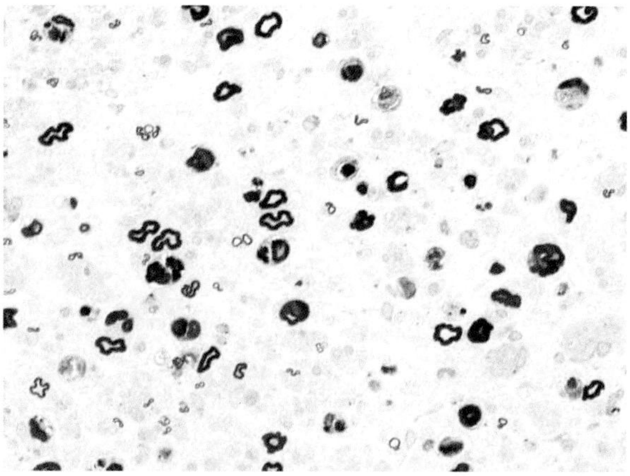

Figure 7.7 Alcoholic neuropathy. Severe loss of myelinated nerve fibers and many myelin breakdown products are indicative of rapid progression. Semithin section, paraphenylenediamine.

Changes in myelin sheaths

There is a large spectrum of myelin alterations of varying severity, especially at the node of Ranvier [6] and at Schmidt–Lanterman incisures [7]. Table 7.1 shows a classification of the main developmental, pathological, and artificial changes of myelin sheaths most of which are illustrated in an atlas [3]. The fine structure of myelin is particularly sensitive to mechanical and chemical or freezing artifacts (Fig. 7.11 vs Fig. 7.12).

Demyelination and remyelination

The most common and most severe myelin change is designated as *segmental demyelination* (Fig. 7.3, 7.4). This is the basic reaction of nerve fibers in all conditions primarily or secondarily affecting the myelin sheath. If demyelination is limited to the paranode (*paranodal demyelination*), characteristic short and thinly myelinated internodes, called *intercalated discs*, may ensue. Because of their short length, these structures can only be identified in teased fiber preparations or on optimally oriented longitudinal, semi- and ultrathin sections.

Segmental demyelination may be followed by *remyelination*. The regenerated myelin sheath does not reach the dimensions of the original myelin sheath. Myelin thickness and internodal length especially of the largest remyelinated fibers remain reduced. Thus, on cross sections the ratios between myelin thickness and axon caliber and between axon diameter and total fiber diameter are decreased, or increased, respectively. The latter is called the *g ratio* with a normal value of 0.5–0.7. As measured on longitudinal sections or teased fiber preparations; the

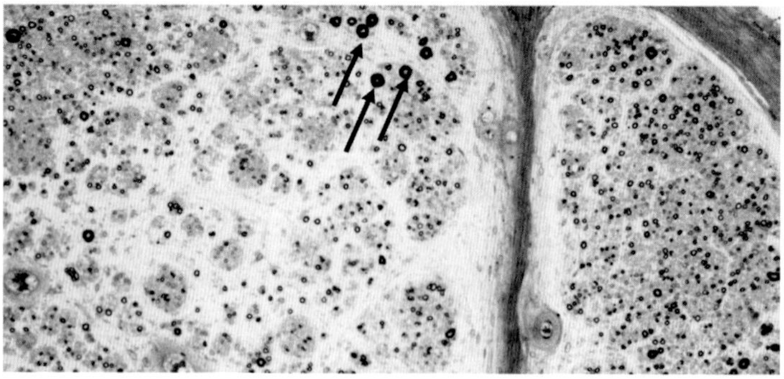

Figure 7.8 Extensive retrograde fiber degeneration in a 46-year-old man whose leg had been amputated when aged 4. The arrows indicate thickly myelinated atrophic axons that have nevertheless survived. Source: Schröder, 1987 [130]. Reproduced with permission of VCH Publishers.

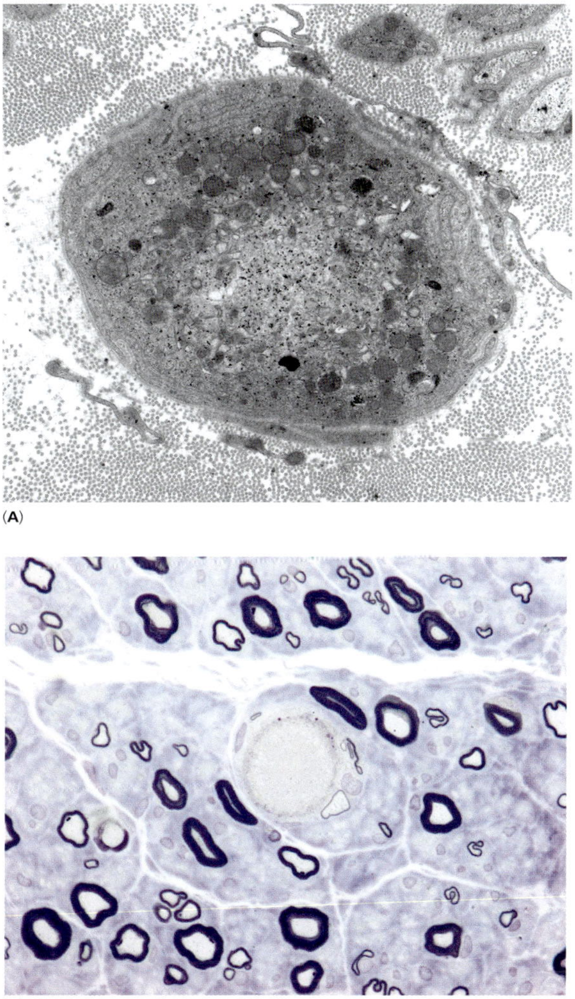

(A)

(B)

Figure 7.9 (**A**) Giant growth cone within a cluster of regenerating nerve fibers. Semithin section, Toluidine blue. (**B**) Prominent axonal swelling with accumulation of organelles, probably a growth cone. EM.

internodal length of remyelinated segments is reduced (250–300 μm). These features are of diagnostic importance especially for identifying chronic, slowly progressive demyelinating neuropathies.

During development the axon/myelin ratio changes towards thicker myelin; adult values are not reached until about age 15 [8]. It is important to note that for this reason, myelin sheaths in infants and children are relatively thin in relation to the axonal caliber and should not be regarded as pathologically *hypomyelinated* (see next: developmental disturbances of myelination).

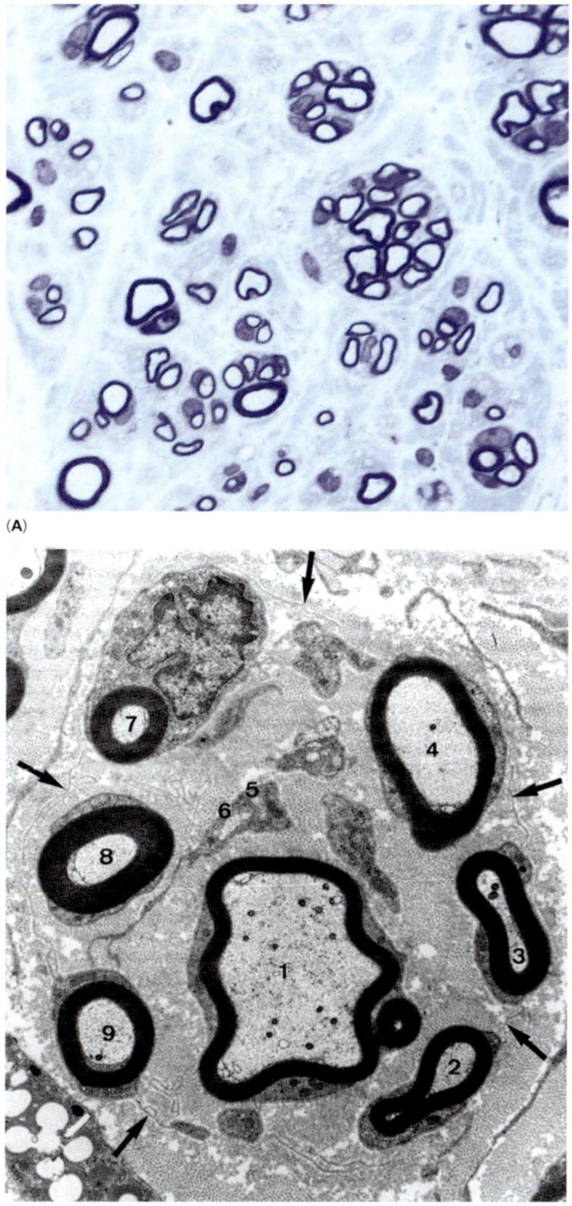

(A)

(B)

Figure 7.10 (**A**) Clusters of regenerating nerve fibers in neuropathy due to *Mitofusin-2* mutation. Semithin section, Toluidine blue. (**B**) Representative cluster of nine regenerated nerve fibers. Only No. 1 has reached a near normal size. The others, including two unmyelinated axons (Nos. 5 and 6), have presumably not reached an adequate target and have remained hypotrophic or atrophic (Nos. 2–4 and 7–9). The basal lamina of the original nerve fiber has remained intact surrounding the whole cluster (arrows) indicating that all axons are sprouts of the same, proximally degenerated nerve fiber ("hyperneurotization" of a band of Büngner). Source: Schröder und Krücke, 1970 [16]. Reproduced with permission of Springer.

Table 7.1 Myelin changes.

Non-progressive, developmental abnormalities

At the paranode

- Non-connection of terminal myelin loops to the axon

Of the internode

- Amyelination
- Hypomyelination
- Hypermyelination
- Dysmyelination; "complex" paranodes; "very short" internodes

Progressive pathological alterations

- **Segmental demyelination**; sequelae:
  - Secondary axonal atrophy (before remyelination)
  - Remyelination with reduced internodal length (250–300 μm) and disproportionately thin myelin sheaths with increased numbers of Schmidt–Lanterman incisures
  - Transnodal remyelination
  - Asymmetric node; hemi-node
  - Hypomyelination
  - Incomplete compaction of myelin lamellae
  - Myelin ovoids at various stages of degradation
  - Onion bulb formation with excess Schwann cells and increased collagen
  - Basal lamina onion bulbs

- **Paranodal demyelination;** sequelae:
  - Very short internodes ("intercalated discs")
  - Heminodes if unilaterally not myelinated

- **Others**
  - Detachment of paranodal myelin loops from the axon ("axoglial" dysjunction)
  - Undercoating of terminal myelin loops by Schwann cell processes
  - Displacement of terminal myelin loops
  - Pseudonodes
  - Disproportionate, concentric "hypertrophy" of myelin due to axonal atrophy (shrinkage) and adaptive slippage of myelin lamellae
  - Microvesicular disintegration and swelling of paranodal myelin loops (e.g., in ethylene oxide intoxication, uremic neuropathy, glomerulonephritis)
  - Vacuolar swelling of terminal myelin loops (e.g., in Marfan syndrome)
  - Precipitation of multilamellar membranous ("myelinoid", phospholipid) bodies at the paranode and at Schmidt–Lanterman incisures (e.g., in chloroquine intoxication)
  - Hypertrophy/hypotrophy with focally folded myelin (e.g., due to genetic defects in HNPP; CMT4B2)
  - Non-compaction of myelin lamellae or widening of the major dense line (e.g., in CMT1B; HNPP)
  - Loosening of myelin lamellae by widening of the intraperiod line (e.g., in paraproteinemic neuropathies)
  - Deposition of granular material at the intraperiod line (e.g., in CIDP [6])
  - Invasion by mononuclear cells (e.g., macrophages, lymphocytes in GBS; EAN; CMT X)
  - Nodal deposition of MAG antibodies (e.g., in AMAN)
  - Axonal outpouching into the paranode
  - Irregularities of the adaxonal network
  - Adaxonal amorphous material (e.g., in paraneoplastic neuropathy and spasmodic torticollis)
  - Adaxonal pleomorphic deposits (e.g., in paraneoplastic neuropathy)
  - Adaxonal homogeneous osmiophilic bodies presumably of lysosomal origin (e.g., in HMSN VI)

Artificial alterations

- **Distortion**
- **Swelling or shrinkage** due to malfixation,
- **Vacuolation** (may not be artificial)

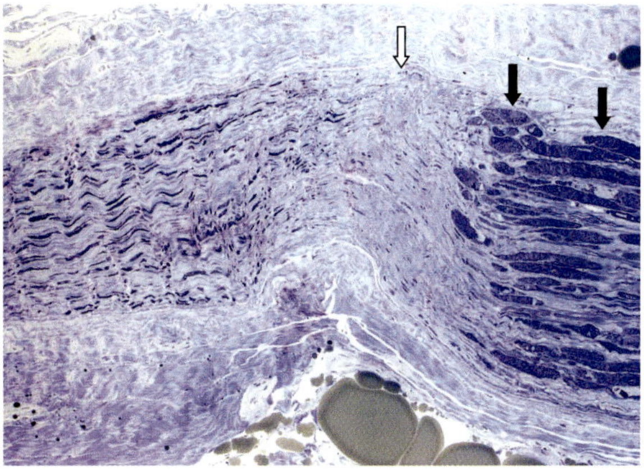

Figure 7.11 Artificial compression of this nerve fascicle lead to squeeze-out of myelin in the center and "hypermyelination" on the right. Semithin section, Toluidine blue.

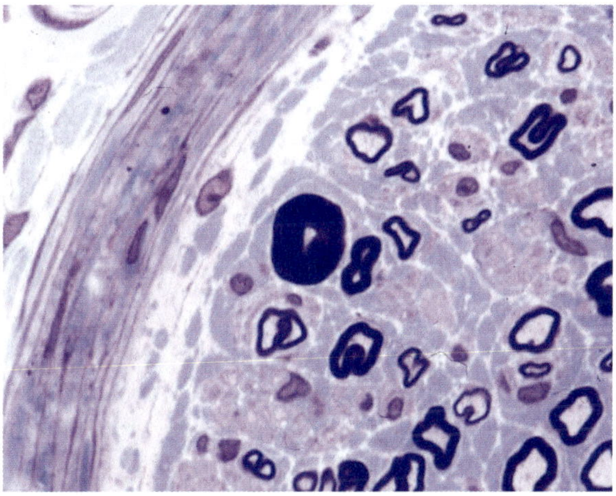

Figure 7.12 Tomaculous fiber in hereditary neuropathy with liability to pressure palsy. Note the disproportionately thin myelin sheaths of adjacent nerve fibers. Semithin section, Toluidine blue.

In addition, following *axonal degeneration and regeneration* myelin sheaths especially ven of the largest nerve fibers do not regain their original thickness or a normal axon/myelin ratio [9]. Thus, an increased axon/myelin ratio does not necessarily indicate developmental delay or preceding segmental demyelination and remyelination; it may also be the outcome of axonal degeneration and regeneration. This is particularly important to realize when isolated nerve fibers have degenerated and regenerated without apparent formation of typical clusters/bundles of regenerated fibers of uneven size. These clusters indicate redundant regeneration ("hyperneurotization" of bands of Büngner) [10].

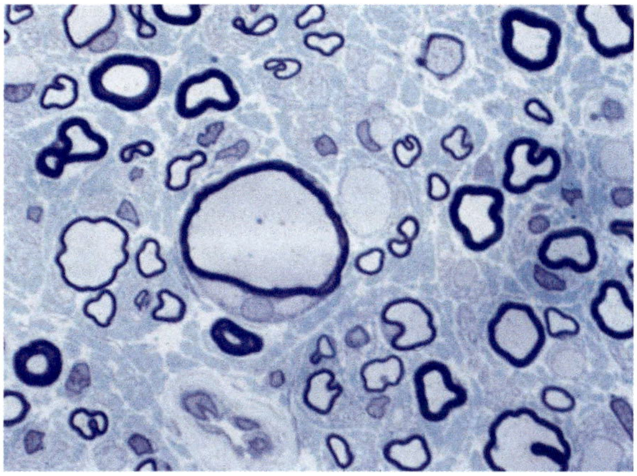

Figure 7.13 Giant axonal neuropathy with distended myelinated and non-myelinated axons. Note the thinning of myelin sheaths due to the expansion of the axons. Semithin section, Toluidine blue.

Myelin sheaths may also become disproportionately thin when axons increase in diameter as seen in polyglucosan body or giant axonal neuropathy [11] (Fig. 7.13, 7.14). It is of interest that axonal neuregulin-1 (NRG-1) type III and NRG-1 type I appear to play a role in regulating myelin thickness; when they were overexpressed in transgenic mice, normal myelin thickness was restored [12].

Onion bulb formation

Repeated demyelination and remyelination usually results in *onion bulb formation* and pseudohypertrophy of peripheral nerves. This is seen in its most severe form in *hypertrophic neuropathy* due to chronic inflammatory demyelinating polyneuropathy (CIDP) and in CMT1A. On cross sections of peripheral nerves at the electron microscopic level *onion bulb formations* were shown to be composed of proliferated Schwann cells [13–15] concentrically arranged around demyelinated and remyelinated axons (Fig. 7.3, 7.4). Schwann cells proliferate during de- and remyelination while the basal lamina of the demyelinated nerve fiber acts as a scaffold keeping the Schwann cells in place close to the central axon, resulting in their semi-circular or circular arrangement. Schwann cell numbers increase by a factor of 8–14, depending on the extent of demyelination, for example,

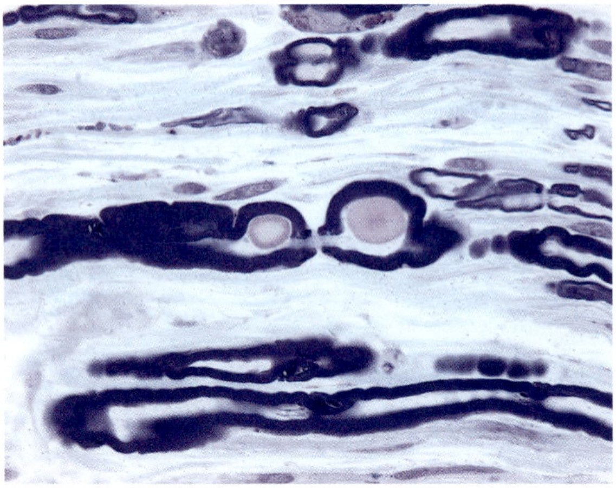

(A)

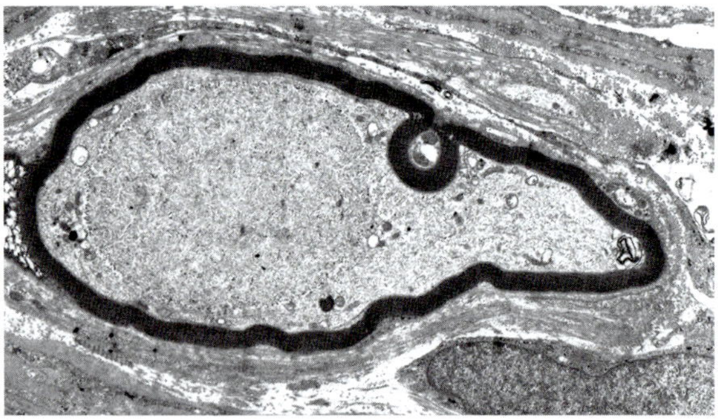

(B)

Figure 7.14 (**A**) Two polyglucosan bodies proximal and distal to a node of Ranvier. Small numbers of polyglucosan bodies are a normal feature in nerve biopsies of older people; large numbers may be indicative of polyglucosan body disease. Semithin section, Toluidine blue. (**B**) Electron micrograph of a polyglucosan body consisting of non-membrane bound granules and filaments located in an axon of an intramuscular nerve fascicle. At this site polyglucosan bodies are encountered relatively often.

in experimental allergic neuritis [14, 16], and during Wallerian degeneration (approx. 8-fold) [17]. This probably equates the numbers found after segmental demyelination in hereditary human neuropathies. However, typical onion bulb formations may be modified if CMT1A, usually a typical demyelinating neuropathy with onion bulb formation, is combined with chronic diabetic neuropathy or other, for example, toxic conditions; this can ultimately lead to a severe neuronal type of neuropathy with loss of myelinated nerve fibers without recognizable onion bulb formation [18, 19].

The *collagen* between the layers of proliferated Schwann cells also increases. The amount of collagen and the thickness of collagen filaments tend to be directly related to the duration of the disease and, possibly, the number of fibroblasts.

Typical onion bulb formations are also seen in autoimmune disorders such as Guillain–Barré syndrome (GBS) and CIDP leading in its extreme form to *multifocal hypertrophic neuropathy* with palpably enlarged nerves [15]. Typical onion bulb formations do not occur in more severe, early manifesting, genetically determined neuropathies such as *congenital hypomyelination neuropathy* (CHN). By contrast, these result in so-called *basal lamina onion bulb formations* in which only the basal lamina of Schwann cells but not the Schwann cells themselves persist (see Chapter 11). Schwann cells in CHN are obviously more liable to waste away leaving empty basal lamina onion bulbs.

In contrast to the wasting of Schwann cells in CHN, there is obvious cell "viability" in a more complex disorder such as *neurofibromatosis type 2* where onion bulb formations are more cellular and larger in size than in any other peripheral neuropathy. Their onion bulbs tend to have more prominent nuclei with irregular size and shape [20] (see Chapter 23).

Disorders characterized by demyelination

Other disorders characterized by demyelination comprise intoxications (e.g., by lead, diphtheria toxin, lysophophatidyl cholin); traumatic lesions (tourniquet, compression [21]); inflammatory disorders (GBS = acute inflammatory demyelinating polyneuropathy; and its experimental analog, experimental allergic neuritis (EAN) [16]; AIDP [22]; and Miller–Fisher syndrome (MFS) [22]. In addition, acute motor axonal neuropathy (AMAN) [23–27], with macrophage infiltration between axon and myelin sheath as the only sign of inflammation, as well as certain paraneoplastic disorders (paraproteinemias and dysglobulinemias, for example, Waldenström's macroglobulinemia) are characterized by demyelination with additional aspects [28]. The following changes may be indicative for specific, genetically determined diseases.

In *periaxin neuropathy* (CMT4F) dissociation of terminal myelin loops from the axon and loss of transverse bands was defined as the initial change [29]. In this type of congenital hypomyelination neuropathy (CHN) *immunohistochemistry* allows a specific diagnosis by lack of staining of defined periaxin subunits [29]. So far, immunohistochemistry leading to a definite diagnosis has not been achieved in other hereditary neuropathies of the CHN, CMT, and hereditary sensory and autonomic neuropathy (HSAN) type (excluding amyloid neuropathies; see Chapter 16).

In dominantly inherited X-linked Charcot–Marie–Tooth neuropathy (CMTX) the onset of demyelination at the paranode is particularly impressive. Microvesiculation of terminal myelin loops is one of the major changes before other, more pleomorphic changes at this site lead to segmental demyelination (see Chapter 13).

It is important to keep in mind that some paranodal myelin loops are normally not attached to the axon. This may cause the erroneous impression of pathological *axoglial dysjunction* [30]. The number of these "detached" loops increases in proportion to the growing thickness of the developing myelin sheath forming the so-called bracelets of Nageotte while the *paranodal myelin attachment zone* does not proportionately increase in length. Its length is about 2.3 µm at birth and no longer than 4–7.8 µm at 2–17 months of age despite an increase of the number of myelin lamellae from 40–125 during this period of development in human sural nerves [31]. This needs to be considered when assessing changes of the paranode in any type of neuropathy.

In CMT4C, caused by *KIAA1985* mutations, thin extended Schwann cell processes, in particular of Schwann cells of unmyelinated axons, are a distinguishing ultrastructural feature [32–34] (see Chapter 11) whereas other signs, such as thoracic scoliosis, are less reliable.

Myelin alterations in axonal disorders

The myelin sheath may appear disproportionately thick in relation to the reduced size of atrophic axons. The mechanism underlying this *disproportionate increase of myelin thickness* is not certain, but can best be explained by a model of concentric slippage of the spiral of the myelin lamella around an atrophic axon following reduction of the axonal perimeter. It is frequently seen in nearly all neuropathies with chronic axonal atrophy and may be due to primary neuronal or axonal disorders, or retrograde atrophy (Fig. 7.8).

Axonal atrophy may cause so-called *secondary segmental demyelination*, which can only be verified morphometrically using statistical analysis of teased fiber preparations as exemplified in uremic neuropathy and Friedreich's disease [35, 36]. Because this method needs laborious verification of many subsequent demyelinated or remyelinated segments on *long teased nerve fibers* (several mm in length) in primarily axonal types of neuropathy, it is not widely used. Nevertheless, secondary segmental demyelination must be considered when disproportionately thin myelin sheaths are seen on cross sections in primarily neuronal or axonal neuropathies.

Hypertrophy of myelin sheaths

By contrast, *hypertrophy* of myelin sheaths as seen in *tomaculous neuropathy* ("hereditary neuropathy with liability to pressure palsies," HNPP; Fig. 7.12) (see Chapter 15) is usually caused by *PMP22 deletion* [37] and tends to be less severe than CMT1A caused by *PMP22 duplication* [19]. Typical tomaculous fibers are due to an intussusception or invagination of a hypertrophic myelin sheath by an additional, double, complete ring of myelin around itself resulting in three complete myelin sheaths on cross section [38]. This produces focal, cylindrical, tomaculous (= sausage-like) thickening of the myelin sheath at the paranode or at other, circumscribed portions of the internode, best visualized on longitudinal sections or in teased fiber preparations. Tomaculous fibers are not absolutely specific for HNPP; they may also occur in *PMP22* duplication (CMT1A) or other conditions; but even so, a single typical tomaculous fiber can lead to the correct diagnosis of a *PMP22* deletion [19].

Tomacula must be distinguished from the very common traumatic (artifactual) damage resulting in severe distortion of the myelin sheath, usually in a large number of adjacent fibers (Fig. 7.11); the focal accumulation of distorted myelin sheaths usually allows distinction between artifacts and real tomaculous fibers. This artifact is frequently misinterpreted as real pathology on a nerve biopsy.

Tomaculous myelin sheaths must also be distinguished from *focally folded myelin* originally described in "globular neuropathy" [39], "congenital hypo- and hypermyelination neuropathy" [40], and autosomal recessive motor and sensory *neuropathy with excessive myelin outfolding* [41]. Autosomal recessive inheritance was also noted in other families with similar myelin changes [42–45] initially linked to chromosome 11q23 [46]. Focally folded myelin has been found in several forms of CMT4 (see Chapter 11 on AR CMT), including CMT4B due to mutations in the myotubularin-related protein-2 gene on chromosome 11q22 [47, 48]. Extensive myelin folds may also occur in paraproteinaemic neuropathy [49–51] (see Chapter 31) although not typically intussuscepted like in tomaculous fibers, nor as excessive as in CMT4B.

Other characteristic myelin changes

Loosening of myelin lamellae

Other important and characteristic myelin changes consist of *"loosening" of myelin lamellae* (= widening of the double layered *intermediate line* representing the original extracellular space between two major dense lines), or *deficient compaction of the major dense line.* (The latter consists of the fused surface membranes of individual Schwann cell processes after losing the intervening cytoplasm). The latter is typically seen in *P0 (MPZ)* mutations (CMT1B) (see Chapter 9) [52] whereas the former may occur in (paraneoplastic) IgM neuropathy and related conditions [28, 51] (see Chapter 31).

Developmental disorders of the myelin sheath

Developmental disorders of the myelin sheath are rare. There may be complete absence of myelin confined to the peripheral nervous system [53, 54], or involving the peripheral *and* central nervous systems [55]. The latter has been attributed to a neurological variant of Waardenburg syndrome with the acronym PCWH (*p*eripheral demyelinating neuropathy, *c*entral dysmyelinating leukodystrophy, *W*aardenburg syndrome, and *H*irschsprung disease) caused by mutations in the *SOX10* gene [56–59] (Fig. 7.2).

Disproportionately thin myelin sheaths

Finally, disproportionately thin myelin sheaths with little or no evidence of progressive neuropathy have also been reported in systemic disorders with presumed metabolic disturbance of myelination such as Leigh's syndrome [60–63], Cockayne syndrome [3, 64, 65], and muscle phosphoglycerate kinase deficiency [66]. Disproportionately thin myelin sheaths seen in these disorders and in certain cases of CMTX and CHN may be caused by a developmental disturbance leading to hypomyelination, or by early demyelination and subsequent remyelination.

Alterations of axons

"Axonal" or "neuronal" types of neuropathies were 3.2-fold more frequent than "demyelinating" types in a data base of more than 8000 sural nerve biopsies collected over 40 years; the ratio was 4500 : 1406 [67]. Of these, 578 were classified as "mixed axonal and demyelinating"; the remainder were not classified using this "classic" scheme.

The excess of axonal over demyelinating forms of neuropathy is presumably due to the extraordinary length of the axon. An axon depends basically on the integrity of its perikaryon, its connection to the target, and a proper endoneurial milieu, which includes an adequate blood supply along its whole length.

The distinction between an axonal and a neuronal type of neuropathy is not arbitrary. Both result in Wallerian degeneration of distal portions of fibers with the formation of bands of Büngner. These bands or tubes consist of proliferated Schwann cells that are reprogrammed by c-Jun and considered essential for regeneration [68]. We consider neuropathies as *axonal* rather than *neuronal* in type when there is evidence of regeneration, that is, when there are clusters of regenerated or regenerating fibers (Fig. 7.10); these clusters indicate a viable cell body (= "soma" or "perikaryon" of a neuron). When there is loss of nerve fibers without evidence of regeneration, a *neuronal* type of neuropathy is assumed suggesting degeneration or lack of viability of the proximal axon and neuron.

Wallerian degeneration

A common type of axonal lesion is interruption of its continuity followed by Wallerian degeneration. Within 48–72 hours after a nerve is cut, axons in mammals degenerate distal to the lesion (Fig. 7.6). Proximally, retrograde reactions subsequently lead to multiple axonal sprouts, Schwann cell proliferation, and endoneurial and perineurial changes if there is no retrograde atrophy and finally retrograde degeneration (Fig. 7.6). In the so-called WldS (for "slow Wallerian degeneration") or "Ola" mouse line, nerve fibers survive for a prolonged period of time and are able to conduct action potentials for up to 4 weeks after separation from their cell bodies; this is caused by expression of a chimeric protein, WldS, that inhibits axonal degeneration [69]. Onset of microscopically evident Wallerian degeneration is similarly delayed [70].

There are several other examples of animal models of neurodegenerative diseases where axonal independence from the cell body has been demonstrated, for example, the mutant *SOD1* model of familial amyotrophic lateral sclerosis [71] altogether justifying the distinction of an *axonal* from a *neuronal* variety of neuropathy.

Developmental disturbances of peripheral neurons

Before discussing further pathological changes of axons, rare *developmental disturbances of peripheral neurons* have to be taken into consideration (Table 7.2; if not quoted otherwise, the changes listed herein are illustrated in an atlas [3]). The most severe form comprises total *absence of myelinated fibers* which differs from primary total *absence of myelin* ("amyelination") (see previously and Table 7.1). Selective involvement of certain neuronal systems is apparent in some diseases and usually needs to be ascertained using morphometry. An example is autosomal recessive *deficiency of large myelinated nerve fibers* in the sural nerve [72] with a corresponding deficiency of large neurons in dorsal root ganglia and in the spinal cord [73] (Fig. 7.1). This rather non-progressive condition is associated with epilepsy, deafness, and mental retardation. Its molecular genetic background has, as far as we know, not yet been established.

Table 7.2 Axonal changes.

Non-progressive, developmental abnormalities

- **Aplasia** of all myelinated fibers
  - **Aplasia** of large myelinated nerve fibers
  - **Aplasia** of small myelinated nerve fibers
  - **Aplasia** of unmyelinated fibers (e.g. in Riley–Day syndrome: HSAN III)
- **Hypoplasia and hypotrophy** (e.g., associated with primary amyelination)
- **Primary hypertrophy**: not known

Progressive pathological alterations

- **Atrophy** (<7–8 μm of the largest fibers after the age of about 5 years): innumerable conditions
- **Hypertrophy**, enlargement: e.g., in giant axonal neuropathy; regenerative end bulbs; proximal to compression (tourniquet)
- **Swelling** in Wallerian degeneration etc., with loss of microtubules and filaments; artificial swelling
- **Regeneration with multiplication of axonal sprouts** ("hyperneurotization" of bands of Büngner)
- **Shrinkage due to atrophy or demyelination**
- **Deformation**
- **Axolemmal disruption/Wallerian degeneration**
- **Inclusions**
  - Membranous cytoplasmic bodies of various shapes
    - Pleomorphic, complex structures
    - Cup-shaped curvilinear bodies
    - Dystrophic membranous corpuscles
  - Vacuoles of the axoplasmic reticulum etc. (e.g., in Friedreich's disease)
  - Lysosomes, autophagic vacuoles, phospholipids (e.g., in type IV glycogenosis)
  - Amorphous and microvesicular inclusions
  - Glycogen granules
  - Glycogenosomes
  - Polyglucosan bodies
  - Double membrane-bound granular inclusions
  - Alterations of mitochondria
    - Accumulation
    - Paracrystalline inclusions
    - Dissolution (e.g., in CMT2A[92])
    - Swelling or shrinkage
  - Abnormal tubules (e.g., following taxol intoxication)
  - Condensation
  - Accumulation of filaments (e.g., in giant axonal neuropathy; IDPN, 2,5-hexandion, aluminium intoxications, etc.)
  - Peroxisomes, not identified in axons

A hereditary sensory neuropathy with selective *reduction of small myelinated nerve* fibers has also been described [74]. This condition may be difficult to distinguish from cases with non-hereditary "small fiber neuropathy" which is increasingly studied using skin biopsies (see Chapter 3).

Almost complete *absence of unmyelinated fibers* is seen in hereditary sensory autonomic neuropathy type III (HSAN III; Riley–Day syndrome); some unmyelinated axons may still develop and survive in this condition as demonstrated by electron microscopy [2].

Inherited axonal neuropathies

Dying back neuropathies

Inherited (nontoxic, ischemic, inflammatory, or traumatic) axonal neuropathies primarily tend to initially involve the most distal portions of a nerve fiber ("dying back" type of neuropathy). The prototype of an axonal type of neuropathy is *neuroaxonal dystrophy* that, however, affects the central nervous system as well (see Chapter 19).

Neuropathies in disorders affecting specific organelles

Other disorders affecting certain organelles in the neuronal perikaryon and/or the axon can cause axonal or neuronal neuropathies. CMT2E is an interesting example of a neuropathy caused by a primary disorder of *neurofilaments,* one of the main components of the axoplasmic cytoskeleton. It is allelic to CMT1F which is a more demyelinating than axonal type of neuropathy. Both phenotypes are caused by mutations in the *NEFL* gene [75, 76]. There is phenotypic variation of axonal changes in CMT2E. Some cases have typical giant axons characteristic for giant axonal neuropathy may occur [77]. Yet giant axonal neuropathy [11, 78] is a disorder affecting also other, non-axonal intermediate filaments as well caused by mutations in the gene gigaxonin (*GAN1*) (Fig. 7.13; see Chapter 18).

Microtubules were also considered as a primary target of CMT2A due to mutations in *KIF1B* [79], but not be confirmed by others [80]. Microtubules are always involved when axons degenerate due to any type of lesion causing distal (Wallerian type) degeneration. The impressive changes in tubular structures seen in experimental taxol neuropathy [81] have, thus far, not been recorded in human nerves. Commonly, neurofilaments may accumulate as described in a variety of neurotoxic conditions including hexacarbons (n-hexane), vincristine/vinblastine, acrylamide, aluminum, carbon disulfide, and IDPN toxicity (see Chapter 30) [82].

Neuropathies in mitochondrial disorders

Other examples of axonal neuropathies are those caused by *mitochondrial disorders.* These may be due either to mutations in the mitochondrial DNA such as NARP, MELAS, MERRF, KSS [83–87], or mutations in the nuclear DNA such as MNGIE [88–90], and the mitofusin 2 gene (*MFN2*) in CMT 2A [91] (see Chapter 17; and Fig. 7.10A).

Fine structural changes of *mitochondria* due to *MFN2* mutations in CMT2A are of special interest because CMT2A comprises about 20% of all axonal CMT neuropathies and because mitochondria are essential for energy supply. The neuropathy is characterized by progressive axonal degeneration and ultimate severe axonal loss. There are large bands of Büngner with variable evidence of axonal regeneration (Fig. 7.10B). Aggregates of abnormal mitochondria showing swelling, shrinkage, and irregularities of the outer and inner mitochondrial membranes occur at paranodal protrusions of the axon and at sites of axonal degeneration [92–94]. Defective mitochondrial fusion was suggested because the longest mitochondria in CMT2A were only 1.35 μm in length on electron micrographs of longitudinally oriented myelinated axons; in CMTX cases, used as (pathological) controls, the maximal length was 5.31 μm [95]. Paracrystalline or homogeneous globular inclusions similar to those in muscle fibers in cases with mtDNA mutations were not detectable [84].

In dominantly inherited neuropathies with optic atrophy of the Vizioli type (HMSN VI) abnormal cristae with paracrystalline material have been described in some Schwann cells of myelinated fibers in addition to rare abnormal mitochondria in axons with needle-like inclusions (presumably of hydroxyapatite) [83, 84, 96]. The Vizioli type of neuropathy is assumed to be caused by mitofusin 2 mutations such as in CMT2A [97]. Mitochondrial changes in perikarya of human motor neurons of spinal cord or sensory dorsal root ganglia neurons have not yet been studied although this would be of major interest (cf. Chapter 10).

In Leber's hereditary optic neuropathy (LHON) which is known to be caused by mutations in the mtDNA, paracrystalline inclusions were noted only in Schwann cells of unmyelinated fibers where they had already been seen in various other neuropathies [98] including Refsum's disease [99] and mitochondrial myopathy of undefined cause [84, 100].

It would be worthwhile studying DNA in archival material from these cases to classify these disorders with molecular genetic techniques as has been done in other cases [19, 101, 102]. Whether early alterations of mitochondria illustrated in isoniazid neuropathy [103] indicate the primary site of the lesions is debatable.

Intermediate (axonal and demyelinating) forms of neuropathy

An increasing number of neuropathies are neither typically demyelinating (conduction velocities <38 m/s) nor typically axonal (conduction velocities ranging from normal to 38 m/sec). These are designated as "intermediate" and comprise cases due to mutations, for example, in *Cx32* [104, 105], *NEFL* [76], and *GDAP1* [106]. They also include other dominant intermediate forms of CMT (DI-CMT) such as those caused by mutations of the pleckstrin homology domain of dynamin 2 (*DNM2*) [107] (see Chapter 14). Biopsies in cases with *GDAP1* mutations revealed evidence of axonal degeneration and regeneration and segmental demyelination and remyelination with a moderate degree of onion bulb formation [106]. Interestingly, P0 mutations may result in a predominantly axonal type of neuropathy [108] although P0 is the major component of peripheral myelin sheaths.

Alterations of unmyelinated nerve fibers

Bundles of collagen fibers ensheathed by processes of non-myelinating Schwann cells are called "collagen pockets" (Fig. 7.15). They increase in number with age and are considered a sign of unmyelinated nerve fiber degeneration if they are unusually numerous. Complete denervation of Remak bundles results in large denervated Schwann cell bands devoid of myelin breakdown products (Fig. 7.16).

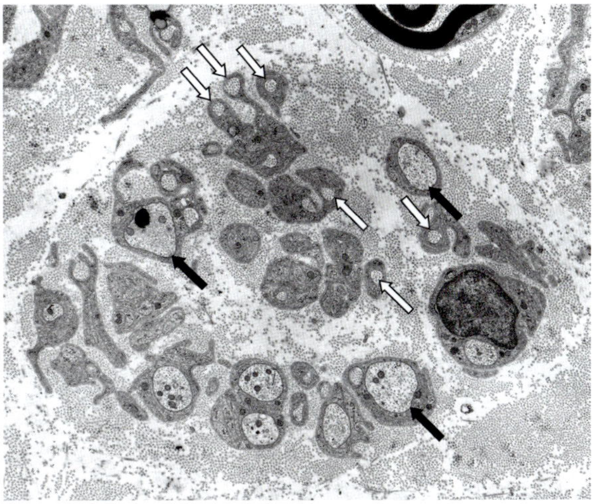

Figure 7.15 Remak bundle containing bundles of collagen fibers ensheathed by Schwann cell processes (so-called "collagen pockets"; white arrows). Some of the preserved unmyelinated axons are labeled with black arrows. EM.

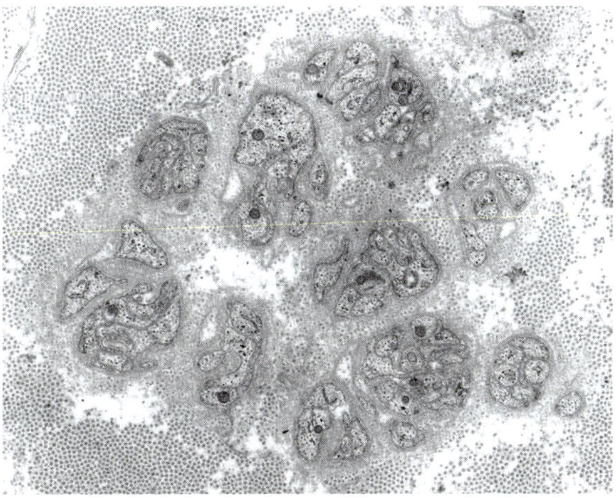

Figure 7.16 Denervated Remak bundle devoid of any unmyelinated axon. EM.

Endoneurial connective tissue changes

The endoneurial connective tissue is regularly affected in all types of peripheral neuropathy, usually secondarily. Primary involvement occurs in inflammatory disorders. The most common change is endoneurial edema associated with leakage of endoneurial capillaries in inflammatory, traumatic, toxic, allergic, hereditary, or any other disorder. Disturbances of the endoneurial environment will ensue [109]. Other endoneurial alterations may also occur in paraglobulinemias, dysglobulinemias, and various forms of sporadic or hereditary *amyloidosis* (see Chapters 18 and 33). These can frequently be identified

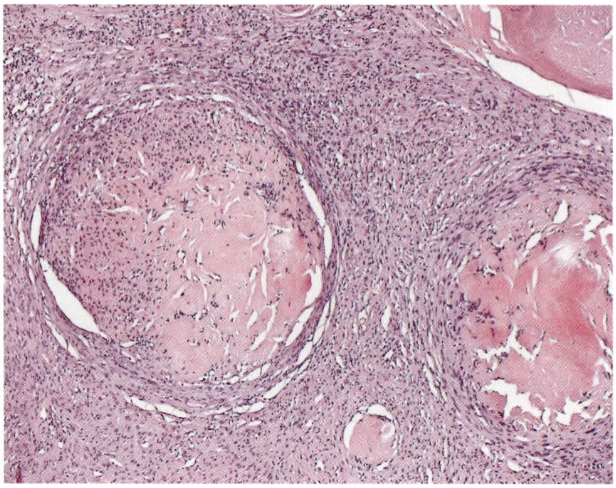

Figure 7.17 The endoneurium of several nerve fascicles is largely replaced by collagen in this case of severe chronic neuritis. H&E.

immunohistochemically or electron microscopically by their characteristic fibrillar and other endoneurial deposits [110].

The endoneurial *collagen* is greatly increased in chronic "hypertrophic" neuropathies, possibly due to an interaction between proliferated Schwann cells and fibroblasts. As mentioned previously, in chronic cases collagen fibers are a major component of onion bulb formations, and are particularly prominent in multifocal hypertrophic neuropathy [15]. Complete endoneurial, collagenous fibrosis may result when all parenchymal elements (axons and Schwann cells) have disappeared [102] (Fig. 7.17).

Mutations of collagen VI subtypes cause severe forms of congenital muscular dystrophy. Structural details of peripheral nerves have seemingly not been analyzed in this group of early, genetically determined collagen diseases. Severe nerve fiber changes (hyper- and hypomyelination, widening of nodes, non-compaction of myelin lamellae etc.) have, however, been reported in *congenital muscular dystrophy with merosin deficiency* (MDC1A) [111, 112].

Degenerating endoneurial cells are common in a large spectrum of peripheral neuropathies including inherited neuropathies. They are particularly frequent in vasculitic neuropathy [113]. Neuropathies due to *neurofibromatosis type 2* also involve endoneurial connective tissue although Schwann cells, regarded as parenchymal cells, appear to be more severely affected than *fibroblasts* [20] (cf. Chapter 23).

Quiescent or active endoneurial *monocytes/macrophages* may be regarded as a component of the connective tissue. They play a major role in various storage diseases and in removing debris from degenerating nerve fibers (Fig. 7.3). Direct cell-to-cell contacts between endoneurial macrophages and fibroblasts have been described in various conditions including Wallerian degeneration [114] and hereditary neuropathies [115]. Rare but definite broad contacts to lymphocytes in cryoglobulinemia, or to mast cells in panarteritis, have also been reported [3, 113]. Large vacuolated macrophages occur in chronic hereditary neuropathies and are non-specific indicators of chronicity.

Perineurial changes

A rare presumably heterogeneous autosomal recessive "complicated" type of neuropathy is associated with mental retardation and cataract. The histopathological hallmarks are abnormally proliferated, indented perineurial cells in the endoneurium [117–119]. These are unlike those seen in posttraumatic *minifascicles* [120, 121], or *minifascicular neuropathy* [122], or in *perineuriomas* (see Chapter 37) (Table 7.3).

Sural nerve biopsy of a case with *Cogan's syndrome*, a special type of systemic vasculitis with non-infectious keratitis, showed either subperineurial, or perivascular cells engulfing bundles of collagen [123]. These cells were immunohistochemically positive with epithelial membrane antibodies (EMA) and were therefore classified as being derived from the perineurium. Other perineurial alterations include thickenening of basal laminae, which in diabetes mellitus was shown to be reversible [124], accumulation of vacuoles, lipids, debris, and calcospherites.

Table 7.3 Perineurial alterations.

Hypertrophic perineurial dysplasia ("perineuriosis")
Minifascicular neuropathy in 46 X,Y partial gonadal dysgenesis due to mutation of the desert hedgehog gene
Minifascicle formation due to neuromatous reinnervation
Calcification, e.g., in diabetic neuropathy, or chronic polyradiculoneuritis **perineuritis**, e.g., Cogan syndrome
Reactive hypertrophy: e.g., in homologous nerve grafts
Perineurioma

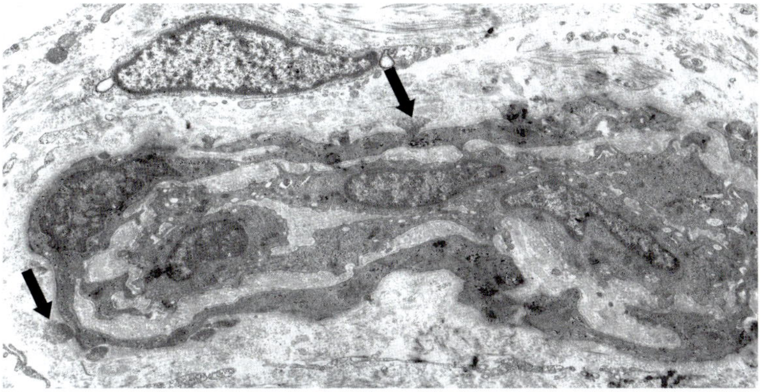

(A)

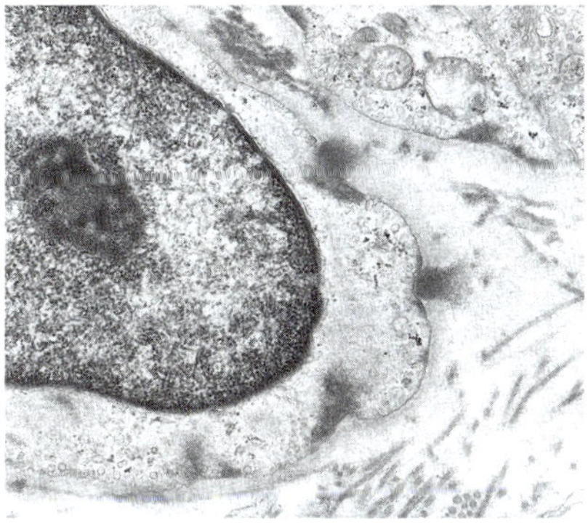

(B)

Figure 7.18 CADASIL (**A**) Blood vessel showing the typical extracellular deposits of granular osmiophilic material (arrows) associated with smooth muscle cells in CADASIL. EM (**B**) Deposits of granular osmiophilic material in CADASIL at higher magnification. Note the close association of the deposits with the bulged plasma membrane of the smooth muscle cell. EM.

Vascular changes

Certain hereditary diseases are associated with characteristic vascular changes in endothelial, smooth muscle, or perivascular cells and can be diagnosed on peripheral nerve biopsy. These diseases include neuraminidase A and B deficiency (Sandhoff's disease) [3], CADASIL [125] (Fig. 7.18), and ferritinopathy [126, 127]. Thickening of endo- and epineurial blood vessel walls due to basal lamina reduplication and endothelial hyperplasia is a hallmark of diabetic neuropathy, but can also occur in patients without a history of diabetes (Fig. 7.19; see also Chapter 30). Focally accentuated loss of nerve fibers varying within and between fascicles is typical for any angiopathic neuropathy. This phenomenon is usually most prominent in vasculitic neuropathy in which inflammatory infiltration and fibrinoid necrosis of vessel

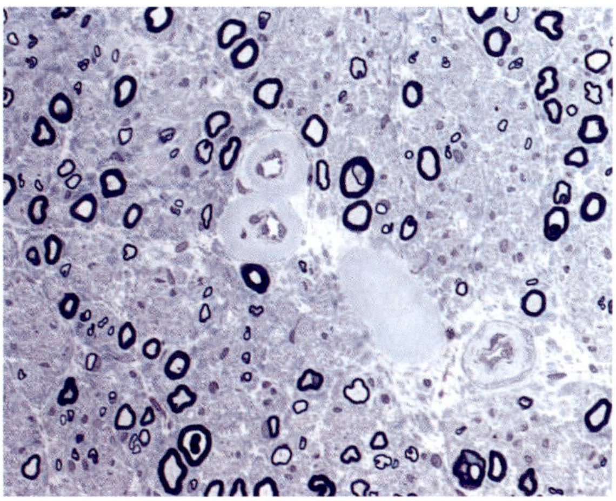

Figure 7.19 Endoneurial blood vessels in microangiopathic neuropathy show thickened, hyalinized walls. Semithin section, Toluidine blue.

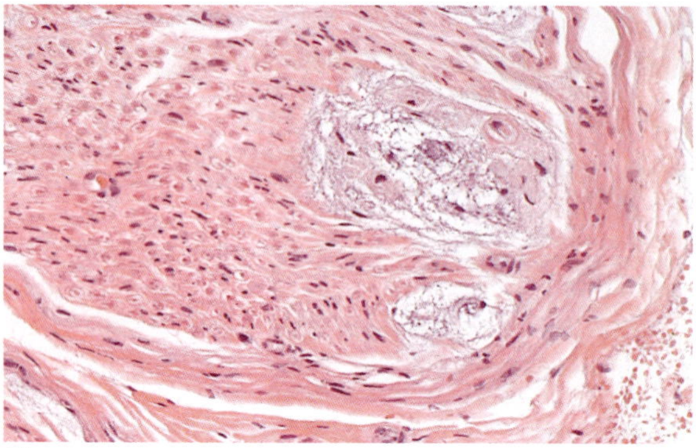

(A)

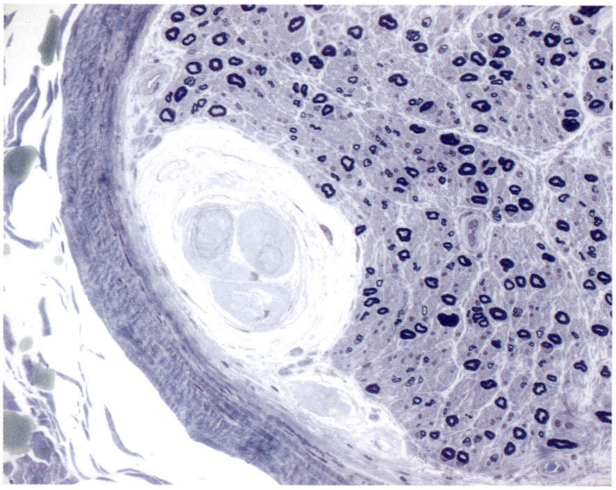

(B)

Figure 7.20 Subperineurial Renaut bodies in a paraffin section, H&E (**A**), and in a semithin section, Toluidine blue (**B**).

walls, as well as vascular occlusion and recanalization are found (see Chapter 26). Disruption of the normal vessel wall architecture, especially of the lamina elastica, is still detectable in chronic cases even if acute changes such as inflammatory infiltrates have already resolved. Epineurial blood vessel numbers in sural nerves increase from a normal mean value of 57.7 to 196 in chronic occlusive, especially inflammatory angiopathies [128]. Aberrant outgrowth of neuromatous minifascicles in the peri- and epineurium is sometimes seen as a sequel of focal inflammatory, especially vasculitic, ischaemic and traumatic nerve lesion (see Chapters 24, 35, and 36).

Epineurial hemosiderin-laden macrophages in vasculitic neuropathy should be searched for in every biopsy by iron staining. Fresh hemorrhage is infrequent and has to be distinguished from bleeding during excision. Both old and fresh hemorrhages can occur as a consequence of traumatic nerve injury. Endoneurial, mostly subperineurial Renaut bodies (Fig. 7.20) develop at sites of chronic nerve compression and contain elastic fiber precursors [129]. They are not rare in sural nerve biopsies and may be misinterpreted as nerve infarcts.

References

1 Dyck PJ, Thomas PK. *Peripheral Neuropathy*. 4th edn. Philadelphia: Elsevier Saunders; 2005.

2 Schröder JM. *Pathologie Peripherer Nerven*. 1st edn. Seifert G (ed.). Berlin Heidelberg New York: Springer; 1999.

3 Schröder JM. *Pathology of Peripheral Nerves. An Atlas of Structural and Molecular Pathological Changes*. Berlin-Heidelber-New York: Springer; 2001.

4 King RHM. *Atlas of Peripheral Nerve Disorders*. London, Sydney, Auckland: Arnold; 1999.

5 Midroni G, Bilbao JM. *Biopsy Diagnosis of Peripheral Neuropathy*. Boston Oxford Melbourne: Butterworth-Heinemann; 1995.

6 Schröder JM. Developmental and pathological changes at the node and paranode in human sural nerves. *Microsc Res Tech*. 1996;34(5):422–435.

7 Schröder JM, Himmelmann F. Fine structural evaluation of altered Schmidt-Lanterman incisures in human sural nerve biopsies. *Acta Neuropathol* (Berl). 1992;83(2):120–133.

8 Schröder JM, Bohl J, von Bardeleben U. Changes of the ratio between myelin thickness and axon diameter in human developing sural, femoral, ulnar, facial, and trochlear nerves. *Acta Neuropathol* (Berl). 1988;76(5):471–483.

9 Schröder JM. Altered ratio between axon diameter and myelin sheath thickness in regenerated nerve fibers. *Brain Res*. 1972;45(1):49–65.

10 Schröder JM. Die Hyperneurotisation Büngnerscher Bänder bei der experimentellen Isoniazid-Neuropathie: Phasenkontrast- und elektronenmikroskopische Untersuchungen. *Virch Arch Abt B Zellpath*. 1968;1:131–156.

11 Asbury AK, Gale MK, Cox SC, *et al*. Giant axonal neuropathy – a unique case with segmental neurofilamentous masses. *Acta Neuropathol (Berl)*. 1972;20(3):237–247.

12 Stassart RM, Fledrich R, Velanac V, *et al*. A role for Schwann cell-derived neuregulin-1 in remyelination. *Nat Neurosci*. 2013 Jan;16(1):48–54.

13 Schröder JM. The role of Schwann cells in the formation of onion bulbs found in chronic neuropathies. *J Neuropathol Exp Neurol*. 1967;26(1):135–136.

14 Schröder JM. Überzählige Schwannzellen bei der Remyelinisation regenerierter und segmental demyelinisierter Axone im peripheren Nerven. *Verh Dtsch Ges Pathol*. 1968;52:222–228.

15 Webster HD, Schröder JM, Asbury AK, Adams RD. The role of Schwann cells in the formation of "onion bulbs" found in chronic neuropathies. *J Neuropathol Exp Neurol* 1967;26: 276–299.

16 Schröder JM, Krücke W. Zur Feinstruktur der experimentell-allergischen Neuritis beim Kaninchen. *Acta Neuropathol (Berl).* 1970;14(4):261–283.

17 Seiler N, Schröder JM. Beziehungen zwischen Polyaminen und Nucleinsäuren. II. Biochemische und feinstrukturelle Untersuchungen am peripheren Nerven während der Wallerschen Degeneration. *Brain Res.* 1970;22(1):81–103.

18 Beckmann A, Schröder JM. Screening for Charcot–Marie–Tooth type 1A and hereditary neuropathy with liability to pressure palsy in archival nerve biopsy samples by direct-double-differential PCR. *Acta Neuropathol.* 2000; 100:459–463.

19 Thiex R, Schröder JM. PMP-22 gene duplications and deletions identified in archival, paraffin-embedded sural nerve biopsy specimens: correlation to structural changes. *Acta Neuropathol* 96: 13–21. 1998.

20 Sperfeld AD, Hein C, Schröder JM, *et al.* Occurrence and characterization of peripheral nerve involvement in neurofibromatosis type 2. *Brain.* 2002;125(Pt 5):996–1004.

21 Ochoa J, Fowler TJ, Gilliatt RW. Anatomical changes in peripheral nerves compressed by a pneumatic tourniquet. *J Anat.* 1972;113(3):433–455.

22 Yuki N, Takahashi M, Tagawa Y, *et al.* Association of *Campylobacter jejuni* serotype with antiganglioside antibody in Guillain–Barré syndrome and Fisher's syndrome. *Ann Neurol.* 1997;42(1):28–33.

23 Yuki N, Yoshino H, Sato S, *et al.* Severe acute axonal form of Guillain–Barré syndrome associated with IgG anti-GD1a antibodies. *Muscle Nerve.* 1992;15(8):899–903.

24 McKhann GM, Cornblath DR, Griffin JW, *et al.* Acute motor axonal neuropathy: a frequent cause of acute flaccid paralysis in China. *Ann Neurol.* 1993;33(4):333–342.

25 Yuki N, Kuwabara S, Koga M, Hirata K. Acute motor axonal neuropathy and acute motor-sensory axonal neuropathy share a common immunological profile. *J Neurol Sci.* 1999; 168(2):121–126.

26 Yuki N, Kuwabara S. Axonal Guillain–Barre syndrome: carbohydrate mimicry and pathophysiology. *J Peripher Nerv Syst.* 2007 Dec;12(4):238–2349.

27 Willison HJ. The translation of the pathological findings described in humans to experimental models of acute motor axonal neuropathy. *J Peripher Nerv Syst.* 2012 Dec;17 Suppl 3:3–8.

28 Jacobs JM. Morphological changes at paranodes in IgM paraproteinaemic neuropathy. *Microsc Res Tech.* 1996;34(6):544–553.

29 Takashima H, Boerkoel CF, De Jonghe P, *et al.* Periaxin mutations cause a broad spectrum of demyelinating neuropathies. *Ann Neurol.* 2002;51(6):709–715.

30 Thomas PK, Beamish NG, Small JR, *et al.* Paranodal structure in diabetic sensory polyneuropathy. *Acta Neuropathol* (Berl). 1996;92(6):614–620.

31 Bertram M, Schröder JM. Developmental changes at the node and paranode in human sural nerves: morphometric and fine-structural evaluation. *Cell Tissue Res.* 1993;273(3):499–509.

32 Gabreels-Festen A, van Beersum S, Eshuis L, *et al.* Study on the gene and phenotypic characterisation of autosomal recessive demyelinating motor and sensory neuropathy (Charcot–Marie–Tooth disease) with a gene locus on chromosome 5q23-q33. *J Neurol Neurosurg Psychiatry.* 1999 May;66(5):569–574.

33 Senderek J, Bergmann C, Stendel C, *et al.* Mutations in a gene encoding a novel SH3/TPR domain protein cause autosomal recessive Charcot–Marie–Tooth type 4C neuropathy. *Am J Hum Genet.* 2003 Nov;73(6):1106–1119.

34 Weis J, Nolte K, Mader H, *et al.* Late sporadic CMT4C – A new KIAA1985 mutation. In: Dyck PJ, Dyck PJB, Engelstad JK, Low PA, Amrani KK, Spinner RJ, *et al.* (eds). *Companion to Peripheral Neuropathy Illustrated Cases and Developments,* p. 171–173. Philadelphia: Saunders Elsevier; 2010.

35 Dyck PJ, Johnson WJ, Lambert EH, O'Brien PC. Segmental demyelination secondary to axonal degeneration in uremic neuropathy. *Mayo Clin Proc.* 1971;46(6):400–431.

36 Thomas PK, Hollinrake K, Lascelles RG, *et al.* The polyneuropathy of chronic renal failure. *Brain.* 1971;94(4):761–780.

37 Chance PF, Alderson MK, Leppig KA, *et al.* DNA deletion associated with hereditary neuropathy with liability to pressure palsies. *Cell.* 1993;72(1):143–151.

38 Madrid R, Bradley WG. The pathology of neuropathies with focal thickening of the myelin sheat (tomaculous neuropathy). Studies on the formation of the abnormal myelin sheath. *J Neurol Sci.* 1975;25:415–448.

39 Dayan AD, Graveson GS, Robinson PK, Woodhouse MA. Globular neuropathy. A disorder of axons and Schwann cells. *J Neurol Neurosurg Psychiatry.* 1968;31(6):552–560.

40 Vallat JM, Gil R, Leboutet MJ, *et al.* Congenital hypo- and hypermyelination neuropathy. Two cases. *Acta Neuropathol (Berl).* 1987;74(2):197–201.

41 Ohnishi A, Murai Y, Ikeda M, *et al.* Autosomal recessive motor and sensory neuropathy with excessive myelin outfolding. *Muscle Nerve.* 1989;12(7):568–575.

42 Gabreels-Festen AA, Joosten EM, Gabreels FJ, *et al.* Congenital demyelinating motor and sensory neuropathy with focally folded myelin sheaths. *Brain.* 1990;113(Pt 6): 1629–1643.

43 Sabatelli M, Mignogna T, Lippi G, *et al.* Autosomal recessive hypermyelinating neuropathy. *Acta Neuropathol (Berl).* 1994;87(4):337–342.

44 Quattrone A, Gambardella A, Bono F, *et al.* Autosomal recessive hereditary motor and sensory neuropathy with focally folded myelin sheaths: clinical, electrophysiologic, and genetic aspects of a large family. *Neurology.* 1996;46(5): 1318–1324.

45 Gambardella A, Bolino A, Muglia M, *et al.* Genetic heterogeneity in autosomal recessive hereditary motor and sensory neuropathy with focally folded myelin sheaths (CMT4B). *Neurology.* 1998 Mar;50(3):799–801.

46 Salih MA, Maisonobe T, Kabiraj M, *et al.* Autosomal recessive hereditary neuropathy with focally folded myelin sheaths and linked to chromosome 11q23: a distinct and homogeneous entity [In Process Citation]. *Neuromuscul Disord.* 2000;10(1):10–15.
47 Bolino A, Muglia M, Conforti FL, *et al.* Charcot–Marie–Tooth type 4B is caused by mutations in the gene encoding myotubularin-related protein-2. *Nat Genet.* 2000;25(1):17–19.
48 Previtali SC, Zerega B, Sherman DL, *et al.* Myotubularin-related 2 protein phosphatase and neurofilament light chain protein, both mutated in CMT neuropathies, interact in peripheral nerve. *Hum Mol Genet.* 2003 Jul 15;12(14): 1713–1723.
49 Rebai T, Mhiri C, Heine P, *et al.* Focal myelin thickenings in a peripheral neuropathy associated with IgM monoclonal gammopathy. *Acta Neuropathol (Berl).* 1989;79(2):226–232.
50 Vital A, Vital C, Julien J, *et al.* Polyneuropathy associated with IgM monoclonal gammopathy. Immunological and pathological study in 31 patients. *Acta Neuropathol (Berl).* 1989; 79(2):160–167.
51 Lach B, Rippstein P, Atack D, *et al.* Immunoelectron microscopic localization of monoclonal IgM antibodies in gammopathy associated with peripheral demyelinative neuropathy. *Acta Neuropathol (Berl).* 1993;85(3):298–307.
52 Gabreels-Festen AA, Hoogendijk JE, Meijerink PH, *et al.* Two divergent types of nerve pathology in patients with different P0 mutations in Charcot–Marie–Tooth disease. *Neurology.* 1996;47(3):761–765.
53 Palix C, Coignet J. Un cas de polyneuropathie péripherique neo-natale par amyélinisation. *Pediatrie.* 1978;33:201–207.
54 Charnas L, Trapp B, Griffin J. Congenital absence of peripheral myelin: abnormal Schwann cell development causes lethal arthrogryposis multiplex congenita. *Neurology.* 1988; 38(6):966–974.
55 Schröder JM, Bohl J. Altered ratio between axon caliber and myelin thickness in sural nerves of children. In: Peripheral neuropathies. In: Canal N (ed.). *Peripheral Neuropathies.* Amsterdam: Elsevier; 1978. p. 49–62.
56 Inoue K, Ohyama T, Sakuragi Y, *et al.* Translation of SOX10 3′ untranslated region causes a complex severe neurocristopathy by generation of a deleterious functional domain. *Hum Mol Genet.* 2007 Dec 15;16(24):3037–3046.
57 Lupski JR. Interruption of SOX10 function in myelinopathies. *Ann Neurol.* 2010 Aug;68(2):121–123.
58 Pingault V, Bondurand N, Kuhlbrodt K, *et al.* SOX10 mutations in patients with Waardenburg–Hirschsprung disease. *Nat Genet.* 1998;18(2):171–173.
59 Pingault V, Girard M, Bondurand N, *et al.* SOX10 mutations in chronic intestinal pseudo-obstruction suggest a complex physiopathological mechanism. *Hum Genet.* 2002 Aug;111(2): 198–206.
60 Schröder JM. Feinstrukturell-morphometrische Analyse anaboler Myelinisationsstörungen im peripheren Nerven. In: Hübner H (ed.) *Verh Dtsch Ges Pathol Stuttgart,* New York.
61 Goebel HH, Bardosi A, Friede RL, *et al.* Sural nerve biopsy studies in Leigh's subacute necrotizing encephalomyelopathy. *Muscle Nerve.* 1986;9(2):165–173.
62 Peiffer J, Kustermann-Kuhn B, Mortier W, *et al.* Mitochondrial myopathies with necrotizing encephalopathy of the Leigh type. *Pathol Res Pract.* 1988;183(6):706–716.
63 Jacobs JM, Harding BN, Lake BD, *et al.* Peripheral neuropathy in Leigh's disease. *Brain.* 1990;113(Pt 2):447–462.
64 Moosa A, Dubowitz V. Peripheral neuropathy in Cockayne's syndrome. *Arch Dis Child.* 1970;45(243):674–677.
65 Ohnishi A, Mitsudome A, Murai Y. Primary segmental demyelination in the sural nerve in Cockayne's syndrome. *Muscle Nerve.* 1987;10(2):163–167.
66 Schröder JM, Dodel R, Weis J, *et al.* Mitochondrial changes in muscle phosphoglycerate kinase deficiency. *Clin Neuropathol.* 1996;15(1):34–40.
67 Schröder JM. Neuropathology of Charcot–Marie–Tooth and related disorders. *Neuromolecular Med.* 2006;8(1–2):23–42.
68 Arthur-Farraj PJ, Latouche M, Wilton DK, *et al.* c-Jun reprograms Schwann cells of injured nerves to generate a repair cell essential for regeneration. *Neuron.* 2012 Aug 23;75(4):633–647.
69 Wang JT, Medress ZA, Barres BA. Axon degeneration: molecular mechanisms of a self-destruction pathway. *J Cell Biol.* 2012 Jan 9;196(1):7–18.
70 Lunn ER, Perry VH, Brown MC, *et al.* Absence of Wallerian degeneration does not hinder regeneration in peripheral nerve. *Eur J Neurosci.* 1989;1:27–33.
71 Glass JD. The ultimate question: why do axons degenerate? A tribute to the work and mentorship of John W. Griffin, MD. *J Peripher Nerv Syst.* 2012 Dec;17 Suppl 3:24–29.
72 Sabatelli M, Mignogna T, Lippi G, *et al.* Hereditary motor and sensory neuropathy with deafness, mental retardation, and absence of sensory large myelinated fibers: confirmation of a new entity. *Am J Med Genet.* 1998;75:309–313.
73 Müller HD, Mugler M, Ramaekers VT, Schröder JM. Hereditary motor and sensory neuropathy with absence of large myelinated fibers due to absence of large neurons in dorsal root ganglia and anterior horns, clinically associated with deafness, mental retardation, and epilepsy (HMSN-ADM). *J Peripher Nerv Syst.* 2000 Sep;5(3):147–157.
74 Donaghy M, Hakin RN, Bamford JM, *et al.* Hereditary sensory neuropathy with neurotrophic keratitis. Description of an autosomal recessive disorder with a selective reduction of small myelinated nerve fibres and a discussion of the classification of the hereditary sensory neuropathies. *Brain.* 1987;110(Pt 3):563–583.
75 Jordanova A, De Jonghe P, Boerkoel CF, *et al.* Mutations in the neurofilament light chain gene (NEFL) cause early onset severe Charcot–Marie–Tooth disease. *Brain.* 2003 Mar;126(Pt 3):590–597.
76 Züchner S, Vorgerd M, Sindern E, Schröder JM. The novel neurofilament light (NEFL) mutation Glu397Lys is associated with a clinically and morphologically heterogeneous type of Charcot–Marie–Tooth neuropathy. *Neuromuscul Disord.* 2004 Feb;14(2):147–157.

77 Fabrizi GM, Cavallaro T, Angiari C, *et al.* Giant axon and neurofilament accumulation in Charcot–Marie–Tooth disease type 2E. *Neurology.* 2004 Apr 27;62(8):1429–1431.

78 Sabatelli M, Bertini E, Servidei S, *et al.* Giant axonal neuropathy: report on a case with focal fiber loss. *Acta Neuropathol (Berl).* 1992;83(5):543–546.

79 Zhao C, Takita J, Tanaka Y, *et al.* Charcot–Marie–Tooth disease type 2A caused by mutation in a microtubule motor KIF1Bbeta. *Cell.* 2001;105(5):587–597.

80 Bissar-Tadmouri N, Nelis E, Züchner S, *et al.* Absence of KIF1B mutation in a large Turkish CMT2A family suggests involvement of a second gene. *Neurology.* 2004 May 11;62(9): 1522–1525.

81 Röyttä M, Raine CS. Taxol-induced neuropathy: chronic effects of local injection. *J Neurocytol.* 1986;15(4):483–496.

82 Griffin JW, Gold BG, Cork LC, *et al.* IDPN neuropathy in the cat: coexistence of proximal and distal axonal swellings. *Neuropathol Appl Neurobiol.* 1982;8(5):351–364.

83 Schröder JM, Sommer C. Mitochondrial abnormalities in human sural nerves: fine structural evaluation of cases with mitochondrial myopathy, hereditary and non-hereditary neuropathies, and review of the literature. *Acta Neuropathol (Berl).* 1991;82(6):471–482.

84 Schröder JM. Neuropathy associated with mitochondrial disorders. *Brain Pathol.* 1993;3(2):177–190.

85 Molnar M, Neudecker S, Schröder JM. Increase of mitochondria in vasa nervorum of cases with mitochondrial myopathy, Kearns–Sayre syndrome, progressive external ophthalmoplegia and MELAS. *Neuropathol Appl Neurobiol.* 1995;21(5):432–49.

86 Molnár M, Zanssen S, Buse G, Schröder JM. A large-scale deletion of mitochondrial DNA in a case with pure mitochondrial myopathy and neuropathy. *Acta Neuropathol* (Berl). 1996;91(6):654–658.

87 Zanssen S, Molnar M, Buse G, Schröder JM. Mitochondrial cytochrome b-gene deletion in Kearns Sayre syndrome associated with a mild type of peripheral neuropathy. *Clin Neuropathol.* 1998;17:291–296.

88 Bardosi A, Creutzfeldt W, DiMauro S, *et al.* Myo-, neuro-, gastrointestinal encephalopathy (MNGIE syndrome) due to partial deficiency of cytochrome-c-oxidase. A new mitochondrial multisystem disorder. *Acta Neuropathol (Berl).* 1987;74(3):248–258.

89 Papadimitriou A, Comi GP, Hadjigeorgiou GM, *et al.* Partial depletion and multiple deletions of muscle mtDNA in familial MNGIE syndrome. *Neurology.* 1998;51(4):1086–1092.

90 Nishino I, Spinazzola A, Hirano M. MNGIE: from nuclear DNA to mitochondrial DNA. *Neuromuscul Disord.* 2001;11(1): 7–10.

91 Züchner S, Mersiyanova IV, Muglia M, et al. Mutations in the mitochondrial GTPase mitofusin 2 cause Charcot–Marie–Tooth neuropathy type 2A. *Nat Genet.* 2004 May;36(5):449–451.

92 Verhoeven K, Claeys KG, Züchner S, et al. MFN2 mutation distribution and genotype/phenotype correlation in Charcot–Marie–Tooth type 2. *Brain.* 2006 May 19;129: 2093–2102.

93 Vallat JM, Ouvrier RA, Pollard JD, *et al.* Histopathological findings in hereditary motor and sensory neuropathy of axonal type with onset in early childhood associated with mitofusin 2 mutations. *J Neuropathol Exp Neurol.* 2008 Nov; 67(11):1097–1102.

94 Sole G, Ferrer X, Vital C, et al. Ultrastructural mitochondrial modifications characteristic of mitofusin 2 mutations (CMT2A). *J Peripher Nerv Syst.* 2009 Sep;14(3):206–207.

95 Schröder JM, Verhoeven K, Van Hul M, et al. Alterations of axonal mitochondria in CMT2A due to mitofusin 2 mutation: caparison to cases with mitochondrial DNA mutation. *J Periph Nerv Syst.* [Abstract]. 2005;10(Suppl. 1):84–85.

96 Sommer C, Schröder JM. Hereditary motor and sensory neuropathy with optic atrophy. Ultrastructural and morphometric observations on nerve fibers, mitochondria, and dense-cored vesicles. *Arch Neurol.* 1989;46(9):973–977.

97 Yiu EM, Ryan MM. Genetic axonal neuropathies and neuronopathies of pre-natal and infantile onset. *J Peripher Nerv Syst.* 2012 Sep;17(3):285–300.

98 Lyon G, Evrard P. Sur la présence d'inclusions cristalline dans les cellules d Schwann dans diverses neuropathies périphériques. *CR des Sciences (Paris) D Sci Nat D.* 1970;272:1000–1002.

99 Fardeau M, Engel WK. Ultrastructural study of a peripheral nerve biopsy in Refsum's disease. *J Neuropathol Exp Neurol.* 1969,28:278–294.

100 Yiannikas C, McLeod JG, Walsh JC. Peripheral neuropathy associated with polycythemia vera. *Neurology.* 1983;33(2): 139–143.

101 Senderek J, Bergmann C, Quasthoff S, *et al.* X-linked dominant Charcot–Marie–Tooth disease: nerve biopsies allow morphological evaluation and detection of connexin32 mutations (Arg15Trp, Arg22Gln). *Acta Neuropathol (Berl).* 1998;95(5):443–439.

102 Züchner S, Sperfeld AD, Senderek J, *et al.* A novel nonsense mutation in the ABC1 gene causes a severe syringomyelia-like phenotype of Tangier disease. *Brain.* 2003;126(Pt 4): 920–927.

103 Schröder JM. Zur Pathogenese der Isoniazid-Neuropathie. I. Eine feinstrukturelle Differenzierung gegenüber der Wallerschen Degeneration. *Acta Neuropathol.* 1970b;16: 301–323.

104 Rouger H, LeGuern E, Birouk N, *et al.* Charcot–Marie–Tooth disease with intermediate motor nerve conduction velocities: characterization of 14 Cx32 mutations in 35 families. *Hum Mutat.* 1997;10(6):443–452.

105 Senderek J, Hermanns B, Bergmann C, *et al.* X-Linked dominant Charcot–Marie–Tooth neuropathy: clinical, electrophysiological, and morphological phenotype in four families with different connexin32 mutations. *J Neurol Sci.* 1999;167:90–101.

106 Senderek J, Bergmann C, Ramaekers VT, *et al.* Mutations in the ganglioside-induced differentiation-associated protein- 1

(GDAP1) gene in intermediate type autosomal recessive Charcot–Marie–Tooth neuropathy. *Brain.* 2003;126(Pt 3): 642–649.

107 Züchner S, Noureddine M, Kennerson M, *et al.* Mutations in the pleckstrin homology domain of dynamin 2 cause dominant intermediate Charcot–Marie–Tooth disease. *Nat Genet.* 2005 Mar;37(3):289–294.

108 Senderek J, Hermanns B, Hartmann C, Schröder JM. P0 point mutations in Charcot–Marie–Tooth neuropathy type 2: Two novel amino acid substitutions (TYR119CYS; ASP61GLY) and a possible "hot spot" on THR124MET – Abstract. *J Peripher Nerv Syst.* 1999;4:301–302.

109 Mizisin AP, Weerasuriya A. Homeostatic regulation of the endoneurial microenvironment during development, aging and in response to trauma, disease and toxic insult. *Acta Neuropathol.* 2011 Mar;121(3):291–312.

110 Sommer C, Schröder JM. Amyloid neuropathy: immunocytochemical localization of intra- and extracellular immunoglobulin light chains. *Acta Neuropathol (Berl).* 1989; 79(2):190–199.

111 Deodato F, Sabatelli M, Ricci E, et al. Hypermyelinating neuropathy, mental retardation and epilepsy in a case of merosin deficiency. *Neuromuscul Disord.* 2002;12(4):392–398.

112 Feltri ML, Wrabetz L. Laminins and their receptors in Schwann cells and hereditary neuropathies. *J Peripher Nerv Syst.* 2005 Jun;10(2):128–143.

113 Grehl H, Schröder JM. Significance of degenerating endoneurial cells in peripheral neuropathy. *Acta Neuropathol (Berl).* 1991;81(6):680–685.

114 Ohara S, Takahashi H, Ikuta F. Specialised contacts of endoneurial fibroblasts with macrophages in wallerian degeneration. *J Anat.* 1986 Oct;148:77–85.

115 Groh J, Weis J, Zieger H, *et al.* Colony-stimulating factor-1 mediates macrophage-related neural damage in a model for Charcot–Marie–Tooth disease type 1X. *Brain.* 2012 Jan;135(Pt 1):88–104.

116 Schröder JM. Zur Pathogenese der Isoniazid-Neuropathie. II. Phasenkontrast- und elektronenmikroskopische Untersuchungen am Rückenmark, an den Spinalganglien und Muskelspindeln. *Acta Neuropathol.* 1970c;16:324–341.

117 Schröder JM, Rollnik JD, Schubert M, Dengler R. Demyelinating sensorimotor neuropathy with congenital cataract, mental retardation, and unique, dysplastic perineurial cells within the endoneurium. *Acta Neuropathol (Berl).* 1999;98(4):421–426.

118 Thomas PK, King RHM, Workman JM, Schröder JM. Hypertrophic perineurial dysplasia in multifocal and generalized peripheral neuropathies. *Neuropathol Appl Neurobiol.* 2000;26:536–543.

119 Wolfe GI, Brower RD, Burns DK. Perineurial cell hyperplasia in early-onset polyneuropathy with multiple cranial neuropathies [In Process Citation]. *Neuromuscul Disord.* 2000;10(7):503–506.

120 Schröder JM, Seiffert KE. Die Feinstruktur der neuromatösen Neurotisation von Nerventransplantaten. Virchows *Arch B Cell Pathol.* 1970;5(3):219–235.

121 Popovic M, Bresjanac M, Sketelj J. Regenerating axons enhance differentiation of perineurial-like cells involved in minifascicle formation in the injured peripheral nerve. *J Neuropathol Exp Neurol.* 1994;53(6):590–597.

122 Umehara F, Tate G, Itoh K, *et al.* A novel mutation of desert hedgehog in a patient with 46,XY partial gonadal dysgenesis accompanied by minifascicular neuropathy. *Am J Hum Genet.* 2000 Nov;67(5):1302–1305.

123 Nolte KW, Hans VJ, Schattenfroh C, *et al.* Perineurial cells filled with collagen in "atypical" Cogan's syndrome. *Acta Neuropathol.* 2008 May;115(5):589–596.

124 Beggs JL, Johnson PC, Olafsen AG, *et al.* Regression of perineurial cell basement membrane in a human diabetic following isogenic pancreas transplant. *Acta Neuropathol (Berl).* 1989;79(1):108–112.

125 Schröder JM, Sellhaus B, Jörg J. Identification of the characteristic vascular changes in a sural nerve biopsy of a case with cerebral autosomal dominant arteriopathy with subcortical infarcts and leukoencephalopathy (CADASIL). *Acta Neuropathol (Berl).* 1995;89(2):116–121.

126 Schröder JM, Krämer KG, Hopf HC. Granular nuclear inclusion body disease: fine structure of tibial muscle and sural nerve. *Muscle Nerve.* 1985;8(1):52–59.

127 Schröder JM. Ferritinopathy: diagnosis by muscle or nerve biopsy, with a note on other nuclear inclusion body diseases. *Acta Neuropathol (Berl).* 2005 Jan;109(1):109–114.

128 Schütz G, Schröder JM. Number and size of epineurial blood vessels in normal and diseased human sural nerves. *Cell Tissue Res.* 1997;290(1):31–37.

129 Weis J, Alexianu ME, Heide G, Schröder JM. Renaut bodies contain elastic fiber components. *J Neuropathol Exp Neurol.* 1993;52(5):444–451.

130 Schröder JM. Pathomorphologie der peripheren Nerven. In: *Polyneuritiden und Polyneuropathien Weinheim: D. Edition Medizin,* Neundörfer B, Schimrigk K, Soyka K (eds). VCH; 1987. p. 11–104.

CHAPTER 8

Introduction to the hereditary neuropathies

Joachim Weis[1] and Jan Senderek[2]

[1] Institute of Neuropathology, RWTH Aachen University Hospital and JARA Brain Translational Medicine, Aachen, Germany

[2] Friedrich Baur Institute, Department of Neurology, Ludwig Maximilians University, Munich, Germany

The non-syndromic hereditary peripheral nerve disorders comprise four major subgroups, hereditary motor and sensory neuropathies (HMSN; Charcot–Marie–Tooth diseases, CMT), hereditary sensory and autonomic neuropathies (HSAN), hereditary motor neuropathies (HMN), and hereditary recurrent focal neuropathies (hereditary neuropathy with liability to pressure palsies, HNPP, and hereditary neuralgic amyotrophy, HNA). Moreover, peripheral neuropathy is a prevailing or prominent clinical feature in a heterogeneous group of other diseases, which includes familial amyloid neuropathy (FAP), giant axonal neuropathy (GAN), polyglucosan body disease, metabolic conditions such as metachromatic leukodystrophy, and Refsum disease. Most of these entities are covered in the present book with the exception of the HMNs. The latter are closely linked to the group of hereditary motor neuron diseases such as familial amyotrophic lateral sclerosis and spinal muscular atrophy, which are not part of this volume. Moreover, biopsy or autopsy studies on HMNs are exceedingly rare.

Mutations in certain genes may lead to more than one phenotype, including different forms of neuropathies and disorders of other organ systems such as the CNS, sensory organs, and skeletal muscle. The following chapter focuses on the PNS manifestations and, more specifically, on the nerve biopsy features of gene defects that predominantly manifest as peripheral neuropathies.

The prevalence of the largest group of hereditary neuropathies, the HMSNs/CMTs, was estimated to be 1:2.500 [1, 2] and the prevalence of all hereditary neuropathies including the other groups mentioned previously should be even higher. Moreover, the number of patients with inherited neuropathies is likely to grow as ever-improving molecular genetic testing strategies will continue to assign cases previously labeled "sporadic" or "idiopathic" to distinct gene defects. Due to the growing elderly population, this might be particularly relevant for so-far etiologically unexplained peripheral neuropathies in the group of aging people. We should also expect to witness discovery of an increasing number of gene alterations that predispose to clinical manifestation of a neuropathy when they occur together with other genetic factors or other endogenous and exogenous influences (e.g., hypomorphic mutations in neuropathy genes, treatment with neurotoxic drugs, or aging).

The freely available website of the Neuromuscular Disease Center of Washington University lists more than 100 different hereditary neuropathy entities that fall into the previously mentioned disease groups. A slightly lower, but rapidly increasing number of neuropathy genes have been discovered so far. The proteins encoded by these genes are related to diverse molecular and cellular functions (listed in Table 8.1 and illustrated in Fig. 8.1). Some of these functions can easily be linked to peripheral nerve development, function, and maintenance. Axonal transport is vital for nerve fibers and most hereditary neuropathies affect nerve fibers in a length-dependent manner. Therefore, it was not surprising that mutations in several genes, which encode proteins that are involved in the complex mechanisms maintaining axonal transport, were found to lead to hereditary neuropathies. It is also easy to conceive that mutations in the neurotrophic factor *NGF* and its receptor TrkA, and genetic defects in major myelin genes such as *PMP22* and *MPZ* can cause hereditary neuropathies. On the contrary, we are just beginning to understand why mutations in proteins involved in central biological mechanisms such

Peripheral Nerve Disorders: Pathology and Genetics, First Edition. Edited by Jean-Michel Vallat, Joachim Weis, Francoise Gray, and Katy Keohane.

Table 8.1 Functional categories of genes involved in HMSN and related neuropathies.

Gene	Disease
1. Myelin proteins	
PMP22	CMT1A, HNPP, DSS, CHN
MPZ/PO	CMT1B, DSS, CHN, CMT2I, CMT2J, CMT DID
2. Nucleotide and nucleic acid processing/metabolism	
PRPS1	CMTX5
GARS	CMT2D
AARS	CMT2N
YARS	CMT DIC
KARS	CMT RIB, HNPP
3. Transcriptional regulation	
EGR2	CMT1D, DSS, CMT4E, CHN
SOX10	PNS and CNS hypomyelination
MED25	AR-CMT2B
IGHMBP2	HMN6, SMARD
DNMT1	HSAN
IKBKAP	HSAN3
SETX	HMN, AOA2
4. Mitochondrial dynamics	
GDAP1	CMT4A, CMT2K, CMT RIA
MFN2	CMT2A, HMSN V, HMSN VI, AR CMT2
5. Intracellular transport	
SH3TC2/KIAA1985	CMT4C
RAB7	CMT2B, HSAN
GJB1	CMTX1
DNM2	CMT2M, CMT DIB
ATL1	HSAN
DCTN1	HMN
LRSAM1	AR-CMT2
6. Phosphoinositide metabolism	
MTMR2	CMT4B1
SBF2/MTMR13	CMT4B2
FIG4	CMT4J
7. Cytoskeleton, nucleoskeleton, and cytoskeleton remodeling	
NEFL	CMT1F, CMT2E
ARHGEF10	slow NCV, thin myelin, no clinical manifestation
FGD4	CMT4H
LMNA	AR-CMT2A
PLEKHG5	HMN
CCT5	HSAN
8. Interaction with the cellular environment (ECM, ion channels)	
PRX	CMT4F, DSS
TRPV4	CMT2C
FBLN5	CMT1
9. Heat shock proteins	
HSPB1	CMT2F, HMN2A
HSPB8	CMT2L, HMN2B
HSPB3	HMN2C
10. Protein degradation	
Gigaxonin	giant axonal neuropathy
11. Neurotrophin signaling	
NGFB	HSAN
NTRK1	CIPA, HSAN IV
12. Sphingolipid biosynthesis	
SPTLC1	HSAN
SPTLC2	HSAN
13. Unknown (or known function unlikely/not clearly related to the disease mechanism)	
LITAF	CMT1C
NDRG1	CMT4D
BSCL2	HMN 5B
HK1	HMSNR
FAM134B	HSAN
WNK1	HSAN

as mitochondrial dynamics, nuclear envelope structure, phosphoinositide metabolism, Rho GTPase signaling, and transcriptional regulation selectively affect the peripheral nervous system.

Over the last decades, the study of peripheral nerve fiber pathology has provided a detailed record of lesion and reaction patterns in peripheral neuropathies. The neuropathy genes discovered so far add to this picture a fascinating catalogue of genetic mechanisms and gene functions that are needed for building and maintaining peripheral nerves. Functional consequences of mutations causing hereditary neuropathy in human patients can be conveniently studied in nerve and skin biopsies. Such insights are expected to improve our understanding of the pathomechanisms of neurodegeneration in the PNS with every new gene defect discovered. From a practice oriented, clinical point of view, correlation of gene alterations found in a patient's exome, or even genome, by the new large scale DNA sequencing methods with nerve and skin biopsy findings may also help to decide which of the many variants is truly pathogenic. Moreover, biopsy diagnosis may reveal concomitant

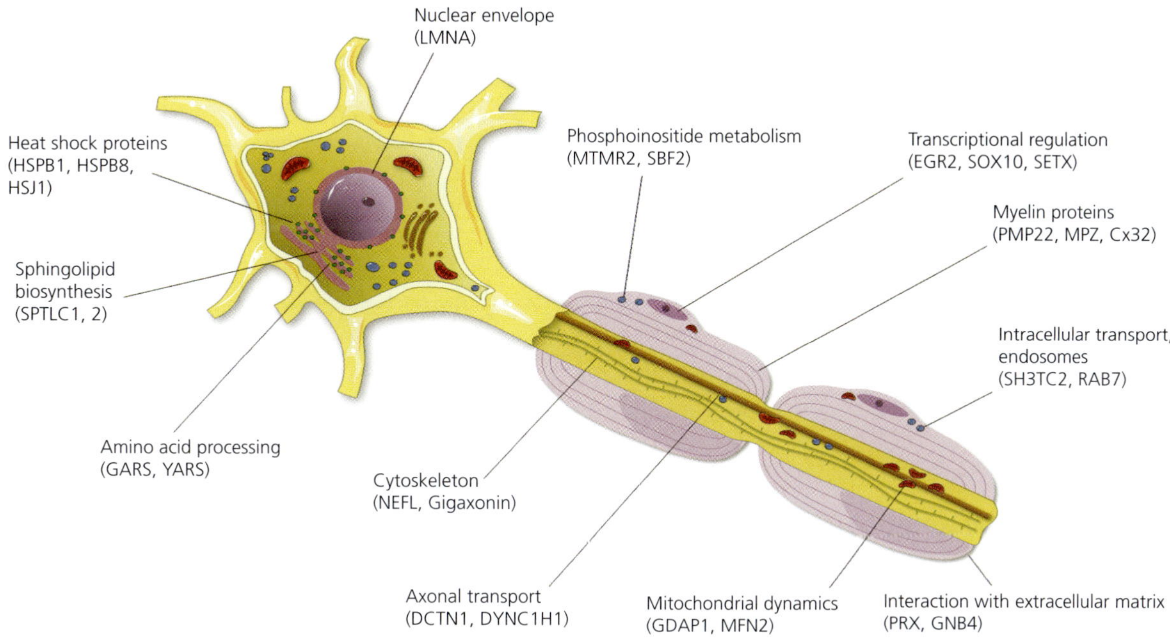

Figure 8.1 Schematic overview of Schwann cells and axon, highlighting the subcellular localization of proteins mutated in peripheral neuropathies.

pathology, for example, vascular or inflammatory changes, which contribute to the manifestation of a hereditary neuropathy. Biopsy studies also provide important clues which of the manifold pathophysiological aspects observed in cell culture and mouse models are actually relevant for the human disease.

Studying the pathology of hereditary neuropathies in nerve and skin biopsies may also promote the understanding of the pathomechanisms of the much more frequent non-hereditary neuropathies which are likely to involve secondary and acquired alterations of similar pathways that are targeted by gene mutations in the hereditary forms. A comprehensive understanding of the normal and disturbed physiology of the PNS will foster the targeted development of therapeutic approaches for both hereditary and non-hereditary neuropathies. Finally, the pathophysiologies of PNS and CNS disorders largely overlap, and many gene defects affect both the PNS and the CNS. Thus, the study of peripheral neuropathies may also provide valuable insight into etiology and pathogenesis of CNS disorders. Nerve biopsies and the analysis of nerve fibers in skin biopsies present a unique opportunity to study such pathomechanisms in biologically relevant human tissue.

CHAPTER 9

Autosomal dominant demyelinating Charcot–Marie–Tooth (CMT1)* neuropathies

Jean-Michel Vallat[1] and Stéphane Mathis[2]

[1] *Neurology Laboratory, National Referral Center for Rare Peripheral Neuropathies, University Hospital, Limoges, France*

[2] *Department of Neurology, La Milétrie University Hospital, Poitiers, France*

Definition

Charcot–Marie–Tooth (CMT) disease (MIM 118300), also called "hereditary motor and sensory neuropathy" (HMSN), is the commonest inherited neuromuscular disorder, and one of the most common groups of human hereditary disorders. It was first described in the late 1800s [1]. In Western countries most CMT are autosomal-dominant (CMT 1 and 2), but others are X-linked (CMTX) or autosomal-recessive (AR, CMT4), mainly in Mediterranean countries [2]. Many cases are sporadic. Since the duplication of the *PMP22* gene in CMT1A was identified [3], more than 40 responsible gene mutations have been found. CMT1A corresponds to an autosomal-dominant inherited demyelinating CMT.

Epidemiology

The prevalence of CMT is estimated between 1/1214 to 1/2500 in Norway, however, other epidemiological studies from Spain, Italy, Iceland, and Japan reported a prevalence of 1/3500 to 1/9200 [4]. CMT1A is the most frequent form of inheritable neuropathy, and represents 80.4% of all CMT [5].

Clinical features

Diagnosis of CMT requires a combination of clinical, genetic and electrophysiological features. Although it can be caused by mutations in many different genes, the clinical phenotype of CMT is relatively homogeneous, with wasting and weakness of distal limb muscles usually associated with distal sensory loss, skeletal deformities including high arched feet (*pes cavus*), and decreased or absent deep tendon reflexes [2].

Symptoms may appear in the first decade, but CMT is usually diagnosed later [6]. The clinical severity varies widely from classical mild or moderate forms to severe forms, such as Déjérine–Sottas disease (DSD) or CMT3 [2]. Congenital hypomyelinating neuropathy (CHN), responsible for hypotonia and muscle weakness at birth and in infancy, is usually recessive merging into DSD [7].

Nowadays, CMT is classified into subtypes based on inheritance and electrophysiological features [1] that separate demyelinating and axonal forms. A cut-off of 38 m/s for the median nerve conduction velocity (NCV) is accepted: value <38 m/s favors CMT1 (demyelinating form) and >38 m/s favors CMT2 (axonal forms) [8]. An "intermediate group" of CMT disease with NCV between 30 and 40 m/s has also been reported [9]. One-third of CMT appears to be primary axonal [1]. CMT1 is

* (CMT1 = Hereditary motor and sensory neuropathy = HMSNI)

Peripheral Nerve Disorders: Pathology and Genetics, First Edition. Edited by Jean-Michel Vallat, Joachim Weis, Francoise Gray, and Katy Keohane.

associated with uniformly slow NCV, unlike CIDP in which slow NCVs are mostly multifocal [10]. Any chronic demyelinating neuropathy induces significant axonal loss [7], probably secondary to long-standing abnormal axon-Schwann cell interactions [11]; the degree of axonal loss determines the patient's functional disability [12] that can be evaluated by a CMT neuropathy score [13]. Nerve biopsy is not routinely carried out in CMT, but pathological findings can help determine the morphological pattern of the neuropathy and narrow down the potential disease gene [14].

Pathology

In CMT1, the primary genetic defect affects the myelin-forming Schwann cell causing abnormalities of the myelin sheath. The main histopathological characteristics of CMT1 are listed in Table 9.1. Pathological hallmarks are loss of large myelinated fibers, and demyelinating-remyelinating lesions surrounded by numerous and proliferating onion-bulbs (Figure 9.1); thin myelin sheaths relative to axon size are frequent, but aspects of hypermyelinization such as tomaculae may be seen (Figure 9.2). In advanced cases, onion-bulb formations are usually associated with abnormal proliferation of the endoneurial collagen [7]. These characteristic lesions are best detected by electron microscopy. Rarely, coexisting hereditary (CMT1) and inflammatory (CIDP) features with typical macrophage-related demyelination can be observed, suggesting a cryptic mild inflammatory process [15]. Tomaculae, a hallmark of hereditary neuropathy with liability to pressure palsies (HNPP), are sometimes found in CMT1. Degenerating axons are often associated with tomaculae and myelin sheaths, which are too thick for their axonal diameters. Most of these pathological

Table 9.1 Correlations between genotype and pathological features on nerve biopsy in CMT1patients

Genes	Type of CMT	Microscopical anomalies
PMP22 duplication or mutations	CMT 1A CMT1E	Onion bulbs (Schwann cell cytoplasms, basal lamina)
MPZ mutations	CMT 1B	Uncompacted myelin; myelin outfoldings Onion bulbs
LITAF mutations	CMT1C	Onion bulbs (Schwann cell cytoplasms, basal lamina)
EGR2 (*KROX20*) mutations	CMT 1D CHN	Very severe demyelination, dysmyelination, or no myelination
NEFL mutations	CMT1F	Giant axons

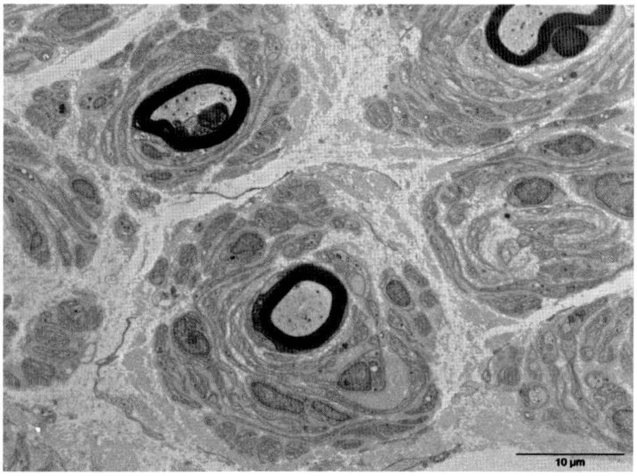

Figure 9.1 Electron micrograph. Transverse section. CMT1A. Several typical onion bulbs; they have numerous whorls of Schwann cell cytoplasmic processes in most cases, surrounding myelinated fibers.

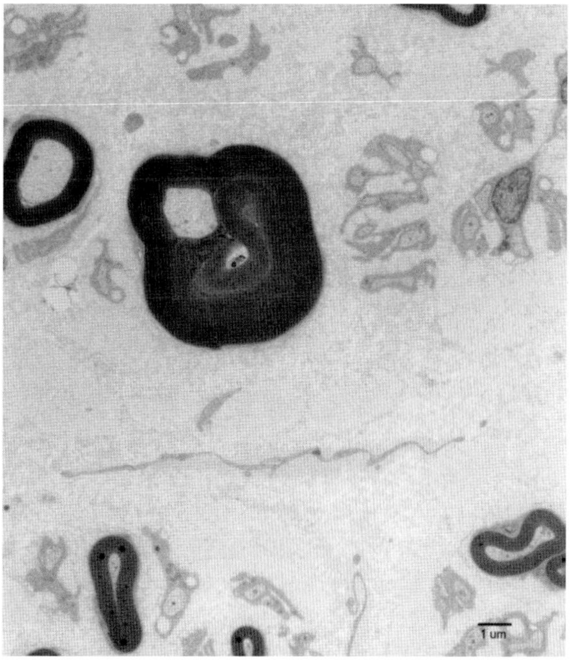

Figure 9.2 Electron micrograph. Transverse section. CMT1A. Outfolded redundant myelin loops surround the axon, which appears constricted.

signs are more severe in DSD or CHN. In these entities, onion-bulbs often consist of intense proliferations of basal lamina [7].

Pathological features of CMT1A (duplication of *PMP22*)

Pathological hallmarks are numerous multilayered onion bulbs, usually consisting of Schwann cell processes and more rarely of basement membranes (or both) and axons encircled with abnormally thin or relatively thick myelin sheaths [7]. These are the common features of "hypertrophic neuropathies," such as CMT1 or DSD, but may also be present in 10 to 43% of cases of CIDP [16]. There are some differences between onion-bulbs in CMT1A and in CIDP. In CMT1A, most myelinated fibers are surrounded by onion-bulbs, whereas in CIDP myelinated fibers surrounded by onion bulbs are interspersed with myelinated fibers without onion-bulbs [17]. Specific immunoreactivity for PMP22 can be shown in onion bulbs in CMT1A, but not in other CMT subtypes or in CIDP [18]. The demyelinating process in CMT1A appears more severe in patients under 15 than in older patients [19]. Segmental demyelination, thinly remyelinated internodes and an increase of Schwann cell nuclei can be observed on teased-nerve preparations, sometimes with markedly reduced density of myelinated fibers in advanced disease. In CMT1A (and in CMT1B), demyelination seems to be stable although axonal loss may increase concomitantly with advancing disease [7]. In CMT1A, tomaculae can also be observed: their mean diameter is 14.1 µm (SD 3.5), and their mean length is 77.4 µm (SD 16.1) [20]. Vital *et al.* reported a CMT1A case with macrophage-associated demyelination [21]. As previously mentioned, this supports an inflammatory demyelinating process superimposed on a chronic genetic disease. In our experience, such an inflammatory process may also be encountered in other CMT subtypes.

Pathological features of CMT1B (*MPZ* mutations)

Pathological features are a marked decrease in the density of myelinated fibers, segmental demyelination, numerous onion-bulb formations, and no involvement of unmyelinated fibers [7]. Two main changes in myelin sheaths have been described: non-compaction and focal folding of myelin lamellae [22]. Some cases with focally folded myelin mimic multiple entrapment neuropathies [23]. Disturbed myelin compaction (Figure 9.3) and focal myelin foldings (Figures 9.4 and 9.5) can be found in the same biopsy [24]. In CMT1B with *MPZ* mutations involving the extra-cellular domain of P0 (codon 98 in particular), uncompacted myelin lamellae have been described involving the inner and outer myelin lamellae or, occasionally, the whole myelin sheath [25]. They consist of widening between dense lines, due to a dissociation of the paired intraperiod lines. The widenings

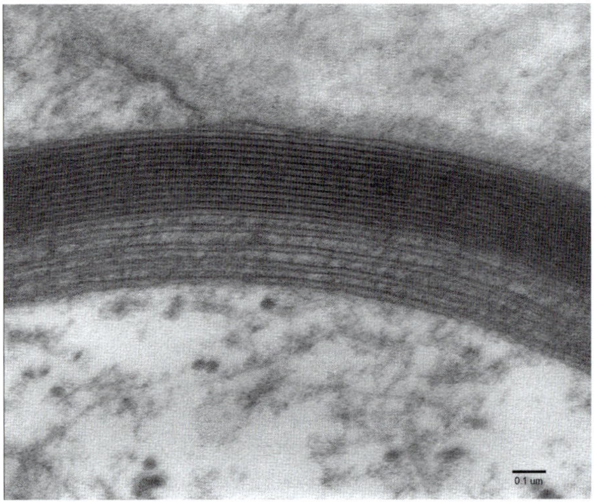

Figure 9.3 Electron micrograph. Transverse section. CMT 1B. The inner myelin lamellae of this myelin sheath are regularly and abnormally widened. Note the normal compaction of the other myelin lamellae.

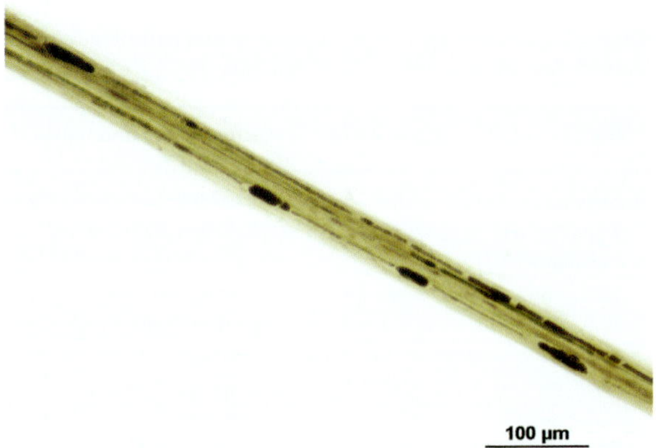

Figure 9.4 Teased fiber preparation. CMT1B. Numerous hypermyelinated lesions which look like tomaculae; between them, most axons are demyelinated.

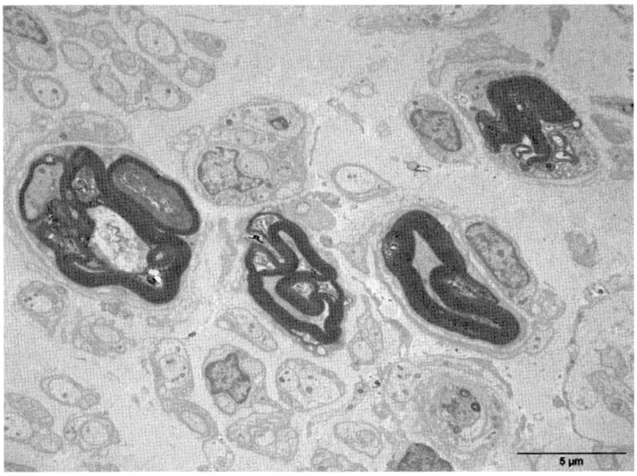

Figure 9.5 Electron micrograph. CMT1B. All the myelin sheaths have numerous in- and outfoldings. The axons are all constricted and seem very abnormal.

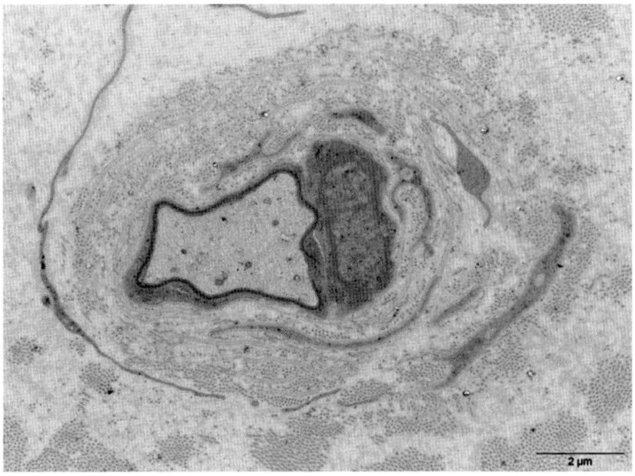

Figure 9.6 Electron micrograph. CMT1E. Onion bulbs are characterized by intense concentric proliferations of basal laminae, which are intermingled with cytoplasmic Schwann cell processes. They surround an axon with a disproportionately thin myelin sheath, favoring a remyelinating process.

are the same size in an individual patient, but vary between patients; they resemble those found in the *P0* KO mouse model [26]. Other types of widened myelin lamellae are also described in POEMS (Polyneuropathy, Organomegaly, Endocrinopathy, M-protein, Skin changes) syndrome [27], in IgM monoclonal gammopathy with anti-MAG activity, and very rarely in IgA or IgG monoclonal gammopathy [28].

In CMT1B, the folding corresponds to an aberrant proliferation of myelin sheaths and is present along all large and small myelinated fibers in teased fiber preparations. Numerous folds give a pattern called "globular neuropathy" [29]. They can be detected easily on semithin sections and by electron microscopy, and are a mixture of infoldings extending towards the axon (which can distort the transverse profile of the axon) and outfoldings extending into the Schwann cell cytoplasm [30]. They are quite different to tomaculae, which have smooth external contours [31]. Similar myelin foldings are also observed in AR-CMT4B.

A few cases of CMT1B (with *MPZ* mutation Ile99Thr) have both clinical and electrophysiological features of CIDP, and may respond to corticosteroid treatment [32]. Inflammatory signs are often detected in nerves of old heterozygous (P0+/−) mice.

Pathological features of CMT1C (*LITAF* mutations)

In CMT1C, microscopic lesions are identical to those observed in CMT1A [7].

Pathological features of CMT1D (*EGR2* mutations)

Nerve biopsy usually shows a severe loss of myelinated fibers with numerous onion-bulbs [33]. Complete absence of *EGR2*, recessively transmitted, induces a congenital amyelinating neuropathy [34].

Pathological features of CMTIE (*PMP22* mutations)

Severe and early phenotypes of CMT1E mimic CMT1A, with profound loss of myelinating fibers and abundant onion-bulbs often characterized by intense concentric proliferations of basal laminae (Figure 9.6) [35]. In cases of *PMP22* frameshift mutations or HNPP-like presentation, the nerve biopsy also shows large tomaculae [36]. In cases with missense mutations and a mild HNPP phenotype, in spite of reduction in myelin thickness and abundance of large myelinated fibers, no onion-bulbs were observed [37].

Pathological features of CMT1F (*NEFL* mutations)

Mutations were first described as causing the axonal autosomal dominant CMT2E [38]. However, some of these patients have NCV in a demyelinating range with pathological lesions characterized by small onion bulbs and thinly myelinated axons [39], resulting in a diagnosis of CMT1F [2]: for this reason, this entity has been also called CMT2E/1F.

Giant axons with focal accumulation of neurofilaments have also sometimes been observed, and *NEFL* mutations cause profound alterations of the cytoskeleton [40]. Rarely, *NEFL* mutations can be associated with an AR-CMT2 [41].

Genetics

CMT type 1A (CMT1A)

Up to 90% of CMT1A are associated with a submicroscopic 1.5-megabase duplication on the short arm of the chromosome 17p11.2 (in the region p11.2-p12) which contains *PMP22* [35]. This neuropathy expresses itself in early life, varies clinically in severity and remains relatively stable in adulthood [19]. In most cases, motor NCV in the median nerve is < 30 m/s, and distal latencies are usually >5 ms [42].

PMP22 is a small hydrophobic tetraspan membrane glycoprotein (22 kDa) of compact myelin of the PNS: it is composed of 160 amino acids, and contains four transmembrane domains TM1–4, two short cytoplasmic tails, a short intracellular loop, and two extracellular loops (the first loop bearing the L2/HNK1 epitope, a mediator of adhesive process): PMP22 is expressed in myelinating Schwann cells, as well as in other neural and non-neural tissues. It localizes in the compact myelin and accounts for 2–5% of the total myelin protein. PMP22 is not present in the central nervous system, but shares structural features with PLP (proteolipid protein), a major protein of central nervous system myelin [35]. The biological functions of PMP22 are largely unknown. Saporta *et al.* reported a 7-year-old boy with a *PMP22* homozygous deletion and suggested PMP22 is important for the normal function of neurons that express PMP22 during early development making a comparison with *PMP22* null mice [43]. We now know that the CMT1A phenotype is caused by a gene dosage effect [35]. Immunocytochemical quantitative analysis showed an increased expression of PMP22 levels in myelin sheaths compared with controls [7].

CMT type 1B (CMT1B)

CMT1B results from mutations in the *P0 glycoprotein* (*myelin protein zero*, or *MPZ*) gene, in the q22-q23 region of chromosome 1 [44]. *MPZ* mutations are due to various mechanisms involving gain of function, dominant negative effects, partial loss of function, and hyperglycosylation [44].

MPZ, expressed predominantly in Schwann cells, represents up to 50% of the protein content of the PNS myelin [45]. It is a transmembrane protein (29 kDa) of 219 amino acid residues, and consists of three domains: a glycosylated immunoglobulin-like extracellular domain, a membrane, and a highly basic intracellular domain [45]. MPZ is a member of the immunoglobulin super-family, acting as a homophilic adhesion protein essential for normal myelin structure and function: it maintains compact myelin at the intraperiod line by adhesion between apposed *MPZ* tetramers at the outer membrane surface. During myelination, MPZ seems to induce myelin compaction by excluding MAG [7].

CMT type 1C (CMT1C)

CMT1C is linked to the chromosome 16p13.1 and mutations in *LITAF* (*lipopolysaccharide-induced TNF factor*), also known as *SIMPLE* (*small integral membrane protein of lysosome/late endosome*) or *PIG-7* (*p53 inductible gene-7*) gene [46]. Initially, two transcripts, encoding different proteins (LITAF and *SIMPLE*), were reported [2]. The *LITAF* transcript seems to result from a DNA sequencing error, and the *SIMPLE* transcript appears to be the only true transcript of this gene [47]. SIMPLE is an early endosomal membrane protein (18 kDa), highly expressed in Schwann cells [48]. Lack of *SIMPLE* accelerates myelin destruction and the emergence of axonal sprouts, and increases the number of macrophages during Wallerian degeneration [49]. It is hypothesized that CMT1C can be due to a combination of loss of function and toxic gain of function mechanisms, with an important role for both the proteosome and autophagy pathways [48].

CMT type 1D (CMT1D)

CMT1D is a rare form of CMT1 resulting from mutations in the *early growth response 2* (*EGR2*) gene mapped on the 10q21-q22 chromosome [50]. These mutations can also be recessive [51]. *EGR2* (*Krox20*), with *Sox10* (that regulates *EGR2*), play a key role in the formation and maintenance of myelin [52]. *EGR2* is a Cys2-His2 zinc-finger transcription factor that regulates the expression of peripheral myelin protein genes such as *MPZ, Cx32, MBP*, and *PMP22* [53]. Even in patients with an identical mutation, there is a wide clinical spectrum of CMT1D, from a moderate late onset form to severe early onset DSD or CHN [50].

CMT type 1E (CMT1E)

CMT1E, representing 1–5% of the CMT1 neuropathies, are associated with point mutations in *PMP22* [35]. Initially, *PMP22* mutation cases were considered to be clinically more severely affected in comparison to patients with a *PMP22* duplication [54]. In fact, CMT1E shows a wide phenotypic spectrum, and the clinical manifestations range from mild HNPP-like neuropathy to severe DSS-like neuropathy and CHN [35]. It seems that R159C mutation can also lead to an "axonal CMT1E" [55].

CMT type 1F (CMT1F)

NEFL (*Neurofilament protein light polypeptide*) encodes the neurofilament light chains (NF-L), a major constituent of intermediate filaments that play a crucial function in the assembly and maintenance of axonal cytoskeleton [40].

Other autosomal dominant inherited neuropathies with a CMT1 pattern

Roussy– Levy syndrome (*RLS*)

This syndrome was first described in 1926 by Gustave Roussy and Gabrielle Levy as an AD hereditary ataxia with tremor [56]. Patients have slow NCV and demyelination of nerve fibers with onion-bulb formations, reasons why RLS is considered to be a variant of CMT1: clinically, these patients have gait ataxia, *pes cavus*, areflexia, and sometimes postural tremor and minor sensory loss. Some patients have focally hypertrophic myelin sheaths and major loss of myelinated fibers [57]. Hypertrophic roots can be observed rarely [58].

A *MPZ* mutation has been found in members of the original RLS family [57]. However, identical phenotypes were also associated with duplication [56] or point mutations [59] of *PMP22*.

CMT1 and *Fibulin-5* mutations

Recently, missense mutations of *Fibulin-5* (*FBLN5*) were found in chromosome 14q32.12, in two CMT1 families [60]. *FBLN5*, a matricellular calcium-binding glycoprotein, is also a key regulator of development and maintenance of elastic fiber-rich tissues; mutations of *FBLN5* usually causes cutis laxa [60]. *FBLN5* appears to be indispensable for elastogenesis [60].

Clinical and electrophysiological findings of patients with *FBLN5* mutations are consistent with a late-onset CMT1 neuropathy, but a spinal pattern was found in one patient, and a late-onset axonal neuropathy in another. CMT with *FBLN5* mutations usually manifest with skin hyperlaxity and age-related macular degeneration, sometimes concurrent [60].

To date, nerve biopsy of this CMT subtype has not been reported.

CMT1 and *GJB3* mutations

Dominantly inherited mutations in the *GJB3* gene, encoding Connexin 31 (Cx31), cause the skin disease "erythrokeratodermia variabilis" and sensorineural hearing loss, with or without neuropathy [61]. Connexins are major components of gap-junctions, and Cx31 is highly expressed in epidermals stratum granulosum, cochlea, and nerves [61].

Although pathological features are consistent with a demyelinating process, sometimes with onion bulbs, patients with *GJB3* mutations and neuropathy have electrophysiological features favoring an axonal neuropathy [62].

Animal models and future perspectives

The spontaneous mouse mutants trembler and trembler-J both carry point mutations in the *PMP22* gene and share pathological features with CMT1A. To date, five trembler mouse spontaneous mutations in the *PMP22* gene have been identified: trembler, trembler-J, trembler-NCnp, trembler m2H. However, these mice cannot be considered as typical models for the human gene dosage disorder CMT1A [63].

The first animal models of CMT1A (CMT rats) were generated by pronuclear injection of cosmid-derived 43 Kb DNA fragments, harboring the entire *PMP22* gene [63]. There is also a murine model of CMT1B (where a mutation encoding R98C was targeted to the mouse *MPZ* gene): the R98C mouse [64].

CMT1A is an incurable disease necessitating active treatment. One treatment aimed at slowing the progression of CMT1A is the use of a synthetic antagonist of the nuclear progesterone receptor, which reduced *PMP22* overexpression and lessened the severity of disease in animal models [63]. Another interesting molecule is ascorbic acid, known to be necessary to induce myelin formation in neuron-Schwann cell co-cultures [63]. However, if ascorbic acid reduces the severity of neuropathy in transgenic mice overexpressing *PMP22*, it has no significant effect on CMT1A neuropathy after 2 years of treatment in humans [63]. Recently, curcumin (one of the major component of *Curcuma longa*) was shown to improve the peripheral neuropathy in R98C mice by alleviating endoplasmic reticulum stress. The mechanism is by reducing the activation of unfolded protein response and by promoting Schwann cell differentiation [64].

Future identification of biomarkers for disease severity would be crucial. Recently, in *PMP22* transgenic rats, a German study demonstrated that transcriptional analysis of skin biopsy is suitable to identify biomarkers of CMT1A [65].

Conclusion

CMT1, a demyelinating and autosomal dominant hereditary neuropathy, is the most common form of CMT and is linked to several different genes (Figure 9.7). The

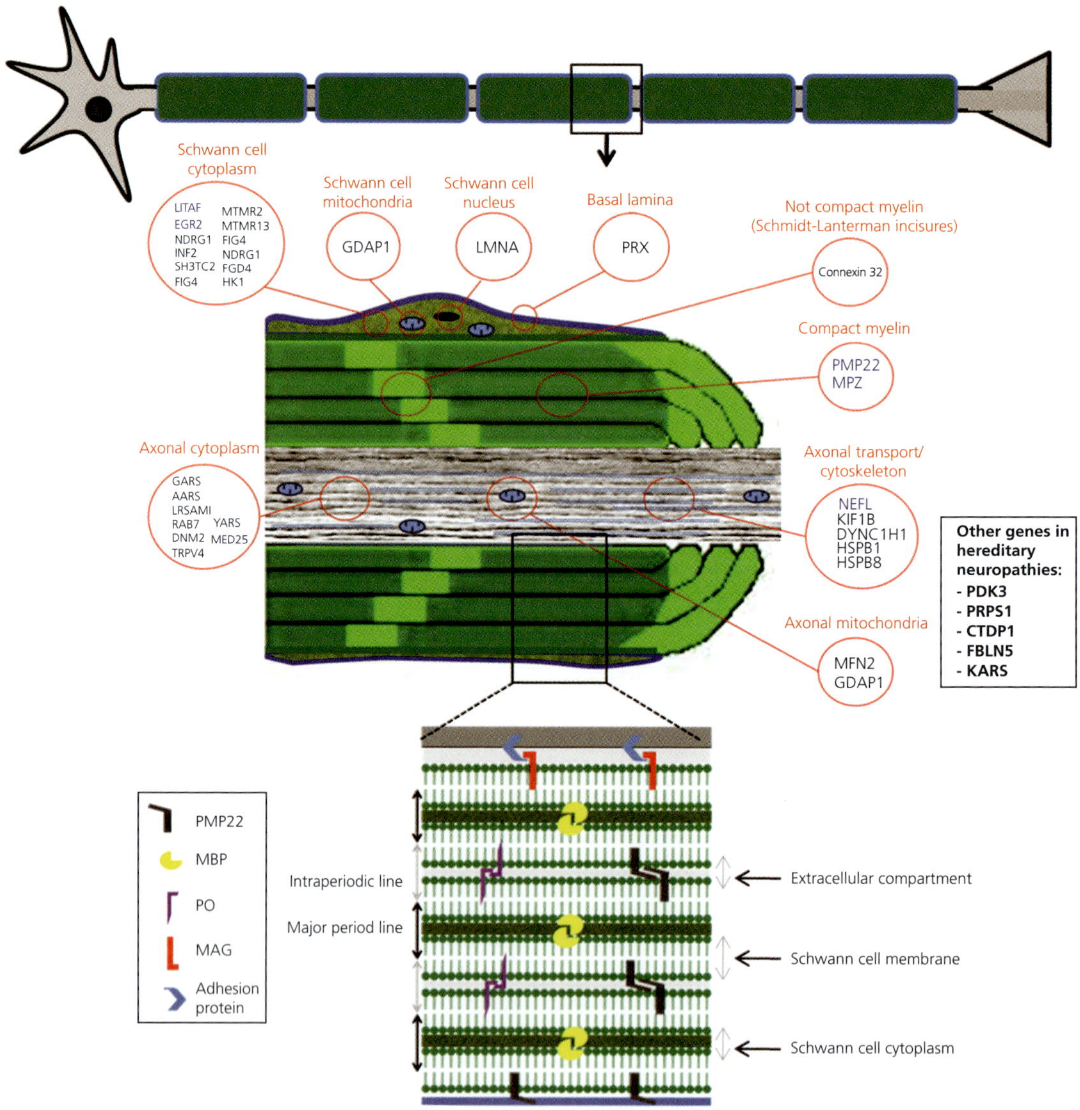

Figure 9.7 This figure shows the various localizations of the proteins present in axons and Schwann cells. Those written in blue are abnormal (duplicated or mutated) in CMT1.

clinical features are similar to other forms of CMT, and electrophysiological and pathological studies confirm a demyelinating process. On nerve biopsy, some signs are more frequent in CMT1, such as onion-bulb formations (different from those in CIDP), tomaculae, and foldings. There is no current successful therapy, but new treatments may be possible using animal models to identify potential pharmacological targets.

References

1 Saporta AS, Sottile SL, Miller LJ, *et al.* (2011) Charcot–Marie–Tooth disease subtypes and genetic testing strategies. *Ann Neurol*;69:22–33.

2 Houlden H, Reilly MM. (2006) Molecular genetics of autosomal-dominant demyelinating Charcot–Marie–Tooth disease. *Neuromolecular Med*;8:43–62.

3 Lupski JR, de Oca-Luna RM, Slaugenhaupt S, *et al.* (1991) DNA duplication associated with Charcot–Marie–Tooth disease type 1A. *Cell*;66:219–232.

4 Braathen GJ, Sand JC, Lobato A, *et al.* (2011) Genetic epidemiology of Charcot–Marie–Tooth in the general population. *Eur J Neurol*;18:39–48.

5 Murphy SM, Laura M, Fawcett K, *et al.* (2012) Charcot–Marie–Tooth disease: frequency of genetic subtypes and guidelines for genetic testing. *J Neurol Neurosurg Psychiatry*; 83:706 710.

6 Souayah N, Seltzer WK, Brannagan TH, *et al.* (2007) Rare myelin protein zero sequence variant in late onset CMT1B. *J Neurol Sci*;263:177–179.

7 Vallat JM. (2003) Dominantly inherited peripheral neuropathies. *J Neuropathol Exp Neurol*;62:699–714.

8 Harding AE, Thomas PK. (1980) The clinical features of hereditary motor and sensory neuropathy types I and II. *Brain*;103:259–280.

9 Bouche P, Gherardi R, Cathala HP, *et al.* (1983) Peroneal muscular atrophy. Part 1. Clinical and electrophysiological study. *J Neurol Sci*;61:389–399.

10 Lewis R, Sumner A. (1999) Electrophysiological features of inherited demyelinating neuropathies: a reappraisal. *Ann N Y Acad Sci*;883:321–35.

11 Maier M, Berger P, Suter U. (2002) Understanding Schwann cell-neurone interactions: the key to Charcot–Marie–Tooth disease? *J Anat*;200:357–366.

12 Hattori N, Yamamoto M, Yoshihara T, *et al.* (2003) Demyelinating and axonal features of Charcot–Marie–Tooth disease with mutations of myelin-related proteins (PMP22, MPZ and Cx32): a clinicopathological study of 205 Japanese patients. *Brain*;126:134–151.

13 Murphy SM, Herrmann DN, McDermott MP, *et al.* (2011) Reliability of the CMT neuropathy score (second version) in Charcot–Marie–Tooth disease. *J Peripher Nerv Syst*;16:191–198.

14 Weis J, Brandner S, Lammens M, *et al.* (2012) Processing of nerve biopsies: a practical guide for neuropathologists. *Clin Neuropathol*;31:7–23.

15 Gabriel CM, Gregson NA, Wood NW, Hughes RA. (2002) Immunological study of hereditary motor and sensory neuropathy type 1a (HMSN1a). *J Neurol Neurosurg Psychiatry*;72: 230–235.

16 Oh SJ. (1990) Diagnostic usefulness and limitations of the sural nerve biopsy. *Yonsei Med J*;31:1–26.

17 Dyck P, Engelstad J. (1999) Pattern of onion-bulb distribution predicts acquired versus inherited hypertrophic neuropathy. *Ann Neurol*;46:482.

18 Nishimura T, Yoshikawa H, Fujimura H, *et al.* (1996) Accumulation of peripheral myelin protein 22 in onion bulbs and Schwann cells of biopsied nerves from patients with Charcot–Marie–Tooth disease type 1A. *Acta Neuropathol*; 92:454–460.

19 Fabrizi GM, Simonati A, Morbin M, *et al.* (1998) Clinical and pathological correlations in Charcot–Marie–Tooth neuropathy type 1A with the 17p11.2p12 duplication: a cross-sectional morphometric and immunohistochemical study in twenty cases. *Muscle Nerve*;21:869–877.

20 Sander S, Ouvrier RA, McLeod JG, *et al.* (2000) Clinical syndromes associated with tomacula or myelin swellings in sural nerve biopsies. *J Neurol Neurosurg Psychiatry*;68:483–488.

21 Vital A, Vital C, Lagueny A, *et al.* (2003) Inflammatory demyelination in a patient with CMT1A. *Muscle Nerve*;28: 373–376.

22 Gabreels-Festen AA, Hoogendijk JE, Meijerink PH, *et al.* (1996) Two divergent types of nerve pathology in patients with different P0 mutations in Charcot–Marie–Tooth disease. *Neurology*;47:761–765.

23 Iida M, Koike H, Ando T, *et al.* (2012) A novel MPZ mutation in Charcot–Marie–Tooth disease type 1B with focally folded myelin and multiple entrapment neuropathies. *Neuromuscul Disord*;22:166–169.

24 Vallat JM, Magy L, Lagrange E, *et al.* (2007) Diagnostic value of ultrastructural nerve examination in Charcot–Marie–Tooth disease: two CMT 1B cases with pseudo-recessive inheritance. *Acta Neuropathol*;113:443–439.

25 Lagueny A, Latour P, Vital A, *et al.* (1999) Peripheral myelin modification in CMT1B correlates with MPZ gene mutations. *Neuromuscul Disord*;9:361–367.

26 Xu W, Manichella D, Jiang H, *et al.* (2000) Absence of P0 leads to the dysregulation of myelin gene expression and myelin morphogenesis. *J Neurosci Res*;60:714–724.

27 Vital C, Gherardi R, Vital A, *et al.* (1994) Uncompacted myelin lamellae in polyneuropathy, organomegaly, endocrinopathy, M-protein and skin changes syndrome. Ultrastructural study of peripheral nerve biopsy from 22 patients. *Acta Neuropathol*;87:302–307.

28 Vallat JM, Magy L, Richard L, *et al.* (2008) Contribution of electron microscopy to the study of neuropathies associated with an IgG monoclonal paraproteinemia. *Micron*;39:61–70.

29 Vallat JM, Gil R, Leboutet MJ, *et al.* (1987) Congenital hypo- and hypermyelination neuropathy. Two cases. *Acta Neuropathol*;74:197–201.
30 Umehara F, Takenaga S, Nakagawa M, *et al.* (1993) Dominantly inherited motor and sensory neuropathy with excessive myelin folding complex. *Acta Neuropathol*;86: 602–608.
31 Nakagawa M, Suehara M, Saito A, *et al.* (1999) A novel MPZ gene mutation in dominantly inherited neuropathy with focally folded myelin sheaths. *Neurology*;52:1271–1275.
32 Donaghy M, Sisodiya SM, Kennett R, *et al.* (2000) Steroid responsive polyneuropathy in a family with a novel myelin protein zero mutation. *J Neurol Neurosurg Psychiatry*;69: 799–805.
33 Szigeti K, Wiszniewski W, Saifi GM, *et al.* (2007) Functional, histopathologic and natural history study of neuropathy associated with EGR2 mutations. *Neurogenetics*;8:257–262.
34 Funalot B, Topilko P, Arroyo MA, *et al.* (2012) Homozygous deletion of an EGR2 enhancer in congenital amyelinating neuropathy. *Ann Neurol*;71:719–723.
35 Li J, Parker B, Martyn C, Natarajan C, *et al.* (2013) The PMP22 gene and its related diseases. *Mol Neurobiol*;47: 673–698.
36 Lenssen PP, Gabreels-Festen AA, Valentijn LJ, *et al.* (1998) Hereditary neuropathy with liability to pressure palsies. Phenotypic differences between patients with the common deletion and a PMP22 frame shift mutation. *Brain*;121: 1451–1458.
37 Luigetti M, Conte A, Madia F, *et al.* (2008) A new single-nucleotide deletion of PMP22 in an HNPP family without recurrent palsies. *Muscle Nerve*;38:1060–1064.
38 Mersiyanova IV, Perepelov AV, Polyakov AV, *et al.* (2000) A new variant of Charcot–Marie–Tooth disease type 2 is probably the result of a mutation in the neurofilament-light gene. *Am J Hum Genet*;67:37–46.
39 Jordanova A, De Jonghe P, Boerkoel CF, *et al.* (2003) Mutations in the neurofilament light chain gene (NEFL) cause early onset severe Charcot–Marie–Tooth disease. *Brain*; 126:590–597.
40 Fabrizi GM, Cavallaro T, Angiari C, *et al.* (2007) Charcot–Marie–Tooth disease type 2E, a disorder of the cytoskeleton. *Brain*;130:394–403.
41 Yum SW, Zhang J, Mo K, *et al.* (2009) A novel recessive NEFL mutation causes a severe, early-onset axonal neuropathy. *Ann Neurol*;66:759–770.
42 Deymeer F, Matur Z, Poyraz M, *et al.* (2011) Nerve conduction studies in Charcot–Marie–Tooth disease in a cohort from Turkey. *Muscle Nerve*;43:657–664.
43 Saporta MA, Katona I, Zhang X, *et al.* (2011) Neuropathy in a human without the PMP22 gene. *Arch Neurol*;68: 814–821.
44 Prada V, Passalacqua M, Bono M, *et al.* (2012) Gain of glycosylation: a new pathomechanism of myelin protein zero mutations. *Ann Neurol*;71:427–431.
45 Liu Z, Wang Y, Yedidi RS, *et al.* (2012) Crystal structure of the extracellular domain of human myelin protein zero. *Proteins*;80:307–313.
46 Eaton HE, Desrochers G, Drory SB, *et al.* (2011) SIMPLE/LITAF expression induces the translocation of the ubiquitin ligase itch towards the lysosomal compartments. *PLoS One*;6:e16873.
47 Saifi GM, Szigeti K, Wiszniewski W, *et al.* (2005) SIMPLE mutations in Charcot–Marie–Tooth disease and the potential role of its protein product in protein degradation. *Hum Mutat*;25:372–383.
48 Lee SM, Olzmann JA, Chin LS, *et al.* (2011) Mutations associated with Charcot–Marie–Tooth disease cause SIMPLE protein mislocalization and degradation by the proteasome and aggresome-autophagy pathways. *J Cell Sci*;124:3319–3331.
49 Somandin C, Gerber D, Pereira JA, *et al.* (2012) LITAF (SIMPLE) regulates Wallerian degeneration after injury but is not essential for peripheral nerve development and maintenance: implications for Charcot–Marie–Tooth disease. *Glia*;60:1518–1528.
50 Safka Brozkova D, Nevsimalova S, Mazanec R, *et al.* (2012) Charcot–Marie–Tooth neuropathy due to a novel EGR2 gene mutation with mild phenotype – usefulness of human mapping chip linkage analysis in a Czech family. *Neuromuscul Disord*;22:742–746.
51 Boerkoel CF, Takashima H, Garcia CA, *et al.* (2002) Charcot–Marie–Tooth disease and related neuropathies: mutation distribution and genotype-phenotype correlation. *Ann Neurol*; 51:190–201.
52 Decker L, Desmarquet-Trin-Dinh C, Taillebourg E, *et al.* (2006) Peripheral myelin maintenance is a dynamic process requiring constant Krox20 expression. *J Neurosci*;26: 9771–9779.
53 Srinivasan R, Sun G, Keles S, *et al.* (2012) Genome-wide analysis of EGR2/SOX10 binding in myelinating peripheral nerve. *Nucleic Acids Res*;40:6449–6460.
54 Scherer SS, Chance PF. (1995) Myelin genes: getting the dosage right. *Nature Genet*;11:226–228.
55 Gess B, Jeibmann A, Schirmacher A, *et al.* (2011) Report of a novel mutation in the PMP22 gene causing an axonal neuropathy. *Muscle Nerve*;43:605–609.
56 Auer-Grumbach M, Strasser-Fuchs S, Wagner K, *et al.* (1998) Roussy–Levy syndrome is a phenotypic variant of Charcot–Marie–Tooth syndrome IA associated with a duplication on chromosome 17p11.2. *J Neurol Sci*;154:72–75.
57 Plante-Bordeneuve V, Guiochon-Mantel A, Lacroix C, *et al.* (1999) The Roussy–Levy family: from the original description to the gene. *Ann Neurol*;46:770–773.
58 Haubrich C, Krings T, Senderek J, *et al.* (2002) Hypertrophic nerve roots in a case of Roussy–Levy syndrome. *Neuroradiology*; 44:933–937.
59 Zubair S, Holland NR, Beson B, Parke JT, Prodan CI. (2008) A novel point mutation in the PMP22 gene in a family with Roussy–Levy syndrome. *J Neurol*;255:1417–1418.

60 Auer-Grumbach M, Weger M, Fink-Puches R, *et al.* (2011) Fibulin-5 mutations link inherited neuropathies, age-related macular degeneration and hyperelastic skin. *Brain*;134: 1839–1852.
61 Tattersall D, Scott CA, Gray C, *et al.* (2009) EKV mutant connexin 31 associated cell death is mediated by ER stress. *Hum Mol Genet*;18:4734–4745.
62 Lopez-Bigas N, Olive M, Rabionet R, *et al.* (2001) Connexin 31 (GJB3) is expressed in the peripheral and auditory nerves and causes neuropathy and hearing impairment. *Hum Mol Genet*;10:947–952.
63 Fledrich R, Stassart RM, Sereda MW. (2012) Murine therapeutic models for Charcot–Marie–Tooth (CMT) disease. *Br Med Bull*;102:89–113.
64 Patzko A, Bai Y, Saporta MA, *et al.* (2012) Curcumin derivatives promote Schwann cell differentiation and improve neuropathy in R98C CMT1B mice. *Brain*;135: 3551–3566.
65 Fledrich R, Schlotter-Weigel B, Schnizer TJ, *et al.* (2012) A rat model of Charcot–Marie–Tooth disease 1A recapitulates disease variability and supplies biomarkers of axonal loss in patients. *Brain*;135:72–87.

CHAPTER 10

Autosomal dominant neuropathy of the axonal Charcot–Marie–Tooth type 2*

J. Michael Schröder,[1] Joachim Weis,[1] and Jan Senderek[2]

[1] Institute of Neuropathology, RWTH Aachen University Hospital and JARA Brain Translational Medicine, Aachen, Germany

[2] Friedrich Baur Institute, Department of Neurology, Ludwig-Maximilians University, Munich, Germany

Definition

Dominantly inherited axonal or neuronal forms of motor and sensory neuropathy type II (HMSN II) are a heterogeneous group of peripheral polyneuropathies characterized by predominantly distal degeneration (and regeneration) of axons, usually without demyelination and onion bulb formation. Geneticists classify these as CMT2; this term is now more generally used. This group is subdivided according to the affected gene or gene locus into type CMT2A–CMT2P. Some of these are allelic to predominantly demyelinating neuropathies (type CMT1) such as those caused by mutations of the genes *NEFL* and *MPZ*. Mutations in the *GDAP1* gene may occur in autosomal dominant as well as in autosomal recessive diseases (CMT2K and CMT4A, respectively). There may also be intermediate, partly axonal, partly demyelinating disease types (ID-CMT = CMTID A–E; and in X-linked CMT, CMTX). In addition to CMT2 cases, other dominantly inherited axonal forms of peripheral neuropathy occur in the setting of hereditary sensory and autonomic neuropathies (HSANs), and neuropathies associated with motor neuron diseases (ALS, SMA), spinocerebellar atrophies (ADCA), mitochondrial disorders, and complex syndromic diseases.

General characteristics of CMT2

Clinical presentation

Many clinical signs and symptoms, or histopathological changes are common for the different axonal forms of hereditary neuropathy caused by mutations in various genes. Clinical symptoms and signs in CMT2 cases resemble those in dominantly inherited demyelinating forms of CMT (CMT1) but generally become manifest later and show less severe involvement of upper limbs and only minor ataxia, reduction in tendon reflexes and sensory loss [1]. Skeletal deformities are also less prominent, presumably due to later onset of the disease. Nerve conduction velocity is in the normal range or only moderately reduced (>38 m/s for the motor part of the median nerve) [2]. Certain forms show special clinical features such as foot ulcers, diaphragm and vocal cord paresis, or onset in small hand muscles. Autosomal dominant (AD) cases of the axonal type are generally less severely affected than autosomal recessive (AR) ones. This is especially so in cases manifesting in childhood [3]. Intermediate, partly axonal, partly demyelinating types, and X-chromosomal forms are discussed separately (see Chapters 12–13).

*(CMT2 = Hereditary motor and sensory neuropathy type II, HMSN II)

Peripheral Nerve Disorders: Pathology and Genetics, First Edition. Edited by Jean-Michel Vallat, Joachim Weis, Francoise Gray, and Katy Keohane.

Epidemiology

In a Norwegian population, one in 1214 people had CMT: CMT1 was found in 48.2%, CMT2 in 49.4%, and intermediate CMT in 2.4% of patients. Mutations of the *MNF2* gene were found in 6.2% of the families [4]. Genomic data from 36 unrelated Taiwanese CMT2 patients revealed 10 independent mutations in 14 patients: one each in *AARS, HSPB1*, and *GDAP*1, three in *NEFL* (six patients), and four in *MFN2* (five patients). Despite an extensive survey, the genetic causes of CMT2 remained elusive in the remaining 22 CMT2 patients (61.1%) [5]. Next generation sequencing ("massively parallel sequencing") is now widely used to disclose most of the suspected remaining unidentified mutations in hereditary neuromuscular disorders (approx. 50%) [6].

General histopathology of CMT2

Many histopathological changes are not distinctive for certain CMT2 or other axonal forms of hereditary neuropathy.

Nerve biopsy reveals predominant loss of nerve fibers with minor evidence of secondary segmental demyelination due to axonal atrophy. Yet at the site of degenerated nerve fibers there are usually bands of Büngner with or without bundles of closely adjacent regenerated nerve fibers due to supernumerary axonal sprouts (see Chapter 7). The endoneurial connective tissue is almost normal, edematous, or moderately increased in amount. Cellular loss in bands of Büngner is slowly progressive occurring over months to years; complete loss of all bands of Büngner with total or subtotal endoneurial fibrosis is extremely rare (cf. Fig. 7.17). Nerve fascicles nevertheless persist. The number of unmyelinated axons is usually also reduced, most clearly established by electron microscopy. Typical onion bulb formations ("hypertrophic" changes) are not seen although regenerated nerve fibers in bands of Büngner may mimic onion bulb formation when regenerated fibers degenerate again, especially if this process occurs repeatedly (*pseudo-onion bulbs*). During the usual chronic course of inherited axonal neuropathies, there is typically simultaneous Wallerian degeneration and regeneration of fibers (see Chapter 7). Their number depends on how chronic the process is, that is, its progression and duration. In contrast to progressive neuropathies, *developmental disturbances* of large, small, or all-myelinated or unmyelinated fibers, are characterized by a non-progressive stable state without products of degeneration; these need to be distinguished from disturbances of the development of myelin sheaths (amyelination, hypomyelination). Conversely, simultaneous occurrence of numerous degenerating fibers in the same stage of degeneration and/or marked focal nerve fiber loss is evidence against a (purely) hereditary type of neuropathy; in those situations (additional) toxic, mechanical, or immunologic factors should be considered.

Anterior horn cells, at autopsy, may show *chromatolysis* and finally *neuronophagia*. Similar neuronal changes are seen in dorsal root ganglia (DRG) along with distally accentuated loss of axons in spinal roots and peripheral nerves. Loss of axons in the dorsal columns may occur due to wasting of neurons in DRGs. These changes are most prominent in the lumbosacral region, namely in the fasciculi graciles [7]. More specific changes are described in the following subsections.

CMT2A (MIM 609260)

Definition, epidemiology, genetics, and pathogenesis

Neuropathies caused by mutations of the *MFN2* gene [8] are classified as CMT2A and account for 3% of infantile neuropathies [9], and 5–30% of CMT2 cases [10]. Thus CMT2A represents the most frequent autosomal dominantly inherited axonal neuropathy.

Neuropathies caused by *MFN2* mutations are sometimes classified as CMT2A2 because of a single family with a *KIF1B* mutation previously classified as CMT2A [11], and now listed as CMT2A1 (MIM 118210). *KIF1B* mutations have thus far not been confirmed in studies of CMT2 cases by others [12].

MFN2 encodes a protein, mitofusin-2, of the outer mitochondrial membrane. Hence CMT2A is a mitochondriopathy transmitted not by the mitochondrial, but by the nuclear genome. Mutations of *MFN2* alter the equilibrium between fusion and fission of the mitochondrial net and are thought to affect intra-axonal mitochondrial transport and cellular bioenergetics including the OXPHOS system [13]. They may also be related to a decrease of mitochondrial DNA (mtDNA) replication [14].

Clinical presentation

Rapid progression following onset in early childhood and, less commonly, adult onset with slow progression may be seen [10], [15–17], occasionally with optic

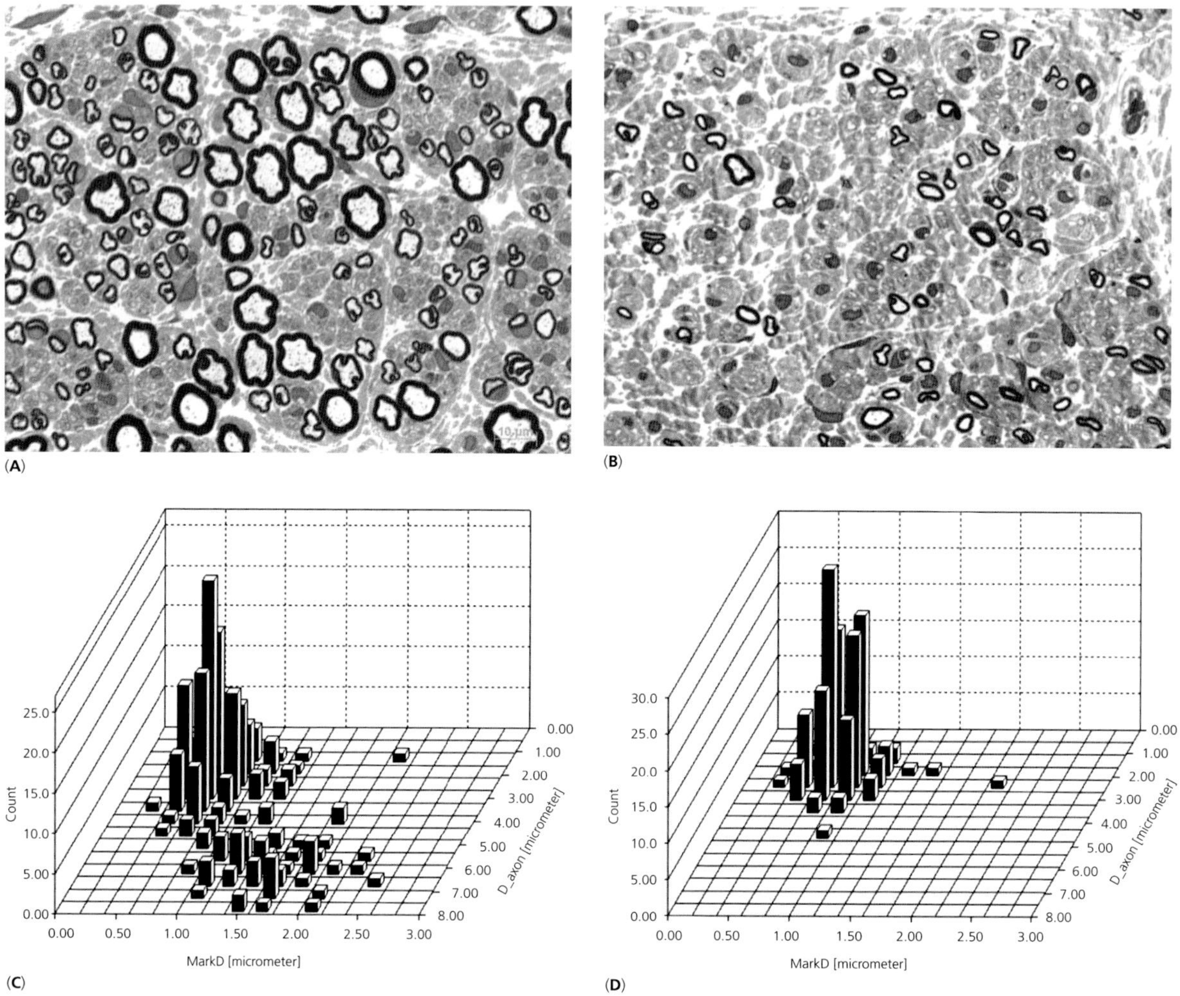

Figure 10.1 Sural nerve in a 7-year-old boy with CMT 2A due to a mutation in the Mitofusin2 (*Mfn2*) gene (**B**) compared to an age-matched control (**A**). The number of large myelinated fibers is severely reduced, which is more apparent in a three-dimensional diagram simultaneously illustrating the number of fibers per endoneurial area, the axonal diameters, and their myelin thickness (**D**), compared to an age-matched control (**C**).

atrophy, pyramidal features, tremor and Parkinsonism [18, 19]. The combination of CMT with optic atrophy was previously classified as HMSN VI [10], and that with pyramidal features as HMSN V [20]. Typically there is distal sensory loss, distal weakness and muscle atrophy, pes cavus, and scoliosis, but nerve conduction velocity (NCV) remains relatively well preserved (electrophysiologically "axonal" type of neuropathy). Asymptomatic mutation carriers have been reported in some families with *MFN2* mutations [21].

Histopathology

The number of myelinated nerve fibers is reduced depending on the onset and duration of the disease (Fig. 10.1B,D). In early childhood, as in other types of axonal neuropathy, the most impressive finding is the coexistence of degenerating and regenerating axons. The regenerating axons may be located in large clusters (Fig. 7.10A; 10.2). *EM* reveals distinct changes of axonal mitochondria including condensations, swellings, and interruptions of the outer mitochondrial membrane, predominantly at the

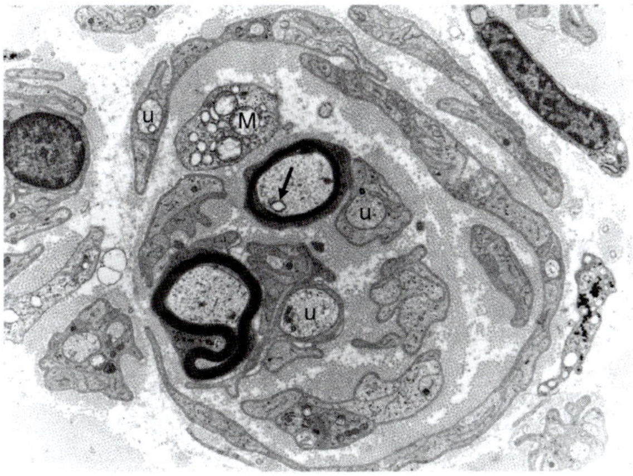

Figure 10.2 Same case as in Figure 10.1. Typical band of Büngner ("pseudo-onion bulb") with two regenerated myelinated and several unmyelinated axons (u) as well as multiple interdigitating, circularly arranged Schwann cell processes. The outer membranes of a mitochondrion appear fused forming an abnormal vacuole (arrow). One of at least five fibroblasts or their processes shows an increased number of large, swollen mitochondria in addition to several small vacuoles (M). The collagen fibrils inside this band of Büngner have similar diameters as those outside indicating early formation. Source: Verhoeven *et al.*, 2006 [15]. Reproduced with permission of Oxford University Press.

site of paranodal axonal protrusions where mitochondria may accumulate [15]. Occasional mitochondria contain homogeneous or filamentous material [22]. The changes were more pronounced in three out of nine cases who had a second biopsy, 7–19 years after the first biopsy; axonal mitochondria were smaller than normal, rounded, and abnormally aggregated [23]. There were no paracrystalline inclusions similar to those seen in muscle fibers in certain mitochondrial myopathies. However, needle-like, crystalline intramitochondrial inclusions (spiculae) were seen in a case of HSMN VI (Hereditary motor and sensory neuropathy type VI, Vizioli; AD with optic atrophy) [24], which would nowadays presumably be classified as CMT2A [10]. In addition swollen, enlarged mitochondria were noted in endoneurial fibroblasts (Fig. 10.2) [15], and atypically branched mitochondrial cristae were observed in Schwann cells [25].

Experimental animals

Transgenic mice expressing a pathogenic *Mfn2* T105M mutation in peripheral motor neurons developed clinical key features of CMT2A in a dose-dependent manner [26]. Yet both Mfn1- and Mfn2-deficient mice died in midgestation [27]. In the canine *Mfn2* gene, homozygous 3-bp deletion was identified as causative of a severe autosomal recessive form of fetal-onset neuroaxonal dystrophy [28].

CMT2B (MIM 600882)

Definition, genetics, and pathogenesis

This AD axonal type neuropathy is caused by mutations in the *RAB7A* gene on chromosome 3q21 [29, 30]. Rab7 belongs to the Ras superfamily of small GTPases and is a master regulator of early to late endocytic membrane transport. In neurons, Rab7 regulates retrograde axonal transport and is important for endosomal trafficking and signaling of neurotrophins [31]. Rab7 mutations lead to dysregulation of TrkA and other growth factor receptor signaling [32, 33]. In addition, altered interaction between disease-causing Rab7A mutants and the neuronal intermediate filament peripherin could be involved in Rab7A-related neuropathies [30].

Clinical presentation

CMT2B is clinically characterized by severe symmetric distal sensory loss, reduced ankle tendon reflexes, weakness in the lower limbs and muscle atrophy, complicated by ulcerations that often lead to amputations [29]. Patients may also present with ulcero-mutilating lesions without motor changes [34].

Histopathology

A sural nerve biopsy showed chronic sensory axonal neuropathy with axonal degeneration and prominent regeneration [34]. Skin biopsy, sudomotor, and cardiovascular tests revealed both pathological and functional evidence of autonomic nervous system involvement [35].

CMT2C (MIM 606071)

Definition, genetics, and pathogenesis

This neuropathy is caused by heterozygous missense mutations in the *t*ransient *r*eceptor *p*otential cation channel, subfamily *V*, member *4* gene (*TRPV4*) on chromosome 12q23-q24 [36–38]. Congenital distal spinal muscular atrophy and scapuloperoneal spinal muscular atrophy (SPSMA) are allelic disorders with overlapping phenotypes [41]. Other mutations in *TRPV4* have been described in separate families with various skeletal dysplasias and short stature [39].

Mutations of *TRPV4* result in a neurotoxic gain-of-function effect from increased Ca2+ influx [36]. The reversibility of neuronal cell death by channel blockade in cell culture may be therapeutically relevant [38].

Clinical presentation

The cardinal features of this neuropathy comprise distal muscle wasting and weakness with additional diaphragmatic and vocal cord paralysis, and mild sensory impairment [40, 41].

Histopathology

Nerve biopsy revealed moderate loss of myelinated fibers and clusters of regenerating axons [40, 42]. Autopsy in SPSMA showed a normal population of motor neurons in the spinal cord suggesting distal motor neuropathy [43].

CMT2D (MIM 601472)

Definition, genetics, and epidemiology

This AD neuropathy is caused by missense mutations in the glycyl tRNA synthetase (*GARS*) gene on 7p15 [44]. It is allelic to distal spinal muscular atrophy type V (dSMA V) and distal hereditary motoneuronopathy type VA (dHMN VA). No mutations in the *GARS* gene were found in 109 Japanese patients with axonal CMT, suggesting that *GARS* mutations are a rare cause of the disorder, at least in this population [45].

Clinical presentation

The clinical picture is different from other axonal CMT2 types in that weakness and atrophy as well as sensory deficits are more severe in the hands than in the feet [46]. Sambuughin *et al.* [47] diagnosed dSMA V based on the presence of hand and peroneal muscle weakness and atrophy without sensory deficits, whereas CMT2D was diagnosed when there were weakness and atrophy in the same muscle groups, hypoactive knee and ankle reflexes, glove and stocking distribution of sensory loss, and reduced sensory nerve action potential amplitudes.

Histopathology

A sural nerve biopsy revealed mild to moderate, selective loss of small and medium-sized myelinated and unmyelinated axons while sensory nerve action potentials were not significantly decreased [48].

Animal models

Mutant mice showed neurodegenerative changes at the neuromuscular junction, with more severe changes in distal muscles [49]. Nerve conduction velocities were severely decreased and peripheral nerves showed reduced axonal diameters and loss of large-diameter axons, but no evidence of demyelination.

CMT2E (MIM 607684)

Definition, genetics, epidemiology, and pathogenesis

CMT2E is a predominantly axonal type of neuropathy caused by mutations in the neurofilament light (*NEFL* or *NF-L*) gene on 8q21 [50–53]. It is allelic to the demyelinating variant CMT1F. In CMT2E significant demyelinating changes may occur resulting in an intermediate type of neuropathy [54] although the underlying mutations occur in a gene that codes for a cytoskeletal protein expressed in neurons.

Epidemiology: In a cohort of 323 CMT patients, 7 (2%) had identified *NF-L* mutations [55]. In 36 Taiwanese families of Han Chinese descent with CMT2, *NEFL* mutations were identified in six (16.7%) [5].

Pathogenesis: It is suggested that disruption of the neurofilament network with aggregation of *NEFL* is a common triggering event of neuronal degeneration in CMT2E and CMT1F [56].

Histopathology

The changes usually correspond to an axonal type of neuropathy [55]. Like in most hereditary neuropathies, acutely degenerating fibers are rarely observed in neuropathies due to *NEFL* mutations. In two patients with an intermediate type of disease (Fig. 10.3A, B) [54], the number of large myelinated fibers was more severely reduced than that of small myelinated ones resulting in loss of the bimodal fiber spectrum. Morphometry revealed the percentage of endoneurial myelin area was reduced from a normal range of 20–30% in controls to 12–16%. A considerable proportion of thickly myelinated fibers showed decreased axonal diameters. Other fibers showed external or internal myelin loops. Clusters of regenerated fibers and small onion bulb formations were equally frequent in both patients. Tomacula or focally folded myelin sheaths were absent.

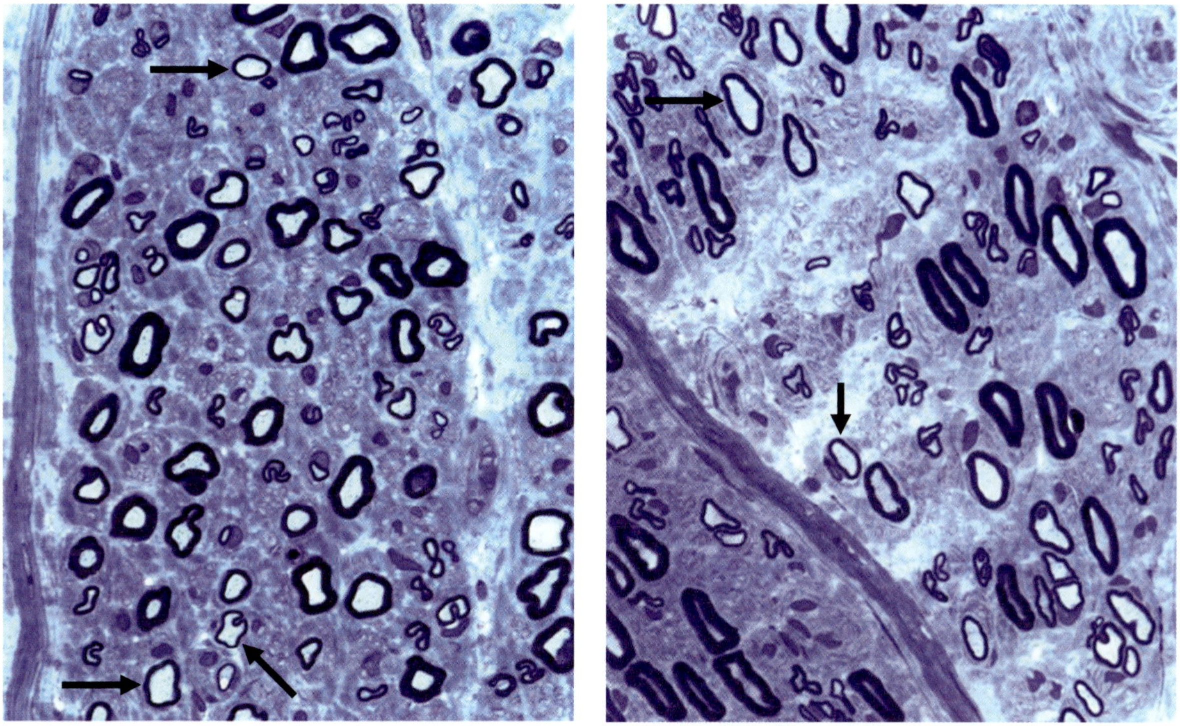

(A) (B)

Figure 10.3 Sural nerve of a mother (**A**) with a point mutation of the neurofilament light gene (*NEFL*) at the age of 53 years and her daughter (**B**) at the age of 25 years. In the selected area, loss of nerve fibers and endoneurial edema appears more pronounced in the daughter's nerve. (Flattened fibers in **B** indicate artificial compression.) Clusters of regenerated fibers are repeatedly seen as are thinly remyelinated fibers with incipient onion bulb formation (arrows).

EM revealed bands of Büngner derived from myelinated and unmyelinated fibers in addition to clusters of regenerated fibers and onion bulb formations of moderate size [57]. Collagen pockets in Schwann cells indicated loss of unmyelinated fibers. Fibers undergoing acute Wallerian degeneration were rare. Occasional π-granules showed unusually fine granular components. The paranodes were distorted. Glycogen granules were apparent in the axoplasm at nodes and paranodes.

Both myelinated and unmyelinated axons in neuropathy due to *NEFL* mutation include a variety of focally accumulated organelles such as mitochondria, small vesicular structures, neurosecretory vesicles, neurofilaments, microtubules, amorphous substances, and autophagic material. The density of neurofilaments within axons can vary considerably: some axons may be condensed and show much closer arrangements of neurofilaments than normal; other axons are swollen. Occasional giant axons show an accumulation of disorganized neurofilaments [58]. Degenerating endoneurial fibroblasts (or macrophages) are found repeatedly [54].

CMT2F (MIM 606595)

This usually autosomal dominant, sometimes recessive axonal neuropathy is allelic to distal hereditary motor neuronopathy type IIB (dHMN2B) caused by mutations in the alpha-crystalline domain of the heat shock 27-kDa protein1 (*HSPB1*) gene on chromosome 7q11–12 [59, 60].

In the AD and AR families, there were no clinically apparent sensory findings. Nevertheless, reduced sural nerve action potential amplitudes were found in some affected individuals, indicating that long sensory axons were mildly affected in this predominantly motor disorder.

CMT2G (MIM 608591)

This AD neuropathy is caused by mutations in an unknown gene on chromosome 12q12–13 [61]. Nerve biopsy showed some loss of myelinated fibers with regenerating ones and atrophic axons.

CMT2H (MIM 607731)

This is an AR neuropathy with pyramidal features linked to chromosomal locus 8q21.3 [62], the same region where the *GDAP1* gene is located, and therefore possibly allelic to CMT4A.

CMT2I (MIM 607677)

Definition and genetics

Mutations in the (*P0*) gene more frequently cause demyelinating than axonal forms of neuropathy (cf. CMT1B, DSS); yet allelic, predominantly axonal forms (CMT2I), or intermediate forms (ID-CMT) may occur [63–67].

Histopathology

In *semithin sections*, large myelinated nerve fibers are reduced in number and multiple clusters of regenerated axonal sprouts occur [65]. Typical, large onion bulb formations are absent. Infrequently, myelin sheaths are disproportionately thin while other fibers have disproportionately thick myelin sheaths. In a patient who was biopsied twice, at ages 47 and 51, the neuropathy progressed and large myelinated fibers were depleted (Fig. 10.4B,D) [65].

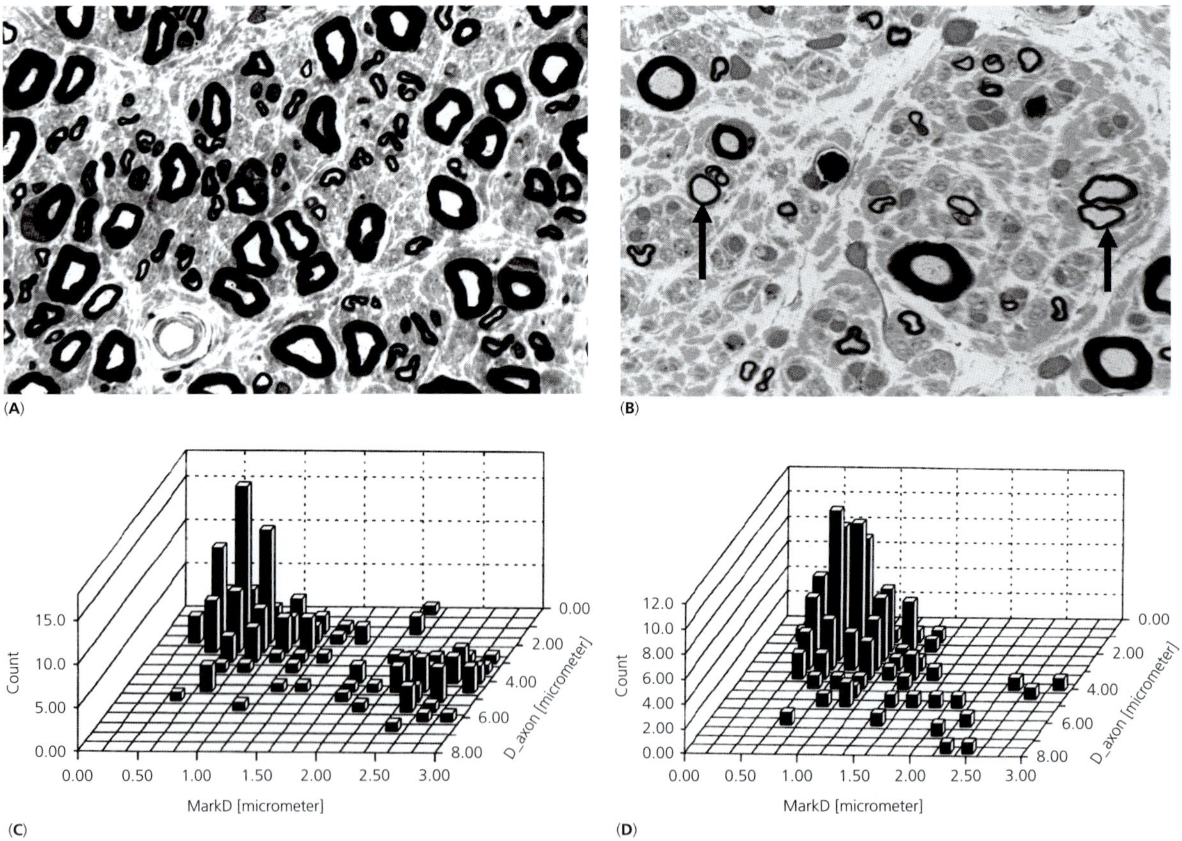

Figure 10.4 Severe loss of myelinated nerve fibers in a 65-year-old woman with an Ala237Thr mutation in the coding region of exon 6 in *P0* (*MPZ*) resulting in a neuronal/axonal type of neuropathy (**B, D**) compared to an age-matched control (**A, C**). Minor clusters of regenerated fibers are indicated by arrows.

EM reveals degenerating axons, bands of Büngner with and without myelin degradation products, and many groups of regenerated or regenerating axons. These clusters may be surrounded by Schwann cell processes forming onion bulb-like structures ("pseudo-onion bulbs"). Incipient onion bulbs with single layers of Schwann cells can be present. Some myelin sheaths form abnormally thin paranodal loops extending into the abaxonal cytoplasm [65]. Paranodal and segmental demyelination is absent. Analysis of myelin periodicity may not reveal pathological changes similar to those seen in the demyelinating forms of neuropathy due to P0 mutation [68] (cf. CMT1B or CMT4E).

CMT2J (MIM 607736)

Definition, genetics, and clinical characteristics

This axonal type of neuropathy is also caused by heterozygous mutation in the myelin protein-zero (*MPZ; P0*) gene on chromosome 1q23 (MIM 118200). It is therefore allelic to CMT1B, CMT2I, and Déjérine–Sottas syndrome (DSS) (see Chapter 9). Clinically, pupillary abnormalities and hearing loss are distinguishing features [1].

Histopathology

There is considerable loss of myelinated fibers. In one biopsy, thinly myelinated fibers with or without onion bulbs of flat Schwann cells were present with or without unmyelinated axons [1]. Multiple clusters of thinly myelinated fibers indicated axonal involvement with axonal regeneration. *EM* revealed normal myelin packing and periodicity whereas occasional myelin sheaths were abnormally thick because of redundant loop formation. Another patient [69] showed profound loss of large myelinated fibers, multiple clusters of regenerated axonal sprouts, and no onion bulb formations.

CMT2K (MIM 607831)

Definition, genetics, and pathogenesis

CMT2K designates severe AR as well as rare and mild AD axonal neuropathies [70–72] caused by mutations of the *GDAP1* (*g*anglioside-induced *d*ifferentiation-*a*ssociated *p*rotein *1*) gene. CMT2K is allelic with severe AR demyelinating CMT4A (Chapter 11). An intermediate form (CMTID), either more axonal or more demyelinating in type, may also occur [73, 74]. GDAP1 is expressed in neurons and is associated with mitochondria indicating that CMT2K and CMT4A belong to the category of mitochondrial disorders due to mutations of a nuclear gene [75, 76].

Histopathology

A sural nerve biopsy in a case with an AD *GDAP1* mutation revealed depletion of myelinated fibers, regenerative clusters, and features of mitochondrial degeneration with mitochondrial aggregates [77]. One boy with AR mutation biopsied at the age of 3.5 years showed a similarly marked loss of large myelinated fibers and numerous clusters of small, closely adjacent regenerated fibers [74]. Occasional demyelinated fibers and some isolated, thinly remyelinated fibers with surrounding flat cell processes were also apparent. Another recessive case studied at the age of 2 years showed more isolated, thinly remyelinated fibers with incipient onion bulb formation. Clusters of regenerated fibers were less frequent.

EM revealed numerous degenerating axons, bands of Büngner and groups of regenerated myelinated fibers combined with not-yet remyelinated ones. Some of these clusters were surrounded by supernumerary Schwann cell processes forming onion bulb-like structures [74]. Demyelinated axons and incipient onion bulb formations with up to three Schwann cell layers were encountered in both cases. Few fibers displayed non-compacted innermost myelin lamellae with adaxonal vacuoles. Analysis of myelin periodicity did not reveal further changes. Unmyelinated fibers appeared better preserved than myelinated ones, yet their diameter varied considerably. Specific mitochondrial or other changes were not detected. A peroneal nerve biopsy supported an axonal type neuropathy showing a marked reduction of myelinated fibers and signs of axonal regeneration, including frequent pseudo-onion bulb formations [73]. A skin biopsy, sudomotor, and cardiovascular tests revealed involvement of the autonomic nervous system [35].

CMT2L (MIM 608673)

Definition and clinical characteristics

This AD axonal neuropathy is allelic to distal hereditary motor neuronopathy IIA (dHMN2A) with an overlapping phenotype. In the AD and AR families, there were no clinical sensory findings, but reduced sural nerve action potential amplitudes were found in some affected individuals, indicating that long sensory axons are mildly affected.

Genetics and pathogenesis

CMT2L is caused by mutations in the heat shock 22 kDa protein 8 (*HSPB8*) gene on chromosome 12q24.23 [78–80] (MIM 608014).

Mutations affect a highly conserved residue in the central alpha-crystallin domain of the protein. *In vitro* aggregate formation around nuclei was seen, which may be due to HSPB8 conformational changes leading to self-aggregation and its abnormal interaction with other HSPs, such as HSPB1 (HSP27) [81].

Histopathology

Sural nerve biopsy in a case with linkage to a locus on chromosome 12q24, that is, possible CMT2L, revealed severe loss of large myelinated fibers and clusters with mostly thinly myelinated axons [82].

CMT2M (MIM 602378)

Mutations in the gene encoding dynamin-2 (*DNM2*) may cause dominant intermediate Charcot–Marie–Tooth (CMT) disease and axonal CMT that map to chromosome 19p. It will be discussed in Chapter 10 on CMTDIB.

CMT2N (MIM 613287)

This form of axonal Charcot–Marie–Tooth disease type 2, designated CMT2N, is caused by heterozygous mutation in the alanyl-tRNA-synthetase (*AARS*) gene on chromosome 16q21 [83, 84].

Nerve conduction velocities are within the intermediate range, and audiology shows mild to moderate high frequency sensorineural loss.

Nerve biopsy findings have thus far not been described.

CMT2O (MIM 600112)

Definition and genetics

Autosomal dominant axonal Charcot–Marie–Tooth disease type 2O (CMT2O) is caused by heterozygous mutation in the *DYNC1H1* gene on chromosome 14q32 [85]. In mouse models, mutations in dynein causing motor neuron degeneration appeared to be linked to defects in retrograde transport [86].

Histopathology

To date, nerve biopsies have not been reported.

CMT2P (MIM 610933)

Definition and genetics

This axonal Charcot–Marie–Tooth disease type 2P (CMT2P) can be caused by homozygous or heterozygous mutation in the *LRSAM1* gene on chromosome 9q33 [87].

Histopathology

To date, nerve biopsies have not been reported.

HMSN P (MIM 614436)

Definition and genetics

This AD, axonal motor and sensory neuropathy with proximal predominance (HMSN-P) is an adult-onset disorder, which thus far has only been reported on the Okinawa Islands, Japan. Exome sequencing of the chromosomal region 3q13.1 showed a mutation in the TRK-fused gene (*TFG*) in the families studied [88].

Histopathology

Pathological studies of an autopsied patient revealed fragmentation of the Golgi apparatus, TFG-, TAR DNA-binding protein 43 kDa (TDP-43)-positive, and ubiquitin-immunopositive cytoplasmic inclusions in the spinal and cortical motor neurons. Pathological overlap of proteinopathies involving TFG and TDP-43 obviously highlight a new pathway leading to motor neuron degeneration. Histological findings in DRG and sensory or motor nerves have thus far not been reported.

CMT2Q (MIM 615025)

Definition and genetics

Charcot–Marie–Tooth disease type 2Q(CMT2Q) is caused by a heterozygous loss-of-fu nction mutation in the *DHTKD1* gene on chromosome 10p14. Compound heterozygous mutation in this gene results in 2-aminoadipic 2-oxoadipic aciduria [89].

Histopathology

To date, nerve biopsies have not been reported.

Dominant intermediate neuropathy (CMTDIE) associated with focal segmental glomerulosclerosis (MIM 614455)

This dominant intermediate neuropathy is associated with focal segmental glomerulosclerosis (FSGS-CMT) both of which are caused by mutations of the *INF2* gene [90]. Immunohistochemical studies revealed strong INF2 expression in the cytoplasm of Schwann cells and podocytes. It is discussed together with other dominant intermediate neuropathies of the CMT type (CMTDIA-E) in a separate chapter (see previously).

References

1 De Jonghe P, Timmerman V, Ceuterick C, *et al.* (1999) The Thr124Met mutation in the peripheral myelin protein zero (MPZ) gene is associated with a clinically distinct Charcot–Marie–Tooth phenotype. *Brain*;122:281–290.

2 Harding AE, Thomas PK (1980) Genetic aspects of hereditary motor and sensory neuropathy (types I and II). *J Med Genet*;17:329–336.

3 Ouvrier RA, McLeod JG, Morgan GJ, *et al.* (1981) Hereditary motor and sensory neuropathy of neuronal type with onset in early childhood. *J Neurol Sci*;51:181–197.

4 Braathen GJ (2012) Genetic epidemiology of Charcot–Marie–Tooth disease. *Acta Neurol Scand* Suppl;193:iv–22.

5 Lin KP, Soong BW, Yang CC, *et al.* (2011) The mutational spectrum in a cohort of Charcot–Marie–Tooth disease type 2 among the Han Chinese in Taiwan. *PLoS One*;6:e29393.

6 Vasli N, Laporte J (2013) Impacts of massively parallel sequencing for genetic diagnosis of neuromuscular disorders. *Acta Neuropathol*;125:173–185.

7 Berciano J, Combarros O, Figols J, *et al.* (1986) Hereditary motor and sensory neuropathy type II. Clinicopathological study of a family. *Brain*;109:897–914.

8 Züchner S, Mersiyanova IV, Muglia M, *et al.* (2004) Mutations in the mitochondrial GTPase mitofusin 2 cause Charcot–Marie–Tooth neuropathy type 2A. *Nat Genet*;36:449–451.

9 Baets J, Deconinck T, De Vriendt E, *et al.* (2011)Genetic spectrum of hereditary neuropathies with onset in the first year of life. *Brain*;134:2664–2676.

10 Yiu EM, Ryan MM (2012) Genetic axonal neuropathies and neuronopathies of pre-natal and infantile onset. *J Peripher Nerv Syst*;17:285–300.

11 Zhao C, Takita J, Tanaka Y, *et al.* (2001) Charcot–Marie–Tooth disease type 2A caused by mutation in a microtubule motor KIF1Bbeta. *Cell*;105:587–597.

12 Bissar-Tadmouri N, Nelis E, Züchner S, *et al.* (2004) Absence of KIF1B mutation in a large Turkish CMT2A family suggests involvement of a second gene. *Neurology*;62:1522–1525.

13 Cartoni R, Martinou JC (2009) Role of mitofusin 2 mutations in the physiopathology of Charcot–Marie–Tooth disease type 2A. *Exp Neurol*;218:268–273.

14 Vielhaber S, Debska-Vielhaber G, Peeva V, *et al.* (2013) Mitofusin 2 mutations affect mitochondrial function by mitochondrial DNA depletion. *Acta Neuropathol*;125:245–256.

15 Verhoeven K, Claeys KG, Züchner S, *et al.* (2006) MFN2 mutation distribution and genotype/phenotype correlation in Charcot–Marie–Tooth type 2. *Brain*;129:2093–2102.

16 Chung KW, Kim SB, Park KD, *et al.*(2006) Early onset severe and late-onset mild Charcot–Marie–Tooth disease with mitofusin 2 (MFN2) mutations. *Brain*;129:2103–2118.

17 Ouvrier R, Grew S (2010) Mechanisms of disease and clinical features of mutations of the gene for mitofusin 2: an important cause of hereditary peripheral neuropathy with striking clinical variability in children and adults. *Dev Med Child Neurol*;52:328–330.

18 Banchs I, Casasnovas C, Montero J, *et al.* (2008) Two Spanish families with Charcot–Marie–Tooth type 2A: clinical, electrophysiological and molecular findings. *Neuromuscul Disord*;18:974–978.

19 Feely SM, Laura M, Siskind CE, *et al.* (2011) MFN2 mutations cause severe phenotypes in most patients with CMT2A. *Neurology*;76:1690–1696.

20 Zhu D, Kennerson ML, Walizada G, *et al.* (2005) Charcot–Marie–Tooth with pyramidal signs is genetically heterogeneous: families with and without MFN2 mutations. *Neurology*;65:496–497.

21 Lawson VH, Graham BV, Flanigan KM (2005) Clinical and electrophysiologic features of CMT2A with mutations in the mitofusin 2 gene. *Neurology*;65:197–204.

22 Lv H, Wang L, Li W, *et al.* (2013) Mitofusin 2 gene mutation causing early-onset CMT2A with different progressive courses. *Clin Neuropathol*;32:16–23.

23 Vallat JM, Ouvrier RA, Pollard JD, *et al.* (2008) Histopathological findings in hereditary motor and sensory neuropathy of axonal type with onset in early childhood associated with mitofusin 2 mutations. *J Neuropathol Exp Neurol*;67:1097–1102.

24 Sommer C, Schröder JM (1989) Hereditary motor and sensory neuropathy with optic atrophy. Ultrastructural and morphometric observations on nerve fibers, mitochondria, and dense-cored vesicles. *Arch Neurol*;46:973–977.

25 Sole G, Ferrer X, Vital C, *et al.* (2009) Ultrastructural mitochondrial modifications characteristic of mitofusin 2 mutations (CMT2A). *J Peripher Nerv Syst*;14:206–207.

26 Detmer SA, Vande Velde C, Cleveland DW, Chan DC (2008) Hindlimb gait defects due to motor axon loss and reduced distal muscles in a transgenic mouse model of Charcot–Marie–Tooth type 2A. *Hum Mol Genet*;17:367–375.

27 Chen H, Detmer SA, Ewald AJ, *et al.* (2003) Mitofusins Mfn1 and Mfn2 coordinately regulate mitochondrial fusion and are essential for embryonic development. *J Cell Biol*;160: 189–200.

28 Fyfe JC, Al-Tamimi RA, Liu J, *et al.* (2011) A novel mitofusin 2 mutation causes canine fetal-onset neuroaxonal dystrophy. *Neurogenetics*;12:223–232.

29 Verhoeven K, De Jonghe P, Coen K, *et al.* (2003) Mutations in the small GTP-ase late endosomal protein RAB7 cause Charcot–Marie–Tooth type 2B neuropathy. *Am J Hum Genet*; 72:722–727.30.

30 Cogli L, Progida C, Thomas CL, *et al.* (2013) Charcot–Marie–Tooth type 2B disease-causing RAB7A mutant proteins show altered interaction with the neuronal intermediate filament peripherin. *Acta Neuropathol*;125:257–272.

31 Bucci C, De Luca M (2012) Molecular basis of Charcot–Marie–Tooth type 2B disease. *Biochem Soc Trans*;40:1368–1372.

32 Basuray S, Mukherjee S, Seaman MN, Wandinger-Ness A (2012) Rab7 mutants associated with Charcot–Marie–Tooth disease cause delayed growth factor receptor transport and altered endosomal and nuclear signaling. *J Biol Chem*;288: 1135–1149.

33 Zhang K, Fishel Ben Kenan R, Osakada Y, *et al.*(2013) Defective axonal transport of Rab7 GTPase results in dysregulated trophic signaling. *J Neurosci*;33:7451–7462.

34 Houlden H, King RH, Muddle JR, *et al.* (2004) A novel RAB7 mutation associated with ulcero-mutilating neuropathy. *Ann Neurol*;56:586–90.

35 Manganelli F, Pisciotta C, Provitera V, *et al.* (2012) Autonomic nervous system involvement in a new CMT2B family. *J Peripher Nerv Syst*;17:361–364.

36 Landoure G, Zdebik AA, Martinez TL, *et al.*(2010) Mutations in TRPV4 cause Charcot–Marie–Tooth disease type 2C. *Nat Genet*;42:170–174.

37 Klein CJ, Cunningham JM, Atkinson EJ, *et al.* (2003) The gene for HMSN2C maps to 12q23–24: a region of neuromuscular disorders. *Neurology*;60:1151–1156.

38 Klein CJ, Shi Y, Fecto F, *et al.*(2011) TRPV4 mutations and cytotoxic hypercalcemia in axonal Charcot–Marie–Tooth neuropathies. *Neurology*;76:887–894.

39 Chen DH, Sul Y, Weiss M, *et al.* (2010) CMT2C with vocal cord paresis associated with short stature and mutations in the TRPV4 gene. *Neurology*;75:1968–1975.

40 Dyck PJ, Litchy WJ, Minnerath S, *et al.* (1994) Hereditary motor and sensory neuropathy with diaphragm and vocal cord paresis. *Ann Neurol*;35:608–615.

41 McEntagart ME, Reid SL, Irrthum A, *et al.* (2005) Confirmation of a hereditary motor and sensory neuropathy IIC locus at chromosome 12q23-q24. *Ann Neurol*;57:293–297.

42 Santoro L, Manganelli F, Di Maio L, *et al.* (2002) Charcot–Marie–Tooth disease type 2C: a distinct genetic entity. Clinical and molecular characterization of the first European family. *Neuromuscul Disord*;12:399–404.

43 Deng HX, Klein CJ, Yan J, *et al.* (2010) Scapuloperoneal spinal muscular atrophy and CMT2C are allelic disorders caused by alterations in TRPV4. *Nat Genet*;42:165–169.

44 Antonellis A, Ellsworth RE, Sambuughin N, *et al.* (2003) Glycyl tRNA synthetase mutations in Charcot–Marie–Tooth disease type 2D and distal spinal muscular atrophy type V. *Am J Hum Genet*;72:1293–1299.

45 Abe A, Hayasaka K (2009) The GARS gene is rarely mutated in Japanese patients with Charcot–Marie–Tooth neuropathy. *J Hum Genet*;54:310–312.

46 Ionasescu V, Searby C, Sheffield VC, *et al.* (1996) Autosomal dominant Charcot–Marie–Tooth axonal neuropathy mapped on chromosome 7p (CMT2D). *Hum Mol Genet*;5:1373–1375.

47 Sambuughin N, Sivakumar K, Selenge B, *et al.* (1998) Autosomal dominant distal spinal muscular atrophy type V (dSMA-V) and Charcot–Marie–Tooth disease type 2D (CMT2D) segregate within a single large kindred and map to a refined region on chromosome 7p15. *J Neurol Sci*;161:23–28.

48 Sivakumar K, Kyriakides T, Puls I, *et al.* (2005) Phenotypic spectrum of disorders associated with glycyl-tRNA synthetase mutations. *Brain*;128:2304–2314.

49 Seburn KL, Nangle LA, Cox GA, *et al.* (2006) An active dominant mutation of glycyl-tRNA synthetase causes neuropathy in a Charcot–Marie–Tooth 2D mouse model. *Neuron*; 51:715–726.

50 Mersiyanova IV, Perepelov AV, Polyakov AV, *et al.* (2000) A new variant of Charcot–Marie–Tooth disease type 2 is probably the result of a mutation in the neurofilament-light gene [see comments]. *Am J Hum Genet*;67:37–46.

51 De Jonghe P, Mersivanova I, Nelis E, *et al.* (2001) Further evidence that neurofilament light chain gene mutations can cause Charcot–Marie–Tooth disease type 2E. *Ann Neurol*;49:245–249.

52 Georgiou DM, Zidar J, Korosec M, *et al.* (2002) A novel NF-L mutation Pro22Ser is associated with CMT2 in a large Slovenian family. *Neurogenetics*;4:93–96.

53 Yoshihara T, Yamamoto M, Hattori N, *et al.* (2002) Identification of novel sequence variants in the neurofilament-light gene in a Japanese population: analysis of Charcot–Marie–Tooth disease patients and normal individuals. *J Peripher Nerv Syst*;7:221–224.

54 Züchner S, Vorgerd M, Sindern E, Schröder JM (2004) The novel neurofilament light (NEFL) mutation Glu397Lys is associated with a clinically and morphologically heterogeneous type of Charcot–Marie–Tooth neuropathy. *Neuromuscul Disord*;14:147–57.

55 Jordanova A, De Jonghe P, Boerkoel CF, *et al.* (2003) Mutations in the neurofilament light chain gene (NEFL) cause early onset severe Charcot–Marie–Tooth disease. *Brain*;126:590–597.

56 Zhai J, Lin H, Julien JP, Schlaepfer WW (2007) Disruption of neurofilament network with aggregation of light neurofilament protein: a common pathway leading to motor neuron

degeneration due to Charcot–Marie–Tooth disease-linked mutations in NFL and HSPB1. *Hum Mol Genet*;16:3103–116.

57 Malandrini A, Ceuterick C, Villanov M, *et al.* (2001) Ultrastructural findings in the peripheral nerve in a family with the intermediate form of Charcot–Marie–Tooth disease. *J Submicrosc Cytol Pathol*;33:59–63.

58 Fabrizi GM, Cavallaro T, Angiari C, *et al.*(2004) Giant axon and neurofilament accumulation in Charcot–Marie–Tooth disease type 2E. *Neurology*;62:1429–1431.

59 Evgrafov OV, Mersiyanova I, Irobi J, *et al.* (2004) Mutant small heat-shock protein 27 causes axonal Charcot–Marie–Tooth disease and distal hereditary motor neuropathy. *Nat Genet*;36:602–606.

60 Houlden H, Laura M, Wavrant-De Vrieze F, *et al.* (2008) Mutations in the HSP27 (HSPB1) gene cause dominant, recessive, and sporadic distal HMN/CMT type 2. *Neurology*; 71:1660–1668.

61 Nelis E, Berciano J, Verpoorten N, *et al.* (2004) Autosomal dominant axonal Charcot–Marie–Tooth disease type 2 (CMT2G) maps to chromosome 12q12-q13.3. *J Med Genet*; 41:193–197.

62 Barhoumi C, Amouri R, Ben Hamida C, *et al.* (2001) Linkage of a new locus for autosomal recessive axonal form of Charcot–Marie–Tooth disease to chromosome 8q21.3. *Neuromuscul Disord*;11:27–34.

63 Marrosu MG, Vaccargiu S, Marrosu G, *et al.* (1998) Charcot–Marie–Tooth disease type 2 associated with mutation of the myelin protein zero gene. *Neurology*;50:1397–401.

64 Schiavon F, Rampazzo A, Merlini L, *et al.* (1998) Mutations of the same sequence of the myelin P0 gene causing two different phenotypes. *Hum Mutat*;Suppl 1:S217–219.

65 Senderek J, Hermanns B, Lehmann U, *et al.* (2000)Charcot–Marie–Tooth neuropathy type 2 and P0 point mutations: two novel amino acid substitutions (Asp61Gly; Tyr119Cys) and a possible "hotspot" on Thr124Met. *Brain Pathol*;10:235–248.

66 Misu K, Yoshihara T, Shikama Y, *et al.*(2000) An axonal form of Charcot–Marie–Tooth disease showing distinctive features in association with mutations in the peripheral myelin protein zero gene (Thr124Met or Asp75Val). *J Neurol Neurosurg Psychiatry*;69:806–811.

67 Boerkoel CF, Takashima H, Garcia CA, *et al.* (2002) Charcot–Marie–Tooth disease and related neuropathies: mutation distribution and genotype-phenotype correlation. *Ann Neurol*;51:190–201.

68 Gabreels-Festen AA, Hoogendijk JE, Meijerink PH, *et al.* (1996) Two divergent types of nerve pathology in patients with different P0 mutations in Charcot–Marie–Tooth disease. *Neurology*;47:761–765.

69 Seeman P, Mazanec R, Huehne K, *et al.* (2004) Hearing loss as the first feature of late-onset axonal CMT disease due to a novel P0 mutation. *Neurology*;63:733–735.

70 Claramunt R, Pedrola L, Sevilla T, *et al.* (2005) Genetics of Charcot–Marie–Tooth disease type 4A: mutations, inheritance, phenotypic variability, and founder effect. *J Med Genet*;42:358–365.

71 Crimella C, Tonelli A, Airoldi G, *et al.* (2010) The GST domain of GDAP1 is a frequent target of mutations in the dominant form of axonal Charcot–Marie–Tooth type 2K. *J Med Genet*;47:712–716.

72 Zimon M, Baets J, Fabrizi GM, *et al.* (2011) Dominant GDAP1 mutations cause predominantly mild CMT phenotypes. *Neurology*;77:540–548.

73 Birouk N, Azzedine H, Dubourg O, *et al.* (2003) Phenotypical features of a Moroccan family with autosomal recessive Charcot–Marie–Tooth disease associated with the S194X mutation in the GDAP1 gene. *Arch Neurol*;60:598–604.

74 Senderek J, Bergmann C, Ramaekers VT, *et al.* (2003) Mutations in the ganglioside-induced differentiation-associated protein- 1 (GDAP1) gene in intermediate type autosomal recessive Charcot–Marie–Tooth neuropathy. *Brain*;126:642–649.

75 Niemann A, Ruegg M, La Padula V, *et al.* (2005) Ganglioside-induced differentiation associated protein 1 is a regulator of the mitochondrial network: new implications for Charcot–Marie–Tooth disease. *J Cell Biol*;170:1067–1078.

76 Pedrola L, Espert A, Wu X, *et al.* (2005) GDAP1, the protein causing Charcot–Marie–Tooth disease type 4A, is expressed in neurons and is associated with mitochondria. *Hum Mol Genet*;14:1087–1094.

77 Sivera R, Espinos C, Vilchez JJ, *et al.* (2010) Phenotypical features of the p.R120W mutation in the GDAP1 gene causing autosomal dominant Charcot–Marie–Tooth disease. *J Peripher Nerv Syst*;15:334–344.

78 Timmerman V, Raeymaekers P, Nelis E, *et al.* (1992) Linkage analysis of distal hereditary motor neuropathy type II (distal HMN II) in a single pedigree. *J Neurol Sci*;109:41–48.

79 Tang BS, Luo W, Xia K, *et al.* (2004) A new locus for autosomal dominant Charcot–Marie–Tooth disease type 2 (CMT2L) maps to chromosome 12q24. *Hum Genet*;114:527–533.

80 Tang BS, Zhao GH, Luo W, *et al.* (2005) Small heat-shock protein 22 mutated in autosomal dominant Charcot–Marie–Tooth disease type 2L. *Hum Genet*;116:222–224.

81 Zhang RX, Tang BS, Zi XH, *et al.* (2006) [Study on aggregate formation mechanism of HSPB8 gene mutation resulting in CMT2L]. *Zhonghua Yi Xue Yi Chuan Xue Za Zhi*;23:601–604.

82 Luo W, Tang YL, Tang BS, *et al.*(2005) [Clinical, pathological and genetic studies in a Chinese Charcot–Marie–Tooth disease type 2 family]. *Zhejiang Da Xue Xue Bao Yi Xue Ban*;34:529–533.

83 Latour P, Thauvin-Robinet C, Baudelet-Mery C, *et al.* (2010) A major determinant for binding and aminoacylation of tRNA(Ala) in cytoplasmic Alanyl-tRNA synthetase is mutated in dominant axonal Charcot–Marie–Tooth disease. *Am J Hum Genet*;86:77–82.

84 McLaughlin HM, Sakaguchi R, Giblin W, *et al.* (2012) A recurrent loss-of-function alanyl-tRNA synthetase (AARS) mutation in patients with Charcot–Marie–Tooth disease type 2N (CMT2N). *Hum Mutat*;33:244–253.

85 Weedon MN, Hastings R, Caswell R, *et al.* (2011) Exome sequencing identifies a DYNC1H1 mutation in a large pedigree with dominant axonal Charcot–Marie–Tooth disease. *Am J Hum Genet*;89:308–312.

86 Hafezparast M, Klocke R, Ruhrberg C, *et al.* (2003) Mutations in dynein link motor neuron degeneration to defects in retrograde transport. *Science*;300:808–812.
87 Weterman MA, Sorrentino V, Kasher PR, *et al.* (2012) A frameshift mutation in LRSAM1 is responsible for a dominant hereditary polyneuropathy. *Hum Mol Genet*;21:358–370.
88 Ishiura H, Sako W, Yoshida M, *et al.* (2012) The TRK-fused gene is mutated in hereditary motor and sensory neuropathy with proximal dominant involvement. *Am J Hum Genet*;91:320–329.
89 Xu WY, Gu MM, Sun LH, *et al.* (2012) A nonsense mutation in DHTKD1 causes Charcot–Marie–Tooth disease type 2 in a large Chinese pedigree. *Am J Hum Genet*;91:1088–1094.
90 Boyer O, Nevo F, Plaisier E, *et al.* (2011) INF2 mutations in Charcot–Marie–Tooth disease with glomerulopathy. *N Engl J Med*;365:2377–2388.

CHAPTER 11

Autosomal recessive demyelinating or axonal Charcot–Marie–Tooth neuropathy*

Kristl G. Claeys,[1,2] Martin Lammens,[3] Jan Senderek,[4] and Joachim Weis[1]

[1] *Institute of Neuropathology, RWTH Aachen University Hospital and JARA Brain Translational Medicine, Aachen, Germany*

[2] *Department of Neurology, RWTH Aachen University Hospital and JARA Brain Translational Medicine, Aachen, Germany*

[3] *Department of Pathology, Antwerp University Hospital Edegem, and University of Antwerp, Antwerp, Belgium*

[4] *Friedrich Baur Institute, Department of Neurology, Ludwig Maximilians University, Munich, Germany*

Introduction

Charcot–Marie–Tooth disease (CMT) or hereditary motor and sensory neuropathy (HMSN) comprises a group of clinically and genetically heterogeneous hereditary neuropathies. CMT is the most common inherited neuromuscular disorder, with a prevalence of 17–40 per 100,000 individuals [1]. To date, more than 50 causative genes are known but in a considerable number of hereditary neuropathies the genetic defect remains to be identified. Next generation sequencing ("massively parallel sequencing") is now widely used to uncover most of the suspected remaining (approximately 50%) so far unidentified mutations in hereditary neuromuscular disorders [2].

The clinical features of HMSN include progressive distal muscle weakness and atrophy starting in the lower limbs and later affecting the upper limbs, steppage gait, foot deformities, distal sensory loss, and decreased or absent deep tendon reflexes [3]. Hereditary neuropathies are classified as motor and sensory neuropathies (HMSN) if muscle weakness is predominant with mild sensory deficits, as distal hereditary motor neuropathy (HMN) if the motor deficit is predominant, and as hereditary sensory and autonomic neuropathy (HSAN) if sensory deficits and/or autonomic dysfunction predominate.

According to electrophysiological criteria, HMSN is classified into two main subgroups: demyelinating type (HMSN I or CMT1, and CMT4), which is a primarily demyelinating neuropathy with severely reduced motor nerve conduction velocities (MNCV in upper limbs <38 m/s), and axonal type (HMSN II or CMT2) with primarily axonal loss characterized by normal or slightly reduced MNCV (MNCV in upper limbs >38 m/s) but decreased amplitudes [4]. Furthermore, a genetically heterogeneous, autosomal dominant, intermediate HMSN (CMT DI) subgroup with median MNCV between 25 and 45 m/s has been identified [5, 6]. Déjérine–Sottas syndrome (DSS) or HMSN III or hypertrophic neuropathy is an early-onset, clinically severe, demyelinating motor and sensory neuropathy with MNCV below 12 m/s, and can be considered as a severe subtype of HMSN I [7]. Similarly, congenital amyelination neuropathy (CAN) and congenital hypomyelinating neuropathy are part of the demyelinating neuropathy spectrum [8, 9].

Further subdivisions within HMSN (CMT) are based on the inheritance pattern and molecular genetic defects. Inheritance in CMT can be autosomal dominant (AD), X-linked or autosomal recessive (AR). In Western countries, the dominant forms of CMT are the most frequent, but in countries with a high prevalence of consanguineous families, such as in North-Africa or the

*(AR CMT1 = CMT4 = Autosomal recessive hereditary motor and sensory neuropathy type I, AR HMSN I; AR CMT2 = Autosomal recessive hereditary motor and sensory neuropathy type II, AR HMSN II)

Peripheral Nerve Disorders: Pathology and Genetics, First Edition. Edited by Jean-Michel Vallat, Joachim Weis, Francoise Gray, and Katy Keohane.

Middle-East, autosomal recessive cases may account for 30–50% of all CMT cases [10].

In general, histopathological studies in demyelinating CMT show segmental demyelination and remyelination with prominent onion bulb formation, and in axonal CMT show signs of axonal degeneration with regenerative sprouting [11, 12].

General characteristics of AR CMT

In comparison with AD CMT, patients with AR CMT usually have an earlier disease onset (before the age of 3 years) and a more rapid clinical progression, resulting in a severe polyneuropathy and more marked deformities such as pes equinovarus, claw-like hands, and often major spinal deformities. Within AR CMT, the age at onset in axonal AR CMT subtypes is generally later and the disease is usually less severe compared to the demyelinating AR CMT subtypes.

In recent years many genes have been identified as the underlying cause of AR CMT, based on the clinical, morphological, and molecular findings in CMT families with autosomal recessive inheritance. To date, 11 different subtypes (CMT4A-J) of demyelinating forms of AR CMT (AR CMT1 or CMT4), corresponding to 11 different genes, have been identified: *GDAP1, MTMR2, SBF2 (MTMR13), SBF1, SH3TC2(KIAA1985), NDRG1, EGR2, PRX, HK1, FGD4,* and *FIG4.* The nine genes known to cause axonal AR CMT (AR CMT2) are *LMNA, MED25, GDAP1, HINT1, LRSAM1, TRIM2, HSPB1, MFN2,* and *NEFL.* Some of these genes, such as *GDAP1* and *NEFL,* are implicated in axonal, demyelinating, and intermediate CMT (see Chapters 10, 9, and 12) and can follow both an autosomal dominant and autosomal recessive inheritance pattern. However, many patients remain without a genetic diagnosis, making further investigations into AR CMT families necessary in order to discover new genes and common pathways.

Many histopathological changes are non-specific and not distinctive for certain AR CMT. However, some characteristics in the nerve tissue can point towards the specific AR CMT subtype and might guide molecular diagnosis. These features are discussed in more detail in the following paragraphs. In this chapter, we review the recent developments regarding the genotypes and the corresponding clinical and pathological phenotypes of both demyelinating and axonal AR CMT.

Demyelinating forms of autosomal recessive CMT (CMT4 or AR CMT1)

CMT4A (AR CMT1A; MIM 214400)

Definition, genetics, and epidemiology

CMT4A is the most frequent recessive subtype of demyelinating CMT. CMT4A was originally mapped to chromosome 8q21.3 in four Tunisian consanguineous families with a severe CMT phenotype [13]. This locus accounted for approximately 25% of AR CMT cases [14, 15]. Later, the causative ganglioside-induced differentiation-associated protein 1 encoding gene (*GDAP1*) was identified [16, 17]. Mutations in the *GDAP1*-gene cause not only CMT4A [14, 18–20], but also axonal AR CMT with hoarseness (AR CMT2K) [17], intermediate AR CMT A (CMT RIA) [21], AR CMT with pyramidal involvement [22] and the rare AD CMT2K [20, 23–25].

Clinical presentation

Patients with CMT4A show severe early childhood-onset, rapidly progressive neuropathy with prominent weakness beginning in the lower limbs. Weakness then spreads proximally and affects the distal upper limbs within the first decade of life. Independent ambulation is lost at the beginning of the second decade. Sensory disturbances are less prominent, but foot deformities are frequently present [15–17].

Histopathology

Peripheral nerve biopsy in CMT4A shows features of demyelination, such as hypomyelination, segmental demyelination, onion bulb formation, and sometimes mild focal folding of the outer myelin lamellae, as well as axonal degeneration with early loss especially of large myelinated axons [14, 15, 26].

Pathogenesis

The GDAP1 protein regulates mitochondrial dynamics that are critical for the proper function of myelinated peripheral nerves [27, 28]. GDAP1 is an integral membrane protein of the outer mitochondrial membrane and is expressed in both Schwann cells and motor and sensory neurons of human and rat peripheral nerves, as well as in the brain and spinal cord. GDAP1 is involved in the control of the intracellular antioxidant glutathione content and mitochondrial activity, indicating a possible involvement of oxidative stress in the pathogenesis of CMT4A [29].

CMT4 with focally folded myelin sheaths or CMT4B

CMT4B1 AR CMT1B1; MIM 601382)

Definition, genetics, and epidemiology

CMT4B1 is an autosomal recessive demyelinating CMT caused by mutations in the myotubularin-related protein 2 encoding gene (*MTMR2*), located at chromosome 11q22 [30, 31]. CMT4B1 has been reported in Italian, Japanese, and Saudi Arabian families. The myotubularin-related protein 13 (MTMR13) and the myotubularin-related protein 5 (*MTMR5*) are other members of the myotubularin family and cause autosomal recessive demyelinating CMT4B2 and CMT4B3, respectively. Myotubularin 1 (*MTM1*) also belongs to the myotubularin protein family and causes X-linked myotubular myopathy [32].

Clinical presentation

Patients with CMT4B1 have early onset of disease (before 4 years of age, mean 2 years). They develop progressive symmetrical weakness in the distal and proximal lower limbs, become wheelchair-dependent in adolescence or as young adults, and eventually develop weakness in the hands and forearms. Facial weakness and respiratory failure due to diaphragmatic involvement can occur [33–35]. CMT4B1 patients have panmodal sensory loss in the distal legs, absent deep tendon reflexes and pes equinovarus.

Histopathology

Peripheral nerve biopsy in CMT4B1 shows focally folded myelin sheaths [36]. Ultrastructural study of a superficial peroneal nerve biopsy showed a significant loss of myelinated fibers and prominent myelin in- and outfoldings in the majority of large-diameter fibers [37]. This finding has been considered as the pathological hallmark of CMT4B1 and CMT4B2. However, similar focally folded myelin sheaths were found, although to a lesser extent, in *FGD4, PRX, MPZ,* and *SH3TC2* associated CMT [38–40]. Secondary axonal loss is usually observed in CMT4B1.

Pathogenesis

Myotubularin-related protein 2 (*MTMR2*) is expressed at high levels in myelinating and non-myelinating Schwann cells and in neurons. MTMR2 is one of the approximately 20 known dual specificity phosphatases (DSP), which interact with proteins containing a SET domain that associates with chromatin. Loss of the phospholipid phosphatase MTMR2 causes CMT4B1 in human and mouse peripheral nerves [41]. MTMR2 might have a role in membrane trafficking, which is important for myelin membrane biogenesis and homeostasis [42].

Animal model

A mouse model of CMT4B1 has been developed by introducing an E276X mutation in exon 9 of *MTMR2* and deleting the chromosomal region immediately downstream of the stop codon up to within exon 13 [43]. The resulting allele closely mimicked the mutation found in a Saudi Arabian patient with CMT4B1. Animals homozygous for the mutation showed various degrees of complex myelin infoldings and outfoldings exclusively in peripheral nerves. This pathology progressed with age. Axonal damage was occasionally observed. Distal nerve regions were more severely affected than proximal parts; however, there were no significant electrophysiologic changes, even in aged (16-month-old) mice. This suggests that myelin infoldings and outfoldings per se are not invariably associated with detectable electrophysiologic abnormalities [43].

CMT4B2 (AR CMT1B2; MIM 604563)

Definition, genetics, and epidemiology

CMT4 with focally folded myelin sheaths (CMT4B) is genetically heterogeneous. This was demonstrated in consanguineous Tunisian families by absence of linkage to the 11q22 locus, and subsequent mapping to chromosome 11p15 [44]. The gene responsible for CMT4B2 encodes the SET binding factor 2 (SBF2) [45], also called the myotubularin-related protein 13 (MTMR13) [46].

Clinical presentation

Symptoms in patients with CMT4B2 are less severe than in CMT4B1 and start in the first two decades of life. Delayed motor development in childhood does not occur. Weakness predominates in the intrinsic foot and anterior leg muscles. Years after disease onset, progression to proximal weakness with loss of ambulation occurs in some patients. Severe distal sensory loss, absent deep tendon reflexes in the legs, reduced reflexes in the arms, pes cavus, and hammer toes were noted in CMT4B2 patients [44–46]. In some families, the CMT4B2 phenotype segregates with a congenital or juvenile-onset glaucoma [46–48].

Histopathology

Nerve biopsy in CMT4B2 reveals irregular folding and redundant loops of myelin or focally folded myelin sheaths, segmental demyelination, and the presence of onion bulbs. Axonal loss, especially of large myelinated axons is also seen.

Pathogenesis

Whereas the MTMR2 protein has a phosphatase domain, SBF2/MTMR13 has a catalytically inactive pseudophosphatase domain due to replacement of a catalytic cysteine residue with leucine. SBF2 interacts with MTMR2, and loss of SBF2 function causes loss of MTMR2 function, leading to accumulation of phosphatidylinositol 3-phosphate and phosphatidylinositol 3,5-biphosphate. This results in dysfunctional membrane trafficking and endocytic/exocytic processes and altered neuron-Schwann cell interactions [49]. Recent studies indicated that MTMR2 and MTMR13/SBF2 play critical roles in the modulation of cellular signaling which are disturbed in CMT4B [50].

Animal model

The *Sbf2*-null mouse is a mouse model of CMT4B2 in which the mice progressively developed myelin outfoldings and infoldings in motor and sensory peripheral nerves concomitant with decreased motor performance. The number and complexity of myelin misfoldings increased with age and was associated with axonal degeneration. There was mild impairment of nerve conduction velocities, but no significant alteration in myelin thickness or axon diameter [51].

A targeted disruption of the *Sbf2*-gene in mice resulted in a peripheral neuropathy characterized by reduced nerve conduction velocity, myelin outfoldings and infoldings, and progressive dysmyelination, similar to that observed in CMT4B2 patients. Mtmr2 levels were decreased by approximately 50% in Sbf2-deficient sciatic nerves, suggesting a regulatory relationship between the two proteins [52].

CMT4B3 (AR CMT1B3; MIM 615284)

Definition, genetics, and epidemiology

This AR demyelinating CMT subtype is caused by compound heterozygous mutations in the SET binding factor 1 encoding gene (*SBF1*), also called *MTMR5*, and has thus far been identified in only one Korean family, using whole exome sequencing [53].

Clinical presentation

In the single reported CMT4B3 family, the disease started between 5 and 11 years of age, with distal leg weakness resulting in a gait disorder. Pes planus and scoliosis were present. Progression was slow and most patients remained ambulatory.

Histopathology

Peripheral nerve pathology showed focally folded myelin and occasional onion bulbs, loss of large myelinated axons, and a few regenerating clusters consisting of two or more adjacent myelinated axons surrounded by flattened Schwann cell processes [53].

Pathogenesis

SBF1 is structurally similar to SBF2 and interacts with MTMR2 and SBF2. The function of SBF1 is largely unknown.

CMT4C (AR CMT1C; MIM 601596)

Definition, genetics, and epidemiology

CMT4C represents a frequent cause of AR CMT and is due to homozygous or compound heterozygous mutations in the SH3 domain and tetratricopeptide repeat domain 2 encoding gene (*SH3TC2*), also called *KIAA1985*, situated on chromosome 5q32 [54–56]. A mutation hot spot in exon 11 of *SH3TC2* was identified. The R954X mutation frequently occurs in French Canadian and English families [57], whereas the R1190X mutation is often found in Spanish Gypsies [58].

Clinical presentation

CMT4C is less severe than other AR CMT. The disease usually starts in childhood or adolescence and is generally characterized by a relatively slow progression of the motor deficit. There is considerable intra- and interfamilial variability in CMT4C and patients with infantile onset neuropathy and early loss of ambulation and respiratory problems have also been described. Foot deformities and early severe scoliosis requiring surgery was present in all patients [59]. Hypoacusis and facial paresis can be found in some CMT4C patients [56], as well as nystagmus, unresponsive pupils, or unilateral tongue atrophy. An increased frequency of carpal tunnel syndrome in heterozygotes has been reported [60].

Histopathology

Nerve biopsies (Fig. 11.1) showed severe depletion of large myelinated axons, small and large focal myelin thickenings, wide nodes of Ranvier, and onion bulbs that are smaller than those seen in CMT1A. Schwann cells, especially those of unmyelinated nerve fibers, show peculiar extended processes [56, 61, 62]. Nerve fibers are often surrounded by excess basal laminae. Giant axons have been reported in some CMT4C cases [59]. Inflammatory CD4-positive T-lymphocyte infiltration has been reported in the biopsy of one patient with CMT4C, suggesting a possible predisposition to peripheral nerve inflammation associated with *SH3TC2* mutations [61].

Pathogenesis and animal model

The SH3TC2/KIAA1985 protein is expressed in neural tissues and in peripheral nerve Schwann cells. Sh3tc2-null mice manifested a progressive peripheral neuropathy with decreased motor and sensory nerve conduction velocity and hypomyelination. The protein localized to the plasma membrane and the perinuclear endocytic recycling compartment. Myelin in the peripheral nerve of mutant mice showed abnormal organization of the nodes of Ranvier, a phenotype that was confirmed in CMT4C patient nerve biopsies. Thus, the SH3TC2/KIAA1985 protein might have a role in myelination and maintenance of nodes of Ranvier through axo-glial interaction [62]. Mistargeting of the protein away from the recycling endosome has also been shown as a fundamental molecular defect leading to CMT4C [63].

CMT4D (AR CMT1D; MIM 601455)

Definition, genetics, and epidemiology

CMT4D was previously called hereditary motor and sensory neuropathy of Lom type (HMSNL) and is caused by mutations in the N-myc Downstream-Regulated Gene 1 (*NDRG1*) on chromosome 8q24 [64, 65]. The disease was identified in Bulgarian gypsies and named after the town of Lom where the initial cases were found. The disorder was subsequently found also in other gypsy communities.

Clinical presentation

CMT4D consistently begins in the first decade of life with gait difficulties and foot deformities (50%), followed by upper limb weakness in the second decade. Most patients develop deafness, most often first noticed in the third decade [64]. There is sensory loss for all modalities and deep tendon reflexes are absent. Scoliosis is present in 20% of the patients and tongue atrophy can occur. The disease progresses to severe disability in the fifth decade.

Histopathology

CMT4D nerve pathology reveals signs of demyelination with onion bulbs, especially in younger patients. In older patients Schwann cell processes with a circular pattern and uncompacted myelin are described. Pleomorphic inclusions in Schwann cells at the adaxonal cytoplasm, and axonal inclusions of irregularly arranged curvilinear profiles are present, resembling the findings in experimental vitamin E deficiency. Nerve biopsy shows severe loss of large myelinated axons and a markedly increased amount of endoneurial collagen. Some endoneurial blood vessels showed non-specific basal lamina reduplication [64–66].

Pathogenesis

The NDRG1 protein is ubiquitously expressed and present at high levels in Schwann cells. NDRG1 has been proposed to play a role in growth arrest and cell differentiation, possibly as a signaling protein shuttling between cytoplasm and the nucleus [65]. Another possible mechanism in NDRG1 deficiency might be due to impaired intracellular trafficking in Schwann cells, which fail to meet the demands of the nerve fiber [66].

CMT4E (AR CMT1E; MIM 605253)

Mutations in the early growth response 2 gene (*EGR2*), also called *KROX20*, localized to chromosome 10q21, cause CMT4E [67]. EGR2 gene mutations cause a broad spectrum of CMT phenotypes, ranging from early onset severe congenital hypomyelination neuropathy (CHN) to late onset demyelinating CMT1D [67–69]. *EGR2* associated diseases can be transmitted in an autosomal dominant (CMT1D) or autosomal recessive (CMT4E) manner. Nerve pathology revealed absent or greatly reduced myelin on most axons, occasional occurrence of onion bulbs, and mild to moderate axonal loss [67].

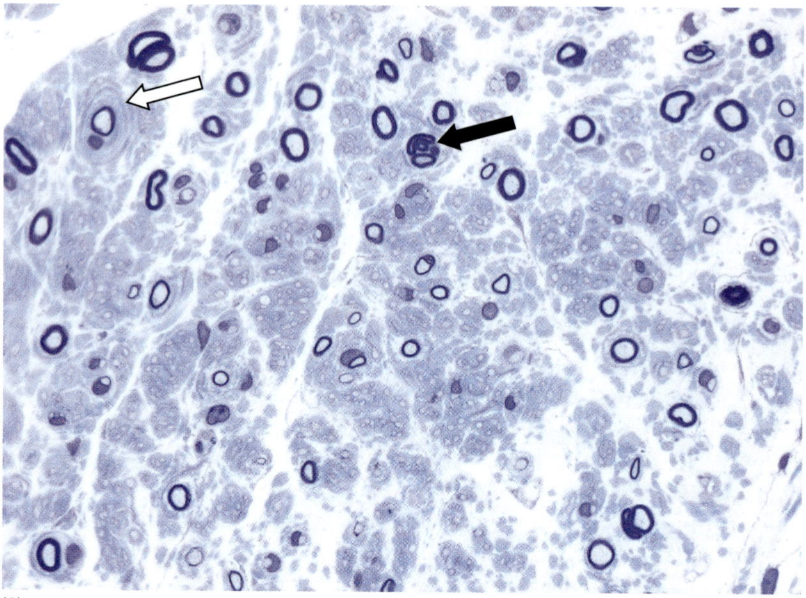

(A)

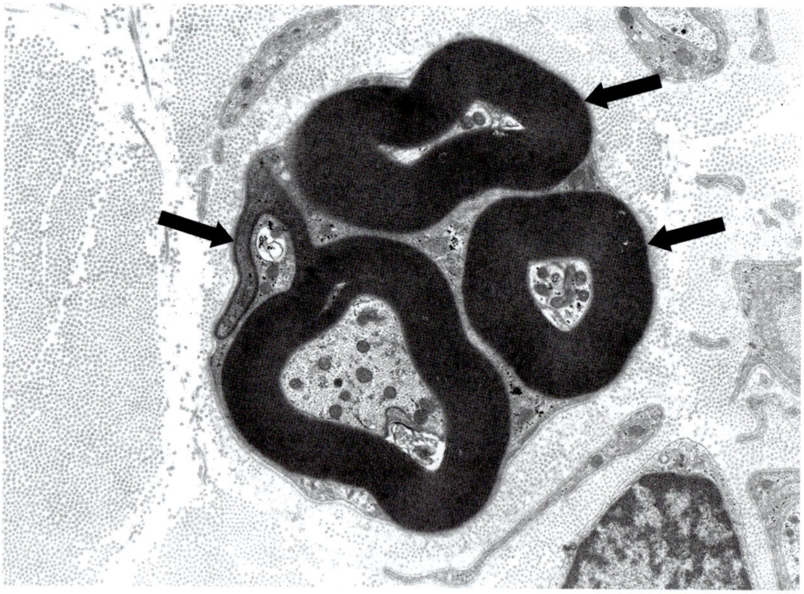

(B)

Figure 11.1 Sural nerve biopsy findings in CMT4C due to mutation of the *SH3TC2/KIAA1985* gene. (**A**) Loss of myelinated nerve fibers, disproportionately thin myelin sheaths and onion bulb formations (white arrow) as well as occasional focally folded myelin (black arrow). Semithin section, Toluidine blue. (**B**) Abnormal myelin foldings (arrows). EM. (**C**) Thinly myelinated and non-myelinated large axons and abnormally long processes of Schwann cells of unmyelinated nerve fibers (arrows). EM. (**D**) Onion bulb formation containing excess basal lamina (arrows). EM. (**E**) Abnormal branching of Schwann cell processes of unmyelinated nerve fibers and excess Schwann cell basal laminae. EM.

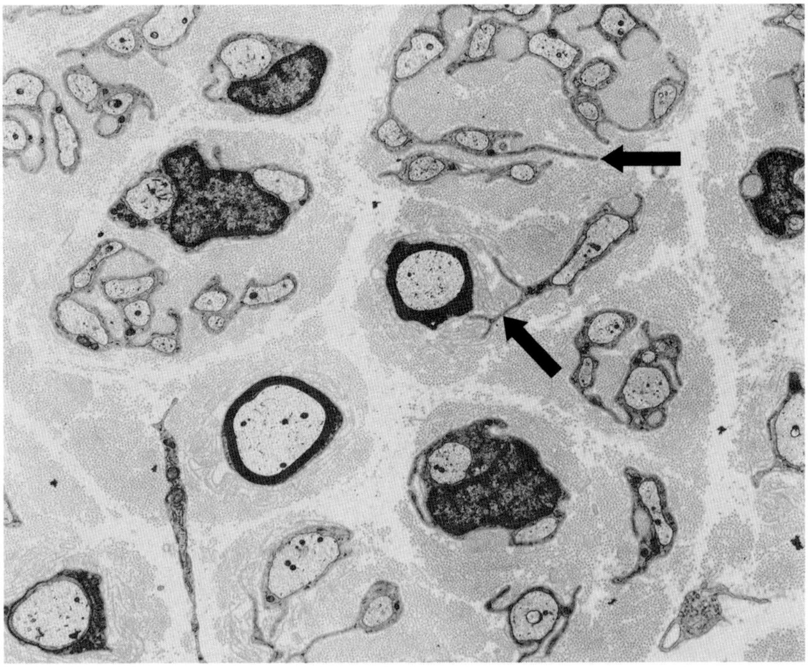

(C)

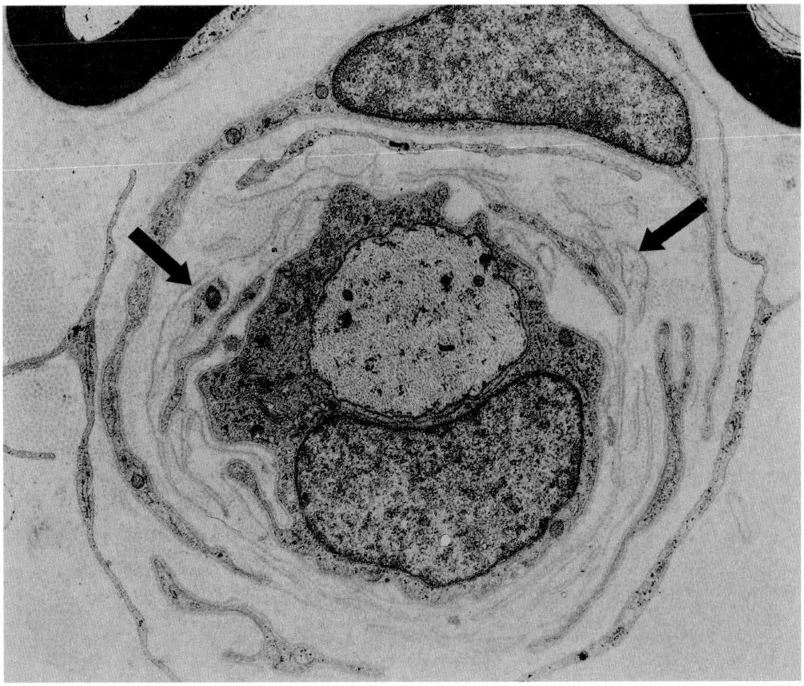

(D)

Figure 11.1 (*Continued*)

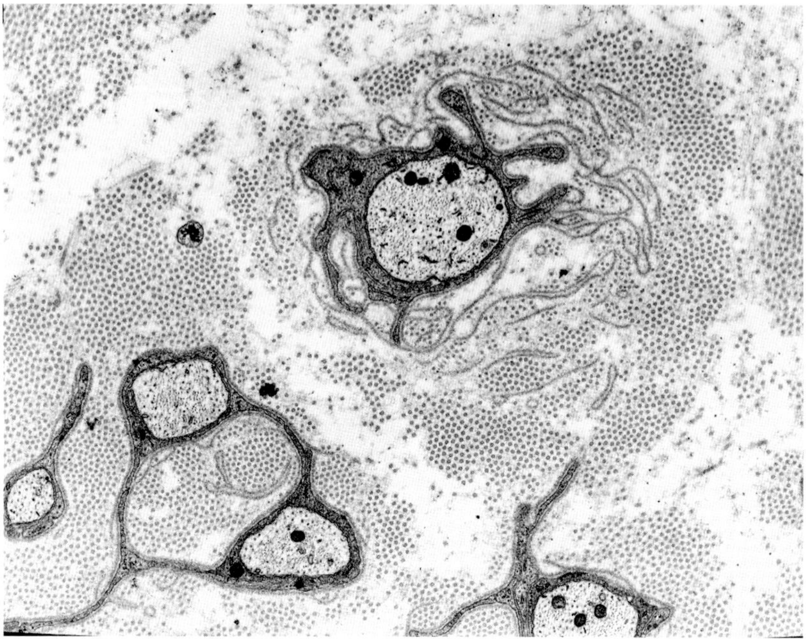

(E)

Figure 11.1 *(Continued)*

The congenital amyelination neuropathy (CAN) is an autosomal recessive variant caused by *EGR2* mutations with oligohydramnios, hypotonia, respiratory failure, reduced movements, and arthrogryposis at birth and death before 1 year of age. Nerve biopsy showed a complete absence of PNS myelin, large axons ensheathed by Schwann cell processes and absent EGR2 immunoreactivity in Schwann cells [70].

CMT4F (AR CMT1F; MIM 614895)

Definition, genetics, and epidemiology

Autosomal recessive Charcot–Marie–Tooth disease type 4F (CMT4F) is caused by homozygous or compound heterozygous mutation in the periaxin gene (*PRX*) located on chromosome 19q13 [71–73]. CMT4F has been diagnosed in several ethnic groups, such as Lebanese Shiite Muslim, North American Hispanic, Northern European, and Vietnamese patients.

Clinical presentation

CMT4F usually presents with early onset (4 weeks to 7 years), although some later onset variants also exist. Motor milestones are delayed. Patients showed a wide-based ataxic gait, slowly progressive severe weakness in the distal legs at 9–10 years and in the hands at 14 to 15 years [74–77]. Pansensory loss in arms and legs in CMT4F is more severe than the motor involvement and sensory impairment is more severe than in other CMT subtypes. Ataxia occurs in 80% of the cases, pes cavus in 75%, and mild kyphoscoliosis is frequent. Deep tendon reflexes are absent.

Histopathology

The peripheral nerve in CMT4F showed severe loss of myelinated and unmyelinated fibers, hypomyelination, and occasionally abnormal myelin folding. Residual fibers were surrounded by Schwann cell onion bulb formations [73, 74, 77].

Pathogenesis and animal model

The periaxin gene encodes two PDZ-domain proteins, L- and S-periaxin that are expressed in myelinating Schwann cells. Both periaxins are probably essential for the formation and maintenance of peripheral nerve myelin [72]. During myelination, L-periaxin is located near the adaxonal membrane, whereas in mature myelin sheaths the protein is situated close to the abaxonal membrane, Schmidt–Lanterman incisures and paranodal membranes [78]. Periaxins interact through the PDZ-domains with dystrophin-related protein 2 complex linking the Schwann cell cytoskeleton to the extracellular matrix [79]. The homozygous periaxin-null mice display extensive demyelination of myelinated fibers in the PNS [73].

CMT4G (AR CMT1G, HMSN R usse, HMSNR; MIM 605285)

Definition, genetics, and epidemiology

HMSN Russe or CMT4G has been identified in Bulgarian, Romanian, and Spanish gypsies and mapped to chromosome 10q23, close to the *EGR* gene [80–82]. The hexokinase 1 encoding gene (*HK1*) was identified as the causative gene of CMT4G [82].

Clinical presentation

CMT4G patients present with onset of distal lower limb weakness at 8–16 years of age, and upper limb involvement between 10 and 43 years. The disease is continuously progressive leading to severe disability and total paralysis of muscles below the knees and in many cases also below the elbows by the fourth or fifth decade of life [80, 83]. Panmodal loss is a prominent feature. Deep tendon reflexes are absent. Pes cavus and clawed toes are present in all patients, and clawed hands in 80% of the cases. Occasionally, neuropathic joints, ptosis, facial weakness, or dysphonia are noted.

Histopathology

Nerve biopsy findings are axonal loss, especially of large myelinated axons, abundant regeneration with many small caliber axons, and hypomyelination with uniformly reduced thickness of the myelin sheaths [81].

Pathogenesis

The HK1 protein is ubiquitously expressed and the enzyme catalyzes the first step in the glucose metabolism. The specific effects and pathogenic mechanisms in peripheral nerve remain unknown.

CMT4H (AR CMT1H; MIM 609311)

Definition, genetics, and epidemiology

CMT4H is caused by mutations in the *frabin/FGD4* gene, encoding a Rho GTPase guanine nucleotide exchange factor and localized to chromosome 12p11 [84, 85]. The disease was first reported in two consanguineous families, one from Lebanon and the other from Algeria.

Clinical presentation

Onset is in the first or second year, with delayed walking, severe scoliosis, pes equinus, and toe retraction [84–87]. Thenar and hypothenar atrophy is observed in some patients. Disease progression is slow.

Histopathology

Nerve biopsies (Fig. 11.2) show severe loss of myelinated fibers. The remaining fibers are often surrounded by Schwann cell and basal lamina onion bulbs. Abnormal folding of myelin sheaths (focally folded myelin) is frequent [84, 86, 88].

Pathogenesis

The *FGD4* gene encodes the FGD4 or frabin protein (FGD1-related F-actin binding protein), which is a GDP/GTP nucleotide exchange factor, specific to Cdc42, a member of the Rho family of small guanosine triphosphatase (GTP)-binding proteins (Rho GTPases). Rho GTPases play a key role in regulating signal-transduction pathways in eukaryotes [85]. Mutations in FGD4/frabin might lead to impaired Rho GTPase signaling and alterations of Schwann cell shape, suggesting that Rho GTPase signaling is essential for proper myelination in the peripheral nervous system [88].

CMT4J (ARCMT1J; MIM 611228)

Definition, genetics, and epidemiology

This demyelinating type of AR CMT is caused by compound heterozygous mutations in the polyphosphoinositide phosphatase FIG4 encoding gene (*FIG4*), also called the SAC domain containing inositol phosphatase 3 gene (*SAC3*), situated on chromosome 6q21 [89]. FIG4 mutations causing CMT4J have been described in four unrelated Caucasian patients as well as in the pale tremor mouse [89]. *FIG4* mutations also cause autosomal dominant amyotrophic lateral sclerosis of type 11 (ALS11).

Clinical presentation

CMT4J patients present with motor delay and congenital, childhood or adult onset occurs. Weakness is severe, involves distal and proximal muscles, and can be asymmetrical. Sensory loss is mild. Disease progresses over 5–10 years, leading to quadriparesis and wheelchair dependency. In contrast to the allelic ALS11 disease, in CMT4J there are no upper motor signs.

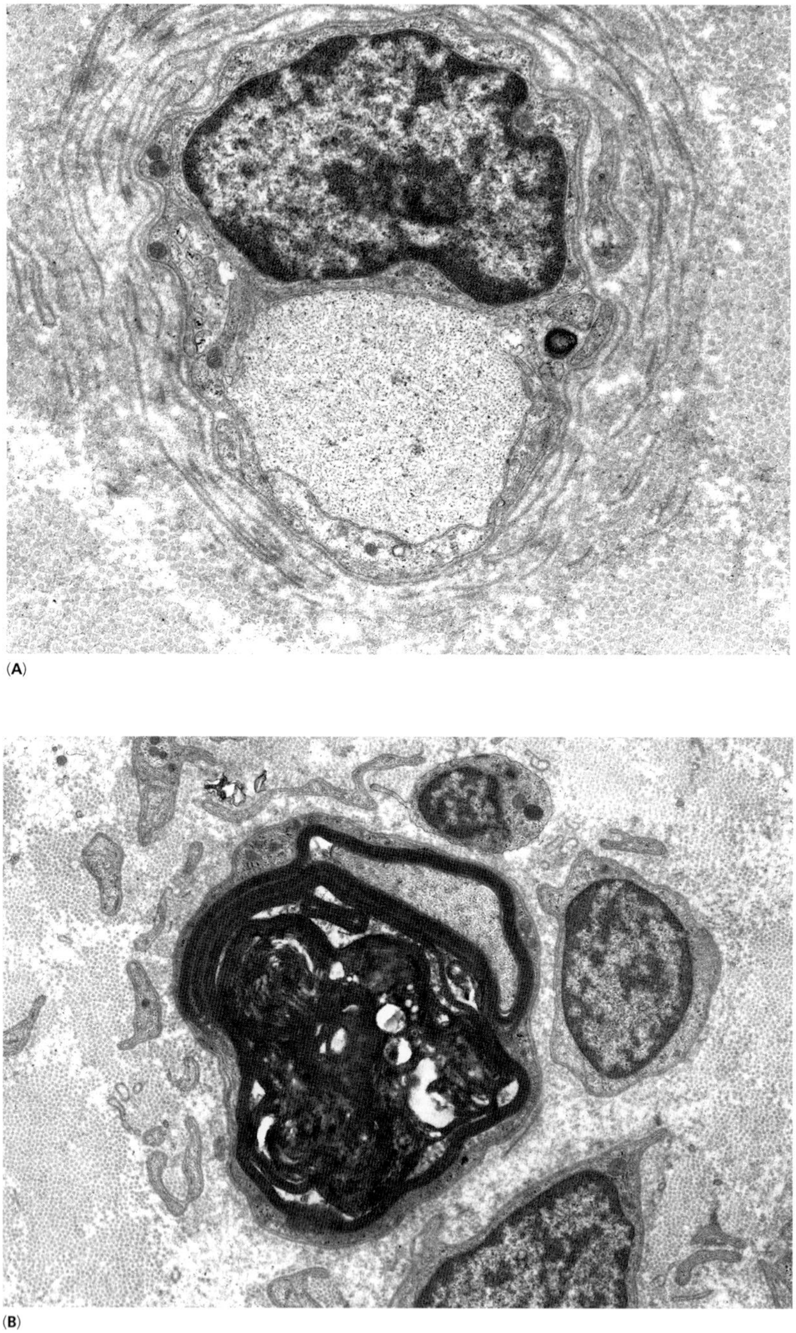

Figure 11.2 Ultrastructure of the sural nerve of a Frabin/FGD4 mutation patient. (**A**) Basal lamina onion bulb. (**B–D**) Different forms of abnormal myelin outfoldings/focally folded myelin.

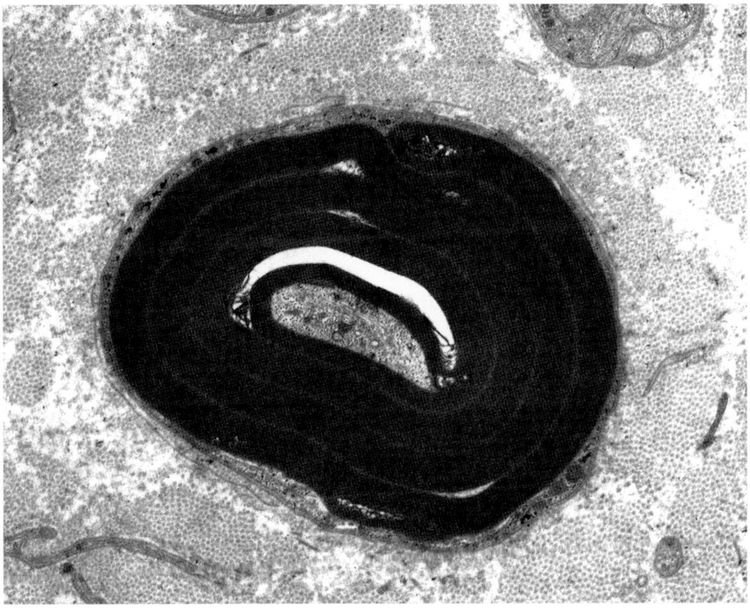

(**C**)

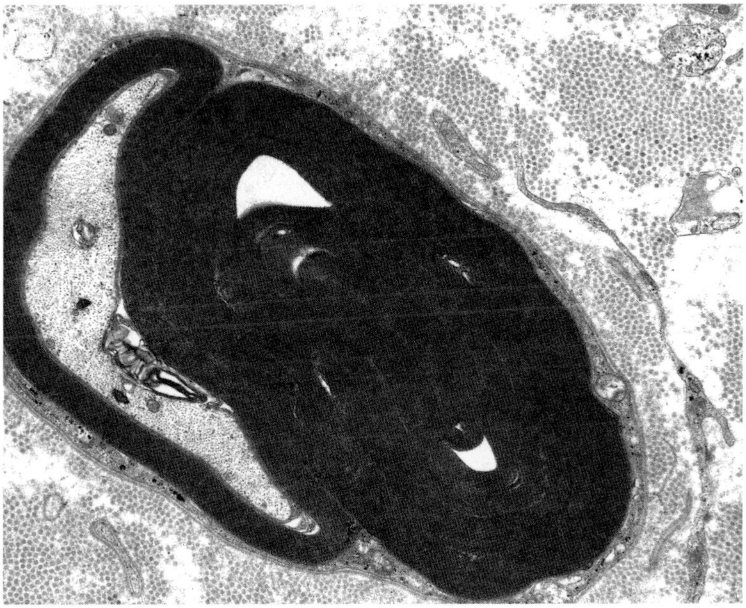

(**D**)

Figure 11.2 (*Continued*)

Histopathology

Nerve biopsy showed axonal loss, especially of large axons, signs of demyelination such as scattered thinly myelinated axons and small onion bulbs, and increased collagen in the extracellular matrix [89].

Pathogenesis and animal model

The FIG4 phosphatase activity specifically removes the 5-phosphate from the inositol ring of $PI(3,5)P_2$, a membrane-bound phospholipid that acts as a molecular signal for trafficking and fusion of intracellular vesicles. In mammals, this complex is localized in the lysosomal/endosomal vesicle system [90]. *FIG4* mutations might lead to an abnormal transport of intracellular organelles. MTMR2 and FIG4 act on the same phospholipid substrate, but with predicted opposite effects. A generated double Mtmr2/Fig4-null mouse showed that Mtmr2 and Fig4 interact in neurons and Schwann cells to control phospholipid metabolism [91].

Mice with *FIG4* mutations ("pale tremor" mice) develop a multi-organ disorder with impaired motor coordination, muscle weakness, "swimming" gait, CNS neuronal degeneration and peripheral neuronopathy and reduced pigmentation [89]. Extensive neuronal vacuolization and degeneration is seen.

Axonal forms of autosomal recessive CMT (AR CMT2)

AR CMT2A (CMT2B1; MIM 605588)

Definition, genetics, and epidemiology

The first autosomal recessive CMT of axonal type was described in consanguineous Moroccan and Algerian families, all showing linkage to chromosome 1q22 [92, 93]. AR CMT2A was caused by homozygous mutations in the *LMNA* gene, encoding the lamins A/C [93]. Mutations in *LMNA* not only cause AR CMT2A, but a whole spectrum of diseases including muscular dystrophy, cardiac disorders, lipodystrophy, and premature aging disorders [94, 95].

Clinical presentation

AR CMT2A usually starts in the second decade of life with distal weakness in the legs. Disease is usually rapidly progressive, with development of proximal weakness in the lower limbs resulting in prominent disability. Patients with a less severe phenotype and slower progression have also been described [96]. Distal muscle atrophy is present and deep tendon reflexes are reduced or absent in the legs. Distal sensory loss is mild (especially large fiber), but worsens with disease progression. Pes cavus is seen in 80% and mild kyphoscoliosis in 30% of the patients [92, 93, 96, 97]. Furthermore, four patients in one family showed scapular and pelvic girdle atrophy and weakness [97].

Histopathology

Nerve biopsies revealed a severe reduction of myelinated fibers, especially of the large diameter fibers [93, 96]. A significant increase in unmyelinated fibers has been reported [96, 98]. There were no signs of fiber degeneration and no regenerative clusters. Signs of demyelination and remyelination, such as onion bulbs, were lacking.

Pathogenesis and animal model

Lamins A/C are major components of the nuclear lamina, which has numerous roles such as transcriptional regulation, heterochromatin organization and maintenance of nuclear shape and structure [99]. These diverse functions of the nuclear lamina proteins might explain the large variability of clinical presentations in case of mutations.

A knock-in mouse model for the Lmna p.Arg298Cys mutation has been generated. This model revealed a significant upregulation of Pmp22, specifically in the sciatic nerves of Lmna (R298C/R298C) mice [100].

AR CMT2B (CMT2B2; MIM 605589)

Definition, genetics, and epidemiology

AR CMT2B is an axonal CMT subtype, described in a large consanguineous Costa Rican family with adult onset. Homozygous mutations (Ala335Val) in the mediator complex subunit 25 gene (MED25) on chromosome 19q13 were identified as its underlying cause [101–103].

Clinical presentation

AR CMT2B is characterized by adult onset (28–42 years) CMT with weakness starting in the ankles and hands. Patients manifested distal symmetrical weakness and atrophy and panmodal sensory deficits in all four limbs. Deep tendon reflexes were often absent at the ankles, and reduced to absent elsewhere [101, 102]. Foot deformities were mild or absent. Cramps and paresthesias in distal extremities may occur. There is slow progression and most patients remain ambulatory.

Histopathology

Nerve biopsy findings in AR CMT2B have, thus far, not been published.

Pathogenesis and animal model

MED25 is a subunit of the human activator recruited cofactor, a family of large transcriptional coactivator complexes related to the yeast mediator. The exact physiological function of MED25 in transcriptional regulation is not known. The expression of *MED25* correlates with the expression of the *PMP22* gene in transgenic mice and rats [103].

AR CMT2P (MIM 614436)

Definition and genetics

AR CMT2P is caused by mutations in the leucine rich repeat and sterile alpha motif containing 1 gene (LRSAM1), mapped to locus 9q33 [104]. Inheritance can occur in a recessive (AR CMT2P) or dominant manner (CMT2P).

Clinical presentation

Disease onset varied from the second to the fifth decade, with distal weakness and panmodal sensory loss in the four extremities. Cramps in the extremities and trunk, and erectile dysfunction as a sign of autonomic involvement have been described. Disease course was slow, with wheelchair dependency in some patients [104].

Histopathology

Nerve biopsy results have thus far not been reported in patients with LRSAM1 mutations.

Pathogenesis

The LRSAM1 protein is a RING finger protein with multiple functions that has a role in receptor endocytosis.

AR CMT2R (MIM 615490)

Definition, genetics, and epidemiology

This AR axonal CMT subtype has been described in only one Finnish patient so far and was caused by compound heterozygous mutations in the gene that encodes the tripartite motif containing protein 2 (TRIM2) located at chromosome 4q31 [105].

Clinical presentation

AR CMT2R is characterized by early disease onset (8 months of age), with poor growth, hypotonia, wide-based gait, small hand and feet muscles, pes cavus, and absent deep tendon reflexes.

Histopathology

Sural nerve biopsy in AR CMT2R revealed reduced numbers of myelinated axons and intra-axonal accumulations of neurofilaments, similar to the findings in mice with *TRIM2* mutations [105].

Pathogenesis

TRIM2 is an E3 ubiquitin ligase that ubiquitinates neurofilament light chain, a component of the intermediate filament in axons. Loss of function mutations in *TRIM2* cause an axonopathy probably as a consequence of axonal accumulation of neurofilaments, secondary to lack of its ubiquitination by TRIM2 [105, 106].

AR CMT2 with neuromyotonia (ARAN-NM, NMAN; MIM 137200)

This AR axonal CMT is associated with neuromyotonia and is caused by mutations in the histidine triad nucleotide binding protein 1 encoding gene (*HINT1*) on chromosome 5q31 [107]. In 11% of 33 heterogeneous AR CMT2 families, homozygous or compound heterozygous mutations in *HINT1* were identified [107]. AR CMT2 with neuromyotonia showed a variable disease onset between 3 and 25 years of age, with gait imbalance. The disease is characterized by distal weakness, foot deformities, toe contractures, and neuromyotonia, especially in the hands, increasing with action, leg stiffness, and cramps. Patients with HINT1 mutations manifested a predominantly motor neuropathy. Sensory loss occurred in some patients. Most patients remained ambulatory [107, 108]. Sural nerve biopsy confirmed an axonal neuropathy.

AR CMT2F (MIM 606595) and other forms with both recessive and dominant occurrence of CMT

This form is caused by mutations in the heat shock 27kD protein 1 encoding gene (*HSPB1; HSP27*) localized to chromosome 7q11 [109]. Heterozygous mutations in *HSPB1* result in the autosomal dominant axonal CMT2F, whereas homozygous mutations cause AR CMT2F [110]. *HSPB1* mutations also cause distal HMN. We refer to the corresponding chapters on AD CMT2 and distal HMN for further details (Chapter 10).

Mutations in other genes such as *GDAP1*, *MFN2*, and *NEFL* can cause both recessive and dominant CMT (see Chapters 9–12).

References

1 Skre H. (1974) Genetic and clinical aspects of Charcot–Marie–Tooth's disease. *Clin Genet* 6, 98–118.

2 Vasli N, Laporte J. (2013) Impacts of massively parallel sequencing for genetic diagnosis of neuromuscular disorders. *Acta Neuropathol* 125, 173–185.

3 Harding AE, Thomas PK. (1980) The clinical features of hereditary motor and sensory neuropathy types I and II. *Brain* 103, 259–280.

4 Dyck PJ, Chance P, Lebo R, *et al.* (1993). Hereditary motor and sensory neuropathies. In: Dyck PJ, Thomas PK, Griffin JW, Low PA and Poduslo JF (eds) *Peripheral Neuropathy*, 3rd edn, pp. 1094–1136. WB Saunders, Philadelphia.

5 Davis CJF, Bradley WG, Madrid R. (1978) The peroneal muscular atrophy syndrome. Clinical, genetic, electrophysiological and nerve biopsy studies. Part 1 (Clinical, genetic and electrophysiological findings). *J Genet Hum* 26, 311–349.

6 Nicholson G, Myers S. (2006) Intermediate forms of Charcot–Marie–Tooth neuropathy: a review. *Neuromolecular Med* 8, 123–130.

7 Plante-Bordeneuve V, Said G. (2002) Dejerine-Sottas disease and hereditary demyelinating polyneuropathy of infancy. *Muscle Nerve* 26, 608–621.

8 Charnas L, Trapp B, Griffin J. (1988) Congenital absence of peripheral myelin: abnormal Schwann cell development causes lethal arthrogryposis multiplex congenita. *Neurology* 38, 966–974.

9 Gabreels-Festen A, Thomas PK. (2005) Autosomal recessive hereditary motor and sensory neuropathies. In: Dyck PJ and Thomas PK (eds) *Peripheral Neuropathy*, 3rd edn, pp. 1769–1790. WB Saunders, Philadelphia.

10 Dubourg O, Azzedine H, Verny C, *et al.* (2006). Autosomal-recessive forms of demyelinating Charcot–Marie–Tooth disease. *Neuromolecular Med* 8, 75–86.

11 Schröder JM. (2001) *Pathology of Peripheral Nerves*. Springer-Verlag, Berlin.

12 Schröder JM. (2006) Neuropathology of Charcot–Marie–Tooth and related disorders. *Neuromolecular Med* 8, 23–42.

13 Ben Othmane K, Hentati F, Lennon F, *et al.* (1993) Linkage of a locus (CMT4A) for autosomal recessive Charcot–Marie–Tooth disease to chromosome 8q. *Hum Mol Genet* 2, 1625–1628.

14 Nelis E, Erdem S, Van Den Bergh PY *et al.* (2002) Mutations in GDAP1: autosomal recessive CMT with demyelination and axonopathy. *Neurology* 59, 1865–1872.

15 Senderek J, Bergmann C, Ramaekers VT *et al.* (2003) Mutations in the ganglioside-induced differentiation-associated protein-1 (GDAP1) gene in intermediate type autosomal recessive Charcot–Marie–Tooth neuropathy. *Brain* 126, 642–649.

16 Baxter RV, Ben Othmane K, Rochelle JM *et al.* (2002) Ganglioside-induced differentiation-associated protein-1 is mutant in Charcot–Marie–Tooth disease type 4A/8q21. *Nat Genet* 30, 21–22.

17 Cuesta A, Pedrola L, Sevilla T *et al.* (2002) The gene encoding ganglioside-induced differentiation-associated protein 1 is mutated in axonal Charcot–Marie–Tooth type 4A disease. *Nat Genet* 30, 22–25.

18 Birouk N, Azzedine H, Dubourg O *et al.* (2003) Phenotypical features of a Moroccan family with autosomal recessive Charcot–Marie–Tooth disease associated with the S194X mutation in the GDAP1 gene. *Arch Neurol* 60, 598–604.

19 Claramunt R, Pedrola L, Sevilla T *et al.* (2005) Genetics of Charcot–Marie–Tooth disease type 4A: mutations, inheritance, phenotypic variability, and founder effect. *J Med Genet* 42, 358–365.

20 Cassereau J, Chevrollier A, Gueguen N *et al.* (2009) Mitochondrial complex I deficiency in GDAP1-related autosomal dominant Charcot–Marie–Tooth disease (CMT2K). *Neurogenetics* 10, 145–150.

21 Kabzinska D, Drac H, Rowinska-Marcinska K *et al.* (2006) Early onset Charcot–Marie–Tooth disease caused by a homozygous Leu239Phe mutation in the GDAP1 gene. *Acta Myol* 25, 34–37.

22 Barhoumi C, Amouri R, Ben Hamida C *et al.* (2001) Linkage of a new locus for autosomal recessive axonal form of Charcot–Marie–Tooth disease to chromosome 8q21.3. *Neuromuscul Disord* 11, 27–34.

23 Chung KW, Kim SM, Sunwoo IN (2008) A novel GDAP1 Q218E mutation in autosomal dominant Charcot–Marie–Tooth disease. *J Hum Genet* 53, 360–364.

24 Crimella C, Tonelli A, Airoldi G *et al.* (2010) The GST domain of GDAP1 is a frequent target of mutations in the dominant form of axonal Charcot–Marie–Tooth type 2K. *J Med Genet* 47, 712–716.

25 Zimoń M, Baets J, Fabrizi GM *et al.* (2011) Dominant GDAP1 mutations cause predominantly mild CMT phenotypes. *Neurology* 77, 540–548.

26 Boerkoel CF, Takashima H, Nakagawa M *et al.* (2003) CMT4A: identification of a Hispanic GDAP1 founder mutation. *Ann Neurol* 53, 400–405.

27 Niemann A, Ruegg M, La Padula V *et al.* (2005) Ganglioside-induced differentiation associated protein 1 is a regulator of the mitochondrial network: new implications for Charcot–Marie–Tooth disease. *J Cell Biol* 170, 1067–1078.

28 Pedrola L, Espert A, Wu X *et al.* (2005) GDAP1, the protein causing Charcot–Marie–Tooth disease type 4A, is expressed in neurons and is associated with mitochondria. *Hum Mol Genet* 14, 1087–1094.

29 Noack R, Frede S, Albrecht P *et al.* (2012) Charcot–Marie–Tooth disease CMT4A: GDAP1 increases cellular glutathione and the mitochondrial membrane potential. *Hum Mol Genet* 21, 150–162.

30 Bolino A, Brancolini V, Bono F *et al.* (1996) Localization of a gene responsible for autosomal recessive demyelinating neuropathy with focally folded myelin sheaths to chromosome 11q23 by homozygosity mapping and haplotype sharing. *Hum Mol Genet* 5, 1051–1054.

31 Bolino A, Muglia M, Conforti FL *et al.* (2000) Charcot–Marie–Tooth type 4B is caused by mutations in the gene encoding myotubularin-related protein-2. *Nat Genet* 25, 17–19.

32 Laporte J, Hu LJ, Kretz C *et al.* (1996) A gene mutated in X-linked myotubular myopathy defines a new putative tyrosine phosphatase family conserved in yeast. *Nat Genet* 13, 175–182.

33 Quattrone A, Gambardella A, Bono F *et al.* (1996) Autosomal recessive hereditary motor and sensory neuropathy with focally folded myelin sheaths: clinical, electrophysiologic, and genetic aspects of a large family. *Neurology* 46, 1318–1324.

34 Houlden H, King RH, Wood NW *et al.* (2001) Mutations in the 5′ region of the myotubularin-related protein 2 (MTMR2) gene in autosomal recessive hereditary neuropathy with focally folded myelin. *Brain* 124, 907–915.

35 Verny C, Ravisé N, Leutenegger AL *et al.* (2004) Coincidence of two genetic forms of Charcot–Marie–Tooth disease in a single family. *Neurology* 63, 1527–1529.

36 Tazir M, Bellatache M, Nouioua S *et al.* (2013) Autosomal recessive Charcot–Marie–Tooth disease: from genes to phenotypes. *Peripher Nerv Syst* 18, 113–129.

37 Nouioua S, Hamadouche T, Funalot B *et al.* (2011) Novel mutations in the PRX and the MTMR2 genes are responsible for unusual Charcot–Marie–Tooth disease phenotypes. *Neuromuscul Disord* 21, 543–550.

38 Takashima H, Boerkoel CF, De Jonghe P *et al.* (2002) Periaxin mutations cause a broad spectrum of demyelinating neuropathies. *Ann Neurol* 51, 709–715.

39 Fabrizi GM, Taioli F, Cavallaro T *et al.* (2009) Further evidence that mutations in FGD4/frabin cause Charcot–Marie–Tooth disease type 4H. *Neurology* 72, 1160–1164.

40 Baets J, Deconinck T, De Vriendt E *et al.* (2011) Genetic spectrum of hereditary neuropathies with onset in the first year of life. *Brain* 134, 2664–2676.

41 Previtali SC, Quattrini A, Bolino A. (2007) Charcot–Marie–Tooth type 4B demyelinating neuropathy: deciphering the role of MTMR phosphatases. *Expert Rev Mol Med* 9, 1–16.

42 Bolis A, Coviello S, Visigalli I *et al.* (2009) Dlg1, Sec8, and Mtmr2 regulate membrane homeostasis in Schwann cell myelination. *J Neurosci* 29, 8858–8870.

43 Bonneick S, Boentert M, Berger P, *et al.* (2005) An animal model for Charcot–Marie–Tooth disease type 4B1. *Hum Mol Genet* 14, 3685–3695.

44 Othmane KB, Johnson E, Menold M *et al.* (1999) Identification of a new locus for autosomal recessive Charcot–Marie–Tooth disease with focally folded myelin on chromosome 11p15. *Genomics* 62, 344–349.

45 Senderek J, Bergmann C, Weber S *et al.* (2003) Mutation of the SBF2 gene, encoding a novel member of the myotubularin family, in Charcot–Marie–Tooth neuropathy type 4B2/11p15. *Hum Mol Genet* 12, 349–356.

46 Azzedine H, Bolino A, Taïeb T *et al.* (2003) Mutations in MTMR13, a new pseudophosphatase homologue of MTMR2 and Sbf1, in two families with an autosomal recessive demyelinating form of Charcot–Marie–Tooth disease associated with early-onset glaucoma. *Am J Hum Genet* 72, 1141–1153.

47 Kiwaki T, Umehara F, Takashima H *et al.* (2000) Hereditary motor and sensory neuropathy with myelin folding and juvenile onset glaucoma. *Neurology* 55, 392–397.

48 Hirano R, Takashima H, Umehara F *et al.* (2004) SET binding factor 2 (SBF2) mutation causes CMT4B with juvenile onset glaucoma. *Neurology* 63, 577–580.

49 Robinson FL, Dixon JE. (2005) The phosphoinositide-3-phosphatase MTMR2 associates with MTMR13, a membrane-associated pseudophosphatase also mutated in type 4B Charcot–Marie–Tooth disease. *J Biol Chem* 280, 31699–31707.

50 Berger P, Tersar K, Ballmer-Hofer K *et al.* (2011) The CMT4B disease-causing proteins MTMR2 and MTMR13/SBF2 regulate AKT signalling. *J Cell Mol Med* 15, 307–315.

51 Tersar K, Boentert M, Berger P *et al.* (2007) Mtmr13/Sbf2-deficient mice: an animal model for CMT4B2. *Hum Mol Genet* 16, 2991–3001.

52 Robinson FL, Niesman IR, Beiswenger KK *et al.* (2008) Loss of the inactive myotubularin-related phosphatase Mtmr13 leads to a Charcot–Marie–Tooth 4B2-like peripheral neuropathy in mice. *Proc Natl Acad Sci U S A.* 105, 4916–4921.

53 Nakhro K, Park JM, Hong YB *et al.* (2013) SET binding factor 1 (SBF1) mutation causes Charcot–Marie–Tooth disease type 4B3. *Neurology* 81, 165–173.

54 LeGuern E, Guilbot A, Kessali M *et al.* (1996) Homozygosity mapping of an autosomal recessive form of demyelinating Charcot–Marie–Tooth disease to chromosome 5q23-q33. *Hum Mol Genet* 50, 1685–1688.

55 Gabreëls-Festen A, van Beersum S, Eshuis L *et al.* (1999) Study on the gene and phenotypic characterisation of autosomal recessive demyelinating motor and sensory neuropathy (Charcot–Marie–Tooth disease) with a gene locus on chromosome 5q23-q33. *J Neurol Neurosurg Psychiatry* 66, 569–574.

56 Senderek J, Bergmann C, Stendel C *et al.* (2003) Mutations in a gene encoding a novel SH3/TPR domain protein cause autosomal recessive Charcot–Marie–Tooth type 4C neuropathy. *Am J Hum Genet* 73, 1106–1119.

57 Gosselin I, Thiffault I, Tétreault M *et al.* (2008) Founder SH3TC2 mutations are responsible for a CMT4C French-Canadians cluster. *Neuromuscul Disord* 18, 483–492.

58 Colomer J, Gooding R, Angelicheva D *et al.* (2006) Clinical spectrum of CMT4C disease in patients homozygous for

the p.Arg1109X mutation in SH3TC2. *Neuromuscul Disord* 16, 449–53.

59 Azzedine H, Ravisé N, Verny C *et al.* (2006) Spine deformities in Charcot–Marie–Tooth 4C caused by SH3TC2 gene mutations. *Neurology* 67, 602–606.

60 Lupski JR, Reid JG, Gonzaga-Jauregui C *et al.* (2010) Whole-genome sequencing in a patient with Charcot–Marie–Tooth neuropathy. *N Engl J Med* 362, 1181–1191.

61 Houlden H, Laura M, Ginsberg L *et al.* (2009) The phenotype of Charcot–Marie–Tooth disease type 4C due to SH3TC2 mutations and possible predisposition to an inflammatory neuropathy. *Neuromuscul Disord* 19, 264–269.

62 Arnaud E, Zenker J, de Preux Charles AS *et al.* (2009) SH3TC2/KIAA1985 protein is required for proper myelination and the integrity of the node of Ranvier in the peripheral nervous system. *Proc Natl Acad Sci U S A* 106, 17528–17533.

63 Roberts RC, Peden AA, Buss F *et al.* (2010) Mistargeting of SH3TC2 away from the recycling endosome causes Charcot–Marie–Tooth disease type 4C. *Hum Mol Genet* 19, 1009–1018.

64 Kalaydjieva L, Nikolova A, Turnev I *et al.* (1998) Hereditary motor and sensory neuropathy--Lom, a novel demyelinating neuropathy associated with deafness in gypsies. Clinical, electrophysiological and nerve biopsy findings. *Brain* 121, 399–408.

65 Kalaydjieva L, Gresham D, Gooding R *et al.* (2000) N-myc downstream-regulated gene 1 is mutated in hereditary motor and sensory neuropathy-Lom. *Am J Hum Genet* 67, 47–58.

66 King RH, Tournev I, Colomer J *et al.* (1999) Ultrastructural changes in peripheral nerve in hereditary motor and sensory neuropathy-Lom. *Neuropathol Appl Neurobiol* 25, 306–312.

67 Warner LE, Mancias P, Butler IJ *et al.* (1998) Mutations in the early growth response 2 (EGR2) gene are associated with hereditary myelinopathies. *Nat Genet* 18, 382–384.

68 Boerkoel CF, Takashima H, Bacino CA *et al.* (2001) EGR2 mutation R359W causes a spectrum of Dejerine–Sottas neuropathy. *Neurogenetics* 3, 153–157.

69 Yoshihara T, Kanda F, Yamamoto M *et al.* (2001) A novel missense mutation in the early growth response 2 gene associated with late-onset Charcot–Marie–Tooth disease type 1. *J Neurol Sci* 184, 149–153.

70 Funalot B, Topilko P, Arroyo MA *et al.* (2012) Homozygous deletion of an EGR2 enhancer in congenital amyelinating neuropathy. *Ann Neurol* 71, 719–723.

71 Delague V, Bareil C, Tuffery S *et al.* (2000) Mapping of a new locus for autosomal recessive demyelinating Charcot–Marie–Tooth disease to 19q13.1–13.3 in a large consanguineous Lebanese family: exclusion of MAG as a candidate gene. *Am J Hum Genet* 67, 236–243.

72 Boerkoel CF, Takashima H, Stankiewicz P. (2001) Periaxin mutations cause recessive Dejerine–Sottas neuropathy. *Am J Hum Genet* 68, 325–333.

73 Guilbot A, Williams A, Ravisé N *et al.* (2001) A mutation in periaxin is responsible for CMT4F, an autosomal recessive form of Charcot–Marie–Tooth disease. *Hum Mol Genet* 10, 415–421.

74 Takashima H, Boerkoel CF, De Jonghe P *et al.* (2002) Periaxin mutations cause a broad spectrum of demyelinating neuropathies. *Ann Neurol* 51, 709–715.

75 Kijima K, Numakura C, Shirahata E *et al.* (2004) Periaxin mutation causes early-onset but slow-progressive Charcot–Marie–Tooth disease. *J Hum Genet* 49, 376–379.

76 Kabzinska D, Drac H, Sherman DL *et al.* (2006) Charcot–Marie–Tooth type 4F disease caused by S399fsx410 mutation in the PRX gene. *Neurology* 66, 745–747.

77 Marchesi C, Milani M, Morbin M *et al.* (2010) Four novel cases of periaxin-related neuropathy and review of the literature. *Neurology* 75, 1830–1838.

78 Gillespie CS, Sherman DL, Blair GE *et al.* (1994) Periaxin, a novel protein of myelinating Schwann cells with a possible role in axonal ensheathment. *Neuron* 12, 497–508.

79 Sherman DL, Fabrizi C, Gillespie CS *et al.* (2001) Specific disruption of a Schwann cell dystrophin-related protein complex in a demyelinating neuropathy. *Neuron* 30, 677–687.

80 Rogers T, Chandler D, Angelicheva D *et al.* (2000) A novel locus for autosomal recessive peripheral neuropathy in the EGR2 region on 10q23. *Am J Hum Genet* 67, 664–671.

81 Thomas PK, Kalaydjieva L, Youl B *et al.* (2001) Hereditary motor and sensory neuropathy-russe: new autosomal recessive neuropathy in Balkan Gypsies. *Ann Neurol* 50, 452–457.

82 Hantke J, Chandler D, King R *et al.* (2009) A mutation in an alternative untranslated exon of hexokinase 1 associated with hereditary motor and sensory neuropathy -- Russe (HMSNR). *Eur J Hum Genet* 17, 1606–1614.

83 Sevilla T, Martínez-Rubio D, Márquez C et al. (2013) Genetics of the Charcot–Marie–Tooth disease in the Spanish Gypsy population: the hereditary motor and sensory neuropathy-Russe in depth. *Clin Genet* 83, 565–570.

84 De Sandre-Giovannoli A, Delague V, Hamadouche T *et al.* (2005) Homozygosity mapping of autosomal recessive demyelinating Charcot–Marie–Tooth neuropathy (CMT4H) to a novel locus on chromosome 12p11.21-q13.11. *J Med Genet* 42, 260–265.

85 Delague V, Jacquier A, Hamadouche T *et al.* (2007) Mutations in FGD4 encoding the Rho GDP/GTP exchange factor FRABIN cause autosomal recessive Charcot–Marie–Tooth type 4H. *Am J Hum Genet* 81, 1–16.

86 Fabrizi GM, Taioli F, Cavallaro T *et al.* (2009) Further evidence that mutations in FGD4/frabin cause Charcot–Marie–Tooth disease type 4H. *Neurology* 72, 1160–1164.

87 Houlden H, Hammans S, Katifi H *et al.* (2009) A novel Frabin (FGD4) nonsense mutation p.R275X associated with phenotypic variability in CMT4H. *Neurology* 72, 617–620.

88 Stendel C, Roos A, Deconinck T *et al.* (2007) Peripheral nerve demyelination caused by a mutant Rho GTPase guanine nucleotide exchange factor, frabin/FGD4. *Am J Hum Genet* 81, 158–164.

89 Chow CY, Zhang Y, Dowling JJ *et al.* (2007) Mutation of FIG4 causes neurodegeneration in the pale tremor mouse and patients with CMT4J. *Nature* 448, 68–72.

90 Dove SK, Dong K, Kobayashi T *et al.* (2009) Phosphatidylinositol 3,5-bisphosphate and Fab1p/PIKfyve underPPIn endo-lysosome function. *Biochem J* 419, 1–13.

91 Vaccari I, Dina G, Tronchère H *et al.* (2011) Genetic interaction between MTMR2 and FIG4 phospholipid phosphatases involved in Charcot–Marie–Tooth neuropathies. *PLoS Genet* 7, e1002319.

92 Bouhouche A, Benomar A, Birouk N *et al.* (1999) A locus for an axonal form of autosomal recessive Charcot–Marie–Tooth disease maps to chromosome 1q21.2-q21.3. *Am J Hum Genet* 65, 722–727.

93 De Sandre-Giovannoli A, Chaouch M, Kozlov S *et al.* (2002) Homozygous defects in LMNA, encoding lamin A/C nuclear-envelope proteins, cause autosomal recessive axonal neuropathy in human (Charcot–Marie–Tooth disorder type 2) and mouse. *Am J Hum Genet* 70, 726–736.

94 Benedetti S, Menditto I, Degano M *et al.* (2007) Phenotypic clustering of lamin A/C mutations in neuromuscular patients. *Neurology* 69, 1285–1292.

95 Worman HJ, Bonne G. (2007) "Laminopathies": a wide spectrum of human diseases. *Exp Cell Res* 313, 2121–2133.

96 Tazir M, Azzedine H, Assami S *et al.* (2004) Phenotypic variability in autosomal recessive axonal Charcot–Marie–Tooth disease due to the R298C mutation in lamin A/C. *Brain* 127, 154–163.

97 Bouhouche A, Birouk N, Azzedine H *et al.* (2007) Autosomal recessive axonal Charcot–Marie–Tooth disease (ARCMT2): phenotype-genotype correlations in 13 Moroccan families. *Brain* 130, 1062–1075.

98 Vallat JM, Tazir M, Magdelaine C *et al.* (2005) Autosomal-recessive Charcot–Marie–Tooth diseases. *Neuropathol Exp Neurol* 64, 363–370.

99 Capell BC, Collins FS. (2006) Human laminopathies: nuclei gone genetically awry. *Nat Rev Genet* 7, 940–952.

100 Poitelon Y, Kozlov S, Devaux J *et al.* (2012) Behavioral and molecular exploration of the AR-CMT2A mouse model Lmna (R298C/R298C). *Neuromolecular Med* 14, 40–52.

101 Leal A, Morera B, Del Valle G *et al.* (2001) A second locus for an axonal form of autosomal recessive Charcot–Marie–Tooth disease maps to chromosome 19q13.3. *Am J Hum Genet* 68269–68274.

102 Berghoff C, Berghoff M, Leal A *et al.* (2004) Clinical and electrophysiological characteristics of autosomal recessive axonal Charcot–Marie–Tooth disease (ARCMT2B) that maps to chromosome 19q13.3. *Neuromuscul Disord* 14, 301–306.

103 Leal A, Huehne K, Bauer F *et al.* (2009) Identification of the variant Ala335Val of MED25 as responsible for CMT2B2: molecular data, functional studies of the SH3 recognition motif and correlation between wild-type MED25 and PMP22 RNA levels in CMT1A animal models. *Neurogenetics* 10, 275–287.

104 Guernsey DL, Jiang H, Bedard K *et al.* (2010) Mutation in the gene encoding ubiquitin ligase LRSAM1 in patients with Charcot–Marie–Tooth disease. *PLoS Genet* 6, pii: e1001081.

105 Ylikallio E, Pöyhönen R, Zimon M *et al.* (2013) Deficiency of the E3 ubiquitin ligase TRIM2 in early-onset axonal neuropathy. *Hum Mol Genet* 22, 2975–2983.

106 Balastik M, Ferraguti F, Pires-da Silva A *et al.* (2008) Deficiency in ubiquitin ligase TRIM2 causes accumulation of neurofilament light chain and neurodegeneration. *Proc Natl Acad Sci U S A.* 105, 12016–12021.

107 Zimoń M, Baets J, Almeida-Souza L *et al.* (2012) Loss-of-function mutations in HINT1 cause axonal neuropathy with neuromyotonia. *Nat Genet* 44, 1080–1083.

108 Hahn AF, Parkes AW, Bolton CF *et al.* (1991) Neuromyotonia in hereditary motor neuropathy. *J Neurol Neurosurg Psychiatry* 54, 230–235.

109 Evgrafov OV, Mersiyanova I, Irobi J *et al.* (2004) Mutant small heat-shock protein 27 causes axonal Charcot–Marie–Tooth disease and distal hereditary motor neuropathy. *Nat Genet* 36, 602–606.

110 Houlden H, Laura M, Wavrant-De Vrièze F *et al.* (2008) Mutations in the HSP27 (HSPB1) gene cause dominant, recessive, and sporadic distal HMN/CMT type 2. *Neurology* 71, 1660–1668.

CHAPTER 12

Dominant and recessive intermediate CMT (CMTDI and CMTRI)

Joachim Weis,[1] Andreas Roos,[1] Istvan Katona,[1] Kristl G. Claeys,[1,2] and Jan Senderek[3]

[1] *Institute of Neuropathology, RWTH Aachen University Hospital and JARA Brain Translational Medicine, Aachen, Germany*

[2] *Department of Neurology, RWTH Aachen University Hospital and JARA Brain Translational Medicine, Aachen, Germany*

[3] *Friedrich Baur Institute, Department of Neurology, Ludwig Maximilians University, Munich, Germany*

Definition

In 1978, Davis and colleagues suggested a classification of dominantly inherited peroneal muscular atrophy cases based on upper limb motor nerve conduction velocity (NCV) measurements. Cases with NCVs of >25 m/s were assigned to the demyelinating (or hypertrophic) neuropathy group, patients with NCVs between 25 and 45 m/s comprised the intermediate group and cases with NCVs >45 m/s were assigned to the axonal (or neuronal) sensorimotor neuropathy group [1]. Two years later, Harding and Thomas [2] proposed a median nerve motor NCV of 38 m/s as a cut-off value to distinguish between HMSN I (<38 m/s) and HMSN II (>38 m/s). The latter two-tiered system has been used more widely ever since, because it provided a more clear-cut distinction between the patient groups [3, 4]. However, the definition of an intermediate type of CMT has proven useful in the identification of gene defects in patients and families with motor NCVs between 25 and 45 m/s [3]. Gene defects that fall into this group include mutations in *DNM2*, *YARS*, and *INF2*. In addition, certain mutations in genes primarily involved in demyelinating or axonal neuropathies, for instance in *MPZ*, *NEFL*, or *GDAP1*, may be associated with intermediate CMT in some families. Moreover, NCVs may vary within the same family making it difficult to assign to either the HMSN I/CMT-1 or the HMSN II/CMT-2 or the intermediate CMT phenotype. Especially in families with X-linked CMT due to *GJB1/Cx32* mutations sex differences and non-random X-inactivation in females may lead to a wide range of NCV findings. Both demyelinating and axonal lesions may be prominent in nerve biopsies, and large myelinated nerve fibers are selectively affected in many cases. The gene defects leading to intermediate CMT are of special interest, because the same mutation may simultaneously cause axonal and Schwann cell damage. This is in line with the finding that many of the intermediate CMT genes are expressed in both axons and Schwann cells [4].

General clinical characteristics of intermediate CMT

Many clinical signs and symptoms are similar to those found in CMT1 and 2; they vary from mild and slowly progressive in most AD forms of intermediate CMT to severe, early-onset, and rapidly progressive in AR CMT due to Ganglioside-induced differentiation-associated protein-1 (GDAP1) mutation and many cases of AD CMT caused by Inverted Formin 2 (INF2) mutation.

Dominant intermediate CMT type A (CMTDIA; DI-CMTA; MIM 606483)

Hereditary neuropathy in a large Italian kindred was slowly progressive, with minor motor symptoms in childhood and severe walking difficulties in many older patients. Motor median NCVs were between 50 and

Peripheral Nerve Disorders: Pathology and Genetics, First Edition. Edited by Jean-Michel Vallat, Joachim Weis, Francoise Gray, and Katy Keohane.

96% of normal [5]. The disorder was mapped to chromosome 10q24.1-q25.1, but the mutated gene has not yet been identified [6]. In sural nerve biopsies, signs of axonal degeneration and regeneration, including clusters of regenerating nerve fibers, coexisted with Schwann cell onion bulbs and focal Schwann cell hyperplasia as well as myelin splits with uncompacted and irregularly enlarged lamellae, mostly at Schmidt–Lantermann incisures and in the paranodal region [5, 7]. Unmyelinated nerve fibers were also involved [7].

Dominant intermediate CMT type B (CMTDIB; DI-CMTB; MIM 606483); allelic with CMT2M

Definition, genetics, and pathogenesis

Mutations in the pleckstrin homology, middle, and proline-rich domains of the *Dynamin 2* (*DNM2*) gene on chromosome 19p12-p13.2 cause AD distal sensorimotor neuropathy [8–10]. Mutation of DNM2 can also lead to centronuclear myopathy (CNM). The same domains and even two adjacent amino acids have been shown to be involved in both conditions [11]. CNM patients may show reduced compound motor action potentials (CMAPs) [12] and other signs of peripheral nerve involvement [13]. Moreover, intramuscular nerve fibers in a CNM case were altered [14].

Dynamin 2 is a ubiquitously-expressed large GTPase involved in diverse cellular processes including clathrin-dependent and clathrin-independent endocytosis, membrane trafficking, vesicle formation, exocytosis, cytokinesis, phagocytosis, and cell migration [11, 15]. The protein is also involved in centrosome cohesion [16] and in the regulation of actin and microtubule networks [15]. Dynamin 2 binds to the phosphoinositides PtdIns(4,5)*P*2, and to Src-Homology-3 (SH3) domain proteins including amphiphysins [17]. Cultured Schwann cells expressing CMTDI-associated *DNM2* mutants showed defects in clathrin-mediated endocytosis and altered Schwann cell surface protein levels (21).

Clinical presentation

The disease usually starts with gait abnormalities and/or foot deformities in the first or second decade of life and follows a slowly progressive, rather benign course [9, 10]. Occasionally, neuropathy may be combined with cataracts and hematological abnormalities [9, 10]. NCVs range from 24 m/s to normal; CMAP amplitudes are reduced or normal [10].

Histopathology

In sural nerve biopsies there is selective loss of large myelinated axons, but few, if any acutely degenerating nerve fibers [8, 10]. Groups of regenerating fibers are frequent; thus, the overall number of nerve fibers was actually increased in one case [10]. Segmental de- and remyelination with onion bulb formation was sparse in one case [8] and absent in another [10]. In the latter case, occasional myelin sheath thickenings and abnormally widened Schmidt–Lanterman incisures were found [10]. Groups of collagen pockets and of flattened Schwann cell processes indicated that unmyelinated fibers were also affected [10].

CMT2M

Fabrizi and colleagues reported two unrelated families with AD CMT and heterozygous mutations in the *DNM2* gene [18]. NCV analysis was consistent with an axonal neuropathy. Nerve biopsies of two cases revealed loss of large myelinated nerve fibers, an overall reduction in the number of myelinated fibers, numerous clusters of regenerating fibers, and occasional onion bulb formations [18]. No paranodal or segmental demyelination was observed in teased fiber preparations. Numerous collagen pockets were found by EM and indicated loss of unmyelinated fibers [18]. Further patients with axonal CMT due to *DNM2* mutation have been reported [19, 20].

Animal models

Dnm2 knockout in mice resulted in early embryonic lethality [21]. Lentiviral expression of CMTDIB-related *Dnm2* mutants in dorsal root ganglia explants derived from embryos carrying a heterozygous *Dnm2* null allele reduced myelination [22]. Further *drosophila*, *C. elegans*, and mammalian models of pathologies related to *DNM2* mutation have been established [17, 23, 24].

Dominant intermediate CMT type C (CMTDIC; DI-CMTC; MIM 603623)

Definition, clinical presentation, genetics, and pathogenesis

Mutation of the *YARS* gene encoding tyrosyl-tRNA synthetase (TyrRS) caused moderately severe, slowly progressive sensorimotor neuropathy with onset between the age of 10 and 60 years, distal weakness, leg muscle atrophy, and motor median NCVs between 25 and 58 m/s [25, 26]. Functional *in vitro* studies suggested that the mutant proteins partially lose their aminoacylation activity [26]. Mutations in other aminoacyl tRNA synthetase genes lead to further forms of hereditary neuropathies including CMT 2N and CMT 2D (see Chapter 10) and recessive intermediate CMT type B (CMTRIB; see next).

Histopathology

Sural nerve biopsies demonstrated clusters of regenerating nerve fibers and age-dependent reduction in fiber density and myelin thickness, but no onion bulbs [25].

Animal model

Ubiquitous as well as selective neuronal expression of mutant TyrRS caused axonal degeneration and neuronal dysfunction in *Drosophila* [27].

Dominant intermediate CMT type D (CMTDID; DI-CMTD; MIM 607792)

Myelin protein zero (*MPZ*) mutations cause both demyelinating and axonal CMT as well as congenital hypomyelinating neuropathy (see Chapter 10). Therefore it is not surprising that *MPZ* mutations can also lead to intermediate CMT (see, e.g., [28, 29]) with moderately reduced NCV and histological evidence of combined axonal degeneration and segmental myelin sheath degeneration and regeneration [28] (Fig. 12.1A).

Dominant intermediate CMT type E (CMTDIE; DI-CMTE; MIM 614455)

Definition and genetics

Mutations in the *Inverted formin 2* (*INF2*) gene on chromosome 14q32.33 cause isolated dominant focal segmental glomerulosclerosis-5 (FSGS5; MIM 613237) and dominant intermediate Charcot–Marie–Tooth disease with FSGS [30, 31]. Schwann cells strongly express INF2 while axons showed minor INF2-immunoreactivity [30]. Formins mediate actin filament formation and actin-microtubule crosstalk [32]. The INF2 protein interacts with the actin-regulating Rho-GTPase CDC42 and the myelin and lymphocyte protein (MAL), both of which are known to be crucial for myelination and myelin maintenance [33, 34]. Interestingly, mutations causing neuropathy are localized within the CDC42 binding domain of INF2 [31]. In functional studies, INF2 mutation led to altered intracellular MAL distribution and to dysregulated actin-dependent processes including mitochondrial fission [30, 35].

Clinical presentation and epidemiology

INF2-related sensory neuropathy is usually severe starting in the first or second decade of life [30]. Median NCVs were 23–45 m/s [30]. CNS anomalies as well as sensory hearing loss can be present [30, 31]. INF2 mutations are detectable in 75% of FSGS-CMT patients [30].

Histopathology

INF2-related CMT is characterized by age-dependent axonal loss, severe hypomyelination with onion bulb formations, and supernumerary elongated cytoplasmic extensions of many non-myelinating Schwann cells [30] (Fig. 12.1B).

Dominant intermediate CMT type F (CMTDIF; DI-CMTF; MIM 615185)

Definition, genetics, and pathogenesis

This neuropathy is caused by mutation of the *GNB4* gene encoding guanine-nucleotide-binding protein subunit beta-4 ($G\beta_4$)[36, 37]. G proteins interact with cell surface receptors to transmit signals into the cell. *In vitro* studies demonstrated that wild-type $G\beta_4$ facilitates bradykinin-induced G-protein-coupled-receptor (GPCR) signaling, which is impaired by pathogenic $G\beta_4$ mutations [36].

Clinical presentation

The age of onset ranges from 10–45 years and clinical severity varies from being asymptomatic to being wheelchair-bound. Males appear more severely affected than females. Median motor NCVs were between 16 and 46 m/s [36, 37].

Histopathology

$G\beta_4$ is expressed by many cell types. $G\beta_4$ immunoreactivity was abundant in axons and Schwann cells of normal nerves [36]. Sural nerve biopsies revealed

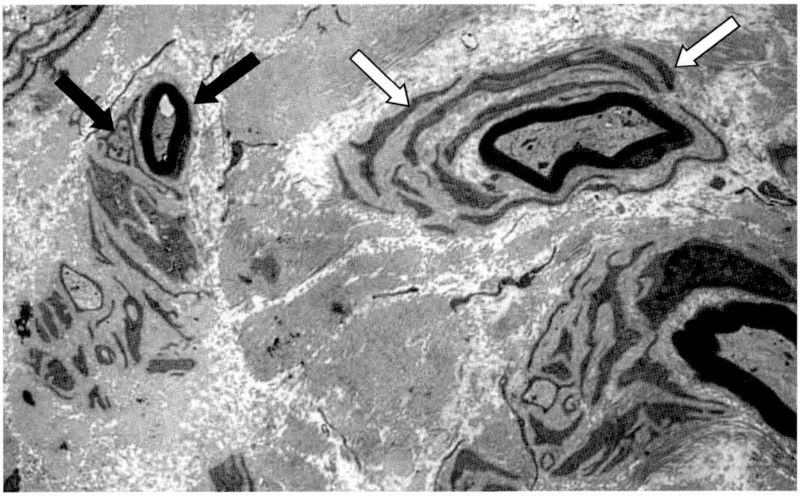

(A)

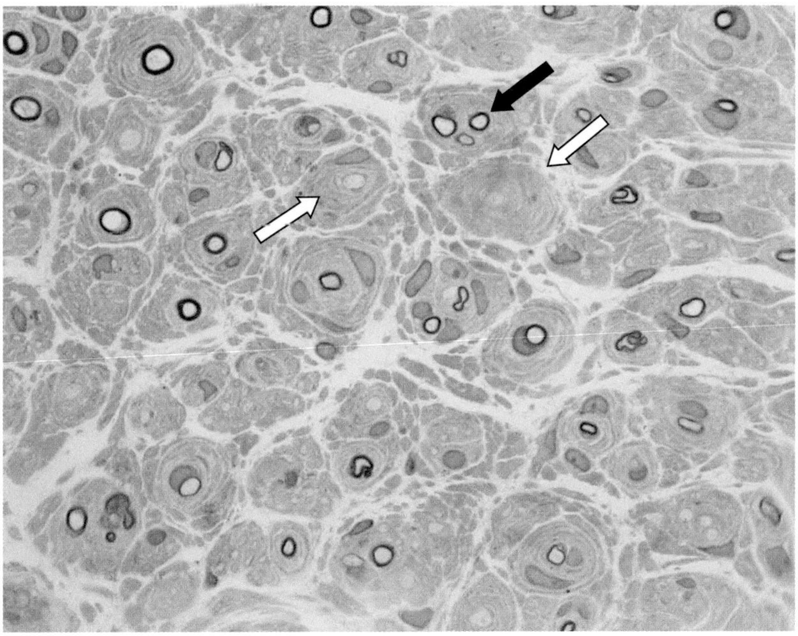

(B)

Figure 12.1 Sural nerve biopsy findings in intermediate CMT. (**A**) Onion bulb formation (white arrows) containing a disproportionately thin myelinated axon indicating de- and remyelination and a cluster of regenerated myelinated and unmyelinated nerve fibers (black arrows) indicative of previous axonal breakdown in intermediate CMT due to *MPZ* mutation. Electron microscopy. (**B**) Prominent onion bulb formations (white arrows) and occasional clusters of regenerating nerve fibers (black arrow) in a case of neuropathy due to *INF2* mutation. Semithin section, Toluidine blue. (**C**) Onion bulb formation, (**D**) cluster of regenerated nerve fibers, one of which shows abnormal myelin folding (arrow) and (**E**) rominent intra-axonal accumulation of organelles in a myelinated nerve fiber in a case of neuropathy due to *NEFL* mutation. Electron microscopy.

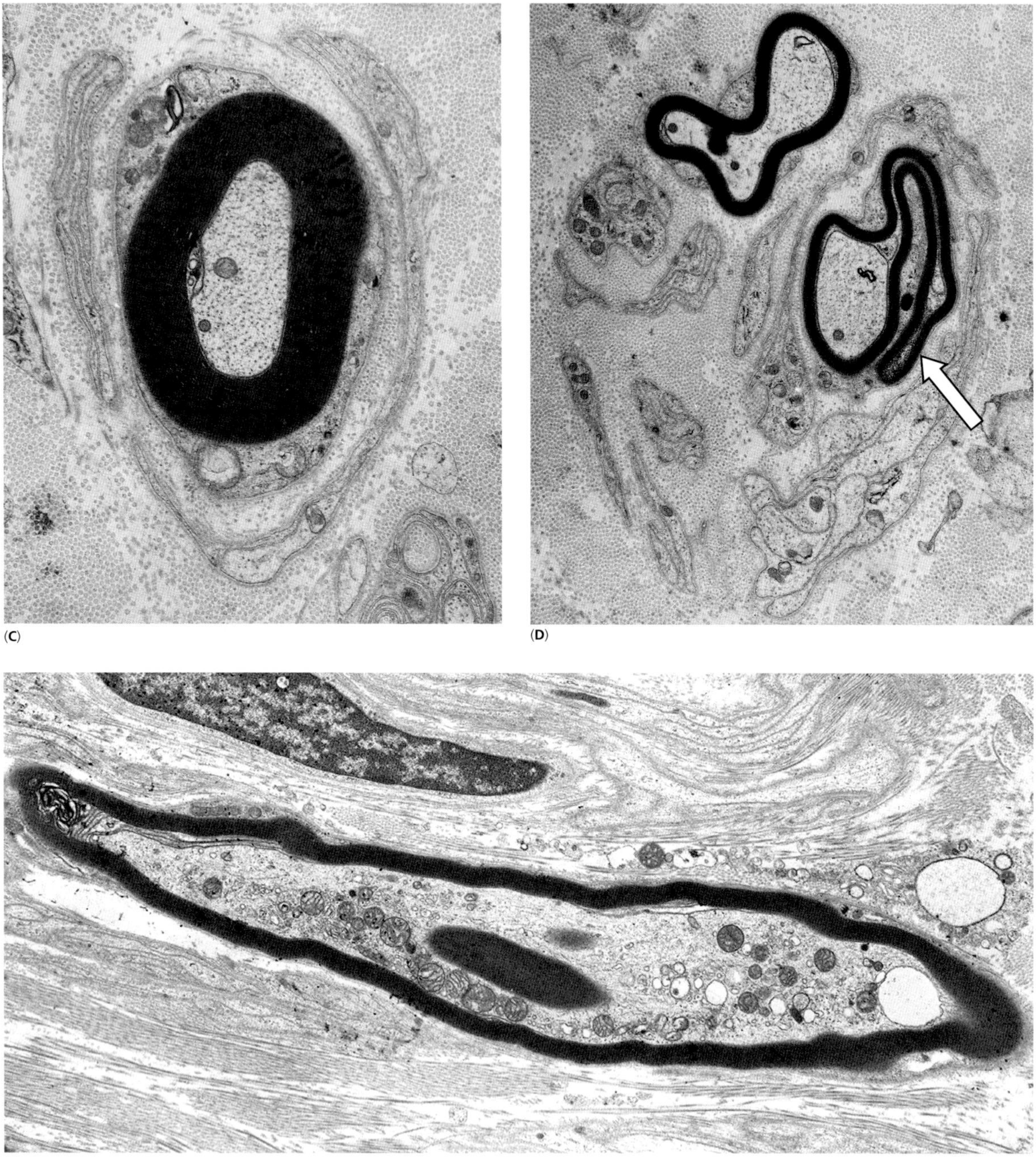

Figuer 12.1 (*Continued*)

loss of myelinated fibers, clusters of regenerating nerve fibers and onion bulb formations [36, 37]. Axon and Schwann cell immunoreactivity for Gβ_4 was reduced in two Gly53Asp Gβ_4 mutation patients [36]; in one patient, the residual Gβ_4 immunoreactivity gave a "rosette" pattern with Gβ4 staining both in the axons and in the cytoplasm of surrounding Schwann cells [36].

Recessive intermediate CMT type A (CMTRIA; RI-CMTA; MIM 608340)

Definition, clinical presentation, genetics, and pathogenesis

Ganglioside-induced differentiation-associated protein-1 (GDAP1) mutation can cause several forms of CMT, including CMT4A (Chapter 13), CMT2K (Chapter 10), and AD CMT (Chapter 10) with pyramidal involvement Functional *in vitro* studies suggest that GDAP1 regulates mitochondrial and peroxisomal fission [38], and mitochondrial movement [39]. An early-onset, severe AR intermediate CMT with variable NCVs and both axonal and demyelinating phenotypes has been observed by several groups [40–43]. NCVs were between 25 and 35 m/s in one study and [40] and highly variable in another [41].

Histopathology

In nerve biopsies, axonal as well as demyelinating changes with predominant loss of large myelinated fibers as well as onion bulb formations were found [40, 41]. A few nerve fibers showed redundant myelin loops and folded myelin sheaths [41]. These findings support the notion that GDAP1 is important for both axonal integrity and Schwann cell maintenance [40, 41]. Interestingly, mitochondrial abnormalities including focal accumulations, enlargement, and disorganized cristae were found in many axons of a recently described case of intermediate CMT due to GDAP1 mutation, consistent with the proposed function of GDAP1 in mitochondrial fission [29]. Unmyelinated fibers appeared to be well preserved in a nerve biopsy studied by EM [41]. A combined axonal and demyelinating phenotype with similar histopathological changes was also found in AD CMT due to GDAP1 mutation [44].

Recessive intermediate CMT type B (CMTRIB; RI-CMTB; MIM 613641)

Compound heterozygosity for two variants of the *lysyl-tRNA synthetase* (*KARS*) gene was found in a single patient with intermediate CMT, developmental delay, self-abusive behavior, dysmorphic features, and vestibular schwannoma [45].

Recessive intermediate CMT type C (CMTRIB; RI-CMTC; MIM 615376)

Definition, clinical presentation, and genetics

A single autosomal recessive mutation of the *Pleckstrin homology domain-containing, family G, member 5* (*PLEKHG5*) gene was initially described as causing lower motor neuron disease with childhood onset/ autosomal recessive distal spinal muscular atrophy-4 [46]. More recently, two different homozygous truncating mutations [47] and compound heterozygosity for two missense mutations [48] in *PLEKHG5* were found to lead to intermediate CMT with moderately decreased NCVs.

Pathogenesis and animal model

PLEKHG5 is expressed by both neuronal and glial cells [47, 48]. *In vitro* assays using transfected cells suggested that the missense mutants show impaired ability to activate the NFKB signaling pathway [46, 48] and form intracellular aggregates [46]. *PLEKHG5* knockout mice showed reduced NCVs [47].

Histopathology

In sural nerve biopsies, marked loss of large nerve fires, axonal atrophy, clusters of regenerating fibers, disproportionately thin myelin sheaths of the remaining large axons, myelin folds, as well as endoneurial fibrosis, were found [47, 48]. Overall lowered levels of PLEKHG5 as well as abnormal accumulation of PLEKHG5 immunoreactivity in Schwann cell nuclei were observed in one biopsy [48].

Miscellaneous

NEFL

Other cases of CMT with intermediate NCV include patients with mutations in the *NEFL* gene encoding neurofilament light chain [49]. Nerve biopsies showed both demyelinating and axonal changes including prominent axonal swellings and focal alterations of the axonal cytoskeleton [49] (Fig. 12.1C–E).

MFN2

Even though *MFN2* (*Mitofusin 2*) mutations lead to axonal CMT in most cases, families with intermediate CMT have been described [50, 51].

Connexin 32/GJB1

Intermediate type CMT is a classical presentation of neuropathy caused by mutation of the *Connexin 32/GJB1* gene (see Chapter 13).

ARHGEF10

The autosomal-dominantly inherited Thr109Ile mutation in the *ARHGEF10* (Rho guanine-nucleotide exchange factor 10) gene caused moderate, non-progressive slowing of NCVs without an overt clinical phenotype in numerous members of a large family [52, 53]. Nerve biopsy revealed disproportionately thin myelin sheaths of many large fibers as well as rare onion bulb formations and clusters of regenerating nerve fibers [52, 53]. These findings are indicative of a congenital disorder of peripheral nerve fiber/myelin sheath development.

References

1 Davis CJ, Bradley WG, Madrid R (1978) The peroneal muscular atrophy syndrome: clinical, genetic, electrophysiological and nerve biopsy studies. I. Clinical, genetic and electrophysiological findings and classification. *J Genet Hum*;26:311–349.

2 Harding AE, Thomas PK (1980) The clinical features of hereditary motor and sensory neuropathy types I and II. *Brain*;103:259–280.

3 Shy ME, Lupski JR, Chance PF *et al.* (2005) Hereditary motor and sensory neuropathies: An overview of clinical, genetic, electrophysiologic, and pathologic features. In: Dyck PJ, Thomas PK (eds). *Peripheral Neuropathy*. Elsevier Saunders, Philadelphia.

4 Nicholson G, Myers S (2006) Intermediate forms of Charcot–Marie–Tooth neuropathy: a review. *Neuromolecular Med*;8: 123–130.

5 Rossi A, Paradiso C, Cioni R *et al.* (1985) Charcot–Marie–Tooth disease: study of a large kinship with an intermediate form. *J Neurol*;232:91–98.

6 Verhoeven K, Villanova M, Rossi A *et al.* (2001) Localization of the gene for the intermediate form of Charcot–Marie–Tooth to chromosome 10q24.1-q25.1. *Am J Hum Genet*;69:889–894.

7 Malandrini A, Ceuterick C, Villanov M *et al.* (2001) Ultrastructural findings in the peripheral nerve in a family with the intermediate form of Charcot–Marie–Tooth disease. *J Submicrosc Cytol Pathol*;33:59–63.

8 Kennerson ML, Zhu D, Gardner RJ *et al.* (2001) Dominant intermediate Charcot–Marie–Tooth neuropathy maps to chromosome 19p12-p13.2. *Am J Hum Genet*;69:883–888.

9 Zuchner S, Noureddine M, Kennerson M *et al.* (2005) Mutations in the pleckstrin homology domain of dynamin 2 cause dominant intermediate Charcot–Marie–Tooth disease. *Nat Genet*;37:289–294.

10 Claeys KG, Zuchner S, Kennerson M, *et al.* (2009) Phenotypic spectrum of dynamin 2 mutations in Charcot–Marie–Tooth neuropathy. *Brain*;132:1741–1752.

11 Bohm J, Biancalana V, Dechene ET, *et al.* (2012) Mutation spectrum in the large GTPase dynamin 2, and genotype-phenotype correlation in autosomal dominant centronuclear myopathy. *Hum Mutat*;33:949–959.

12 Fischer D, Herasse M, Bitoun M, *et al.* (2006) Characterization of the muscle involvement in dynamin 2-related centronuclear myopathy. *Brain*;129:1463–149.

13 Echaniz-Laguna A, Nicot AS, Carre S, *et al.* (2007) Subtle central and peripheral nervous system abnormalities in a family with centronuclear myopathy and a novel dynamin 2 gene mutation. *Neuromuscul Disord*;17:955–959.

14 Jeub M, Bitoun M, Guicheney P, Kappes-Horn K, *et al.* (2008) Dynamin 2-related centronuclear myopathy: clinical, histological and genetic aspects of further patients and review of the literature. *Clin Neuropathol*;27:430–438.

15 Durieux AC, Prudhon B, Guicheney P, Bitoun M. (2010) Dynamin 2 and human diseases. *J Mol Med (Berl)*;88:339–350.

16 Thompson HM, Cao H, Chen J, *et al.* (2004). Dynamin 2 binds gamma-tubulin and participates in centrosome cohesion. *Nat Cell Biol*;6:335–342.

17 Cowling BS, Toussaint A, Muller J, Laporte J (2012) Defective membrane remodeling in neuromuscular diseases: insights from animal models. *PLoS Genet*;8:e1002595.

18 Fabrizi GM, Ferrarini M, Cavallaro T, *et al.* (2007) Two novel mutations in dynamin-2 cause axonal Charcot–Marie–Tooth disease. *Neurology*;69:291–295.

19 Bitoun M, Stojkovic T, Prudhon B, *et al.* (2008) A novel mutation in the dynamin 2 gene in a Charcot–Marie–Tooth type 2 patient: clinical and pathological findings. *Neuromuscul Disord*;18:334–338.

20 Gallardo E, Claeys KG, Nelis E, *et al.*(2008) Magnetic resonance imaging findings of leg musculature in Charcot–Marie–Tooth disease type 2 due to dynamin 2 mutation. *J Neurol*;255:986–992.

21 Ferguson SM, Raimondi A, Paradise S, *et al.* (2009) Coordinated actions of actin and BAR proteins upstream of dynamin at endocytic clathrin-coated pits. *Dev Cell*;17:811–822.
22 Sidiropoulos PN, Miehe M, Bock T, *et al.* (2012) Dynamin 2 mutations in Charcot–Marie–Tooth neuropathy highlight the importance of clathrin-mediated endocytosis in myelination. *Brain*;135:1395–1411.
23 Tinelli E, Pereira JA, Suter U (2013) Muscle-specific function of the centronuclear myopathy and Charcot–Marie–Tooth neuropathy-associated dynamin 2 is required for proper lipid metabolism, mitochondria, muscle fibers, neuromuscular junctions and peripheral nerves. *Hum Mol Genet*;22:4417–4429.
24 Durieux AC, Vassilopoulos S, Laine J, *et al.* (2012) A centronuclear myopathy– dynamin 2 mutation impairs autophagy in mice. *Traffic*;13:869–879.
25 Jordanova A, Thomas FP, Guergueltcheva V, *et al.* (2003) Dominant intermediate Charcot–Marie–Tooth type C maps to chromosome 1p34-p35. *Am J Hum Genet*;73:1423–1430.
26 Jordanova A, Irobi J, Thomas FP, *et al.* (2006) Disrupted function and axonal distribution of mutant tyrosyl-tRNA synthetase in dominant intermediate Charcot–Marie–Tooth neuropathy. *Nat Genet*;38:197–202.
27 Storkebaum E, Leitao-Goncalves R, Godenschwege T, *et al.* (2009) Dominant mutations in the tyrosyl-tRNA synthetase gene recapitulate in *Drosophila* features of human Charcot–Marie–Tooth neuropathy. *Proc Natl Acad Sci U S A*;106: 11782–11787.
28 Mastaglia FL, Nowak KJ, Stell R, *et al.* (1999) Novel mutation in the myelin protein zero gene in a family with intermediate hereditary motor and sensory neuropathy. *J Neurol Neurosurg Psychiatry*;67:174–179.
29 Benedetti S, Previtali SC, Coviello S, *et al.* (2010) Analyzing histopathological features of rare Charcot–Marie–Tooth neuropathies to unravel their pathogenesis. *Arch Neurol*;67: 1498–1505.
30 Boyer O, Nevo F, Plaisier E, *et al.* (2011) INF2 mutations in Charcot–Marie–Tooth disease with glomerulopathy. *N Engl J Med*;365:2377–88.
31 Mademan I, Deconinck T, Dinopoulos A, *et al.* (2013) De novo INF2 mutations expand the genetic spectrum of hereditary neuropathy with glomerulopathy. *Neurology*;81:1953–1958.
32 Breitsprecher D, Goode BL (2013) Formins at a glance. *J Cell Sci*;126:1–7.
33 Madrid R, Aranda JF, Rodriguez-Fraticelli AE, *et al.* (2010) The formin INF2 regulates basolateral-to-apical transcytosis and lumen formation in association with Cdc42 and MAL2. *Dev Cell*;18:814–827.
34 Andres-Delgado L, Anton OM, Madrid R, *et al.* (2010) Formin INF2 regulates MAL-mediated transport of Lck to the plasma membrane of human T lymphocytes. *Blood*;116:5919–5929.
35 Korobova F, Ramabhadran V, Higgs HN (2013) An actin-dependent step in mitochondrial fission mediated by the ER-associated formin INF2. *Science*;339:464–467.
36 Soong BW, Huang YH, Tsai PC, *et al.* (2013) Exome sequencing identifies GNB4 mutations as a cause of dominant intermediate Charcot–Marie–Tooth disease. *Am J Hum Genet*;92:422–430.
37 Lee YC, Lee TC, Lin KP, *et al.* (2010) Clinical characterization and genetic analysis of a possible novel type of dominant Charcot–Marie–Tooth disease. *Neuromuscul Disord*;20:534–539.
38 Huber N, Guimaraes S, Schrader M, *et al.* (2013) Charcot–Marie–Tooth disease-associated mutants of GDAP1 dissociate its roles in peroxisomal and mitochondrial fission. *EMBO Rep*;14:545–552.
39 Pla-Martin D, Rueda CB, Estela A, *et al.* (2013) Silencing of the Charcot–Marie–Tooth disease-associated gene GDAP1 induces abnormal mitochondrial distribution and affects Ca2+ homeostasis by reducing store-operated Ca2+ entry. *Neurobiol Dis*;55:140–151.
40 Senderek J, Bergmann C, Ramaekers VT, *et al.* (2003) Mutations in the ganglioside-induced differentiation-associated protein-1 (GDAP1) gene in intermediate type autosomal recessive Charcot–Marie–Tooth neuropathy. *Brain*;126:642–629
41 Nelis E, Erdem S, Van Den Bergh PY, *et al.* (2002) Mutations in GDAP1: autosomal recessive CMT with demyelination and axonopathy. *Neurology*;59:1865–1872.
42 Kabzinska D, Drac H, Rowinska-Marcinska K, *et al.* (2006) Early onset Charcot–Marie–Tooth disease caused by a homozygous Leu239Phe mutation in the GDAP1 gene. *Acta Myol*;25:34–37.
43 Chung KW, Hyun YS, Lee HJ, *et al.* (2011) Two recessive intermediate Charcot–Marie–Tooth patients with GDAP1 mutations. *J Peripher Nerv Syst*;16:143–146.
44 Chung KW, Kim SM, Sunwoo IN, *et al.* (2008) A novel GDAP1 Q218E mutation in autosomal dominant Charcot–Marie–Tooth disease. *J Hum Genet*;53:360–364.
45 McLaughlin HM, Sakaguchi R, Liu C, *et al.* (2010) Compound heterozygosity for loss-of-function lysyl-tRNA synthetase mutations in a patient with peripheral neuropathy. *Am J Hum Genet*;87:560–566.
46 Maystadt I, Rezsohazy R, Barkats M, *et al.* (2007) The nuclear factor kappaB-activator gene PLEKHG5 is mutated in a form of autosomal recessive lower motor neuron disease with childhood onset. *Am J Hum Genet*;81:67–76.
47 Azzedine H, Zavadakova P, Plante-Bordeneuve V, *et al.* (2013) PLEKHG5 deficiency leads to an intermediate form of autosomal-recessive Charcot–Marie–Tooth disease. *Hum Mol Genet*;22:4224–4232.
48 Kim HJ, Hong YB, Park JM, *et al.* (2013) Mutations in the PLEKHG5 gene is relevant with autosomal recessive intermediate Charcot–Marie–Tooth disease. *Orphanet J Rare Dis*;8:104.
49 Fabrizi GM, Cavallaro T, Angiari C, *et al.* (2007) Charcot–Marie–Tooth disease type 2E, a disorder of the cytoskeleton. *Brain*;130:394–403.
50 Verhoeven K, Claeys KG, Zuchner S, *et al.* (2006) MFN2 mutation distribution and genotype/phenotype correlation in Charcot–Marie–Tooth type 2. *Brain*;129:2093–2102.

51 Braathen GJ, Sand JC, Lobato A, *et al.* (2010) MFN2 point mutations occur in 3.4% of Charcot–Marie–Tooth families. An investigation of 232 Norwegian CMT families. *BMC Med Genet*;11:48.

52 De Jonghe P, Timmerman V, Nelis E, *et al.* (1999) A novel type of hereditary motor and sensory neuropathy characterized by a mild phenotype. *Arch Neurol*;56:1283–1288.

53 Verhoeven K, De Jonghe P, Van de Putte T, *et al.* (2003) Slowed conduction and thin myelination of peripheral nerves associated with mutant rho Guanine-nucleotide exchange factor 10. *Am J Hum Genet*;73:926–932.

CHAPTER 13

X-linked neuropathy of the Charcot–Marie–Tooth type*

J. Michael Schröder[1] and Jan Senderek[2]

[1] Institute of Neuropathology, RWTH Aachen University Hospital and JARA Brain Translational Medicine, Aachen, Germany

[2] Friedrich Baur Institute, Department of Neurology, Ludwig-Maximilians University, Munich, Germany

Introduction

X-linked dominant Charcot–Marie–Tooth neuropathy (CMTX) comprises about 10% of cases with CMT or hereditary motor and sensory neuropathy (HMSN). There is genetic heterogeneity in X-chromosomal CMT neuropathies. They may be inherited as dominant (CMTX1, CMTX6) or recessive traits (CMTX2 – CMTX5).

CMTX1 = HMSN X1 (MIM 304040)

CMTX1 makes up most of the cases with X-linked CMT and has emerged as the second most common form of CMT1.

Clinical aspects

Symptoms and signs resemble those of CMT1, but male patients are usually more severely affected and there is no male-to-male transmission. Although the age of onset varies considerably (6–35 years), most males are clinically affected by 10 years of age. The clinical presentation of male patients ranges from moderate to severe. Female carriers usually have a later onset than men, show milder symptoms at every age or may be only subclinically affected. The mean motor nerve conduction velocity (MNCV) in males is 31 m/s, range: 27.7–33.3 m/s; whereas in females it is 40 m/s, range: 35–49 m/s [1]. The compound muscle action potentials (CMAP) and sensory nerve action potentials (SNAP) show reduced amplitudes. Some patients have been reported with transient CNS phenomena, including dysarthria, ataxia, tetraparesis, or stroke-like episodes. Reversible bilateral white matter lesions and restricted diffusion on magnetic resonance imaging are characteristic features of the CNS phenotype of CMTX1 [2–4]. One individual with the p.Ala39Val mutation had postural upper limb tremor (Roussy–Levy syndrome) [5]. Analysis of brain stem evoked auditory responses (BEAR) revealed changes in central auditory pathways [2, 3].

Genetics

CMTX1 is caused by hemizygous (or heterozygous) mutations in the gap junction protein B1 (GJB1) gene on chromosome Xq13 coding for the gap junction protein B1 with a molecular weight of 32 kDa (Connexin32, Cx32) [1, 5–12]. Cx32 has been localized in the non-compact peripheral myelin sheath presumably forming gap junctions between adjacent myelin loops.

More than 400 genomic variants of the *GJB1 gene* have been detected [13]. Most disease-causing *GJB1* mutations occur in the coding region, however, mutations altering non-coding regions and genomic deletions have also been reported [14, 15]. There was no consistent relationship between the site and type of connexin32 mutation and the severity of the phenotype [5].

*(CMT X = Hereditary motor and sensory neuropathy type X, HMSN X)

Peripheral Nerve Disorders: Pathology and Genetics, First Edition. Edited by Jean-Michel Vallat, Joachim Weis, Francoise Gray, and Katy Keohane.

Coincidental combination of CMTX1 with a *PMP22* duplication (CMT1A) [16], and with Becker's X-chromosomal muscular dystrophy ("double trouble") have been reported [17].

Histopathology

Semithin sections reveal marked loss of predominantly large myelinated nerve fibers and numerous clusters of small, thinly myelinated, and unmyelinated fibers (Figs. 13.1A–D) [1, 5, 18]. There are many axons with disproportionately thin myelin sheaths in relation to the axon caliber. The myelinated nerve fiber histogram is skewed towards smaller and more thinly myelinated fibers. The g ratio is elevated accordingly (0.65+/−0.09). Small onion bulb formations indicating demyelination and subsequent remyelination are less frequent. Teased fiber preparations reveal occasional widened nodal gaps and focal separation of the myelin sheath from the axon or swelling of the non-compacted Schwann cell cytoplasm of paranodal myelin loops [12].

There are several descriptions of ultrastructural changes in sural nerves [5, 12, 18–22]. Non-compacted parts of the myelin sheaths showed disturbances of myelin structure in four biopsy samples [5]: membranous whorls and microvesicular disintegration of myelin lamellae at Schmidt–Lanterman incisures and paranodes. Abnormal widening of the Schwann cell cytoplasm occurred between axons and the compact myelin sheath. The innermost myelin layers frequently displayed partial dissolution and an abnormal arrangement. The "axoglial" attachment zone repeatedly showed extended transverse-band like structures (Fig. 13.2). Abnormal contacts between adjacent membranes of myelin lamellae with disappearance of the extracellular space were focally noted at higher magnification (Fig. 13.2C) [5]. The axons showed abnormal vesicular or electron-dense inclusions and occasional accumulations of mitochondria with calcium-like precipitates. Some axons showed condensation with increased neurofilaments and relative decrease of microtubules [12]. There was ample deposition of endoneurial collagen. Heterozygous female patients showed qualitatively similar, but less prominent changes [1, 12]. In summary, the combination of signs of de- and remyelination and regenerative clusters of thinly myelinated axons together with abnormal widening of the Schwann cell cytoplasm between axons and compact myelin at the ultrastructural level are evocative of this CMT subtype (J.M. Vallat, personal communication).

Experimental models

Cx32-deficient mice have prominent adaxonal Schwann cell alterations ("periaxonal collars") [23] at the ultrastructural level [23, 24] suggesting similar pathological mechanisms in patients and knockout mice [5]. Axonal changes (reduction of axonal diameters, increased neurofilaments with distal slowing of axonal transport) precede signs of demyelination [25]. A nerve segment from a CMTX patient grafted into nude mice caused atrophy of wild-type axons ensheathed by mutant Schwann cells suggesting that *GJB1* mutations may impair modulatory functions of Schwann cells on axons [26].

Pathogenesis

Mutations ablating Cx32 expression in human CMTX1, *Gjb1* knockout mice and the observation that many Cx32 mutants fail to form functional gap junctions indicate that loss of gap function is the fundamental alteration of most CMT1X mutants [13]. Cx32 is located at the non-compacted parts of the myelin sheath, that is, at the nodes of Ranvier and Schmidt–Lanterman incisures [6, 27]. There is growing evidence that the gap junctions, which are known to contain Cx32, allow ions, metabolites, and second messengers to traverse the myelin lamellae on a radial shortcut instead of travelling through the spirals of Schwann cell cytoplasm [6, 27, 28]. Although advanced demyelination and remyelination are rare [1, 5, 20, 29], some of the multiple ultrastructural abnormalities of noncompact myelin observed in CMTX1 sural nerve biopsy specimens might be related to interruptions of this pathway, while others are non-specific [30, 31].

The most apparent clinical manifestation of Cx32 deficiency is peripheral neuropathy although Cx32 is expressed in various cell populations, namely liver cells, epithelial cells, oligodendrocytes, and Schwann cells. Transient CNS symptoms and involvement of central auditory pathways are observed in human patients, and Cx32-deficient mice exhibit impaired glucose release from hepatocytes [32].

Conclusions

The clinical and pathological features of CMTX1 are of an intermediate, predominantly axonal, partly demyelinating neuropathy. *GJB1* mutations are likely to affect

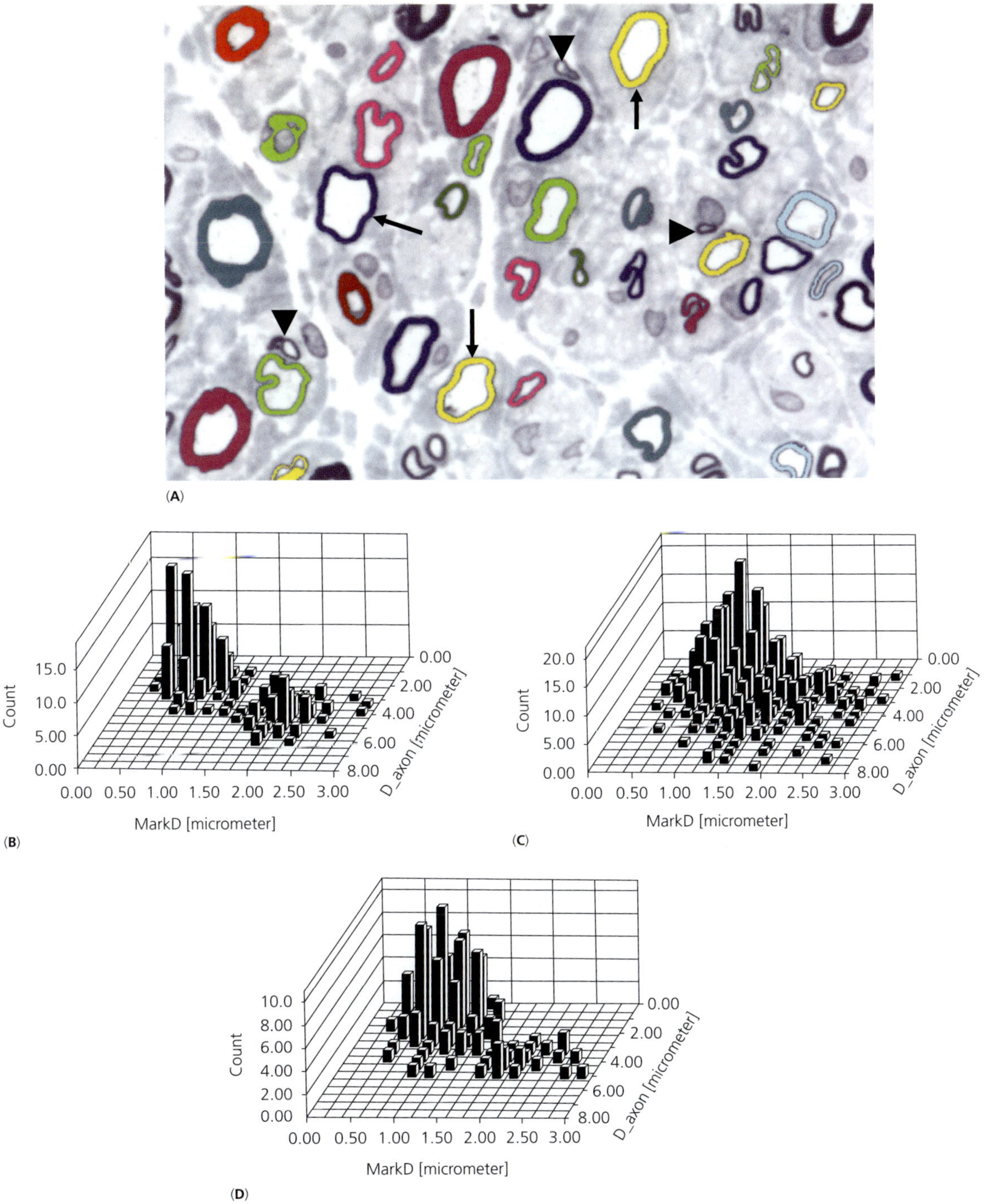

Figure 13.1 Optic-electronic evaluation of a semithin cross section from the sural nerve of a 15-year-old boy (**A, C**) and his 44-year-old mother (**D**) with CMTX1 in comparison to the sural nerve from a 12-year-old control (**B**), using the KS 300 system of Zeiss-Kontron, Oberkochen, Germany [19]. The area is shown at the highest available light microscopic resolution of a planapochromat objective lens (×100). The number of nerve fibers is reduced. Some myelin sheaths are disproportionately thin in relation to the size of their axons (arrows). Most myelinated fibers are matched quite precisely by pseudocolors with the exception of some small myelinated fibers that are closely attached to a neighboring larger, regenerated fiber (arrowheads). The 3D diagrams (**B–D**) illustrate the number of evaluated fibers (*y*-axis), and the wide scatter of myelin thickness (*x*-axis) related to axonal diameters (*z*-axis), especially in the affected boy's nerve (**C**). Source: Schröder, 2006 [47]. Adapted with permission of Humana Press.

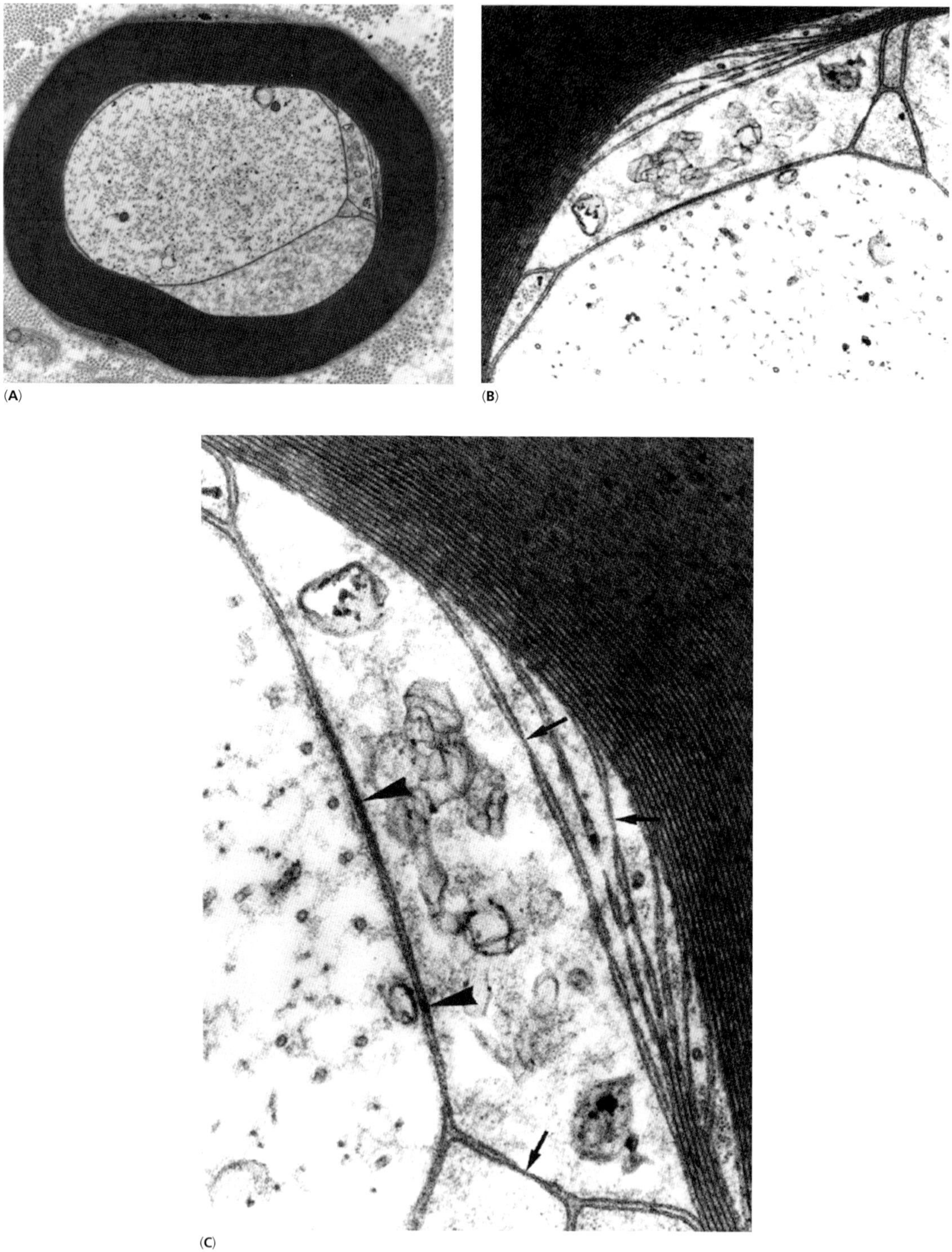

Figure 13.2 Electron micrographs from the same case as in Figure 13.1. The paranodal, adaxonal myelin loops are considerably distended. There are unusual contacts between adjacent membranes that focally form transverse bands similar to those seen in normal paranodes though at an abnormal site (arrowheads). The arrows indicate fusion of adjacent processes of Schwann cells. **A** × 12,600; **B** × 49,000; **C** × 95,000. Source: Senderek *et al.*, 1998 [1]. Reproduced with permission of Springer.

gap junctions between myelin lamellae of Schwann cells where Cx32 is located and where multiple ultrastructural changes were observed. Disturbed (reciprocal) Schwann cell-axon interactions may contribute to secondary axonal changes and complicate the situation in the PNS [33]. The CNS is less prominently affected while other organs expressing high levels of Cx32 are spared in CMTX1 patients.

CMTX2 (MIM 302801) and CMTX3 (MIM 302802)

Clinical aspects

The disease phenotype in one family was characterized by infantile onset, weakness of lower legs, areflexia, pes cavus, and mental retardation (two of five patients). In other families there was late onset, distal weakness, and normal intelligence. Hereditary spastic paraparesis was also present in the CMT patients of one family [34]. Electrophysiological studies were consistent with both demyelination and axonal involvement. Carrier females were unaffected.

Genetics

Ionasescu *et al.* [34, 35] presented data suggesting the existence of two separate loci for X-linked recessive disorders mapping to sites other than CMTX1: CMTX2, which maps to chromosome Xp22.2, and CMTX3, which maps to chromosome Xq26. The genes mutated in these X-linked recessive neuropathies have not yet been identified.

Histopathology

There are no data available.

CMTX4 (MIM 310490)

Synonyms

X-linked recessive Charcot–Marie–Tooth disease (CMTX4); CMT with deafness and mental retardation; neuropathy, axonal motor sensory, with deafness and mental retardation (NAMSD) (NAMDR); Cowchock syndrome.

Cowchock *et al.* described apparently X-linked recessive transmission of a form of axonal motor-sensory neuropathy associated with deafness and mental retardation [36].

Clinical aspects

Males are severely affected with muscle weakness from infancy and most have associated deafness and/or mental retardation. Minor abnormalities in sensory nerve conduction, electromyography, and hearing loss are found in females but are deemed insufficiently consistent to be useful in carrier identification. The patients of Priest *et al.* [37] were severely affected within the first few years of life with distal weakness, muscle atrophy, sensory loss, areflexia, pes cavus, and hammer toes. Motor nerve conduction velocities in affected males were normal to mildly delayed, and sensory conduction was markedly abnormal. Heterozygous females were asymptomatic.

Genetics

CMTX4 maps to chromosome Xq24-q26 [37, 38] and is caused by a mutation in *AIFM1* (OMIM 300169), the gene encoding apoptosis-inducing factor mitochondrion-associated 1 [39].

Histopathology

In a single sural nerve biopsy, the number of myelinated and unmyelinated nerve fibers was severely reduced at the age of 19 years. The endoneurial collagen was somewhat increased in amount.

Electron microscopy revealed stacks of Schwann cell processes which are supposed to indicate loss of unmyelinated axons [36, 37]. In addition there were myelin ovoids indicating progressive degeneration of myelinated fibers.

CMTX5 (MIM 311070)

X-linked recessive Charcot–Marie–Tooth disease-5 (CMTX5) is associated with mutations in the gene encoding phosphoribosylpyrophosphate synthetase I (*PRPS1*) (OMIM 311850) on chromosome Xq22-q24.

Clinical aspects

The phenotype includes peripheral neuropathy, early-onset sensorineural deafness, and visual impairment due to optic neuropathy [40].

Histopathology

A sural nerve biopsy revealed severe loss of myelinated fibers associated with endoneurial fibrosis.

On electron microscopy, concentrically arranged Schwann cell processes were seen forming onion bulb like structures adjacent to abnormally thin myelin sheaths around remyelinating axons [40].

CMTX6 (MIM 300905)

X-linked dominant Charcot–Marie–Tooth disease-6 CMTX6) is caused by a mutation in the gene encoding pyruvate dehydrogenase kinase isoenzyme 3 (PDK3) (OMIM 300906) on chromosome Xp22. One family has been reported [41].

Clinical aspects

Onset of symptoms in affected males was in the first 13 years of life while female carriers in the older generations showed only subtle abnormalities. Neurophysiologic testing revealed predominantly axonal motor and sensory polyneuropathy.

Histopathology

There are no data available.

Differential diagnosis

Particularly in isolated cases, acquired (non-genetic) causes of peripheral neuropathy need to be considered. In addition, *de novo* mutations, variable expressivity, or incomplete recording of the family history may mask autosomal dominant inheritance. Finally, rare autosomal recessive forms of CMT should be considered.

Among 77 families with probable X-linked CMT, only 51% had mutations in *GJB1* suggesting that other forms of X-linked CMT including CMTX2–6 as well as additional unknown loci are affected in a significant number of cases [42]. Kennerson *et al.* [43] described an X-linked form of distal hereditary motor neuropathy with a CMT phenotype linked to Xq13.1–21 and associated with missense mutations in *ATP7A*, the same gene involved in Menkes disease.

Due to the occasional occurrence of CNS manifestations and white matter lesions on MRI, CMTX1 might also be included in the differential diagnosis of transient paralysis in children as well as toxic, inherited metabolic, infectious, and inflammatory diseases of the CNS.

Motor and sensory neuropathy with deafness and mental retardation similar to CMTX4 has been reported combined with absence of large myelinated fibers in the sural nerve [44–46]. Although this condition is transmitted in families probably as an autosomal recessive trait, X-linked inheritance could not be excluded.

References

1 Senderek J, Bergmann C, Quasthoff S, *et al.* (1998) X-linked dominant Charcot–Marie–Tooth disease: nerve biopsies allow morphological evaluation and detection of connexin32 mutations (Arg15Trp, Arg22Gln). *Acta Neuropathol (Berl);* 95(5):443–449.

2 Nicholson G, Corbett A. (1996) Slowing of central conduction in X-linked Charcot–Marie–Tooth neuropathy shown by brain stem auditory evoked responses. *J Neurol Neurosurg Psychiatry;*61(1):43–46.

3 Bähr M, Andres F, Timmerman V, *et al.* (1999) Central visual, acoustic, and motor pathway involvement in a Charcot–Marie–Tooth family with an Asn205Ser mutation in the connexin 32 gene. *J Neurol Neurosurg Psychiatry;*66:202–206.

4 Al-Mateen M, Craig AK, Chance PF. (2014) The central nervous system phenotype of X-Linked Charcot–Marie–Tooth disease: A transient disorder of children and young adults. *J Child Neurol.;*29(3):342–348.

5 Senderek J, Hermanns B, Bergmann C, *et al.* (1999) X-Linked dominant Charcot–Marie–Tooth neuropathy: clinical, electrophysiological, and morphological phenotype in four families with different connexin32 mutations. *J Neurol Sci;*167:90–101.

6 Bergoffen J, Scherer SS, Wang S, *et al.* (1993) Connexin mutations in X-linked Charcot–Marie–Toothdisease. *Science;* 262:2039–2042.

7 Bone LJ, Dahl N, Lensch MW, *et al.* (1995) New connexin32 mutations associated with X-linked Charcot–Marie–Tooth disease. *Neurology;*45:1863–1866.

8 Bone LJ, Deschenes SM, Balice-Gordon RJ, *et al.* (1997) Connexin32 and X-linked Charcot–Marie–Tooth disease. *Neurobiol Dis;*4:221–230.

9 Latour P, Lévy N, Paret M, *et al.* (1997) Mutations in the X-linked form of Charcot–Marie–Tooth disease in the French population. *Neurogenetics;*1:117–123.

10 Birouk N, LeGuern E, Maisonobe T, *et al.* (1998) X-linked Charcot–Marie–Tooth disease with connexin 32 mutations: clinical and electrophysiologic study. *Neurology;*50: 1074–1082.

11 Meggouh F, Benomar A, Rouger H, *et al.* (1998) The first de novo mutation of the connexin 32 gene associated with X linked Charcot–Marie–Tooth disease. *J Med Genet;*35: 251–252.

12 Hahn AF, Ainsworth PJ, Bolton CF, *et al.* (2001) Pathological findings in the x-linked form of Charcot–Marie–Tooth disease: a morphometric and ultrastructural analysis. *Acta Neuropathol;*101:129–139.

13 Kleopa KA, Abrams CK, Scherer SS.(2012) How do mutations in GJB1 cause X-linked Charcot–Marie–Tooth disease? *Brain Res;*1487:198–205.

14 Bergmann C, Zerres K, Rudnik-Schoneborn S, *et al.* (2002) Allelic variants in the 5′ non-coding region of the connexin32 gene: possible pitfalls in the diagnosis of X linked Charcot–Marie–Tooth neuropathy (CMTX). *J Med Genet;*39:e58.

15 Ainsworth PJ, Bolton CF, Murphy BC, *et al.* (1998) Genotype/phenotype correlation in affected individuals of a family with a deletion of the entire coding sequence of the connexin 32 gene. *Hum Genet;*103:242–244.

16 Hodapp JA, Carter GT, Lipe HP, *et al.* (2006) Double trouble in hereditary neuropathy: concomitant mutations in the PMP-22 gene and another gene produce novel phenotypes. *Arch Neurol;*63:112–117.

17 Bergmann C, Senderek J, Hermanns B, *et al.* (2000) Becker muscular dystrophy combined with X-linked Charcot–Marie–Tooth neuropathy. *Muscle Nerve;*23:818–823.

18 Hahn AF, Brown WF, Koopman WJ, Feasby TE. (1990) X-linked dominant hereditary motor and sensory neuropathy. *Brain;*113:1511–1525.

19 Schröder JM (1998) Recommendations for the examination of peripheral nerve biopsies. *Virchows Arch;*432:199–205.

20 Hahn AF (1993) Hereditary motor and sensory neuropathy: HMSN type II (neuronal type) and X-linked HMSN. *Brain Pathol;*3:147–155.

21 Meda P, Pepper MS, Traub O, *et al.* (1993) Differential expression of gap junction connexins in endocrine and exocrine glands. *Endocrinology;*133:2371–2378.

22 Nicholson G, Nash J (1993) Intermediate nerve conduction velocities define X-linked Charcot–Marie–Tooth neuropathy families. *Neurology;*43:2558–2564.

23 Anzini P, Neuberg DH, Schachner M, *et al.* (1997) Structural abnormalities and deficient maintenance of peripheral nerve myelin in mice lacking the gap junction protein connexin 32. *J Neurosci;*17:4545–4551.

24 Scherer SS, Xu YT, Nelles E, *et al.* (1998) Connexin32-null mice develop demyelinating peripheral neuropathy. *Glia;*24:8–20.

25 Vavlitou N, Sargiannidou I, Markoullis K, *et al.* (2010) Axonal pathology precedes demyelination in a mouse model of X-linked demyelinating/type I Charcot–Marie–Tooth neuropathy. *J Neuropathol Exp Neurol;*69:945–958.

26 Sahenk Z, Chen L (1998) Abnormalities in the axonal cytoskeleton induced by a connexin32 mutation in nerve xenografts. *J Neurosci Res;*51:174–184.

27 Scherer SS, Deschenes SM, Xu YT, *et al.* (1995) Connexin32 is a myelin-related protein in the PNS and CNS. *J Neurosci;* 15:8281–8294.

28 Balice-Gordon RJ, Bone LJ, Scherer SS (1998) Functional gap junctions in the Schwann cell myelin sheath. *J Cell Biol;* 142:1095–1104.

29 Sander S, Nicholson GA, Ouvrier RA, *et al.* (1998) Charcot–Marie–Tooth disease: histopathological features of the peripheral myelin protein (PMP22) duplication (CMT1A) and connexin32 mutations (CMTX1). *Muscle Nerve;*21:217–225.

30 Schröder JM, Himmelmann F (1992) Fine structural evaluation of altered Schmidt-Lanterman incisures in human sural nerve biopsies. *Acta Neuropathol (Berl);*83:120–133.

31 Schröder JM (1996) Developmental and pathological changes at the node and paranode in human sural nerves. *Microsc Res Tech;*34:422–435.

32 Nelles E, Butzler C, Jung D, *et al.* (1996) Defective propagation of signals generated by sympathetic nerve stimulation in the liver of connexin32-deficient mice. *Proc Natl Acad Sci U S A;*93:9565–70.

33 Reynolds ML, Woolf CJ (1993) Reciprocal Schwann cell-axon interactions. *Curr Opin Neurobiol;*3:683–693.

34 Ionasescu VV, Trofatter J, Haines JL, *et al.* (1992) X-linked recessive Charcot–Marie–Tooth neuropathy: clinical and genetic study. *Muscle Nerve;*15:368–373.

35 Ionasescu VV, Trofatter J, Haines JL, *et al.* (1991) Heterogeneity in X-linked recessive Charcot–Marie–Tooth neuropathy. *Am J Hum Genet;*48:1075–1083.

36 Cowchock FS, Duckett SW, Streletz LJ, *et al.* (1985) X-linked motor-sensory neuropathy type-II with deafness and mental retardation: a new disorder. *Am J Med Genet;*20:307–315.

37 Priest JM, Fischbeck KH, Nouri N, Keats BJ (1995) A locus for axonal motor-sensory neuropathy with deafness and mental retardation maps to Xq24-q26. *Genomics;*29:409–412.

38 Fischbeck KH, ar-Rushdi N, Pericak-Vance M, *et al.* (1986) X-linked neuropathy: gene localization with DNA probes. *Ann Neurol;*20:527–532.

39 Rinaldi C, Grunseich C, Sevrioukova IF, *et al.* (2012) Cowchock syndrome is associated with a mutation in apoptosis-inducing factor. *Am J Hum Genet;*91:1095–1102.

40 Kim HJ, Sohn KM, Shy ME, *et al.* (2007) Mutations in PRPS1, which encodes the phosphoribosyl pyrophosphate synthetase enzyme critical for nucleotide biosynthesis, cause hereditary peripheral neuropathy with hearing loss and optic neuropathy (cmtx5). *Am J Hum Genet;*81:552–558.

41 Kennerson ML, Yiu EM, Chuang DT, *et al.* (2013) A new locus for X-linked dominant Charcot–Marie–Tooth disease (CMTX6) is caused by mutations in the pyruvate dehydrogenase kinase isoenzyme 3 (PDK3) gene. *Hum Mol Genet;*22:1404–1416.

42 Huttner IG, Kennerson ML, Reddel SW, *et al.* (2006) Proof of genetic heterogeneity in X-linked Charcot–Marie–Tooth disease. *Neurology;*67:2016–2021.

43 Kennerson ML, Nicholson GA, Kaler SG, *et al.* (2010) Missense mutations in the copper transporter gene ATP7A cause X-linked distal hereditary motor neuropathy. *Am J Hum Genet;*86:343–352.

44 Mancardi GL, Di Rocco M, Schenone A, *et al.* (1992) Hereditary motor and sensory neuropathy with deafness, mental retardation and absence of large myelinated fibers. *J Neurol Sci;*110:121–130.

45 Sabatelli M, Mignogna T, Lippi G, *et al.* (1998) Hereditary motor and sensory neuropathy with deafness, mental retardation, and absence of sensory large myelinated fibers: confirmation of a new entity. *Am J Med Genet;*75:309–313.

46 Müller HD, Mugler M, Ramaekers VT, Schröder JM (2000) Hereditary motor and sensory neuropathy with absence of large myelinated fibers due to absence of large neurons in dorsal root ganglia and anterior horns, clinically associated with deafness, mental retardation, and epilepsy (HMSN-ADM). *J Peripher Nerv Syst;*5:147–157.

47 Schröder JM (2006) Neuropathology of Charcot–Marie–Tooth and related disorders. *Neuromolecular Med;*8:23–42.

CHAPTER 14

Hereditary sensory and autonomic neuropathy

Rosalind King
Department of Clinical Neurosciences, Institute of Neurology, University College London, London, UK

Introduction and historical perspective

The hereditary sensory (and autonomic) neuropathies (HSN, HSAN) are clinically heterogeneous but can be separated from other neuropathies by their Mendelian inheritance, primary impairment of sensory and/or autonomic nerves, and atrophy of affected neurons or axons. The onset of dominantly inherited HSANs is usually between the second and fourth decades. The autosomal recessive variants present at birth or during the first decade. In both there may be early death and central nervous system (CNS) involvement including mental retardation. There is often greater morbidity than in hereditary motor and sensory neuropathy (HMSN) (Charcot–Marie–Tooth disease: CMT). Although motor loss can occur in HSAN, especially in older patients, initially symptoms are restricted to sensory and autonomic nerves.

Pathologically HSAN and HSNs show loss of small myelinated and/or unmyelinated fibers but biopsy material is lacking for many sub-types (see Table 14.1). Originally, five subtypes were clinically classified [1]; only HSAN I has autosomal dominant inheritance, the others being autosomal recessive. HSAN is very rare with an incidence of 1 in 25,000 and several genes have been identified and related to specific subtypes. The neuropathy is axonal or neuronal and often involves specific fiber types. The causative genes further subdivide the original five types (Table 14.1) [2]. Twelve genes have so far been identified including those associated with CMT2B and a channelopathy with insensitivity to pain. At least 20% of cases have not been linked to a known gene so more await identification.

HSAN 1 (HSN 1)

Clinical

This is the commonest type with onset typically in the second decade of life or later. Rare cases have earlier onset. Sensory symptoms predominate, are usually symmetrical, mainly in the lower limbs with little proximal involvement. CNS involvement is rare. Clinical presentation varies and includes peroneal muscular atrophy and weakness, mutilating arthropathy, lancinating pain, burning feet, hearing loss, hypohydrosis, and dementia. There may be little or no autonomic involvement. In one series of six families, the age of onset varied between 12 and 70 years. Males presented earlier and had severe neuropathy. The mean age at death was 67 years, probably due to complications of ulcers, amputations, and infection [4].

Additional symptoms sometimes present further subdivide HSANs into five subtypes; in *HSAN1B* there is cough and gastroesophageal reflux in addition to the sensory symptoms plus sensorineural deafness in some patients. HSAN1B lacks motor involvement, acral mutilations, or ulcerations. Autonomic involvement is restricted to reduced sweating [6].

HSAN 1C is difficult to distinguish from CMT2B clinically as both have similar mutilating sensory changes. In CMT2B motor involvement is more prominent, earlier in onset and the spontaneous lancinating pains associated with HSAN1C are absent.

In *HSAN1D* the painless injuries to the extremities, infections and resultant amputations suggest *SPLTC1* mutations, but two families had mutations in the gene for atlastin 1 (ATL1) [8].

Peripheral Nerve Disorders: Pathology and Genetics, First Edition. Edited by Jean-Michel Vallat, Joachim Weis, Francoise Gray, and Katy Keohane.

Table 14.1 Types of HSAN, genes implicated, and pathological alterations.

Type	Inheritance	Gene	Pathology
HSAN I	AD	*SPTLC1*	6 families, axonal loss, [3] 6 families, loss small myelinated fibers [4] 1 biopsy, axonal loss [5]
	De novo	*SPTLC1* *SPTLC2*	
HSAN 1B with cough & gastro-esophageal reflux	AD	Locus 3p22-p24	Loss of large and small myelinated fibers, survivors medium sized. [6]
CMT 2B (HSAN 1C)	AD	*RAB 7*	Loss larger myelin fibs, regeneration with small fibers. Unmyelinated fibers present [7]
HSAN1D	AD?	*ATL 1*	Axonal, demyelinating?, minimal regeneration [8]
HSAN1E c dementia + hearing loss		*DNMT1*	Severe fiber loss [9]
HSAN II	AR	*WNK1/HSN2*	Severe myelinated fiber loss, unmyelinated fibers present; no demyelination [10–12]
		FAM134B	No biopsy
HSAN III	AR	*IKBKAP*	No biopsy
HSAN IV/CIPA	AR	*NTRK1*	Loss small myelinated fibers 3 skin biopsies loss axons [13] Unmyelinated fiber loss, normal LM [14] loss small myelinated & unmyelinated fibers [15] Normal total fiber density (loss small), loss unmyelinated fibers [16]
HSAN V	AR	*NGF B*	No biopsy
HSAN V	AR	*NTRK1*	Loss small myelinated fibers, unmyelinated fibers slightly reduced [17]
HSAN V	AR	*NGF B*	Severe loss unmyelinated fibers, moderate loss small myelinated fibers [18]
HSN with spastic paraplegia	AR	*CCT5*	No biopsy reported
Channelopathy associated with insensitivity to pain	AR	*SCN9A*	Normal nerve [19]

SPTLC 1, serinepalmitoyltransferase, long chain base subunit-1;
RAB7, Member of RAS oncogene family;
WNK1/HS N2, protein kinase with-no-lysine (K)-1/ hereditary sensory neuropathy type 2 gene;
FAM134B, family with sequence similarity 134, member B
ATL1, Atlastin 1
DNMT1 DNA methyltransferase 1
IKBKAP, inhibitor of kappa light polypeptide gene enhancer in B-cells, kinase complex associated protein;
NTRK1, neurotrophic tyrosine kinase receptor type 1;
NGFB, nerve growth factor beta polypeptide
CCT5, cytosolic chaperonin-containing t-complex peptide-1
SCN9A, sodium channel voltage gated, type IX alpha subunit

HSAN1E is rare, with early onset dementia, hearing loss, trophic skin and nail changes, and a mutation in the gene for DNA methyl transferase (DNMT1) [9].

Genetics

At the time of writing, five causative genes have been identified for HSAN1. The first identified was *SPTLC1* (*HSAN1A*). At least seven different mutations have been published. The first (C133W) was found in Australian and British families suggesting a common British founder, but was subsequently reported in a Chinese family [5]. *SPTLC1* encodes the long chain base one (LCB1) of serine palmitoyltranferase, involved in sphingolipid synthesis. This ubiquitously expressed enzyme is located on the endoplasmic reticulum. *SPTLC2* encodes subunit 2 of serine palmitoyltransferase and is phenotypically indistinguishable from *SPTLC1* mutations. Both can be associated with spontaneous lancinating pains. Autonomic symptoms are limited to hypohydrosis [20]. The precise mechanisms by which these mutations lead to predominantly sensory neuropathies are unclear.

HSAN1B is related to the locus 3p22–24 but no causal gene has yet been identified [21].

In 2003, CMT2B (*HSAN1C*) was shown to be caused by two mutations in the small *GTPase late endosomal protein RAB7* gene [22]; the lack of motor involvement makes distinction from HSAN1 problematic. *RAB7* mutations are rare and are associated with sensory loss across all modalities which help differentiation from the more common *SPTLC* mutations. Screening a large number of inherited and sporadic patients with adult onset HSAN I or CMT2B failed to identify any mutations in *RAB7*. RAB7 protein is ubiquitously expressed, binds to early endosomes and helps transport proteins via late endosomes and is also involved in endocytosis.

HSAN1D also overlaps clinically with CMT2B; the gene implicated is *ATL1* that codes for atlastin 1 [8]. This is a dynamin-related GTPase involved in generating the endoplasmic reticulum (ER) network. RAB7 is also involved in ER. Other mutations in *ATL1*, described in early onset spastic paraplegia, affect upper motor neurons in a length-dependent manner. Perhaps the similar diseases resulting from mutations in *SPTLC*, *ATL1*, and *RAB7* result from their related functions but it is also suggested that RAB7 is involved in TrkA signaling.

In *HSAN1E* associated with dementia and hearing loss, the gene is related to mutations in *DNA methyltransferase (DNMT1)* that cause aberrant methylation leading to the complex pathogenesis [9].

Pathology

Nerve biopsies from cases with SPTLC1 mutations (*HSAN1A*) show axonal loss particularly affecting small fibers. In six biopsies there was severe loss of axons of all size possibly sparing some larger fibers, and unmyelinated fiber degeneration [4]; more unmyelinated than myelinated fibers survived. In one autopsy, dorsal root ganglia showed mild/moderate ganglion cells loss, nodules of Nageotte and clusters of fine axonal sprouts, but little to suggest regeneration more distally.

In *HSAN1B* the medium sized fibers are relatively spared.

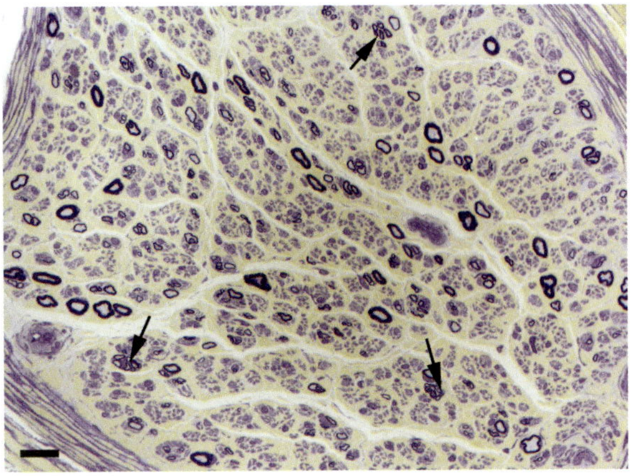

Figure 14.1 Semithin resin section of sural nerve biopsy from a case of CMT2D with a *RAB7* mutation. There is considerable loss of myelinated fibers (3300/mm² myelinated fibers compared to 7000/mm² in a normal control), some regenerative clusters (arrows) and excess collagen in the endoneurium. Bar = 20 µm.

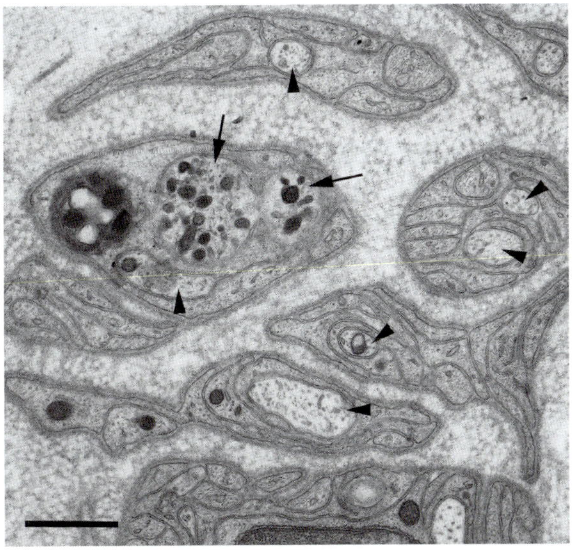

Figure 14.2 Electron micrograph of the same case as in Fig. 14.1. There is a group of Schwann cell processes in which several small unmyelinated axons (arrowheads) are embedded, some of which are degenerating (arrows). Bar = 1 µm.

In *HSAN1C*/CMT2B some of the large fiber damage is replaced by regenerating clusters of small fibers, probably abortive as several unmyelinated fibers were degenerating (Figs 14.1 and 14.2).

Where the gene involved was *ATL1* (*HSAN 1D*), some thinly myelinated fibers suggesting demyelination and remyelination were reported but not illustrated; thin myelin sheaths can also indicate regeneration [8].

In *DNMT1* mutations (*HSAN 1E*) there is extensive myelinated fiber loss of all sizes but there is no report on the status of unmyelinated fibers.

HSAN II

Clinical

This very rare autosomal recessive form related to mutations in *HSN2* was identified in five Canadian families [12]. It presents earlier than HSAN1, with distal numbness and later impairment of pain, temperature, and touch. There is loss of tendon reflexes, plantar, and finger ulcers and spontaneous amputations. Motor weakness is absent or mild and autonomic dysfunction is minimal. Normal mental development distinguishes this disease from HSAN III and IV.

Genetic

HSN2 is a single exon gene located in exon 8 of *protein kinase-with-no-lysine 1* (*PRKWNL*) gene. All nine mutations identified so far result in truncation and presumably loss-of-function but the protein's function is unknown.

Recently another gene, *FAM134B* (*family with sequence similarity 134, member B*) (also called *JK-1*) has been implicated in HSANII [12]. Originally misdiagnosed as leprosy, the disease manifested as early-onset impaired nociception and progressive mutilating ulcerations of hands and feet. The function of the protein produced by this gene is unknown but is thought to be related to the Golgi complex.

Pathology

Sural nerve biopsies showed severe myelinated fiber loss but normal unmyelinated fibers. There was no onion bulb formation or demyelination [10, 11].

HSAN III

Clinical

HSAN III is familial dysautonomia or Riley–Day syndrome. In this congenital progressive condition, patients lack a response to painful stimuli and temperature changes, are unable to produce tears, have absence of fungiform papillae of the tongue, vasomotor instability, hyperhydrosis, and later vibratory sensory loss and impaired coordination. The small fiber atrophy may also affect the cerebellum and optic nerve. Life expectancy is reduced. The majority of cases are in the Ashkenazi Jewish population but rare non-Jewish cases also occur [24].

Genetic

HSANIII is related to mutations in *IKBKAP.* A deficiency in neuronal polarized trafficking was recently suggested as the underlying defect. The mutation reduces splicing efficiency but some wild-type transcript is still produced. Compounds which increase the level of wild-type transcript and hence improved symptoms are being sought.

Pathology

A single peripheral nerve biopsy published in 1971 showed a roughly normal myelinated fiber population, reduced unmyelinated fibers (3617/mm^2 compared to minimum normal of 30,000/mm^2) and was interpreted as implying a developmental defect [25].

The genetically defined cases have not had nerve biopsies.

HSAN IV

Clinical

HSAN IV is congenital with onset at birth, episodic fever, mild mental retardation, skin, and corneal lesions and joint deformities. It is also known as congenital insensitivity to pain with anhydrosis (CIPA). Muscle strength and deep tendon reflexes are usually preserved. The children often show mild mental retardation.

Genetic

HSANIV is related to mutations in *NTRK 1.* The gene encodes neurotrophin receptor 1.

A reported family of five children with the HSAN IV phenotype related to a mutation in *NGFB* throws doubt on the validity of separating HSAN IV and V.

Pathology

Absence or decrease in small myelinated or unmyelinated fibers with possible demyelination was seen in one case [13]. Another with a different mutation was regarded as normal by light microscopy but lacked unmyelinated axons by electron microscopy [14]. The myelinated fiber size distribution was not investigated. Other biopsies showed almost total absence of unmyelinated fibers, reduced numbers of small myelinated fibers or severe loss of myelinated fibers and moderate loss of unmyelinated fibers [26].

Biopsies were not taken from the family with HSAN IV phenotype mentioned previously.

HSAN V

Clinical

This syndrome has early onset, distal loss of pain and temperature sensation, loss of deep pain perception, painless fractures, and joint deformities. It is separated from HSAN IV by the greater severity of anhidrosis in the latter and lack of mental retardation.

Genetic

Both phenotypes may be related to mutations in *NGFB* or rarely to *NTRK*.

Pathology

In a case related to a mutation in *NTRK1*, small myelinated fibers were severely reduced with minor loss of unmyelinated fibers [17] (Figs 14.3 and 14.4), allowing distinction from HSAN IV where unmyelinated axons are virtually absent.

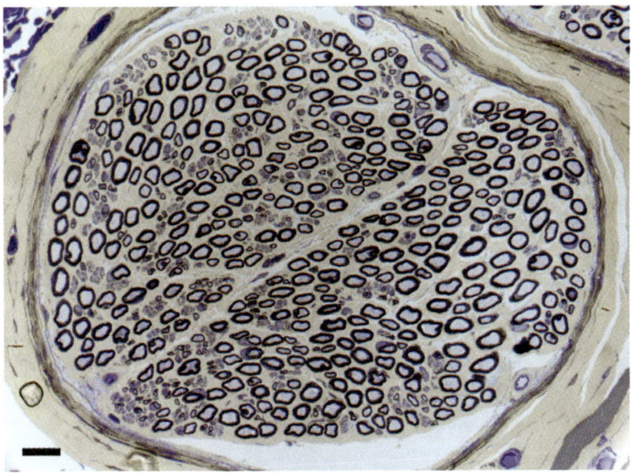

Figure 14.3 Semithin resin section of sural nerve biopsy from a 9-year-old boy with a mutation in NTRKA and the phenotype of HSAN V [27]. The normal fiber size distribution is lost as most of the myelinated fibers are large whereas the small myelinated fiber population is much reduced. There are no regenerative clusters. Bar = 20 μm.

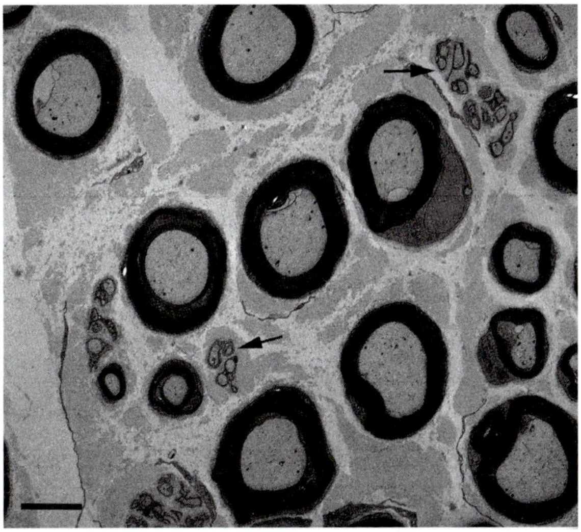

Figure 14.4 Electron micrograph of the same case as in Fig. 14.3. Many of the myelinated fibers are approximately the same size; the unmyelinated fiber population (arrows) is healthy but slightly reduced. Bar = 5 μm.

HSAN with spastic paraplegia

Clinical

This syndrome has onset in early childhood with loss of all sensory modalities, mutilating acropathy, and spastic paraplegia.

Genetic

One family had a mutation in the gene for cytosolic chaparonin-containing t-complex peptide-1 (*CCT5*).

Pathology

Biopsy has not been reported.

Channelopathy associated with insensitivity to pain

Clinical

Three consanguineous families have been reported, all with normal intelligence and complete lack of appreciation of pain leading to painless injuries and fractures. Other sensory modalities and autonomic functions were normal. The condition could be distinguished from indifference to pain by appropriate testing.

Genetic

This syndrome is associated with mutations in the sodium channel voltage gated type IX alpha subunit (*SCN9A*) [19]. Three distinct mutations were discovered resulting in loss of function of the $Na_v1.7$ sodium channel. Mutations in the same gene are associated with hereditary erythromyalgia and paroxysmal extreme pain disorders.

Pathology

Sural nerve biopsies are reported as normal.

Animal models

Syndromes resembling human HSAN have been reported in various dog breeds: French spaniels [27], Doberman, German short-haired pointer dogs, English pointer dogs, English springer spaniels. The disorder is known as "acral mutilation" or "canine sensory neuropathy," and is usually considered as a recessive disease.

A single pathological study of an affected English pointer dog showed a deficiency of primary sensory neurons probably corresponding to a neuronopathy. Neuronal cell bodies were reduced in number and there was degeneration of myelinated and unmyelinated fibers with a reduced fiber density in the dorsolateral fasciculus [28].

Additional studies are needed to characterize and correlate the clinicopathological findings and the genetic aspects of these disorders.

Conclusions and future perspectives

These rare neuropathies are clinically distressing. The involvement of various genes throws some light on their function and peripheral nerve biochemistry. Sensory and autonomic ganglion neurons seem vulnerable to withdrawal of neurotrophins and undergo apoptosis when levels fall. This may explain the association with *NTRK1*, *FAM134B*, and *NGFB* in HSAN.

Most mutations so far identified are associated with some degree of unmyelinated axon loss, except for *WNK1/HSN2* mutations. It is hoped that a greater understanding will lead to treatments of these distressing neuropathies.

References

1 Dyck PJ and Ohta M (1975) Neuronal atrophy and degeneration predominantly affecting peripheral sensory neurons: In: Dyck PJ, Thomas PK, Lambert EH (eds) *Peripheral Neuropathy*, pp. 791–824, WB Saunders, Philadelphia.

2 Verhoeven K Timmerman V, Mauko B, *et al.* (2006) Recent advances in hereditary sensory and autonomic neuropathies, *Current Opinions in Neurology* 19, 474–480.

3 Klein CJ, Wu Y, Kruckeberg KE, *et al.* (2005) SPTLC1 and RAB7 mutation analysis in dominantly inherited and idiopathic sensory neuropathies, *J Neurol Neurosurg Psychiatr* 76, 1022–1024.

4 Houlden H, King R, Blake J, *et al.* (2006) Clinical, pathological and genetic characterization of hereditary sensory and autonomic neuropathy type 1 (HSAN I), *Brain* 129, 411–425.

5 Bi H, Gao Y, Yao S, *et al.* (2007) Hereditary sensory and autonomic neuropathy type I in a Chinese family: British C133W mutation exists in the Chinese, *Neuropathology* 27, 429–433.

6 Spring PJ, Kok C, Nicholson GA, *et al.* (2005) Autosomal dominant hereditary sensory neuropathy with chronic cough and gastro-oesophageal reflux: clinical features in two families linked to chromosome 3p22–p24, *Brain* 128, 2797–2810.

7 Houlden H, King RH, Muddle JR, *et al.* (2004) A novel RAB7 mutation associated with ulcero-mutilating neuropathy, *Ann Neurol* 56, 586–590.

8 Guelly C , Zhu PP, Leonardis L, *et al.* (2011) Targeted high-throughput sequencing identifies mutations in atlastin-1 as a cause of hereditary sensory neuropathy type I, *Am J Hum Genet* 88, 99–105.

9 Klein CJ, Botuyan MV, Wu Y, *et al.* (2011) Mutations in DNMT1 cause hereditary sensory neuropathy with dementia and hearing loss, *Nature Genetics* 43, 595–600.

10 Cho HJ, Kim BJ, Suh YL, *et al.* (2006) Novel mutation in the HSN2 gene in a Korean patient with hereditary sensory and autonomic neuropathy type 2, *J Hum Genet* 51, 905–908.

11 Coen K, Pareyson D, Auer-Grumbach M, *et al.* (2006) Novel mutations in the HSN2 gene causing hereditary sensory and autonomic neuropathy type II, *Neurology* 66, 748–751.

12 Lafreniere RG, MacDonald ML, Dube MP, *et al.* (2004) Identification of a novel gene (HSN2) causing hereditary sensory and autonomic neuropathy type II through the study of Canadian genetic isolates, *Am J Hum Genet* 74, 1064–1073.

13 Rotthier A, Baets J, De Vriendt E, *et al.* (2009) Genes for hereditary sensory and autonomic neuropathies: a genotype-phenotype correlation, *Brain* 132, 2699–2711.

14 Suriu C, Khayat M, Weiler M, *et al.* (2009) Skoura – a genetic island for congenital insensitivity to pain and anhidrosis among Moroccan Jews, as determined by a novel mutation in the NTRK1 gene, *Clinical Genetics* 75, 230–236.

15 Indo Y, Mardy S, Miura Y, *et al.* (2001) Congenital insensitivity to pain with anhidrosis (CIPA): novel mutations of the TRKA (NTRK1) gene, a putative uniparental disomy, and a linkage of the mutant TRKA and PKLR genes in a family with CIPA and pyruvate kinase deficiency, *Human Mutation* 18, 308–318.

16 Goebel HH, Veit S, Dyck PJ (1980) Confirmation of virtual unmyelinated fiber absence in hereditary sensory neuropathy type IV, *J Neuropathol Exp Neurol* 39, 670–675.

17 Houlden H, King RH, Hashemi-Nejad A, *et al.* (2001) A novel TRK A (NTRK1) mutation associated with hereditary sensory and autonomic neuropathy type V, *Ann Neurol* 49, 521–525.

18 Einarsdottir E, Carlsson A, Minde J, *et al.* (2004) A mutation in the nerve growth factor beta gene (NGFB) causes loss of pain perception, *Hum Mol Genet* 13, 799–205.

19 Cox JJ, Reimann F, Nicholas AK, *et al.* (2006) An SCN9A channelopathy causes congenital inability to experience pain, *Nature* 444, 894–898.

20 Rotthier A, Auer Grumbach M, Janssens K, *et al.* (2010) Mutations in the SPTLC2 subunit of serine palmitoyltransferase cause hereditary sensory and autonomic neuropathy type I, *Am J Hum Genet* 87, 513–522.

21 Kok C, Kennerson ML, Spring PJ, *et al.* (2003) A locus for hereditary sensory neuropathy with cough and gastroesophageal reflux on chromosome 3p22–p24, *Am J Hum Genet* 73, 632–637.

22 Verhoeven K, De Jonghe P, Coen K, *et al.* (2003) Mutations in the small GTP-ase late endosomal protein RAB7 cause Charcot–Marie–Tooth type 2B neuropathy, *Am J Hum Genet* 72, 722–727.

23 Kurth I, Pamminger T, Hennings JC, *et al.* (2009) Mutations in FAM134B, encoding a newly identified Golgi protein, cause severe sensory and autonomic neuropathy, *Nature Genetics* 41, 1179–1181.

24 Leyne M, Mull J, Gill SP, *et al.* (2003) Identification of the first non-Jewish mutation in familial Dysautonomia, *Am J Med Genet A* 118A, 305–308.

25 Aguayo AJ, Nair CPV, Bray GM (1971) Peripheral nerve abnormalities in the Riley-Day syndrome: findings in a sural nerve biopsy, *Arch Neurol* 24, 106–116.

26 Huehne K, Zweier C, Raab K, *et al.* (2008) Novel missense, insertion and deletion mutations in the neurotrophic tyrosine kinase receptor type 1 gene (NTRK1) associated with congenital insensitivity to pain with anhidrosis, *Neuromuscular Disorders* 18, 159–166.

27 Paradis M, De Jaham C, Page N *et al.* (2005) Acral mutilation in 13 French spaniels. *Veterinary Dermatology* 16, 87–93.

28 Cummings JF, Lahunta A, Winn SS (1981) Acral mutilation and nociceptive loss in English Pointer dogs. *Acta Neuropathologica* 53, 119-127.

CHAPTER 15

Hereditary neuropathy with liability to pressure palsy

Benjamin Ellezam

Department of Pathology and Cell Biology, Université de Montréal, CHU Sainte-Justine, Montreal, Canada

Definition of the disorder, major synonyms, and historical perspective

A description of hereditary neuropathy with liability to pressure palsy (HNPP) was first published in 1947 by the Dutch neurologist, de Jong, who reported on a family with recurrent episodes of wrist or foot drop associated with kneeling during potato harvests [1]. Hallmark definitive electrophysiological features of this entity were described in the 1960s and included diminished conduction velocities in a number of nerves susceptible to traction or compression, whether currently symptomatic or not, with similar findings in asymptomatic family members [2]. Characteristic histologic features were reported later and included the distinctive myelin thickenings, in the shape of sausages (in Latin: *tomaculum*), which led to the descriptive designation "tomaculous neuropathy" [3, 4]. Genetic characterization and recent experimental data established haploinsufficiency of the gene *PMP22* as the etiology of HNPP [5, 6], adding to the family of *PMP22*-related diseases which together account for more than 50% of hereditary neuropathies.

Epidemiology

Actual prevalence is probably much higher than current estimates of 2–16 in 100,000 [7, 8]. HNPP is more frequent in males than females by a ratio of 4:3 [9–11], possibly due to occupation-related trauma in men, although other unknown gender-specific factors are also probably involved.

Clinical features and investigations

Clinical

Patients first experience symptoms in adolescence or young adulthood as painless focal palsies at usual sites of nerve entrapment, most frequently the peroneal and ulnar nerves, but also the brachial plexus, radial nerve, and at less common sites such as median or facial nerves [9]. Onset is often triggered by positions held for long periods of time but a triggering event is not always evident. Symptoms typically last hours to days, are self-limiting, and may go unreported for years before patients seek medical attention. Less common presentations include recurrent positional paresthesia, chronic sensory polyneuropathy, progressive sensorimotor mononeuropathy, CMT-like neuropathy [9], bilateral hand amyotrophy [12], or recurrent polyradiculoneuropathy [13]. Many completely asymptomatic patients are discovered by electrophysiological and genetic testing of an index case's family members, and only a subset of these have ankle jerk or generalized areflexia on examination [9].

Central nervous system involvement has been reported including a case series describing white matter MRI abnormalities and a recent prospective case-control

Peripheral Nerve Disorders: Pathology and Genetics, First Edition. Edited by Jean-Michel Vallat, Joachim Weis, Francoise Gray, and Katy Keohane.

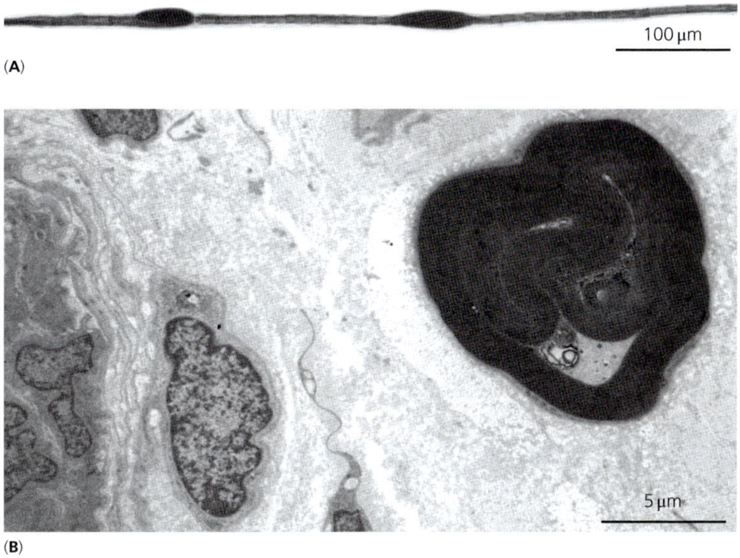

Figure 15.1 **(A)** *Top:* teased nerve fiber preparation showing frequent myelin thickenings (*tomacula*) along a single myelinated axon. **(B)** *Bottom:* electron micrograph of nerve cross-section showing hypermyelination with redundant myelin loops and significant axonal narrowing.

study revealing mild cognitive impairment in 64% of patients, many of whom had significant loss of white matter volume [14].

Electrophysiology

The characteristic electrophysiological findings in HNPP patients are prolonged distal motor latencies with mildly reduced sensory conduction velocities in nerves susceptible to compression, mostly median and peroneal nerves, including those not currently affected by palsy – the same being true in asymptomatic mutation carriers [2, 9, 15]. In symptomatic nerves, conduction blocks may be seen across sites of entrapment (e.g., carpal, cubital, or ulnar tunnel, or across the fibular head). Motor nerve conduction velocities tend to be mildly reduced in the lower limbs but usually remain normal in the upper limbs, in contrast to hereditary demyelinating neuropathies. F-wave latencies are prolonged in HNPP but this feature is less specific [15]. Sensory or motor amplitudes are variably reduced. In a study comparing acquired and hereditary neuropathies, 35% of patients with HNPP versus 57% of patients with CIDP had compound muscle action potential (CMAP) dispersion in at least one nerve, thus limiting this modality as a discriminating tool [16]. In the same study, proximal-distal CMAP dispersion was least frequent in HNPP, compared to other hereditary neuropathies.

Pathology

Histologic features of HNPP have been well-studied but are rarely encountered in modern pathology practice since genetic tests led to a decline in sural nerve biopsy in cases with suspected hereditary neuropathy. The hallmark feature is frequent myelin thickenings (*tomacula* or sausage-shaped structures) in teased nerve preparations (Fig. 15.1A), although they are also conspicuous in cross-sections of resin-embedded specimens [3, 4] (see also Fig. 7.12).

On electron microscopy, the individual lamellae are of normal thickness and are normally spaced but form excessive turns, redundant folded ribbons, and concentric outer layers of myelin, resulting in hypermyelinated fibers with diameters up to twice normal values (Fig. 15.1B). Perfect fixation of these abnormal hypertrophic myelin sheaths is not easy, so myelin can appear cracked without the proper lamellar structure. Although axonal degeneration is not a feature of HNPP, some degree of axonal constriction is often seen within *tomacula* [4]. Rare patients with axonal regeneration and lacking tomacula have also been reported [17].

There has been debate about the specificity of *tomacula* for HNPP as they can also be seen in acquired neuropathies (CIDP, IgM paraproteinemic neuropathy with anti-MAG antibodies) or a few other hereditary neuropathies [18]. However, in no other neuropathy are *tomacula* as numerous as in HNPP where they may be present in about 25% of internodal segments. Exceptionally, CMT1A patients may also have numerous tomacula, although in most cases they are sparse and associated with abundant onion-bulb formations (Vallat JM, personal communication). Focal myelin thickenings with numerous in- and out-foldings ("focally folded myelin," FFM) may be observed in CMT1B and in CMT4B and have been described as *tomacula* [19–21]; however, in those cases myelin sheaths tend to be much more irregular and asymmetric and do not have the smooth external contours of typical *tomacula*.

Onion bulb formations are generally not a feature of HNPP, but teased fiber preparations reveal some degree of demyelination and remyelination in the form of thinly myelinated or unmyelinated internodal segments and irregular shortening of internodal lengths [4, 22]. Another feature is significant loss of large-caliber myelinated axons (>10 µm) leading to a reduction in average fiber diameter [3]. The overall fiber density remains normal because of a corresponding increase in the number of small-caliber myelinated axons. Unmyelinated fibers do not show any significant change.

Genetics

HNPP is an autosomal dominant disorder with incomplete penetrance, which explains the large number of asymptomatic obligate carriers. The genetic locus maps to chromosome 17p11.2–12 where, in approximately 85% of cases, a 1.5 Mb DNA deletion can be found [5, 7]. This deleted region includes the *PMP22* gene, leading to haploinsufficiency at this locus and underexpression of *PMP22* protein. Duplication of the same DNA segment with resulting overexpression of *PMP22* protein is the cause of CMT1A [23]. Despite very different prevalence figures, the two molecular alterations are thought to result from a single unbalanced meiotic recombination event [22]. Underreporting and lower penetrance of HNPP compared to CMT1A probably explains this discrepancy. A small fraction of typical HNPP cases are caused by slightly different 17p11 deletions or by a number of *PMP22* sequence mutations (see [6] for a list). In the latter cases, an expected 50% of functional *PMP22* protein is lacking, effectively leading to haploinsufficiency and a HNPP phenotype. Some point mutations in *PMP22* can also lead to a wide range of clinical phenotypes including mild HNPP-like CMT1 or severe Déjérine–Sottas phenotypes but those are now designated CMT1E.

Pathogenesis and animal models

Several lines of evidence support the hypothesis that PMP22 protein dosage reduction causes the HNPP phenotype. Although the hallmark 17p11 HNPP deletion includes other genes, smaller deletions that cover *PMP22* [24] and small sequence mutations leading to loss-of-function *PMP22* alleles also cause HNPP [6], providing good evidence that *PMP22* is the culprit and not some other gene residing on the locus. Reduction in *PMP22* expression in HNPP patients has been confirmed both at mRNA and protein level [19, 22].

In animal models, knockout mice heterozygous for the deletion (*Pmp22* +/−) have numerous tomacula, little functional impairment, and only develop segmental demyelination in later stages [20, 21]. In comparison, mice with homozygous deletions (*Pmp22* −/−) have early onset demyelination, axonal loss and severe functional impairment. Experimentally, *Pmp22* +/−mice exposed to nerve compression develop conduction block faster than wild-type mice and take longer to recover, indicating that *PMP22* protein somehow protects nerves from mechanical injury [26].

At a molecular level, *PMP22* is a transmembrane protein thought to be involved in Schwann cell interactions with axons and extracellular matrix, and also appears to affect Schwann cell proliferation; however, the cellular function of *PMP22* protein is still poorly understood [6]. How reduced *PMP22* protein dosage leads to *tomacula* formation and demyelination is unknown but appears related to the relative quantities of *PMP22* protein relative to other myelin components. How these morphologic changes relate to compromised action potential propagation and increased susceptibility to mechanical injury is also unknown, although axonal constrictions and poor myelin compaction within *tomacula* have been suggested as potential causes. Windebank [27] reviewed other hypotheses including localized ischemia, mechanical distortion of myelin membranes, defect in Schwann cell-axon interaction leading to hypermyelination, and altered response of myelin to repeated trauma.

Management and future perspectives

Specific treatment for HNPP is not currently available. Correction of *PMP22* protein dosage, either by gene therapy or pharmaceutical intervention, has been considered but lacks experimental confirmation. For the time being, management of HNPP consists in confirming the diagnosis and promoting strategies to prevent palsies. Prevention focuses on avoidance of repetitive movements, excessive force, or any of the fixed positions known to cause nerve compression or traction. Use of tools, orthotics, or occupational aids may also be of help.

References

1 Koehler PJ. (2003) Hereditary neuropathy with liability to pressure palsies: the first publication (1947). *Neurology* 60, 1211–1213.
2 Earl CJ, Fullerton PM, Wakefield GS *et al.* (1964) Hereditary neuropathy, with liability to pressure palsies; a clinical and electrophysiological study of four families. *Q J Med* 33, 481–498.
3 Behse F, Buchthal F, Carlsen F *et al.* (1972) Hereditary neuropathy with liability to pressure palsies. Electrophysiological and histopathological aspects. *Brain* 95, 777–794.
4 Madrid R Bradley WG. (1975) The pathology of neuropathies with focal thickening of the myelin sheath (tomaculous neuropathy). *J Neurol Sci* 25, 415–448.
5 Chance PF, Alderson MK, Leppig KA *et al.* (1993) DNA deletion associated with hereditary neuropathy with liability to pressure palsies. *Cell* 72, 143–151.
6 Li J, Parker B, Martyn C *et al.* (2013) The PMP22 gene and its related diseases. *Mol Neurobiol* 47, 673–698.
7 Meretoja P, Silander K, Kalimo H *et al.* (1997) Epidemiology of hereditary neuropathy with liability to pressure palsies (HNPP) in south western Finland. *Neuromuscul Disord* 7, 529–532.
8 Nelis E, Van Broeckhoven C, De Jonghe P *et al.* (1996) Estimation of the mutation frequencies in Charcot–Marie–Tooth disease type 1 and hereditary neuropathy with liability to pressure palsies: a European collaborative study. *Eur J Hum Genet* 4, 25–33.
9 Mouton P, Tardieu S, Gouider R *et al.* (1999) Spectrum of clinical and electrophysiologic features in HNPP patients with the 17p11.2 deletion. *Neurology* 52, 1440–1440.
10 Rizzuto N, Moretto G, Galiazzo Rizzuto S. (1993) Clinical spectrum of the tomaculous neuropathies. Report of 60 cases and review of the literature. *Ital J Neurol Sci* 14, 609–617.
11 Verhagen WI, Gabreels-Festen AA, Van Wensen PJ *et al.* (1993) Hereditary neuropathy with liability to pressure palsies: a clinical, electroneurophysiological and morphological study. *J Neurol Sci* 116, 176–184.
12 Gochard A, Guennoc AM, Praline J *et al.* (2007) Bilateral hand amyotrophy with PMP-22 gene deletion. *European Journal of Neurology* 14, 115–116.
13 Le Forestier N, Leguern E, Coullin P *et al.* (1997) Recurrent polyradiculoneuropathy with the 17p11.2 deletion. *Muscle Nerve* 20, 1184–1186.
14 Chanson JB, Echaniz-Laguna A, Blanc F *et al.* (2012) Central nervous system abnormalities in patients with PMP22 gene mutations: a prospective study. *J Neurol Neurosurg Psychiatry* doi:10.1136/jnnp-2012-303725.
15 Andersson PB, Yuen E, Parko K *et al.* (2000) Electrodiagnostic features of hereditary neuropathy with liability to pressure palsies. *Neurology* 54, 40–44.
16 Stanton M, Pannoni V, Lewis RA *et al.* (2006) Dispersion of compound muscle action potential in hereditary neuropathies and chronic inflammatory demyelinating polyneuropathy. *Muscle Nerve* 34, 417–422.
17 Sessa M, Nemni R, Quattrini A *et al.* (1997) Atypical hereditary neuropathy with liability to pressure palsies (HNPP): the value of direct DNA diagnosis. *J Med Genet* 34, 889–892.
18 Sander S, Ouvrier RA, Mcleod JG *et al.* (2000) Clinical syndromes associated with tomacula or myelin swellings in sural nerve biopsies. *J Neurol Neurosurg Psychiatry* 68, 483–488.
19 Vallat JM, Sindou P, Preux PM *et al.* (1996) Ultrastructural PMP22 expression in inherited demyelinating neuropathies. *Ann Neurol* 39, 813–817.
20 Adlkofer K, Frei R, Neuberg DH *et al.* (1997) Heterozygous peripheral myelin protein 22-deficient mice are affected by a progressive demyelinating tomaculous neuropathy. *J Neurosci* 17, 4662–4671.
21 Adlkofer K, Martini R, Aguzzi A *et al.* (1995) Hypermyelination and demyelinating peripheral neuropathy in Pmp22-deficient mice. *Nat Genet* 11, 274–280.
22 Pentao L, Wise CA, Chinault AC *et al.* (1992) Charcot–Marie–Tooth type 1A duplication appears to arise from recombination at repeat sequences flanking the 1.5 Mb monomer unit. *Nat Genet* 2, 292–300.
23 Raeymaekers P, Timmerman V, Nelis E *et al.* (1991) Duplication in chromosome 17p11.2 in Charcot–Marie–Tooth neuropathy type 1a (CMT 1a). The HMSN Collaborative Research Group. *Neuromuscul Disord* 1, 93–97.

24 Chapon F, Diraison P, Lechevalier B *et al.* (1996) Hereditary neuropathy with liability to pressure palsies with a partial deletion of the region often duplicated in Charcot–Marie–Tooth disease, type 1A. *J Neurol Neurosurg Psychiatry* 61, 535–536.

25 Schenone A, Nobbio L, Mandich P *et al.* (1997) Underexpression of messenger RNA for peripheral myelin protein 22 in hereditary neuropathy with liability to pressure palsies. *Neurology* 48, 445–449.

26 Bai Y, Zhang X, Katona I *et al.* (2010) Conduction block in PMP22 deficiency. *J Neurosci* 30, 600–608.

27 Windebank AJ. (1984) Inherited recurrent focal neuropathies. In: Dyck PJ *et al.* (eds) *Peripheral Neuropathy*, 2nd edn, pp. 1656–1679. W-B Saunders, Philadelphia.

CHAPTER 16
Familial amyloid polyneuropathy

Manuel Melo Pires, Ricardo Taipa, and António Guimarães
Department of Neuropathology, Hospital de Santo António, Centro Hospitalar do Porto Instituto de Ciências Biomédicas Abel Salazar, Universidade do Porto, Porto, Portugal

Definition

Familial amyloid neuropathy (FAP) is a rare autosomal dominant disease first described in 1952 in Portugal by Andrade [1]. It is a progressive fatal disorder with classical onset before the age of 40 resulting from extracellular deposition of β pleated amyloid fibrils predominantly in the peripheral nerves. It causes severe sensory, motor and autonomic polyneuropathy initially affecting unmyelinated and small diameter myelinated fibers. There is associated systemic amyloidosis, frequently affecting the heart, the vitreous, and the kidney. The commonest fibril protein deposited is a variant form of transthyretin (TTR) [2] and a mutation in which methionine replaces valine in position 30 (TTRVal30Met) is the most frequent genetic defect [3]. Apolipoprotein A-1 and gelsolin are the other amyloid precursor proteins associated with FAP. In this chapter, we describe the characteristics of TTR-FAP, which is by far the most common disease of this group. Most TTR is produced by the liver, so liver transplant (LTx) has been used for 20 years to slow disease progression [4]. Recently, drugs capable of stabilizing TTR or inhibiting fibril formation have been tested, and one is already in use in early-stage disease [5].

Epidemiology

In 1939 Andrade described a patient with a "peculiar form of neuropathy" from a village near Póvoa do Varzim, north of Porto. In 1952 he described 74 further patients [1]. By 1994 there were 1233 cases from 489 pedigrees [6] registered at Unidade Clinica de Paramiloidose in Porto (Hospital Santo António). Currently, 664 families with 2657 patients are known, mainly in Northern Portugal, around Lisbon and in the central mountainous region. 51% of the cases have been diagnosed in the last two decades (Coelho T, unpublished data). The estimated prevalence in Portugal is 1/1000 [7] but prevalence is also significant in Japan and in Northern Sweden [8]. In the USA there is a high prevalence of Val142Ile TTR mutation in Black Americans [9]. FAP has also been reported in Cyprus, Mallorca, France, Greece, Italy, Turkey, Brazil, Ireland, England, and United States. Initially the Val30Met mutation was believed to originate from one founder in Portugal, historically spreading worldwide via the sea-faring Portuguese, and more recently by emigration, particularly to France in the 1960s. Recently, a Portuguese origin for Brazilian patients was suggested, but the Swedish Val30Met carriers have a different founder [10].

Clinical features

The most important clinical feature is a severely disabling ascending autonomic, sensory and motor polyneuropathy, with onset around 30 years of age, although later onset after the fifth decade can occur, particularly in non-endemic areas. Weight loss is a prominent early feature. Autonomic neuropathy occurs early and causes severe gastrointestinal, cardiac, and genitourinary problems [11] including orthostatic hypotension, alternating constipation and diarrhea, gastric retention, sexual impotence, urinary hesitancy, and dry skin. Early loss of pain and temperature are noted in the lower limbs because small fibers are more susceptible, but all sensory

Peripheral Nerve Disorders: Pathology and Genetics, First Edition. Edited by Jean-Michel Vallat, Joachim Weis, Francoise Gray, and Katy Keohane.

modalities soon become impaired. Painless injury to the feet causes ulcers, cellulitis, osteomyelitis and Charcot joints. Locally, the disease is referred to as "doença dos pézinhos," disease of the feet. Motor involvement appears later, causing atrophy, weakness, and loss of reflexes. Patients with late-onset disease tend to have a negative family history, fewer autonomic symptoms, and neuropathic pain requiring treatment is often the presenting symptom [12]. The vitreous and kidneys can be involved. Cardiomyopathy from amyloid deposition in the heart is a prominent feature of the Val122Ile and Leu111Met genotypes [9].

The diagnosis of FAP is based on molecular analysis of the TTR gene. In endemic areas or with a family history of FAP, tissue biopsy is not mandatory. Genetic confirmation of an amyloidogenic TTR mutation should be the first diagnostic step. In patients in non-endemic areas with no family history of FAP (later onset; sporadic presentation), with a nerve length-dependent progressive sensorimotor and autonomic polyneuropathy, often with cardiac involvement, tissue biopsy should be performed [13]. Despite genetic diagnosis, in most centers, biopsy demonstration of amyloid in nerve, skin, or salivary glands remains obligatory prior to liver transplantation or treatment with TTR stabilizers.

Pathology

FAP is a systemic disease with extracellular deposition of amyloid mainly in connective tissue, invariably in peripheral nerves and in some organs (kidney, heart, thyroid, testis, ovary, vitreous, and some exocrine glands, including sweat and salivary). In the brain, there are leptomeningeal, choroid plexus, and subependymal ventricular deposits. The most important lesions are in peripheral nerves, dorsal root ganglia, and the autonomic nervous system [14, 15].

The main pathological features are described in the study of over 1000 nerve, skin, and salivary gland biopsies and 30 autopsies of the Portuguese type of disease, with the Met30Val mutation collected over 40 years in our center. The peripheral nerves show loss of nerve fibers in parallel with the evolution of disease. The earliest lesions are degeneration of unmyelinated fibers, showing a "watery" appearance and dense bodies on electron microscopy (EM), progressing rapidly to severe fiber loss. The next phase starts with obvious loss of small myelinated fibers; large myelinated fibers become progressively affected as the disease evolves, proceeding to an almost complete loss of all nerve fibers in terminal cases. Degenerating myelinated fibers are observed as rows of myelin degenerating material. In teased fiber preparations these have the appearance of Wallerian degeneration or, rarely, segmental demyelination. In typical FAP cases, in patients with no other causes of neuropathy (e.g., diabetes), there are no clusters of regenerating nerve fibers and only rare fibers with disproportionately thin myelin sheaths are present. Onion bulbs are absent [1, 16–20].

Simultaneously and in a somewhat erratic manner, amyloid deposition begins. There is no clear correlation between fiber loss and endoneurial amyloid deposition,

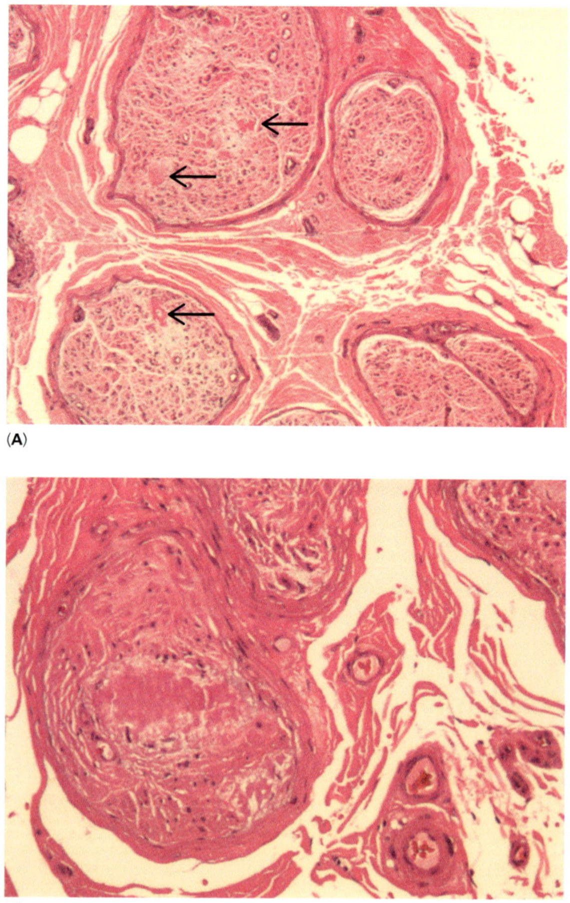

(A)

(B)

Figure 16.1 Transverse sections of sural nerve. (**A**) Several fascicles contain small amounts of amyloid deposits (arrows). Hematoxylin-eosin (H&E). (**B**) Large amyloid deposit in the endoneurium. H&E.

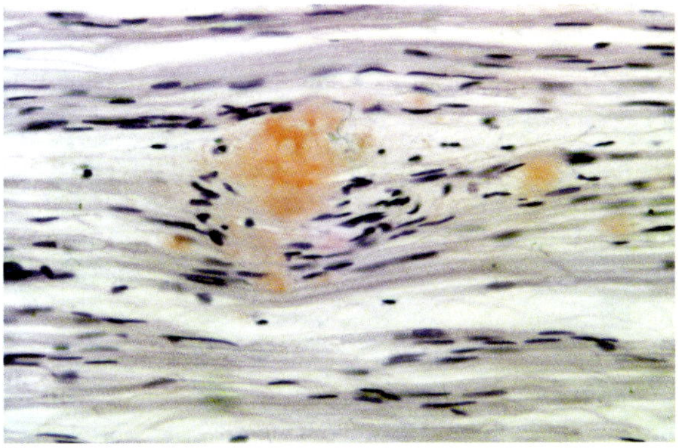

(A)

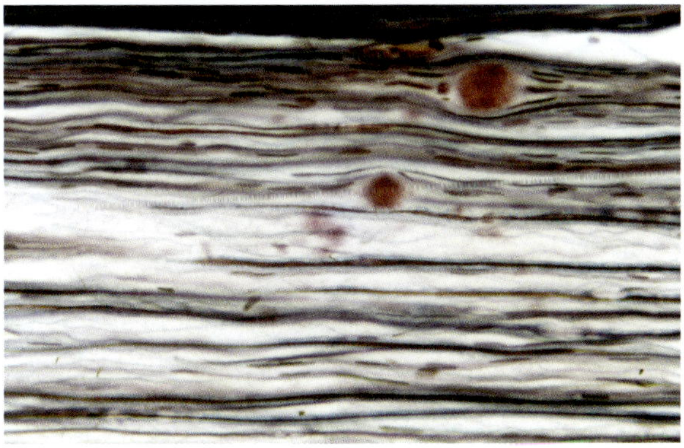

(B)

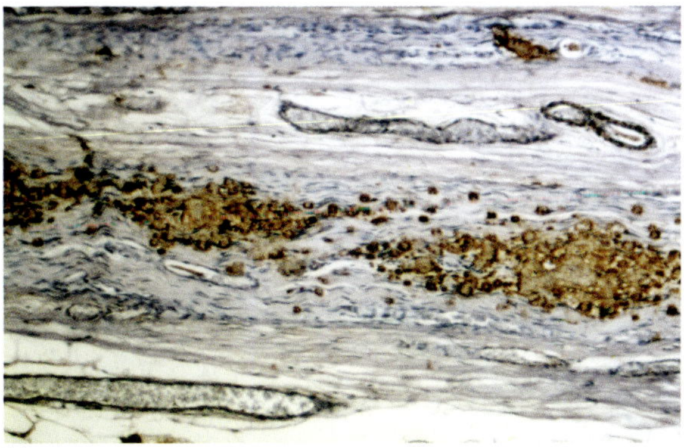

(C)

Figure 16.2 Longitudinal section of sural nerve. (**A**) Several globoid deposits of amyloid. Congo red stain. (**B**) Several globoid deposits of amyloid displace apparently normal myelinated axons. Luxol fast blue-Holmes stain. (**C**) Large anti-TTR immune-positive deposits occupy most of the endoneurium.

especially in later onset cases. The deposits are usually spheroidal, are located between and displace nerve fibers and tend to accumulate at the endoneurial periphery. Amyloid deposition varies from a total absence in very early onset cases to occupation of a large area of the nerve fascicle on transverse section. Sparse deposits maybe found in the epineurium, near the vessels, in connective tissue and around endoneurial capillaries, often infiltrating the vessel wall (Figs 16.1, 16.2A,B, 16.3).

To detect amyloid deposits, Congo red stain is essential, examined under polarized light to detect the typical green birefringence. Even very small deposits are seen by EM as intermingled non-ramified straight filaments 80 nm in diameter, sometimes forming parallel bundles (Fig. 16.4). Immunohistochemistry with antibodies

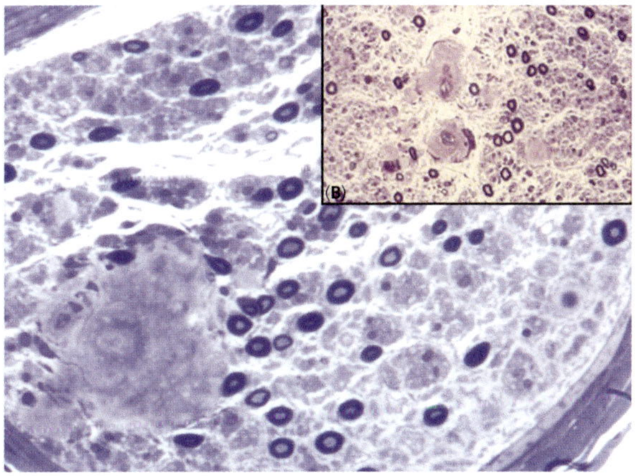

(A)

Figure 16.3 Semi-thin sections. (**A**) Large subperineurial amyloid deposit closely associated with myelinated fibers. Toluidine blue. (**B**) (*insert*) Severe loss of small diameter myelinated fibers with amyloid deposits around capillary walls and a small amount in the endoneurium. Toluidine blue.

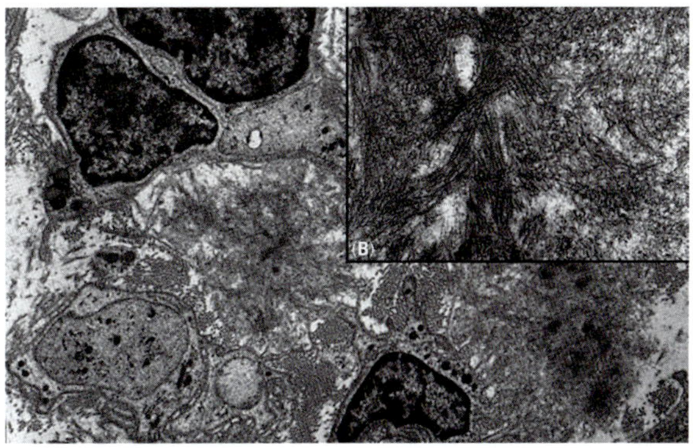

(A)

Figure 16.4 Electron Microscopy (EM). (**A**) Amyloid deposits surrounded by Schwann cell cytoplasm. (**B**) (*insert*) Bundles of amyloid fibrils with typical non-ramified structure surrounding collagen fibers.

against TTR and other amyloidogenic proteins may identify the type of amyloid (e.g., serum amyloid A and amyloid light chain) (Fig. 16.2C).

Progressive fibrosis occurs and in the final stage the endoneurial space is replaced by collagen, fibroblasts, and Schwann cells forming bands of Büngner, with a variable amount of amyloid. In brain autopsy material and biopsies, amyloid deposition occurs in association with leptomeningeal and perforating vessels and the subpial area (Fig. 16.5).

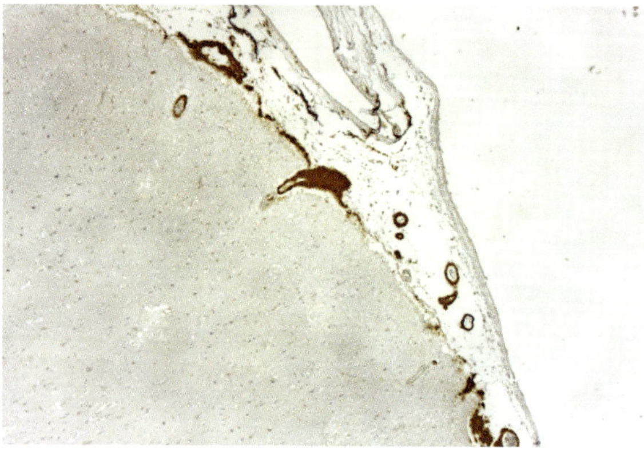

Figure 16.5 TTR immune-positive leptomeningeal amyloid deposition in an ValMet30 *TTR* autopsy case.

Before molecular diagnosis of FAP was available, amyloid deposition in nerve biopsies was required for diagnosis. Skin biopsies are almost as reliable as nerve with amyloid deposition around sweat glands acini and arrector pili muscles. Salivary gland biopsy, a minimally invasive procedure, is a very useful sensitive method to demonstrate amyloid in the basement membrane around gland acini and ducts. It is presently the method of choice in our center [21] and is positive even in early disease and in asymptomatic carriers (Fig. 16.6). Amyloid can also be demonstrated in other biopsy material, for example, colon, kidney, muscle, and abdominal fat.

Genetics

Human TTR is encoded by a single-copy gene on the long arm of chromosome 18. TTR is a homotetrameric plasma protein comprising 127-amino acid monomers produced primarily by the liver. Choroid plexus and retinal cells produce smaller amounts. Normally, TTR transports thyroxin and retinol [22]. FAP associates with point mutations in the *TTR gene*. The commonest molecular abnormality, first described in Portuguese kindreds, is a substitution of methionine for valine at position 30, TTR Val30Met [3]. Over a hundred amyloidogenic mutations

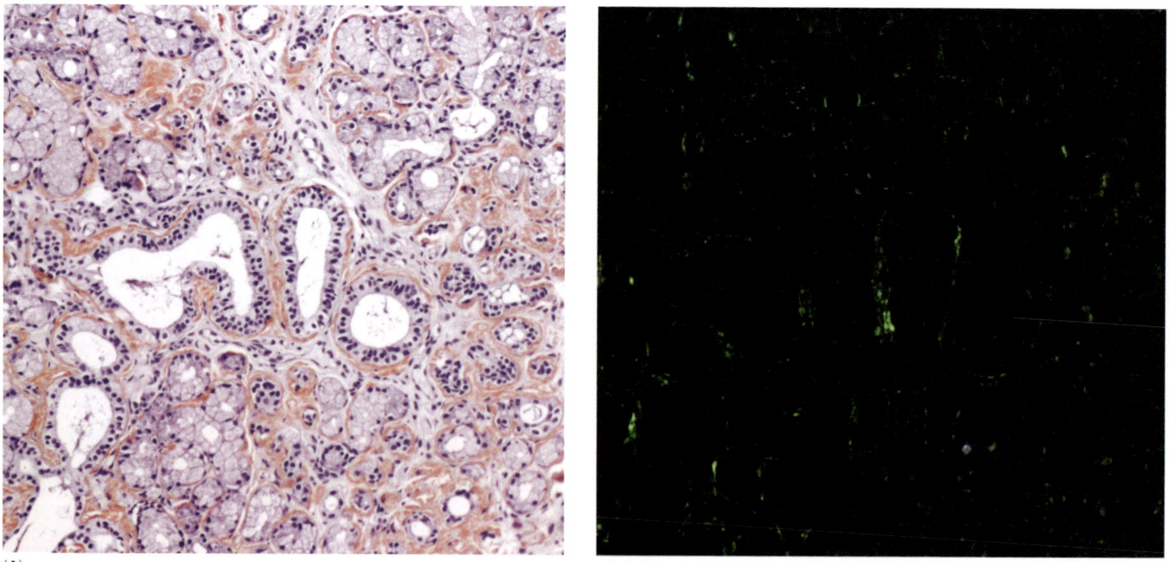

(A) (B)

Figure 16.6 Salivary gland biopsy. (**A**) Large amounts of amyloid surrounding acini and ducts. Congo red stain. (**B**) Green birefringence of amyloid in the salivary gland biopsy. Congo red stain.

in the *TTR* gene have been reported [23] typically presenting with PNS involvement, but some variants give rise to phenotypes that variously include neuropathy, cardiomyopathy, carpal tunnel syndrome, vitreous TTR deposition, and leptomeningeal involvement [24]. Val122Ile is the most common *TTR* mutation in the USA and is associated with cardiac amyloidosis. The Phe64Leu mutation is relatively frequent in Italy and is characterized by a very late onset (65–70 years) and a length-dependent neuropathy in all four limbs [25]. Genetic anticipation is noted in endemic areas [7]. At 80 years of age, penetrance is around 85% in Portugal, Brazil, and France, but only 69% in Sweden [13]. The age of onset of TTR amyloidosis associated with Val30Met varies between populations. The mean age of onset is 56 years in Sweden compared to 34 years in Portugal and Japan [9].

Differential diagnosis

The presumptive diagnosis of FAP is relatively straightforward when sensorimotor and autonomic polyneuropathy is present in a patient with family history of neuropathy. If family history of FAP is absent, a diagnosis of chronic inflammatory demyelinating polyneuropathy (CIDP) is often considered first [26, 27]. CIDP is often associated with elevated CSF protein and nerve conduction studies suggestive of demyelination frequently often accompanied by axonal degeneration (see Chapter 27). CSF protein can be raised also in FAP. Tissue biopsy, including salivary gland biopsy, and/or molecular analysis for TTR mutations can be useful in such cases. Some pathogenic *TTR* mutations lead to prominent bulbar involvement and fasciculations, simulating motor neuron disease, which must be considered in the differential diagnosis [25].

If amyloid is found in biopsies, light-chain amyloidosis is often considered due to the high incidence of monoclonal gammopathies in the elderly. Immunohistochemistry can be difficult to interpret and *TTR* gene sequencing should be done in all such cases [26].

Pathogenesis

The precise molecular mechanism underlying TTR fibrillogenesis is not fully understood. The current hypothesis is that point mutations cause TTR tetramer instability allowing its dissociation to non-native monomers that can self-associate [28]. Soluble monomers aggregate into insoluble multimeric forms leading to amyloid fibrils with the characteristic β pleated-sheet cross structure [28]. Mechanical and toxic effects are proposed as the likely mechanisms whereby endoneurial amyloid deposits cause neuropathy. Single fibers near amyloid deposits show distortion of their myelin sheaths, segmental demyelination and Wallerian degeneration, suggesting multifocal compression [29]. This theory does not explain the symmetrical polyneuropathy found in most FAP patients, the higher susceptibility of unmyelinated fibers [24], fiber degeneration in asymptomatic cases without visible amyloid deposits, or the lack of degeneration of large myelinated fibers displaced by amyloid deposits [17]. Most pathological studies in FAP were performed on sural nerve biopsies which represent a restricted portion of the PNS; TTR deposits more proximally in nerve trunks or in ganglia can lead to distal nerve fiber loss. Mature amyloid fibrils are not toxic to cells, but TTR non-fibrillar aggregates can induce cytoxicity by oxidative and inflammatory stress in neuronal cells, leading to cellular dysfunction and death [30–32].

Most reports of FAP agree that axonal degeneration begins in unmyelinated and small diameter myelinated fibers and large myelinated fibers are only affected in advanced cases [17, 24]. Why unmyelinated fibers are so heavily affected is unclear. There are conflicting data regarding Schwann cells' (SC) susceptibility to amyloid. Susceptibility of SC to endoneurial amyloid could explain the early loss of unmyelinated fibers, because each SC envelops several unmyelinated fibers. Schwann cells in contact with amyloid deposits show degenerative changes [13]. However, in suitably fixed FAP nerves, no morphological changes in SC were found [17, 33]. In our experience, segmental degeneration, onion bulb formation and myelin-axonal disproportion, usually characteristic of Schwannian pathology, are almost always absent and evidence of regeneration is not found in nerve biopsies of patients with FAP.

Animal models

Several groups have generated transgenic mice carrying the human Val30Met *TTR* gene. These mouse models do not show all the features of human disease, since the peripheral nervous tissue is spared. A new mouse model expressing human Val30Met transthyretin in a heat shock transcription factor 1 (Hsf1) null background showed extensive early deposition of non-fibrillar TTR evolving into fibrillar material in specific organs, including the PNS [34].

Conclusions and future perspectives

The most common FAP is caused by mutations in the *TTR* gene. Despite a group of core clinical features and some association of distinct phenotypes with particular genotypes, a wide spectrum of signs and symptoms is observed. The pathology is characterized by systemic amyloid deposits predominantly in the peripheral nervous system. The two treatment options are liver transplantation and the TTR stabilizer tafamidis. The precise molecular mechanism underlying TTR fibrillogenesis remains unclear. A better understanding of FAP pathophysiology and early diagnosis are crucial for the improved management of this severe disorder.

Acknowledgments

The authors thank Isabel Pires and Aurora Rodrigues for technical assistance. We cordially thank Dr Minal Honavar for revising the manuscript. We are also indebted Dr Teresa Coelho and Unidade Clinica de Paramiloidose, Hospital Santo António – Centro Hospitalar do Porto, for many years of clinical collaboration.

References

1 Andrade C. (1952) A peculiar form of peripheral neuropathy: familial atypical generalized amyloidosis with special involvement of the peripheral nerves. *Brain* 75:408–427.
2 Costa PP, Figueira AS, Bravo FR. (1978) Amyloid fibril protein related to prealbumin in familial amyloidotic polyneuropathy. *Proc Natl Acad Sci U S A.* 75:4499–4503.
3 Saraiva MJ, Birken S, Costa PP, *et al.* (1984) Amyloid fibril protein in familial amyloidotic polyneuropathy, Portuguese type. Definition of molecular abnormality in transthyretin (prealbumin). *J Clin Invest.* 74:104–119.
4 Herlenius G, Wilczek HE, Larsson M, *et al.* (2004) Ten years of international experience with liver transplantation for familial amyloidotic polyneuropathy: results from the Familial Amyloidotic Polyneuropathy. *World Transplant Registry Transplantation* 77:64–71.
5 Coelho T, Maia LF, Silva AM, *et al.* (2012) Tafamidis for transthyretin familial amyloid polyneuropathy: a randomized controlled trial. *Neurology* 79:785–792.
6 Coelho T, Sousa A, Lourenço E, *et al.* (1994) A study of 159 Portuguese patients with familial amyloidotic polyneuropathy (FAP) whose parents were both unaffected. *J Med Genet.* 31:293–299.
7 Sousa A, Coelho T, Barros J, *et al.* (1995) Genetic epidemiology of familial amyloidotic polyneuropathy (FAP)-type I in Povoa do Varzim and Vila do Conde (north of Portugal). *Am J Med Genet.* 60:512–521.
8 Andersson, R. (1970) Hereditary amylodosis with polyneuropathy. *Acta Med Scand.* 1–2:85–94.
9 Coelho T, Maurer M, Suhr O. (2013) THAOS – The transthyretin amyloidosis outcomes survey: Inicial report on clinical manifestations in patients with hereditary and wild-type transthyretin amyloidosis. *Curr Med Res Opin* 29:1–14.
10 Zaros C, Genin E, Hellman U, *et al.* (2008) On the origin of the transthyretin Val30Met familial amyloid polyneuropathy. *Annals Human Gen.* 72:478–484.
11 Reilly MM, Staunton H. (1996) Peripheral nerve amyloidosis. *Brain Pathol.* 6:163–77.
12 Conceição I, De Carvalho M. (2007) Clinical variability in type I familial amyloid polyneuropathy (Val30Met): comparison between late- and early-onset cases in Portugal. *Muscle Nerve.* 35:116–118.
13 Planté-Bordeneuve V, Said G. (2011) Familial amyloid polyneuropathy. *Lancet Neurol.* 10:1086–1097.
14 Guimarães A, Monteiro L, Coutinho P. (1980) Pathology of the autonomic nervous system in Andrade type of familial amyloidotic polyneuropathy. Study of 11 postmortem cases. In: Glenner G, Costa P, Freitas A. (eds) *Amyloid and Amyloidosis,* pp. 139–146. Excerpta Medica, Amsterdam-Oxford-Princeton.
15 Ikeda S, Hanyu N, Hongo M, *et al.* (1987) Hereditary generalized amyloidosis with polyneuropathy. Clinicopathological study of 65 Japanese patients. *Brain* 110:315–337.
16 Dick PJ, Lambert EH. (1969) Dissociated sensation in amyloidosis: compound action potential, quantitative histologic and teased-fiber, and electron microscopic studies of sural nerve biopsies. *Arch Neurol* 20:490–507.
17 Guimarães A, Viana Pinheiro A, Leite I (1990) Sural nerve biopsy in familial amyloidotic polyneuropathy: a morphological and morphometric study. In: Natvig JB, Forre O, Husby G, Husenbekk A, Skogen B, Sletten K, Westermark P. (eds) *Amyloid and Amyloidosis,* pp. 493–398. Kluwer Academic Publishers, London.
18 Misu K, Attori N, Nagamatsu M, *et al.* (1999) Late onset familial amyloid polyneuropathy type 1 (transthyretin Met30-associated familial amyloid polyneuropathy) unrelated to endemic focus in Japan. Clinicopathological and genetic features. *Brain* 122:1951–1962.
19 Vital C, Vital A, Bouillot-Eimer S, Brechenmacher *et al.* (2004) Amyloid neuropathy: retrospective study of 35 peripheral nerve biopsies. *J Periph Nervous Syst.* 9:232–241.

20 Said G, Planté-Bordeneuve V (2009) Familial amyloid polyneuropathy. A clinic-pathologic study. *J Neuro Sci.* 284:149–154.
21 Amaral B, Coelho T, Sousa A, *et al* (2009) Usefulness of labial salivary gland biopsy in FAP. *Amyloid* 16:232–238.
22 Saraiva MJ. (2001) Transthyretin mutations in hyperthyroxinemia and amyloid diseases. *Hum Mutat.* 17:493–503.
23 Araki S, Ando Y. (2010) Transthyretin-related familial amyloidotic polyneuropathy-progress in Kumamoto, Japan (1967–2010). *Proc Jpn Acad Ser B Phys Biol Sci.* 86:694–697.
24 Sousa MM, Saraiva MJ. (2003) Neurodegeneration in familial amyloid polyneuropathy: from pathology to molecular signaling. *Prog Neurobiol.* 71:385–400.
25 Cappellari M, Cavallaro T, Ferrarini M, *et al.* (2011) Variable presentations of TTR-related familial amyloid polyneuropathy in seventeen patients. *J Periph Nervous Syst.* 16:199–129.
26 Planté-Bordeneuve V, Ferreira A, Lalu T, *et al.* (2007) Diagnostic pitfalls in sporadic transthyretin familial amyloid polyneuropathy (TTR-FAP). *Neurology* 69:693–698.
27 Mathis S, Magy L, Diallo L, *et al.* (2011) Amyloid neuropathy mimicking chronic inflammatory demyelinating polyneuropathy. *Muscle and Nerve* 45:26–31.
28 Quintas A, Vaz DC, Cardoso I, *et al.* (2001) Tetramer dissociation and monomer partial unfolding precedes protofibril formation in amyloidogenic transthyretin variants. *J Biol Chem* 276:27207–27213.
29 Said G, Ropert A, Faux N. (1984) Length-dependent degeneration of fibers in Portuguese amyloid polyneuropathy: a clinicopathologic study. *Neurology* 34:1025–1032.
30 Sousa MM, Cardoso I, Fernandes R, *et al.* (2001) Deposition of transthyretin in early stages of familial amyloidotic polyneuropathy: evidence for toxicity of nonfibrillar aggregates. *Am J Pathol.* 159:1993–2000.
31 Andersson K, Olofsson A, Niesen EH, *et al.* (2002) Only amyloidogenic intermediates of transthyretin induce apoptosis. *Biochem Biophys Res Commun.* 294:309–314.
32 Sörgjerd K, Klingstedt T, Lindgren M, *et al.* (2005) Prefibrillar transthyretin oligomers and cold stored native tetrameric transthyretin are cytotoxic in cell culture. *Biochem Biophys Res Commun.* 377:1072–1078.
33 Misumi Y, Ueda M, Obayashi K, *et al.* (2012) Relationship between amyloid deposition and intracellular structural changes in familial amyloidotic polyneuropathy. *Hum Pathol.* 43:96–104.
34 Santos SD, Fernandes R, Saraiva MJ. (2010) The heat shock response modulates transthyretin deposition in the peripheral and autonomic nervous systems. *Neurobiol Aging.* 31:280–289.

CHAPTER 17

Peripheral neuropathies in mitochondrial disorders

Benoît Funalot

Departments of Biochemistry, Genetics, and Neurology, National Referral Center for Rare Peripheral Neuropathies, CHU Limoges and EA6309 "Myelin Maintenance and Peripheral Neuropathies," Limoges University Medicine School, Limoges, France

Introduction

Primary mitochondrial disorders are caused by mutations in mitochondrial DNA (mtDNA) or by mutations in nuclear genes encoding proteins involved in mitochondrial function. Each of these mitochondrial disorders is very rare and precise epidemiological data are lacking. In many instances, mitochondrial diseases are multiorgan disorders with multisystem neurological impairment, and peripheral neuropathies (PNP) only represent a minor manifestation with little effect on patient disability [1]. Examples of such disorders are Mitochondrial Encephalomyopathy with Lactic Acidosis and Stroke-like episodes (MELAS), Myoclonic Epilepsy with Ragged Red Fibers (MERRF), or Neuropathy, Ataxia, and Retinitis Pigmentosa (NARP). In some cases however, the peripheral neuropathy can be the first manifestation and/or the main disabling symptom of the disease. The clinical manifestations and neuropathological phenotypes of these diseases will be presented according to the mode of inheritance (mitochondrial or nuclear) and the genes involved.

Peripheral neuropathies associated with mtDNA mutations

PNPs are common in patients harboring mtDNA point mutations but frequently have only few symptoms. They have been repeatedly reported in patients with the following mutations: m.3243A>G (MELAS mutation), m.8344A>G (MERRF mutation), m.8993T>G, and m.8993T>C (NARP mutations). Mitochondrial DNA point mutations are maternally inherited and the level of heteroplasmy (percentage of mutated mtDNA in a given tissue/cell type) is a determinant of the resulting phenotype. In most cases of PNP associated with mtDNA point mutations, clinical examination, and electroneuromyography (ENMG) disclose a sensory or sensorimotor axonal neuropathy [1, 2]. Sural nerve biopsy, when performed, showed a decrease density of myelinated fibers with clusters of regenerating myelinated fibers (indicating chronic axonal degeneration). These alterations were sometimes associated with minimal changes in myelin (disproportionately thin myelin sheaths, few onion bulbs) and subtle mitochondrial alterations in axons and in the Schwann cell cytoplasm [2]. More interestingly, several patients with a Charcot–Marie–Tooth type 2 (CMT2) phenotype were recently found to harbor the m.9185T>C mutation in the *MT-ATP6* gene (representing ~1% of undefined CMT2 cases in a series of 442 patients) [3]. This mutation had previously been associated with maternally-inherited Leigh syndrome or isolated ataxia in several families. To date, nerve biopsy findings have not been reported for this mutation. In a patient with another nearby mutation of the *MT-ATP6* gene, m.9176T>C, nerve biopsy showed features suggestive of a chronic demyelinating neuropathy, with multiple multilayered onion bulbs. In a few other patients with mtDNA point mutations, moderately reduced nerve conduction velocities at ENMG and demyelinating features at nerve biopsy have been reported [2].

Mitochondrial DNA deletions represent the other main type of mtDNA primary mutation. Large deletions

Peripheral Nerve Disorders: Pathology and Genetics, First Edition. Edited by Jean-Michel Vallat, Joachim Weis, Francoise Gray, and Katy Keohane.

are sporadic post-zygotic "accidental" events and are very rarely transmitted maternally. In the setting of a multisystem neurological dysfunction due to mtDNA deletion, such as KSS, PNP can occur and is usually mild or even subclinical. Only one nerve biopsy has been published and showed moderate axonal degeneration [4].

Peripheral neuropathies associated with nuclear DNA mutations

Disorders of mtDNA maintenance

These disorders result from the dysfunction of proteins directly or indirectly involved in the replication and/or repair of mtDNA. They are caused by mutations in nuclear genes, are inherited in a Mendelian fashion as either autosomal dominant or recessive traits and result in mtDNA alterations. The two main types of (secondary) mtDNA abnormalities that have been identified are multiple deletions and depletion of mtDNA (marked decrease of the total amount of mtDNA).

Multiple deletions of mtDNA

These are due to repeated defects of replication and/or repair of mtDNA. They are not present in the blood (leukocyte DNA) but have been found in muscle and sometimes in affected nerves [5]. The most common forms of multiple deletions syndromes combine progressive external ophthalmoplegia with various types of neurologic multisystem involvement. In these syndromes, the peripheral neuropathy can be the initial and/or the most disabling feature [1].

An example of a multiple deletions syndrome is Sensory Ataxic Neuropathy with Dysarthria and Ophthalmoplegia (SANDO), caused by recessive mutations of the *POLG1* gene-encoding the catalytic subunit of the mtDNA polymerase (polymerase gamma). Other *POLG1*-related disorders have been reported under various names: Mitochondrial Recessive Ataxia Syndrome (MIRAS), Ataxia Neuropathy Spectrum (ANS), childhood Myo-Cerebro-Hepatopathy Spectrum (MCHS), Spino-Cerebellar Ataxia with Epilepsy (SCAE), and Myoclonic Epilepsy, Myopathy, and Sensory Ataxia (MEMSA) [6]. Peripheral neuropathy is frequent in these syndromes and can be severe. Most often, it is a sensory ataxic neuropathy (ganglionopathy), but length-dependent sensory or sensorimotor neuropathies (the latter mimicking CMT2) are possible [7]. Neuropathological reports are very scarce and the few published only show features of axonal degeneration in the nerve biopsy (severe loss of myelinated fibers and some clusters of regenerating fibers) and posterior column degeneration [8–10]. The dorsal root ganglia (which might be affected) have not been studied in the two autopsied cases [9, 10].

Mitochondrial Neuro-Gastro-Intestinal Encephalomyopathy (MNGIE) is another multiple deletions syndrome. This autosomal recessive (AR) multisystem mitochondrial disorder is caused by mutations in the *TYMP* gene encoding thymidine phosphorylase [11]. Severe gastrointestinal dysmotility characterizes this disorder and results in progressive cachexia. Additional manifestations include progressive external ophthalmoplegia, retinopathy, myopathy and diffuse leukoencephalopathy (present in all patients). All patients develop a sensorimotor demyelinating PNP but with varying degrees of severity, resulting in distal weakness and atrophy of the lower limb muscles [12]. Nerve biopsies performed in MNGIE patients disclosed demyelinating features, reduction of myelinated fiber density, and clusters of regenerating fibers. Electron microscopy showed dystrophic mitochondria with loss of cristae in axons, Schwann cells and in endothelial cells, with occasional paracrystalline inclusions in several patients [13].

Mitochondrial DNA depletion

Mitochondrial DNA depletion results from a more severe dysfunction of mtDNA maintenance. For this reason, diseases associated with mtDNA depletion usually have early onset and severe clinical presentations [14]. Two AR mtDNA depletion disorders complicated by PNP have been characterized.

Navajo neuro-hepatopathy, an infantile-onset PNP, was reported in 1976 in Native Americans from the Navajo population in the southwestern United States [15]. It is a sensorimotor PNP with distal weakness, areflexia, and loss of sensation that results in corneal ulcers and acral mutilation. Later on, patients develop neurogenic arthropathies. Nerve conduction velocities are reduced and both types of fibers are affected on nerve biopsy, with severe reduction of myelinated fibers associated with marked abnormalities of unmyelinated fibers (reduced axonal diameter, increase of mitochondria and dense bodies, abnormalities of neurofilaments, and microtubules). Affected patients also

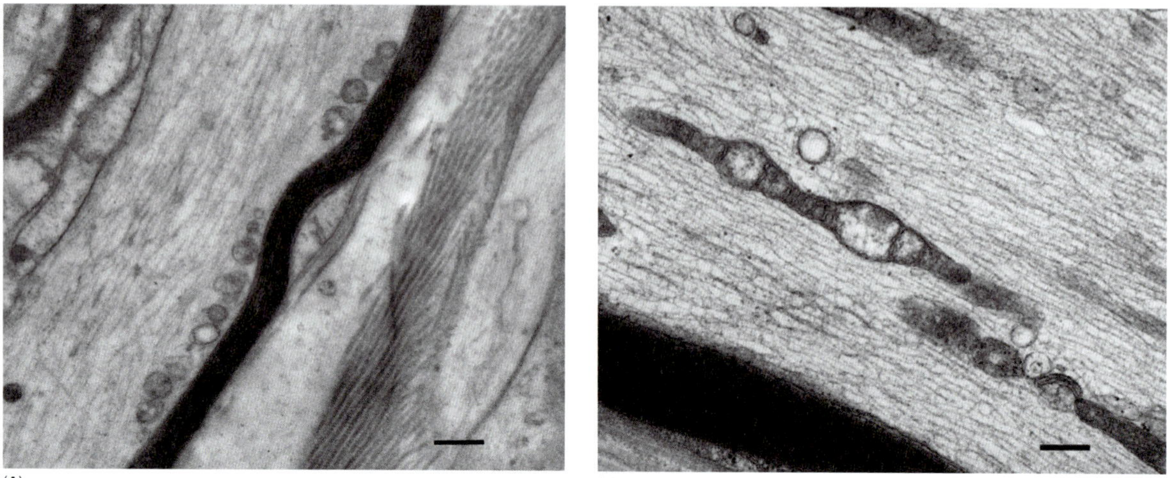

(A) (B)

Figure 17.1 (**A**) Longitudinal section of sural nerve biopsy from a patient with MFN2 mutation, showing a series of small, round, and aggregated mitochondria at the periphery of the axon; bar = 500 nm. (**B**) Longitudinal section from a normal nerve, showing elongated mitochondria scattered within the axon; bar = 500 nm.

have leukoencephalopathy on MRI and liver dysfunction associated with mtDNA depletion in liver tissue. This syndromic PNP is associated with a founder mutation (p.R50Q) in the *MPV17* gene [16].

Infantile-Onset Spinocerebellar Ataxia (IOSCA) is another mtDNA depletion syndrome associated with PN, first reported in the Finnish population [17], in which sensory axonal neuropathy is associated with cerebellar ataxia, epilepsy, athetosis, deafness, and progressive external ophthalmoplegia. This disorder is caused by mutations in the *PEO1* (C10ORF2) gene encoding the mitochondrial helicase Twinkle. Affected patients had mtDNA depletion in the brain and liver [18]. Sural nerve biopsy showed a progressive loss of large myelinated fibers [19].

Primary dysfunction of the mitochondrial respiratory chain

SURF1 mutations represent a major cause of AR Leigh syndrome (LS) associated with cytochrome oxidase deficiency [14]. In patients with SURF1-related LS (usually with infantile onset), PNP could be present in up to 40% of cases [20], even if the most prominent and life-threatening symptoms are related to CNS dysfunction. In these patients, nerve conduction velocities are decreased and nerve biopsy is suggestive of a myelinopathy, with disproportionately thin myelinated fibers and loss of large myelinated fibers [20]. In some patients, the CNS dysfunction is very limited, appears later than the PNP [21], and lifespan is much longer, two of the three patients reported to date being older than 40 years of age. In one patient, nerve biopsy showed features of chronic demyelinating neuropathy, with moderate axonal loss, presence of onion bulbs, and hypomyelinated fibers [21].

Dysfunctions of mitochondrial dynamics

The alteration of mitochondrial fusion and fission processes by mutations in the *MFN2* and *GDAP1* genes are responsible for hereditary sensorimotor neuropathies (CMT). MFN2 mutations cause CMT2A2 and GDAP1 cause CMT4A and CMT2K [1]. The genetics and general neuropathology of these disorders have been described elsewhere in this book (see Chapters 10 and 11). In MFN2-related PN, longitudinal sections of nerve biopsies show marked abnormalities of axonal mitochondria, which appear round and aggregate at the periphery of the axon (Figure 17.1).

Animal models

There is no animal model of peripheral neuropathy associated with a mitochondrial disorder so far.

References

1 Pareyson D, Piscosquito G, Moroni I, *et al.* (2013) Peripheral neuropathy in mitochondrial disorders. *Lancet Neurol* 12, 1011–1024.
2 Bouillot S, Martin-Négrier ML, Vital A, *et al.* (2002) Peripheral neuropathy associated with mitochondrial disorders: 8 cases and review of the literature. *J Peripher Nerv Syst* 7, 213–220.
3 Pitceathly RD, Murphy SM, Cottenie E, *et al.* (2012) Genetic dysfunction of MT-ATP6 causes axonal Charcot–Marie–Tooth disease. *Neurology* 79, 1145–1154.
4 Zanssen S, Molnar M, Buse G, Schröder JM. (1998) Mitochondrial cytochrome b gene deletion in Kearns–Sayre syndrome associated with a subclinical type of peripheral neuropathy. *Clin Neuropathol* 17, 291–296.
5 Fadic R, Russell JA, Vedanarayanan VV, *et al.* (1997) Sensory ataxic neuropathy as the presenting feature of a novel mitochondrial disease. *Neurology* 49, 239–245.
6 Hudson G, Chinnery PF. (2006) Mitochondrial DNA polymerase-gamma and human disease. *Hum Mol Genet* 15, R244–252.
7 Harrower T, Stewart JD, Hudson G, *et al.* (2008) POLG1 mutations manifesting as autosomal recessive axonal Charcot–Marie–Tooth disease. *Arch Neurol* 65, 133–136.
8 Santoro L, Manganelli F, Lanzillo R, *et al.* (2006) A new POLG1 mutation with PEO and severe axonal and demyelinating sensory-motor neuropathy. *J Neurol* 253, 869–874.
9 Van Goethem G, Luoma P, Rantamäki M, *et al.* (2004) POLG mutations in neurodegenerative disorders with ataxia but no muscle involvement. *Neurology* 63, 1251–1257.
10 Hopkins SE, Somoza A, Gilbert DL. (2010) Rare autosomal dominant POLG1 mutation in a family with metabolic strokes, posterior column spinal degeneration, and multi-endocrine disease. *J Child Neurol* 25, 752–756.
11 Nishino I, Spinazzola A, Hirano M. (1999) Thymidine phosphorylase gene mutations in MNGIE, a human mitochondrial disorder. *Science* 283, 689–692.
12 Nishino I, Spinazzola A, Papadimitriou A, *et al.* (2000) Mitochondrial neurogastrointestinal encephalomyopathy: an autosomal recessive disorder due to thymidine phosphorylase mutations. *Ann Neurol* 47, 792–800.
13 Said G, Lacroix C, Planté-Bordeneuve V, *et al.* (2005) Clinicopathological aspects of the neuropathy of neurogastrointestinal encephalomyopathy (MNGIE) in four patients including two with a Charcot–Marie–Tooth presentation. *J Neurol* 252, 655–662.
14 Menezes MP, Ouvrier RA. (2012) Peripheral neuropathy associated with mitochondrial disease in children. *Dev Med Child Neurol* 54, 407–414.
15 Appenzeller O, Kornfeld M, Snyder R. (1976) Acromutilating, paralyzing neuropathy with corneal ulceration in Navajo children. *Arch Neurol* 33, 733–738.
16 Karadimas CL, Vu TH, Holve SA, *et al.* (2006) Navajo neurohepatopathy is caused by a mutation in the MPV17 gene. *Am J Hum Genet* 79, 544–548.
17 Koskinen T, Santavuori P, Sainio K, *et al.* (1994) Infantile onset spinocerebellar ataxia with sensory neuropathy: a new inherited disease. *J Neurol Sci* 121, 50–56.
18 Hakonen AH, Goffart S, Marjavaara S, *et al.* (2008) Infantile-onset spinocerebellar ataxia and mitochondrial recessive ataxia syndrome are associated with neuronal complex I defect and mtDNA depletion. *Hum Mol Genet* 17, 322–335.
19 Koskinen T, Sainio K, Rapola J, *et al.* (1994) Sensory neuropathy in infantile onset spinocerebellar ataxia (IOSCA). *Muscle Nerve* 17, 509–515.
20 Santoro L, Carrozzo R, Malandrini A, *et al.* (2000) A novel SURF1 mutation results in Leigh syndrome with peripheral neuropathy caused by cytochrome c oxidase deficiency. *Neuromuscular disorders* 10, 450–453.
21 Echaniz-Laguna A, Ghezzi D, Chassagne M, *et al.* (2013) SURF1 deficiency causes demyelinating Charcot–Marie–Tooth disease. *Neurology* 81, 1523–1530.

CHAPTER 18
Giant axonal neuropathy

Robert Ouvrier and Manoj Menezes
Department of Neurology, The Children's Hospital at Westmead, Sydney, Australia

Definition

Giant axonal neuropathy (GAN) is an inherited childhood-onset progressive neurodegenerative condition characterized histopathologically by the presence of swollen "giant" axons in nerve and skin biopsies. GAN is caused by recessive mutations in the *GAN* gene that codes for an E3 ligase, gigaxonin, which is a member of the BTB/kelch superfamily of proteins.

Clinical features

GAN is associated with tightly curled hair and progressive neurodegeneration of the peripheral and central nervous system [1]. Parental consanguinity is seen in some families [2].

Onset usually occurs by 7 years of age and children may present with delayed motor milestones and gait abnormalities. The peripheral neuropathy manifests as distal weakness, initially affecting the lower limbs and progressing to involve the upper limbs, though presentation with sensory ataxia has been described [3]. Progressive central nervous system (CNS) involvement may manifest as psychomotor retardation, encephalopathy, severe learning difficulties and seizures. Clinical examination reveals the presence of a large fiber sensory and motor neuropathy with distally predominant weakness, wasting, areflexia, and vibration and proprioceptive sensory loss. CNS involvement is characterized by pyramidal and cerebellar signs, and cranial nerve dysfunction in the form of optic atrophy, nystagmus, ophthalmoplegia, facial weakness, dysarthria and bulbar palsy.

Skeletal deformities may include pes cavus, pes planovalgus, scoliosis, camptodactyly or flexion deformity of the fifth finger [2, 4]. A characteristic, but not universal, feature is the presence of tightly curled hair, described as "frizzy" or "woolly," in many patients irrespective of ethnic background. Morphological examination of the scalp hair shows trichorrhexis nodosa and fringing of the cut ends [5]. Pili torti, characteristic of Menkes disease, are not a feature.

Progressive deterioration results in loss of ambulation and death by the third decade. GAN presenting as an inherited peripheral neuropathy resembling CMT2 with delayed CNS involvement [6] or with severe CNS involvement and mild sensorimotor neuropathy [7] has also been described.

Electrophysiology and imaging

Nerve conduction studies show reduced or absent motor and sensory amplitudes with normal or mildly reduced motor and sensory conduction velocities, consistent with an axonal sensorimotor neuropathy [4]. Visual and auditory evoked potentials and SSEPs may show prolonged latencies, and EEG may show diffuse slow-wave activity but is normal in many cases [4, 8].

MRI may show increased T2 signal in the cerebral and cerebellar white matter, and cortical, cerebellar and brainstem atrophy [4]. Bilateral increase in signal in the globus pallidus and thalamus, and cerebellar tonsillar herniation has been described [9]. MRS shows increased choline/creatinine ratios, increased lactate and decreased N-acetyl aspartate/creatine ratios indicating both myelin and axonal damage [10].

Peripheral Nerve Disorders: Pathology and Genetics, First Edition. Edited by Jean-Michel Vallat, Joachim Weis, Francoise Gray, and Katy Keohane.

Genetics

The *GAN* gene was localized to 16q24 by homozygosity mapping [11] and identified by Bomont and colleagues in 2000 [12]. Different missense, nonsense and frameshift mutations, and microdeletions in the *GAN* gene have been described as causing GAN. There is wide clinical heterogeneity and genotype-phenotype correlation is poor [2]. Manifesting carriers have also been reported [13]. It is postulated that gigaxonin plays a role in degrading cytoplasmic intermediate filaments, which accumulate in neuronal and non-neuronal cells in GAN.

Neuropathology

The initial descriptions of the histopathology on a sural nerve biopsy by Berg [14] and Asbury [15] encapsulate most of the salient features. Transverse sections show large argentophilic cylindrical masses which are distended axons measuring up to 50 μm in diameter. Some nerve fibers have no myelin or thin myelin sheaths and onion bulbs are seen (see Fig. 7.13). There is moderate reduction in the total nerve fiber density. Ultrastructurally, the axonal swellings are due to masses of neurofilaments (Fig. 18.1) and involve both myelinated and unmyelinated fibers. The reduction in nerve fiber density involves all fiber types. There is a mild increase in endoneurial collagen and fibroblasts. The myelin sheath thins out as it stretches out over the axonal swelling due to the sequential peeling of the innermost myelin lamellae. Within the enlarged axons, the individual neurofilament strands, of normal diameter and structure, show a tendency to accumulate into electron-dense masses.

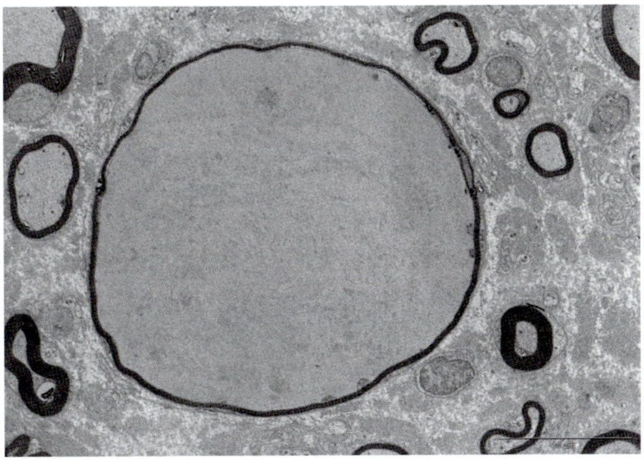

Figure 18.1 Electron micrograph; transverse section. A hugely dilated axon packed with neurofilaments. Its myelin sheath is abnormally thin. Normal sized myelinated axons surround the giant axon. Source: Jean-Michel Vallat, CHU de Limoges, France. Reproduced with permission of Jean-Michel Vallat.

Within the swollen axons, other intracellular organelles like mitochondria, neurotubules, and smooth endoplasmic reticulum are found clustered in neurofilament-free channels in the periphery or in the center of the axonal swellings. Some normal-sized axons show an increase in neurofilaments while other axons have increased neurotubules but no increase in neurofilaments. Discrete masses of filaments have also been reported in other cells including Schwann cells, endoneurial fibroblasts, perineurial cells and endothelial cells in nerve biopsies and in fibroblasts, melanocytes and endothelial cells of capillaries, lymphatic vessels and arterioles of skin biopsies. These cells otherwise appear normal [16, 17]. Histopathological changes similar to those observed in the peripheral nerve biopsy have also been reported in the axons of the myenteric plexus [18].

Teased fibers from the sural nerve show focal axonal swellings, myelin irregularities, paranodal myelin retraction, and segmental demyelination and remyelination. The focal axonal swellings have thin myelin sheaths, can occur within areas of demyelination, and have no relationship to the location of the nodes of Ranvier [19]. In a few cases it has been mentioned that some myelinated fibers are surrounded by basal lamina proliferations with an appearance of onion bulbs.

The muscle biopsy shows changes consistent with denervation. Increase in cytoplasmic microfilaments is not seen in the normal or atrophic fibers, though increased microfilaments may be seen within endomysial fibroblasts [19].

Postmortem examination shows diffuse atrophy throughout the brain and spinal cord including dilated ventricles, thinning of the corpus callosum, atrophy of the cerebellum and thinning of the spinal cord. Microscopy shows axonal spheroids and fusiform swellings in the posterior columns, corticospinal, spinothalamic and spinocerebellar tracts, in the anterior horn cells and less commonly, in the cerebral and cerebellar cortex. There is widespread demyelination. Ultrastructurally, the swollen axons are filled with neurofilaments arranged in an interlacing whorled pattern. Rosenthal fibers are found distributed throughout the CNS, often in areas devoid of axonal swellings, and are most numerous in the cerebellar white matter, walls of the third ventricle, internal capsule and pons [20, 21].

Differential diagnosis

Giant axons in nerves have also been described following exposure to toxins like carbon disulphide, acrylamide, triorthocresylphosphate, iminodipropionitrile, methyl-n-butyl ketone, 2,5-hexanedione and n-hexane [19, 22]. They are also sometimes seen in inherited neuropathies due to mutations in the *NEFL* [23] and *SH3TC2* genes [2, 24] as well as in infantile neuroaxonal dystrophy [25] and in patients with BAG3-associated myofibrillar myopathy [26].

Treatment

No disease-modifying therapy is currently available, and treatment continues to be rehabilitative and supportive.

References

1 Ouvrier RA (1989) Giant axonal neuropathy. A review. *Brain Dev*;11:207–214.

2 Tazir M, Nouioua S, Magy L, *et al.* (2009) Phenotypic variability in giant axonal neuropathy. *Neuromuscul Disord.*;19: 270–24.

3 Ouvrier RA, Prineas J, Walsh JC, *et al.* (1974) Giant axonal neuropathy – a third case. *Proc Aust Assoc Neurol.*;11: 137–144.

4 Koop O, Schirmacher A, Nelis E, *et al.* (2007) Genotype-phenotype analysis in patients with giant axonal neuropathy (GAN). *Neuromuscul Disord.*;17:624–630.

5 Lycklama à Nijeholt J, Koerten HK, de Wolff FA (1994) Giant axonal degeneration: scanning electron microscopic and biochemical study of scalp hair. *Dermatology*;188: 258–262.

6 Zemmouri R, Azzedine H, Assami S, *et al.* (2000) Charcot–Marie–Tooth 2-like presentation of an Algerian family with giant axonal neuropathy. *Neuromuscul Disord.*;10:592–598.

7 Lampl Y, Eshel Y, Ben-David E, *et al.* (1992) Giant axonal neuropathy with predominant central nervous system manifestations. *Dev Med Child Neurol.*;34:164–169.

8 Majnemer A, Rosenblatt B, Watters G, Andermann F (1986) Giant axonal neuropathy: central abnormalities demonstrated by evoked potentials. *Ann Neurol.*;19: 394–396.

9 Ravishankar S, Goel G, Rautenstrauss CP, Nalini A (2009) Spectrum of magnetic resonance imaging findings in a family with giant axonal neuropathy confirmed by genetic studies. *Neurol India.*;57:181–184.

10 Brenner C, Speck-Martins CE, Farage L, Barker PB (2008) 3T MR with diffusion tensor imaging and single-voxel spectroscopy in giant axonal neuropathy. *J Magn Reson Imaging*;28:236–241.

11 Ben Hamida C, Cavalier L, Belal S, *et al.* (1997). Homozygosity mapping of giant axonal neuropathy gene to chromosome 16q24.1. *Neurogenetics.*;1:129–133.

12 Bomont P, Cavalier L, Blondeau F, *et al.* (2000). The gene encoding gigaxonin, a new member of the cytoskeletal BTB/kelch repeat family, is mutated in giant axonal neuropathy. *Nat Genet.*;26:370–374.

13 Houlden H, Groves M, Miedzybrodzka Z, *et al.* (2007) New mutations, genotype phenotype studies and manifesting carriers in giant axonal neuropathy. *J Neurol Neurosurg Psychiatry.*;78:1267–1270.

14 Berg BO, Rosenberg SH, Asbury AK (1972) Giant axonal neuropathy. *Pediatrics.*;49:894–899.

15 Asbury AK, Gale MK, Cox SC, *et al.* (1972) Giant axonal neuropathy--a unique case with segmental neurofilamentous masses. *Acta Neuropathol.*;20:237–247.

16 Prineas JW, Ouvrier RA, Wright RG, *et al.* (1976) Gian axonal neuropathy--a generalized disorder of cytoplasmic microfilament formation. *J Neuropathol Exp Neurol.*;35: 458–470.

17 Takebe Y, Koide N, Takahashi G (1981) Giant axonal neuropathy: report of two siblings with endocrinological and histological studies. *Neuropediatrics.*;12:392–404.

18 Gambarelli D, Hassoun J, Pellissier JF, *et al.* (1977) Giant axonal neuropathy. Involvement of peripheral nerve, myenteric plexus and extra-neuronal area. *Acta Neuropathol.*; 39:261–269.

19 Koch T, Schultz P, Williams R, Lampert P (1977) Giant axonal neuropathy: a childhood disorder of microfilaments. *Ann Neurol.*;1:438–451.

20 Kretzschmar HA, Berg BO, Davis RL. (1987) Giant axonal neuropathy. A neuropathological study. *Acta Neuropathol.*;73: 138–134.

21 Thomas C, Love S, Powell HC, *et al.* (1987) Giant axonal neuropathy: correlation of clinical findings with postmortem neuropathology. *Ann Neurol.*;22:79–84.

22 Carpenter S, Karpati G, Andermann F, Gold R (1974). Giant axonal neuropathy. A clinically and morphologically distinct neurological disease. *Arch Neurol.*;31:312–316.

23 Fabrizi GM, Cavallaro T, Angiari C, *et al.* (2004) Giant axon and neurofilament accumulation in Charcot–Marie–Tooth disease type 2E. *Neurology.*;62:1429–1431.

24 Azzedine H, Ravisé N, Verny C, *et al.* (2006) Spine deformities in Charcot–Marie–Tooth 4C caused by SH3TC2 gene mutations. *Neurology.*;67:602–606.

25 Mahadevan A, Santosh V, Gayatri N, *et al.* (2000) Infantile neuroaxonal dystrophy and giant axonal neuropathy – overlap diseases of neuronal cytoskeletal elements in childhood? *Clin Neuropathol.*;19:221–229.

26 Jaffer F, Murphy SM, Scoto M, *et al.* (2012). BAG3 mutations: another cause of giant axonal neuropathy. *J Peripher Nerv Syst.*;17:210–216.

CHAPTER 19
Neuroaxonal dystrophy

Robert Ouvrier and Manoj Menezes
Department of Neurology, The Children's Hospital at Westmead, Sydney, Australia

Introduction

Infantile neuroaxonal dystrophy (INAD) is an autosomal recessive disorder caused by mutations, in the majority of cases, in the *PLA2G6* gene [1, 2]. *PLA2G6* genes have been linked to two conditions that overlap in their clinical manifestations – infantile neuroaxonal dystrophy and neurodegeneration with brain-iron accumulation (NBIA). INAD is also sometimes classified as NBIA2, with NBIA1 referring to pantothenate-kinase-associated neurodegeneration (PKAN, formerly Hallervorden–Spatz syndrome), a phenotypically separate disorder caused by mutations in the *PANK2* gene. The pathological hallmark of neuroaxonal dystrophy is the presence of axonal swellings, known as spheroids, formed by branched tubular structures and bundles of filaments with mitochondria, in nerve fibers, especially at their terminals.

Clinical features

Onset is usually before three years of age with psychomotor regression. Neurologically, early truncal hypotonia progresses to tetraparesis. The weakness is usually spastic but is sometimes areflexic. Optic atrophy, often with nystagmus, is present in the majority of patients by the age of 3 years. Patients with mutation-positive NBIA have progressive dystonia and dysarthria and neurobehavioral disturbances with impulsivity, distractibility, poor attention span and emotional lability. Seizures have been reported in about one-third of mutation-positive cases but tend to occur later with an average age of onset of 7 years [1]. Slow abnormal limb movements may appear in older patients and death usually occurs by 10 years of age.

Electrophysiology and imaging

EEG characteristically shows high-amplitude, fast (18–24Hz) activity in wakefulness and sleep after 18–30 months of age. Background rhythms are slower than normal and worsen with disease progression. Abnormalities in nerve conduction studies were found in 9 of 13 patients studied by Nardocci *et al.* 1999 [3] and consisted of mild slowing of motor and sensory conduction velocity or reduced CMAPs. Needle electromyography is very frequently abnormal with frequent fibrillations, fasciculations and positive sharp waves. Electroretinography and auditory evoked potentials are usually normal but visual evoked responses are usually abnormal [3].

The characteristic MRI changes consist of progressive cerebellar atrophy, which may not be detectable in the first few years of the illness. Many mutation-positive patients with INAD also have cerebellar hyperintensity on proton density, FLAIR, or T2-weighted MRI studies. Other abnormalities include thinning of the corpus callosum, cerebral cortical atrophy, mega-cisterna magna, thin optic chiasm, enlarged ventricles, vermian atrophy, hyperintensity of the dentate nuclei, and occasional hyperintense putamen and cerebral cortex on T2-weighted imaging [1, 3]. Evidence of iron accumulation in the globus pallidus is rare in INAD but is a common feature of patients classified as NBIA, irrespective of whether they have mutations in *PLA2G6* or not.

Peripheral Nerve Disorders: Pathology and Genetics, First Edition. Edited by Jean-Michel Vallat, Joachim Weis, Francoise Gray, and Katy Keohane.

Neuropathological findings

The neuropathological hallmark of INAD is the presence of spheroid bodies in distal parts of the axons. These can be frequently identified in biopsies of skin, nerve, conjunctiva, areola, rectum and muscle. Similar findings are seen in the brain. Of the peripheral sites available for biopsy, a high yield has been reported for conjunctival and skin biopsies; however, these techniques demand special expertise often not available except in specialized centers. Sural nerve biopsy has a good yield but usually requires availability of electron microscopy for ultrastructural analysis. The yield from muscle biopsy appears to be low [1, 4]. Spheroids are not specific to INAD and may occur in PKAN and in various ill-defined chronic non-progressive or progressive neurological disorders [5].

Central nervous system spheroids are found in the cerebral cortex, the nuclei of Goll and Burdach and in the globus pallidus (which may also contain excessive iron and lipid), cerebellum, brain stem and spinal cord. Spheroids appeared as rounded eosinophilic swellings with a diameter of 30–100 μm that also stain with Bielschowsky silver stain. There is often associated gliosis of the cerebral white matter and degeneration of pyramidal, spinocerebellar and other long tracts.

Spheroids are seen in the axonal endings of subcutaneous nerve fibers and small sympathetic nerves in skin biopsies. Sural nerve biopsies may show focal dilatation of small myelinated axons and some large swollen axons. The rarefaction of myelinated and unmyelinated nerve fibers is mostly mild as the peripheral nervous system is usually only moderately involved. The spheroids (Fig. 19.1) may contain aggregates of mitochondria, neurofilaments, high density granular material, glycogen, vacuoles, and structures known as tubulomembranous or tubulovesicular elements, a term used to describe the appearance of an anastamosing network of delicate membrane structures with a lumen.

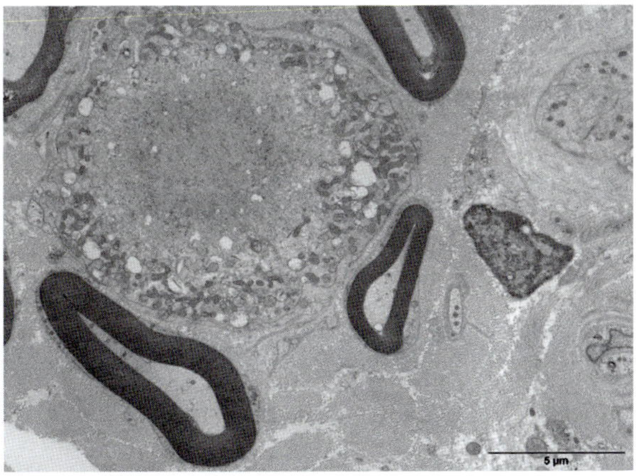

Figure 19.1 Electron micrograph; transverse section. Spheroid body in a widely dilated axon amongst normal myelinated nerve fibers: amorphous granular material, abnormal mitochondria, dense bodies, glycogen aggregates, and neurofilaments fill the axoplasm. Source: Jean-Michel Vallat, CHU de Limoges, France. Reproduced with permission of Jean-Michel Vallat.

Clinical variants

The disorder Schindler disease has been categorized as a neuroaxonal dystrophy but the original reported cases were found to have a deficiency of α-N-acetylgalactosaminidase (α-NAGA). Subsequent investigation has led to the proposition that, while α-NAGA deficiency underlies the abnormal oligosacchariduria found in Schindler disease, its causal role in the neurological phenotype is questioned. Since other patients with α-NAGA deficiency may show a variety of clinical findings or no abnormalities at all, it has been hypothesized that Schindler disease with neuroaxonal dystrophy is the result of an accidental occurrence of two monogenic diseases; Schindler disease and INAD [6].

Early-onset variants (including Seitelberger disease, early-onset INAD with seizures including infantile spasms, congenital hypertonia, and basal ganglia calcification), juvenile onset with myoclonic epilepsy and retinal degeneration, and an association with osteopetrosis have been reported. It is likely that these variants have a different genetic etiology and *PLA2G6* mutations have been excluded in some of these variants.

Genetics and pathogenesis

Most, but not all cases of INAD are caused by mutations in the *PLA2G6* gene on chromosome 22q13.1. Gregory *et al.* [1] found mutations in *PLA2G6* in 80% of a clinically diagnosed cohort of 56 INAD patients compared to only 20% in cases of idiopathic NBIA. *PLA2G6* mutations have also been found in adult-onset Parkinsonism-dystonia syndrome [7].

PLA2G6 encodes i-PLA2G-VIA, a phospholipase catalyzing the release of fatty acids from phospholipids. This entails several functions including phospholipid remodeling, arachidonic release, leukotriene and prostaglandin synthesis, Fas-mediated apoptosis, and transmembrane ion flux in glucose-stimulated B-cells [2].

Animal models

A similar disorder has been observed in several animal species including mice, dogs and horses. The *PLA2G6* knockout mouse shows widespread progressive accumulation of anti-ubiquitin-stained spheroids with numerous tubulovesicular structures on EM [8]. It was suggested that there was protein misfolding and aggregation causing age-dependent impairment of axonal membrane homeostasis and protein degradation pathways, leading to progressive neurological deterioration [8]. Arachidonic acid toxicity may also play a role by increasing apoptosis [4].

Treatment

No disease-modifying therapy is currently available, and treatment continues to be rehabilitative and supportive.

References

1 Gregory A, Westaway SK, Holm IE, *et al.* (2008) Neurodegeneration associated with genetic defects in phospholipase A(2). *Neurology.* 71, 1402–1409.
2 Khateeb S, Flusser H, Ofir R, *et al.* (2006) PLA2G6 mutation underlies infantile neuroaxonal dystrophy. *Am J Human Genetics.* 79, 942–948.
3 Nardocci N, Zorzi G, Farina L, *et al.* (1999) Infantile neuroaxonal dystrophy: clinical spectrum and diagnostic criteria. *Neurology.* 52, 1472–1478.
4 Wu Y, Jiang Y, Gao Z, *et al.* (2009) Clinical study and PLA2G6 mutation screening analysis in Chinese patients with infantile neuroaxonal dystrophy. *Eur J Neurol.* 16, 240–245.
5 Aicardi J, Castelein P. (1979) Infantile neuroaxonal dystrophy. *Brain.* 102, 727–748.
6 Westaway SK, Gregory A, Hayflick SJ. (2007) Mutations in PLA2G6 and the riddle of Schindler disease. *J Med Genetics.* 44, e64.
7 Paisan-Ruiz C, Bhatia KP, Li A, *et al.* (2009) Characterization of PLA2G6 as a locus for dystonia-Parkinsonism. *Ann Neurol.* 65, 19–23.
8 Malik I, Turk J, Mancuso DJ, *et al.* (2008) Disrupted membrane homeostasis and accumulation of ubiquitinated proteins in a mouse model of infantile neuroaxonal dystrophy caused by PLA2G6 mutations. *Am J Pathol.* 172, 406–416.

CHAPTER 20

Peripheral nerve involvement in neurolipidoses

Robert Ouvrier and Manoj Menezes
Department of Neurology, The Children's Hospital at Westmead, Sydney, Australia

Introduction

The neurolipidoses are hereditary metabolic diseases of the nervous system involving lipids and lipoproteins. They are mainly disorders of ceramide derivatives and include certain lysosomal storage diseases (sphingolipidoses and gangliosidoses) as well as some leukodystrophies. Ceramide, which consists of sphingosine coupled with a fatty acid, is a key component of gangliosides and sphingolipids; for example, sphingomyelin that, in contributing to the lipid-protein bilayer of cell membranes, has important signaling as well as structural functions. The lysosomal disorders are due to a deficiency of specific enzymes required for the lysosomal catabolism of the particular lipid (complex lipids such as sphingolipids, cholesterol, and lipoproteins). They are often accompanied by accumulation of the lipid ("storage disease"). Given the high content and importance of lipids in the nervous system, these diseases can result in severe neurologic symptoms and, in some instances, polyneuropathies may be the predominant feature.

Sphingolipidoses

Gaucher disease (glucocerebrosidase deficiency)

Gaucher disease is an autosomal recessive disease due to a deficiency of acid beta-glucosidase (beta-glucocerebrosidase), which catabolizes glucosylceramide into ceramide and glucose. The disease is characterized by the accumulation of glucosylcerebroside within lysosomes, and involves the bone marrow, liver, and spleen. The gene, *GBA*, which encodes glucocerebrosidase is located on chromosome 1q21 and mutations in this gene are responsible for all clinical forms of the disease. Three varieties of Gaucher disease are recognized: the infantile, juvenile, and so-called adult non-neuropathic forms.

Peripheral nerve involvement, which is usually clinically silent, has been described rarely in the infantile form, in which lipid accumulation with glucosylceramide affects histiocytes and Schwann cells without axon loss or demyelination [1]. More recently, an increased prevalence of peripheral neuropathy in the adult variety compared with the normal population has been reported in several series [2].

Krabbe disease (galactocerebrosidase deficiency, globoid cell leukodystrophy)

Definition

This is a rare autosomal recessive neurodegenerative and metabolic disorder due to mutations of the *GALC* gene (located on chromosome 14q31) whose pathophysiology has still not been completely elucidated.

Clinical aspects

The disease incidence is estimated at approximately 1 in 200,000. The "classical" early infantile form is commonest, presents in the first six months of life and death follows within a few years. Although central nervous system symptoms of extreme irritability, developmental regression, hypertonicity, and seizures dominate the clinical picture, the tendon reflexes often disappear

Peripheral Nerve Disorders: Pathology and Genetics, First Edition. Edited by Jean-Michel Vallat, Joachim Weis, Francoise Gray, and Katy Keohane.

despite persistence of hypertonia. Rarely, infants present with an apparently pure progressive or even acute-onset neuropathy with generalized weakness, hypotonia, and areflexia [3]. It is a predominantly motor demyelinating polyneuropathy sometimes with pes cavus and scoliosis [4]. Approximately 10–15% of patients have a later onset, commonly designated as late-infantile (6 months to 3 years) and juvenile (3–8 years). Adult-onset forms also occur. CSF protein is elevated and MRI scans reveal evidence of demyelination and atrophy. Nerve conduction velocity is reduced in the great majority of cases of the classical form of the disease and in about half of the later-onset varieties [5].

Pathology

The pathological hallmark of the disorder, the globoid cell, is a multilamellated macrophage confined to the central nervous system. Sural nerve biopsy, which is not usually indicated except in atypical cases or in those where pseudodeficiency is an issue, reveals a reduced myelinated fiber density, with evidence of segmental demyelination and occasional onion bulb formation. With electron microscopy, unusual elongated or prismatic inclusions of galactosylceramide are seen in the cytoplasm of Schwann cells and brain macrophages [6]. In other reports, widespread hypomyelination with thin myelin sheaths in most myelinated axons has been described [7, 8]

Niemann–Pick disease (sphingomyelin lipidosis)

Definition and genetics

This group of disorders is heterogeneous with at least four major forms currently recognized. All are autosomal recessive conditions. The severe type A form (OMIM 257200) and the allelic visceral, non-neurologic type B are due to mutations of the *SMPD1* gene that causes acid sphingomyelinase deficiency, whereas types C1, C2, and D result from mutations of the *SPC1* and *SPC2* genes involved in cholesterol metabolism. Intermediate forms are also described.

Clinical features

Due to accumulation of sphingomyelin in the reticuloendothelial system and neurons, hepatosplenomegaly with variable central nervous system involvement such as psychomotor retardation, dementia, spasticity, and convulsions results. Peripheral neuropathy, usually of a demyelinating type, occurs mainly in type A cases.

Pathology

Nerve biopsies reveal thin myelin sheaths with occasional onion bulbs and membrane-bound inclusions resembling lipofuscin in Schwann cells and macrophages. Foam cells may invade the endoneurium [9].

Farber lipogranulomatosis (ceramidase deficiency)

This rare autosomal recessive storage disorder, which is usually fatal in infancy, is characterized by multiple granulomatous accumulations of ceramide in subcutaneous tissues, joints, lymph nodes, and viscera, as well as in brain and spinal neurons. Hoarseness, peri-articular swellings and subcutaneous nodules are typical features. Neurological signs, however, are not prominent.

Histopathological examination of peripheral nerves may be diagnostic, revealing axon loss, hypomyelination, optically empty inclusions, and aptly-named "banana bodies" in Schwann cell cytoplasm with variably shaped membrane-bound clefts visible on EM [10, 11].

The disorder is caused by homozygous or compound heterozygous mutations in the gene encoding acid ceramidase (*ASAH1*) on chromosome 8p [12]. Gene therapy is under investigation.

Fabry disease (ceramide trihexoside storage disease; alpha-galactoside A deficiency; angiokeratoma corporis diffusum)

Definition

Fabry disease is an X-linked recessive disorder due to mutations of the *GLA* gene located on Xq21.1 and causing deficiency of the α-galactosidase A enzyme (ceramide trihexosidase) that cleaves the terminal molecule of galactose from ceramide trihexoside, leading to accumulation of trihexoside lipids in various tissues including skin (angiokeratoma corporis), cornea (causing "whorl keratopathy"), kidney, vascular endothelium, heart, and nervous system [13]. Its incidence is about 1/117,000 in males, but could be higher in the general population because of missed asymptomatic forms in females and also misdiagnosed male cases of this disease [14].

Pathophysiology

It is a storage disorder due to the progressive accumulation of the glycolipids ceramide trihexoside, globotriaosylceramide (or Gb3), and galabiosylceramide in various tissues (cornea, vascular endothelium, arterial walls, skin, kidneys, myocardium, but also peripheral nervous system). The mechanism of Fabry neuropathy is poorly understood but could be related to nerve ischemia or dysfunction due to glycolipid accumulation in the vasa nervorum or in dorsal root ganglia [15].

Clinical signs

A small fiber sensory and autonomic neuropathy is a cardinal manifestation, usually without motor and only subtle sensory findings, mostly involving cold perception. Female carriers may be affected but less severely than hemizygotes [14].

The initial clinical manifestations typically commence in late childhood or early adolescence, often with recurrent episodes of severe burning pains in the palms and soles, which may be precipitated by cold, exercise, or fever but last for days or weeks. Autonomic disturbances such as altered sweating, abdominal pain, and diarrhea may also occur [15].

The red-black, flat or raised telangiectatic skin lesions appear in the "bathing costume" region from the chest to the knees and are often most prominent on the buttocks and perineal regions. The corneal deposits are striking but cause little disturbance of vision. Cerebral, renal, cardiac, and vascular disease develops later and may lead to strokes and renal and cardiac failure. Minor manifestations, especially ocular, are not uncommon in female carriers.

Investigations

Conventional nerve conduction studies are unhelpful. Quantitative electrophysiology of peripheral nerves shows a relative preservation of large fiber function with normal nerve conduction velocities, but sometimes with small reductions in sensory nerve amplitude (small axonal loss): the electrophysiological pattern is a length-dependent small fiber neuropathy [16].

Pathology

Biopsies are not usually undertaken but occasionally may unexpectedly lead to the diagnosis. They may reveal lipid deposition in perineurial, endothelial, and smooth muscle cells but not usually in Schwann cells, although axonal degenerative changes may occur. Polarized light examination may demonstrate "Maltese Cross" patterns in perineurium. Electron microscopy demonstrates rounded or comma-shaped inclusions or sometimes "zebra bodies" or regular arrays of circular or hexagonal clumps of storage material [6].

Skin biopsy shows reduction of somatic epidermal and dermal autonomic nerve fibers in male as well as in female patients [17]. Corneal confocal microscopy can also help to detect early nerve fiber damage in Fabry disease [18].

Treatment

Specific enzyme replacement therapy (ERT) with α-Galβ or α-Galα is beneficial in reducing lipid storage and also effective for pain control. Management also involves treatment of the renal, cardiac, and other vascular complications, as well as symptomatic treatment for pain with analgesics, anticonvulsants (including phenytoin, carbamazepine, pregabalin, or gabapentin), and sometimes opioids [19]. The study of murine models of Fabry disease has shown that ERT can improve cardiac function [20] and stabilize the invariant natural killer T cell percentage in the spleen [21].

Gangliosidoses

The gangliosidoses are characterized by the accumulation of gangliosides, which are composed of ceramide linked to an oligosaccharide (up to four hexose saccharides, either galactose or glucose) and one or more sialic acids (N-acetylneuraminic acid, or NANA).

GM_1 gangliosidosis

GM_1 gangliosidosis type I is an autosomal recessive neuronal storage disease caused by a deficiency of β-galactosidase (*GLB1*, chromosome 3p22.3). There is no clinical evidence of neuropathy, but Schwann cell inclusions have been described [1].

GM_2 gangliosidosis (Tay–Sachs disease and variants)

Tay–Sachs disease is an autosomal recessive disease caused by mutations in the α subunit gene of hexosaminidase A (*HEXA*, chromosome 15q23), with deficiencies in hexosaminidase A and S activities.

Infantile Tay–Sachs disease

Classical, infantile Tay–Sachs disease is not associated with clinical evidence of neuropathy [1] but on pathological examination, unmyelinated fibers have occasionally been found to contain multilamellated inclusions and there may be some loss of myelinated axons in the late stages [22].

Late-onset Tay–Sachs disease

In late-onset Tay–Sachs disease (LOTS) caused by partial deficiency of beta-hexosaminidase A, Shapiro and colleagues [23] found neurophysiological evidence of a predominantly axonal degenerative polyneuropathy affecting distal nerve segments in the lower and upper extremities in 8 of 30 patients.

Nerve histology was not described but degenerative changes in the sural nerve were reported by Willner *et al.* [24] in an adult with a chronic form of GM2 gangliosidosis resembling Friedreich's ataxia.

Sulfatidoses, metachromatic leukodystrophies (arylsulfatase A deficiency)

Definition

Metachromatic leukodystrophy (MLD) is a rare autosomal recessive disorder characterized by intra-lysosomal accumulation of the sphingolipid sulfatide in various tissues: nervous system (neurons, oligodendrocytes, Schwann cells), epithelial cells of the bile duct, gallbladder, testes, distal tubules of the kidneys, and urinary sediment [25]. The galactosphingosulfatides that are strongly metachromatic, doubly refractile in polarized light, and pink with PAS are found in excess in the white matter of the central nervous system and in peripheral nerves, as well as in the viscera,.

At least five variants of these conditions have been described and all have peripheral nerve involvement. The late infantile, juvenile, and adult variants are caused by mutations of the *ARSA* gene which encodes the lysosomal enzyme arylsulfatase A. The other variants include multiple sulfatase deficiency (Austin's disease) in which mucopolysaccharides are also stored. It is due to mutations in *SUMF1*, a gene that encodes an activator of several sulfatases. In the AB variant, there is a deficiency of the activator of cerebroside sulfatase, saposin B (*SAP1*).

In most cases of metachromatic leukodystrophy, the diagnosis can be confirmed by assay of aryl sulfatases A and B and cerebroside sulfatase in white cells or cultured skin fibroblasts. Interpretation of nerve biopsies may occasionally be important: (1) when biochemical and/or genetic analyses are not available, (2) in cases presenting with a pure neuropathic syndrome and (3) in the AB variant, where the sulfatase levels are normal, but sulfatide accumulates due to a deficiency of the activator of cerebroside sulfatase [26]. Most of these situations can be resolved now that the genes are cloned.

Pseudoarylsulfatase A deficiency refers to a condition of apparent ARSA enzyme deficiency in persons without neurologic abnormalities leading to an erroneous diagnosis of MLD. It is due to allelic variants of the *ARSA* gene such as the pseudo-deficiency Pd allele which can be recognized by sequencing. It is present in up to 15% of some populations.

Clinical features

The overall incidence is estimated at about 1 in 120,000, but higher rates are seen in certain isolated groups such as Navajo Indians and some Arab communities, both Muslim and Christian. Three forms of MLD are distinguished: late-infantile, juvenile, and adult types. Neurological manifestations include demyelination of the CNS causing hypotonia, ataxia, visual and hearing impairment, seizures, tetraplegia, dementia, and a demyelinating peripheral neuropathy [25].

In the more common late infantile form, there is often a stage of weakness and hypotonia, particularly involving the lower limbs. Later, and in the juvenile forms, the clinical picture in most cases is dominated by dementia, ataxia, spasticity, and hypo- or hyper-reflexia. Except for depressed ankle jerks, the neuropathy is often clinically subtle and best demonstrated electrophysiologically. Some cases, however, present with neuropathic weakness as the dominant clinical feature. In the adult variant, dementia, psychiatric disturbances, and upper motor neuron or extrapyramidal disturbances are usually prominent, but a neuropathy is evident on electrophysiological examination in most cases and occasionally is the cause of presentation. Brain imaging in all variants usually reveals extensive demyelination. CSF protein is often markedly increased.

Nerve conduction velocities are slow in all cases of the late infantile form and almost all early juvenile cases and may be as low as 10–20 m/s. Such abnormalities may be present under the age of 6 months in an otherwise clinically normal infant. Sensory action potentials are usually reduced or absent.

Nerve pathology

There is a reduction in myelinated fiber density, with evidence of chronic demyelination (Fig. 20.1). Many myelin sheaths are thin, their outlines distorted and irregular. Measurement of g-ratios confirms significant reduction of myelin sheath thickness indicating extensive remodeling, particularly in juvenile and adult forms

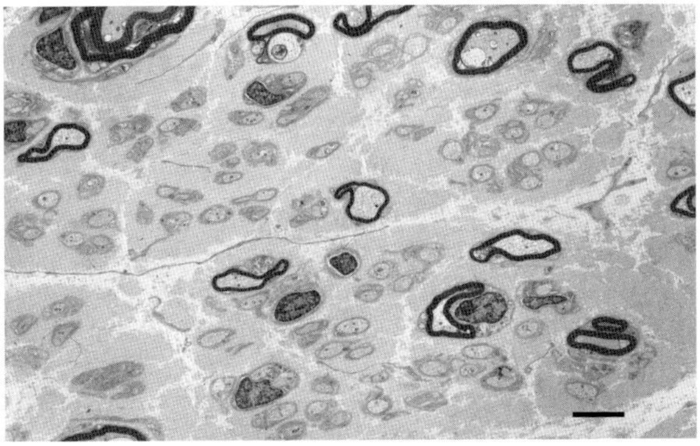

Figure 20.1 Metachromatic leukodystrophy: Electron micrograph; transverse section. Severe rarefaction of myelinated fibers; many of them have a too-thin-for-axon-caliber myelin sheath, which favors a demyelinating process. Bar = 10 μm. Source: Jean-Michel Vallat, CHU de Limoges, France. Reproduced with permission of Jean-Michel Vallat.

[27]. Onion bulbs are seen. Granular material, most dense in the perinuclear regions of the Schwann cell, is visible as brown or brown-yellow metachromasia in cresyl violet or toluidine blue stains (see Fig. 7.3). Electron microscopy demonstrates accumulations of myelin-like material as well as lipid-containing inclusions, known as zebra and "tuffstone" bodies, and prismatic inclusions in the lysosomes of macrophages and Schwann cells (Fig. 20.2A,B) [28].

Management

When pre-symptomatic and early diagnosed cases of the late infantile form are treated with hematopoietic stem cell or bone marrow transplantation, there is clear evidence for amelioration of the CNS manifestations. There is less clear-cut improvement in the peripheral nerve manifestations.

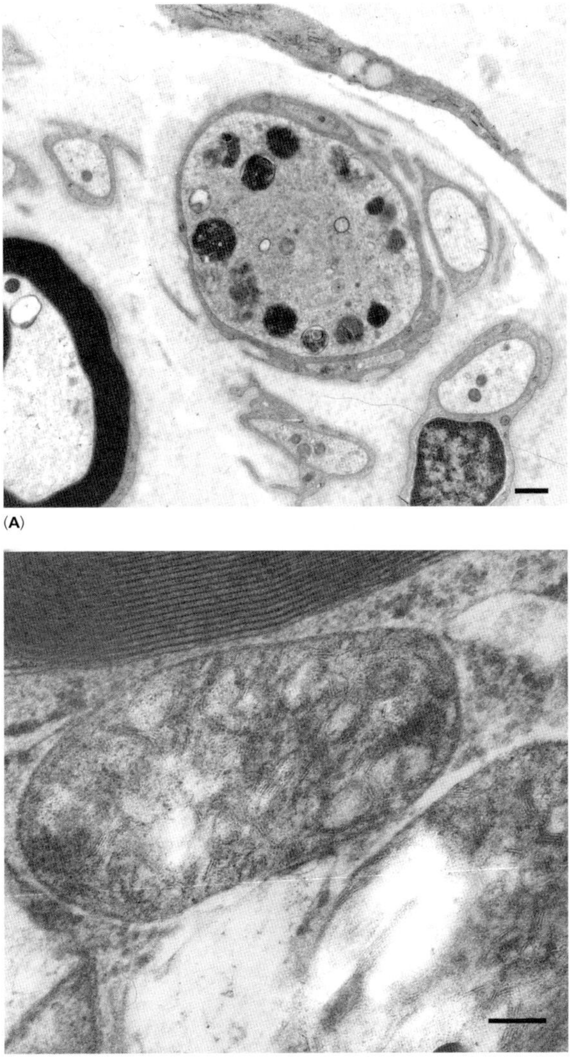

(A)

(B)

Figure 20.2 Metachromatic leukodystrophy. (**A**) Electron micrograph; transverse section. An abnormally dilated unmyelinated axon contains several granular bodies and "tuffstone bodies." Bar = 1 μm. (**B**) Electron micrograph; transverse section. At high magnification, the membrane-bound zebra bodies are composed of groups of lamellae. Bar = 0.3 μm. Source: Jean-Michel Vallat, CHU de Limoges, France. Reproduced with permission of Jean-Michel Vallat.

Deficiency in enzymes involved in metabolism of lipoproteins, other lipids, and cholesterol

Familial high density lipoprotein deficiency (Tangier disease; alpha-lipoprotein deficiency)

Definition and genetics

This very rare autosomal recessive disorder is characterized by (1) an absence of normal high density lipoproteins (HDL); (2) the accumulation of cholesteryl esters in tissue macrophages and prevalent atherosclerosis; and (3) a polyneuropathy with very protean characteristics. Apolipoprotein A1 and A2 levels are very low and serum cholesterol is reduced. The condition is caused by mutations of the *ABCA1* (ATP-Binding Cassette transporter

A1) gene on 9q22–q31 [29], a pivotal gene in the regulation of plasma levels of HDL cholesterol and cellular cholesterol homeostasis.

Pathophysiology and clinical features

The clinical manifestations are secondary to an accumulation of cholesteryl esters in various macrophage-rich tissues such as tonsils, spleen, liver, lymph nodes, thymus, arterial walls, cornea, and also peripheral nerves [30, 31]. Peripheral neuropathy is due to the accumulation of the cholesteryl esters in Schwann cells.

Onset may occur in infancy or in the elderly. The main clinical symptoms are enlarged tonsils (orange-yellow color), hepatosplenomegaly, corneal opacification, and premature coronary disease (about 30% of Tangier disease cases) or stroke, thrombocytopenia, anemia, and gastrointestinal disorder. About half of the reported patients have signs of a neuropathy. Neurological presentations are protean: acute or chronic in onset, relapsing or progressive, proximal or distal, and symmetrical or asymmetrical in distribution. Two main syndromes are seen: (1) a pseudo-syringomyelic syndrome [32, 33], which commences after the second decade and causes dissociated sensory loss particularly for pain in the face, arms, and upper trunk followed by symmetrical progressive facio-brachial wasting and weakness, or (2) a multiple mononeuropathy involving motor and all sensory modalities with a relatively benign, relapsing-remitting course which commences in the first two decades. Cases resembling the Lewis–Sumner syndrome are on record [34].

Less typical presentations are sometimes encountered with cranial nerve disturbances and exceptionally an acute polyneuropathy mimicking Guillain–Barré syndrome [35, 36]. The confusing manifestations may lead to suspicion of autoimmune-mediated neuropathy or even Hansen disease [37, 38].

Investigations

The biological hallmark in plasma of patients with Tangier disease is a deficiency of HDL cholesterol and low level of apoA-I, with low levels of LDL cholesterol and moderate hypertriglyceridemia. Nerve conduction studies generally show absent sensory potentials in the pseudosyringomyelic syndrome with only mild changes in the multiple mononeuropathy cases. They may show evidence of axonal degeneration, demyelination, or a mixed result. Conduction block may be prominent.

Pathology

In the mononeuropathy form sural nerve biopsy shows evidence of demyelination and remyelination with multiple lipid vacuoles particularly concentrated in Remak cells (Figure 20.3) [36]. Axonal degeneration is the predominant feature in the syringomyelia-like neuropathy [39] and at autopsy Schwann cells, spinocerebellar tracts, and dorsal root ganglion cells have been shown to contain numerous lipid inclusions [40]. Redundant

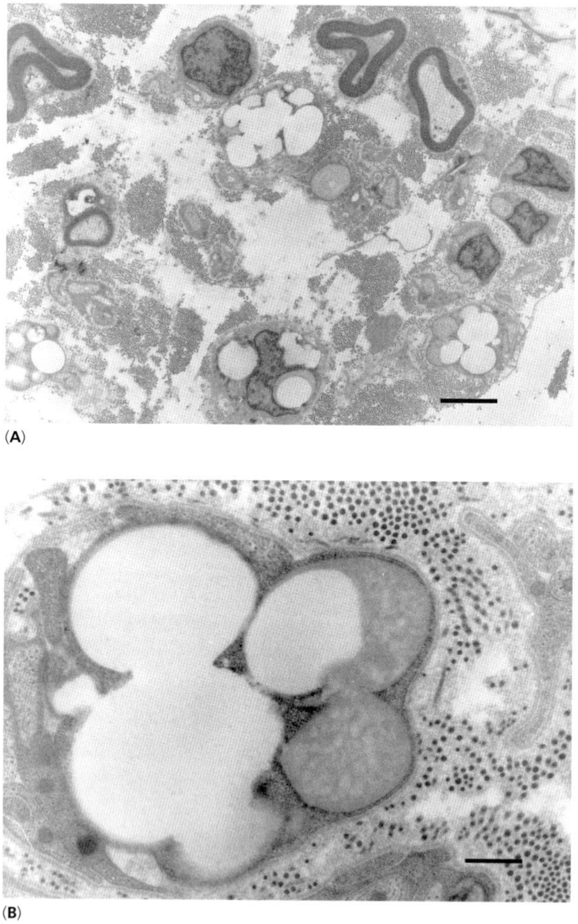

(A)

(B)

Figure 20.3 Tangier disease. (**A**) Electron micrograph; transverse section. The number of myelinated fibers is clearly reduced. Note the presence of multiple intracellular vacuoles which correspond to extracted lipid droplets. Bar = 5 μm. (**B**) High magnification of Figure 20.3A. The distended cytoplasm of a non-myelinating Schwann cell shows partially extracted lipid droplets. Bar = 1 μm. Source: Jean-Michel Vallat, CHU de Limoges, France. Reproduced with permission of Jean-Michel Vallat.

myelin foldings, myelin splitting, vesiculation, and small tomacula are also reported [41]. Electron microscopy reveals lipid vacuoles in myelinated and non-myelinated fibers as well as in pericytes, perineurial, and endothelial cells (Fig. 20.3) [6].

Treatment and future perspectives

Treatment by restriction of dietary fat may be one way to reduce the accumulation of the cholesterol esters in the reticuloendothelial system, possibly resulting in clinical improvement. Drugs known to increase HDL levels have been shown to be ineffective. Recently designed drugs like the cholesteryl ester transfer protein (CETP) inhibitors, dalcetrapib, and anacetrapib, and reconstituted forms of HDL have been proposed until the development of gene therapy [31].

Familial beta-lipoprotein deficiency: Bassen–Kornzweig disease (abetalipoproteinemia) and vitamin E deficiency

Definition

Although abetalipoproteinemia is not a neurolipidosis but a lipid deficiency, its neurological complications are usually described within the hereditary disorders of lipoprotein. Abetalipoproteinemia is a rare autosomal recessive metabolic disorder first described in 1950 by Bassen and Kornzweig [42]. It is a form of neuroacanthocytosis characterized by fat malabsorption, pigmentary degeneration, progressive ataxia, and neuropathy in addition to acanthocytosis (commonly observed when betalipoproteins are absent from the plasma) [43]. It is caused mainly by mutations in the *MTP* gene encoding the microsomal triglyceride transfer protein normally present in liver and intestine [43]. Another entity called "homozygous hypobetalipoproteinemia" has been described with similar clinical symptoms, but this autosomal co-dominant disorder is due to mutations in the *ApoB* gene [44].

Pathophysiology

The absence of apolipoprotein B which contains lipoproteins, VLDL, and LDL, leads to a severe impairment of fat absorption and transport from the intestinal tract, resulting in very low serum triglyceride and cholesterol levels, and also in lipid-soluble vitamin deficiencies (vitamins A, E, and K) [43].

Clinical signs

The clinical presentation is heterogeneous, but the main signs are steatorrhea and growth failure in childhood, and then central (spinocerebellar ataxia) and peripheral (neuropathic) neurological complications as well as ocular manifestations (progressive visual loss due to pigmentary retinopathy, and rarely ophthalmoplegia, ptosis, and nystagmus) due to vitamin E deficiency in young adults [43]. The peripheral nerve disorder consists of a predominantly sensory polyneuropathy. Ataxia could also be partially secondary to proprioceptive abnormalities.

Laboratory studies and electrophysiology

Patients have hypocholesterolemia and hypotriglyceridemia, with low plasma levels of vitamins A and E. The pathognomonic biological sign of the disease is acanthocytosis observed on peripheral blood smear. Electrophysiological studies usually show normal motor conduction with diminution in the amplitude of sensory action potentials and slight-to-moderate slowing in maximum sensory conduction velocity, initially most marked in the distal parts of the nerves [45]. Other electrophysiological features have been described, such as electroretinographic abnormalities or a prolonged P100 latency on visual evoked potentials [45].

Pathology

Sural nerve biopsy shows a decreased number of large fibers (larger than 7 µm), sometimes with clusters of regenerating fibers. In teased fiber preparations, paranodal demyelination may be observed [46]. Central neuropathological changes affect the posterior columns and spinal cerebellar tract, but the cerebellum seems to be spared: these signs are the same as those observed in vitamin E deficiency [47].

Treatment

Early treatment with oral supplementation of the lipid-soluble vitamins A and E can prevent or delay progression of the symptoms, particularly the retinal degeneration [48].

Cerebrotendinous xanthomatosis

Definition

Cerebrotendinous xanthomatosis (CTX) is a rare autosomal recessive lipid-storage disorder caused by a deficiency of the *CYP27A1* gene encoding the mitochondrial sterol 27-hydroxylase: it results in an abnormal deposition of cholestanol and cholesterol in various organs [49].

Clinical presentation

It manifests typically with the triad of juvenile cataracts, tendon xanthomata, and neurological manifestations such as cerebellar ataxia, dementia, and rarely, neuropathy. In CTX, electrophysiological studies may show a mixed axonal and demyelinating sensorimotor polyneuropathy [49].

Pathology

Sural nerve biopsy shows features of axonal neuropathy sometimes with onion-bulb formations [6]. Skin biopsy shows a decrease of intra-epidermal nerve fibers [49].

Treatment

Irreversible neurological damage and permanent disability can be prevented by the early initiation of chenodeoxycholic acid therapy with hydroxymethylglutaryl coenzyme-A (HMG-Co-A) inhibitors.

References

1 Bischoff A (1975) Neuropathy in leukodystrophies. In: Dyck PJ, Thomas PK, Lambert EH, (eds) Peripheral Neuropathy. *Vol* 2, pp. 891–913.W-B Saunders, Philadelphia.

2 Biegstraaten M, Mengel E, Marodi L *et al.* (2010) Peripheral neuropathy in adult type1 Gaucher disease: a 2-year prospective observational study. *Brain;*133:2909–2919.

3 Hagberg B (1984) Krabbe's disease: clinical presentation of neurological variants. *Neuropediatrics;*15 Suppl:11–15.

4 Szymanska K, Lugowska A, Laure-Kamionowska M, *et al.* (2012) Diagnostic difficulties in Krabbe disease: a report of two cases and review of literature. *Folia Neuropathol.;*50:346–356.

5 Zafeiriou DI, Michelakaki EM, Anastasiou AL, *et al.* (1996) Serial MRI and neurophysiological studies in late-infantile Krabbe disease. *Pediatr. Neurol.;*15:240–244.

6 Midroni G, Bilbao JM (eds) (1995), *Biopsy Diagnosis of Peripheral Neuropathy*: Ch. 20, pp. 419–427. Butterworth-Heinemann, Boston.

7 Marks HG, Scavina MT, Kolodny EH *et al.* (1997) Krabbe's disease presenting as a peripheral neuropathy. *Muscle Nerve;*20:1024–1028.

8 Sabatelli M, Quaranta L, Madia F, *et al.* (2002) Peripheral neuropathy with hypomyelinating features in adult-onset Krabbe's disease. *Neuromuscul. Disord.;*12:386–391.

9 Gumbinas M, Larsen M, Mei Liu H (1975) Peripheral neuropathy in classic Niemann-Pick disease: ultrastructure of nerves and skeletal muscles. *Neurology;*25:107–113.

10 Pellissier JF, Berard-Badier M, Pinsard N (1986) Farber's disease in two siblings, sural nerve and subcutaneous biopsies by light and electron microscopy *Acta Neuropathol.;*72: 178–188.

11 Vital C, Vallat J-M (1987) *Ultrastructural Study of the Human Diseased Peripheral Nerve.* 2nd Edn, pp. 219–233. Elsevier, New York.

12 Li, C.-M., Park, J.-H., He, X *et al.* (1999) The human acid ceramidase gene (ASAH): structure, chromosomal location, mutation analysis and expression. *Genomics;*62: 223–231.

13 Schiffmann R. (2009) Fabry disease. *Pharmacol. Ther.;*122:65–77.

14 Mehta A, Ricci R, Widmer U, *et al.* (2004) Fabry disease defined: baseline clinical manifestations of 366 patients in the Fabry Outcome Survey. *Eur. J. Clin. Invest.;*34:236–242.

15 Dutsch M, Hilz MJ. (2010) Neurological complications in Fabry disease. *Rev. Med. Int.* 31; Suppl 2:S243–250.

16 Luciano CA, Russell JW, Banerjee TK, *et al.* (2002) Physiological characterization of neuropathy in Fabry's disease. *Muscle Nerve;*26:622–629.

17 Liguori R, Di Stasi V, Bugiardini E, *et al.* (2010) Small fibre neuropathy in female patients with Fabry disease. *Muscle Nerve;*41:409–412.

18 Tavakoli M, Marshall A, Pitceathly R, *et al.* (2010) Corneal confocal microscopy: a novel means to detect nerve fibre damage in idiopathic small fibre neuropathy. *Exp. Neurol.;*223:245–250.

19 Burlina A P, Sims K, Politei JM *et al.* (2011) Early diagnosis of peripheral nervous system involvement in Fabry disease and treatment of neuropathic pain: the report of an expert panel. *BMC Neurology;*11:61.

20 Nguyen Dinh Cat A, Escoubet B, Agrapart V, *et al.* (2012) Cardiomyopathy and response to enzyme replacement therapy in a male mouse model for Fabry disease. *PLoS One;*7:e33743.

21 Macedo MF, Quinta R, Pereira CS, Sa Miranda MC. (2012) Enzyme replacement therapy partially prevents invariant Natural Killer T cell deficiency in the Fabry disease mouse model. *Mol. Genet. Metab.;*106:83–91.

22 Kristensson K, Olsson Y, Sourander P (1967) Peripheral nerve changes in Tay–Sachs and Batten–Spielmeyer–Vogt disease. *Acta. Pathol. Microbiol. Scand.;*70:630–632.

23 Shapiro BE, Logigian EL, Kolodny EH, Pastores GM (2008) Late-onset Tay–Sachs disease: the spectrum of peripheral neuropathy in 30 affected patients. *Muscle & Nerve;*38: 1012–1015.

24 Willner J P, Grabowski GA, Gordon RE, *et al.* (1981). Chronic GM2 gangliosidosis masquerading as atypical Friedreich ataxia: clinical, morphologic, and biochemical studies of nine cases. *Neurology;*31:787–798.

25 Batzios SP, Zafeiriou DI (2012) Developing treatment options for metachromatic leukodystrophy. *Mol Genet Metab;*105:56–63.

26 Inui K, Emmett M, Wenger DA (1983) Immunological evidence for deficiency in an activator protein for sulfatide sulfatase in a

variant form of metachromatic leukodystrophy. *Proc. Natl. Acad. Sci. U S A*;80:3074–3077.

27 Bardosi A, Friede RL, Ropte S, Goebel HH (1987) A morphometric study on sural nerves in metachromatic leucodystrophy. *Brain.*;110:683–694.

28 Thomas PK, King RH, Kocen RS, Brett EM. (1977) Comparative ultrastructural observations on peripheral nerve abnormalities in the late infantile, juvenile and late onset forms of metachromatic leukodystrophy. *Acta Neuropathol.*;39:237–245.

29 Brooks-Wilson A, Marcil M, Clee SM, *et al.* (1999) Mutations in ABC1 in Tangier disease and familial high-density lipoprotein deficiency. *Nature Genet.*;22:336–345.

30 Hobbs HH, Rader DJ. (1999) ABC1: connecting yellow tonsils, neuropathy, and very low HDL. *J. Clin. Invest.*;104: 1015–1017.

31 Puntoni M, Sbrana F, Bigazzi F, Sampietro T. (2012) Tangier disease: epidemiology, pathophysiology, and management. *Am. J. Cardiovasc. Drugs*;12:303–311.

32 Marbini A, Gemignani F, Ferrarini G *et al.* (1985) Tangier disease. A case with sensorimotor distal polyneuropathy and lipid accumulation in striated muscle and vasa nervorum. *Acta Neuropathol.*;67:121–127.

33 Pietrini V, Rizzuto N, Vergani C *et al.* (1985) Neuropathy in Tangier disease: A clinicopathologic study and a review of the literature. *Acta Neurol. Scand.*;72:495–505.

34 Théaudin M, Couvert P, Fournier E *et al.* (2008) Lewis–Sumner syndrome and Tangier disease. *Arch. Neurol.*;65:968–970.

35 Fazio R, Nemni R, Quattrini A, *et al.* (1993) Acute presentation of Tangier polyneuropathy: a clinical and morphological study. *Acta Neuropathol.*;86:90–94.

36 Pollock M, Nukada H, Frith RW *et al.* (1983) Peripheral neuropathy in Tangier disease. *Brain*;106:911–928.

37 Sinha S, Mahadevan A, Lokesh L *et al.* (2004) Tangier disease – a diagnostic challenge in countries endemic for leprosy. *J. Neurol. Neurosurg. Psych.* ;75:301–304.

38 Gibbels E, Schaefer HE, Runne U *et al.* (1985) Severe polyneuropathy in Tangier disease mimicking syringomyelia or leprosy. Clinical, biochemical, electrophysiological, and morphological evaluation, including electron microscopy of nerve, muscle, and skin biopsies. *J. Neurol.*;232:283–294.

39 Dyck PJ, Ellefson RD, Yao JK, Herbert PN (1978) Adult onset of Tangier disease. I Morphometric and pathological studies suggesting delayed degradation of neutral lipids after fibre degeneration. *J. Neuropathol. Exp. Neurol.*;37:119–137.

40 Schmalbruch H, Stender S, Boysen G (1987) Abnormalities in spinal neurons and dorsal root ganglion cells in Tangier disease presenting with a syringomyelia-like syndrome. *J. Neuropathol. Exp. Neurol.*;46:533–543.

41 Cai Z, Blumbergs PC, Cash K, *et al.* (2006) Paranodal pathology in Tangier disease with remitting-relapsing multifocal neuropathy. *J. Clin. Neuroscience*;13:492–497.

42 Bassen FA, Kornzweig AL (1950) Malformation of the erythrocytes in a case of atypical retinitis pigmentosa. *Blood*;5:381–387.

43 Rampoldi L, Danek A, Monaco AP (2002) Clinical features and molecular bases of neuroacanthocytosis. *J. Mol. Med.*;80:475–491.

44 Linton MF, Farese RV, Jr., Young SG (1993) Familial hypobetalipoproteinemia. *J. Lipid Res.*;34:521–541.

45 Brin MF, Pedley TA, Lovelace RE, *et al.* (1986) Electrophysiologic features of abetalipoproteinemia: functional consequences of vitamin E deficiency. *Neurology*;36: 669–673.

46 Wichman A, Buchthal F, Pezeshkpour GH, Gregg RE. (1985) Peripheral neuropathy in abetalipoproteinemia. *Neurology*; 35:1279–1289.

47 Puri V, Chaudhry N, Tatke M, Prakash V. (2005) Isolated vitamin E deficiency with demyelinating neuropathy. *Muscle Nerve*;32:230–235.

48 Chowers I, Banin E, Merin S, *et al.* (2001) Long-term assessment of combined vitamin A and E treatment for the prevention of retinal degeneration in abetalipoproteinaemia and hypobetalipoproteinaemia patients. *Eye*;15:525–530.

49 Gallus GN, Dotti MT, Federico A, *et al.* (2006) Clinical and molecular diagnosis of cerebrotendinous xanthomatosis with a review of the mutations in the CYP27A1 gene. *Neurol. Sci.*;27:143–149.

CHAPTER 21

Other hereditary neuropathies

Stéphane Mathis,[1] Meriem Tazir,[2] and Jean-Michel Vallat[3]

[1] *Department of Neurology, La Milétrie University Hospital, Poitiers, France*

[2] *Laboratoire de Recherche de Neurosciences, Service de Neurologie, Mustapha Bacha University Hospital, Algiers, Algeria*

[3] *Neurology Laboratory, National Referral Center for Rare Peripheral Neuropathies, University Hospital, Limoges, France*

Introduction

Several hereditary disorders not discussed so far may be responsible for pathological lesions of the peripheral nervous system, which are usually axonal-type, moderate in degree, and non-specific. These diseases may be clinically separated into three groups: isolated (distal hereditary motor neuropathy), neuropathies associated with central nervous system (CNS) involvement (Friedreich's ataxia, spinocerebellar atrophy, spastic paraplegia), and neuropathies associated with systemic involvement in hereditary metabolic diseases.

Distal hereditary motor neuropathies

Definition

Distal hereditary motor neuropathies or neuronopathies (dHMNs) are a group of several clinically and genetically heterogeneous diseases, dominant or recessive, with lower motor neuron (including the axon) length-dependent involvement. About 15 genes are identified at the present time and these genes appear important for axonal transport, for the axonal cytoskeleton, and for neurofilament assembly.

Clinical presentation

Patients develop slowly progressive distal limb muscle weakness and wasting, sometimes associated with pyramidal and sensory signs. The same gene abnormality can be found in both CMT and dHMN [1]. For instance, in CMT2D and dHMN-V there is similar motor predominant hand involvement, but CMT2D patients also have sensory abnormalities.

Investigations

Neurophysiological studies usually show reduced muscle action potentials, secondary to neuronal pathology.

Pathology

Nerve biopsy has rarely been performed and is usually normal [2]. Occasionally, microscopic study of a sensory nerve has detected non-specific mild or moderate loss of both myelinated and unmyelinated axons; these changes are difficult to distinguish from age-related anomalies. We have sometimes observed similar pathological findings in various types of motor neuron diseases.

Hereditary neuropathies with spinal cord involvement

Friedreich's ataxia

Definition

Friedreich's ataxia is an autosomal recessive disease that usually begins in the first two decades of life. The lesions are induced by the expansion of a GAA triplet repeat within the first intron of the frataxin gene, and there is a low level of frataxin in tissues.

Clinical presentation

Progressive gait ataxia, dysarthria, and cardiac abnormalities are characteristic of the disease. Diabetes is also frequent, so a diabetic neuropathy has also to be considered.

Peripheral Nerve Disorders: Pathology and Genetics, First Edition. Edited by Jean-Michel Vallat, Joachim Weis, Francoise Gray, and Katy Keohane.

Mild, moderate, or rarely, severe signs favoring a sensory peripheral neuropathy are present and areflexia is always found. It is accepted that the symptoms and signs are due to a sensory neuronopathy that induces a length-dependent distal axonopathy in peripheral nerves, and on the CNS side an axonopathy of the spinocerebellar, corticospinal, and dorsal column long tracts.

Pathology

There is a marked loss of large myelinated fibers, usually without any increase in regenerating clusters. Onion bulbs are also rare. There are very few changes in unmyelinated fibers. Ouvrier *et al.* stressed that the severity of axonal loss correlates with patient's age [3].

Non Friedreich's inherited spinocerebellar degenerations

Definition

Classification of Spino-Cerebellar Ataxia (SCA) is complex as more than 40 genes are identified at the present time.

Clinical presentation and pathology

Peripheral nervous system involvement is variable. When present, it is usually a sensory neuropathy induced by axonal loss, and confirmed by electrophysiology and nerve biopsy. In some sub-types, such as Machado–Joseph disease (SCA3), neuropathy is usually prominent.

Hereditary spastic paraplegia

Definition

Hereditary spastic paraplegia (HSP or SPG) includes a heterogeneous group of genetic neurodegenerative disorders characterized by lower limb spasticity and weakness (pure phenotype of SPG). More than 50 different genes are identified. SPGs are classified into "pure SPG" (non-syndromic SPG) and "complex SPG" (syndromic SPG) that has a phenotype of SPG with extensive neurological symptoms such as peripheral neuropathy and additional non-neurological symptoms [4].

Clinical presentation

The PNS manifestations can be a disorder of the lower motor neuron called "Silver syndrome," an axonal sensorimotor polyneuropathy, a sensory polyneuropathy or a predominantly motor polyneuropathy. Sensorimotor neuropathy can also be observed in a variant of SPG called SPOAN (with spastic paraplegia and optic atrophy) and in "Japanese SPG" (reminiscent of SPG46). There is also an overlap between SPG and CMT: the same gene (*BSCL2* or *atlastin-1*) can lead to either a CMT/HSAN or a SPG phenotype [5] (see also Chapter 14).

Pathology

Nerve biopsy in three patients from a family with clinical asymptomatic sensory involvement showed decreased numbers of large and medium sized fibers without evidence of demyelination, suggesting an axonal neuropathy [6].

Neuropathies associated with hereditary metabolic diseases

Peroxisomal disorders

Refsum's disease

Definition

Refsum's disease is a rare autosomal recessive peroxisomal disorder of lipid metabolism secondary to a failure of phytanic acid alpha-oxidation and leads to phytanic acid accumulation in tissues. Missense mutations and deletions of the gene *PHYH* encoding for the peroxisomal enzyme phytanoyl-CoA hydroxylase are responsible. *PEX7* (encoding the receptor for the PS2, or type 2 peroxisomal targeting signal) may be mutated in some other cases and also in a severe type of another peroxisomal disorder called "rhizomelic chondrodysplasia punctata type 1" [7]. Two forms of Refsum's disease are distinguished: infantile Refsum's disease (before the age of 20) and adult Refsum's disease (onset between the second and fourth decades) [8].

Pathophysiology

The exact pathomechanisms are debated, as are the relationship between the severity of symptoms and signs, and the accumulation of phytanic acid in various organs. Phytanic acid incorporated in myelin might induce membrane instability.

Clinical signs

The first signs and symptoms usually appear in the first and second decade: visual night blindness due to retinis pigmentosa, followed by a distal symmetrical sensorimotor neuropathy that may manifest as a peroneal muscular atrophy syndrome. Ataxia is also found and was initially thought to be due to cerebellar degeneration but could be induced by the neuropathy, since changes in the cerebellum are very mild. Sometimes peripheral nerves are palpably enlarged. Hearing loss and ichthyosis (scaly skin) are characteristic of the disease, but along with epiphyseal lesions are not always present [9]. These clinical manifestations may worsen, sometimes abruptly, with intercurrent events such as surgery, pregnancy, fever, and so on. Sometimes Guillain–Barré syndrome or CIDP (chronic inflammatory demyelinating polyneuropathy) has to be considered as a differential a diagnosis [10].

Investigations

Phytanic acid serum level is increased and cerebrospinal fluid (CSF) albumin is usually elevated. Electrophysiology detects severe diffuse reduction of nerve conduction velocities.

Pathology

Autopsy studies show that the most prominent lesions are observed proximally in the plexuses and cauda equina. There is significant axon loss, similar to any chronic demyelinating polyneuropathy. Most of the remaining myelinated fibers have too-thin-for-axon-caliber myelin sheaths, secondary to a slow demyelination and remyelination process (Fig. 21.1); active demyelination with macrophages and myelin debris are rarely encountered [11]. Crystalline structures localized in the cytoplasm of Schwann cells were formerly thought to be characteristic of the disease [12], but similar structures have subsequently been observed in several other nerve disorders. The enlargement of nerves is related to the intense proliferation of Schwann cells around the aforementioned too-thin-for-axon-caliber myelin sheaths (Fig. 21.1A,B). Onion bulbs are prominent in adult cases but in infantile cases may be absent. In a few rare cases, normal nerve biopsy or significant axonal loss without any demyelinating lesions has been observed.

Treatment

Plasmapheresis has been useful to decrease serum phytanic acid, and a specific diet is prescribed as phytanic acid exclusively derives from food [13].

Animal models

Ferdinandusse *et al.* have generated and characterized a *PHYH* knockout mouse; they studied the effects of phytanic acid accumulation. Motor nerve conduction revealed a peripheral neuropathy, but the pathological examination of nerves was normal [14].

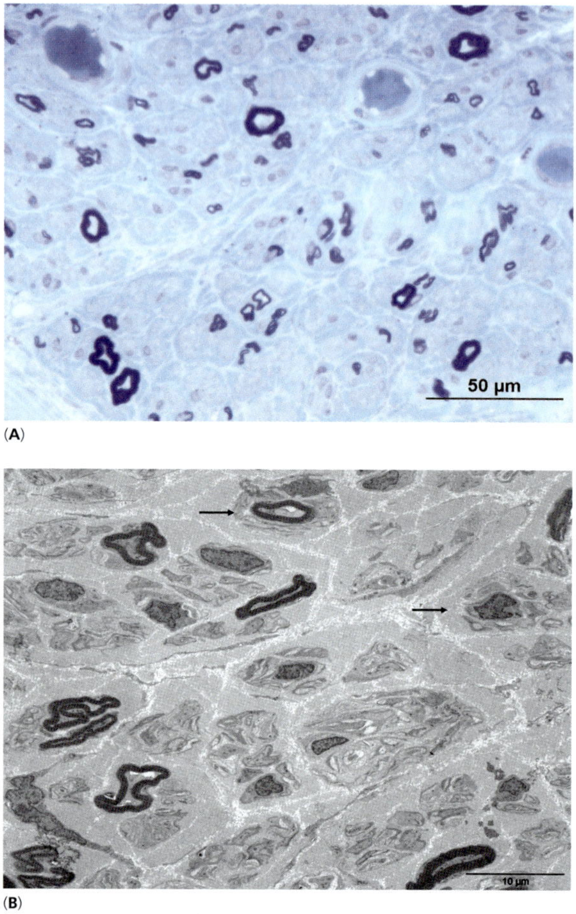

Figure 21.1 Refsum's disease. (**A**) Semi-thin transverse section. Severe reduction of myelinated fibers, predominantly large ones. Onion bulbs are not visible at this magnification. (**B**) Electron micrograph; transverse section. Severe reduction of myelinated fibers; a few onion-bulb proliferations are present (arrows).

Adrenomyeloneuropathy

Definition

Adrenomyeloneuropathy is an X-linked disorder and a variant of adrenoleukodystrophy affecting the nervous system, adrenal cortex, and testis resulting from inactivating mutations in the *ABCD1* gene located on chromosome Xq28 [15].

Clinical presentation

There is predominant spinal cord and peripheral nerve involvement due to an axonopathy. Most but not all patients develop adrenal insufficiency. The prognosis is usually better than for classical adrenoleukodystrophy.

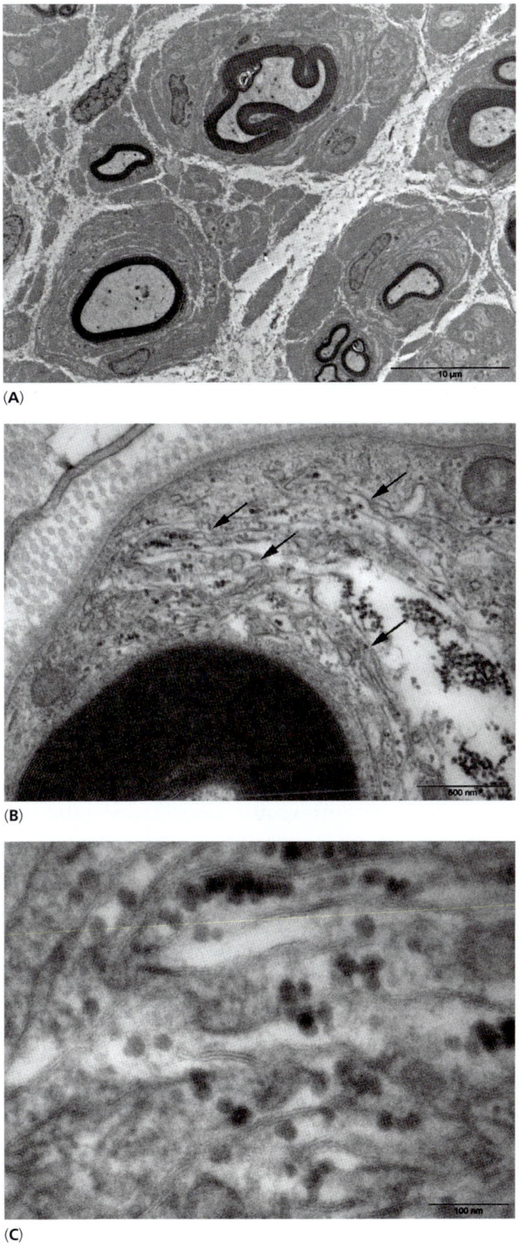

Figure 21.2 Adrenomyeloneuropathy. (**A**) Reduction of myelinated fibers. Proliferation of Schwann cells like onion bulbs around hypomyelinated fibers. (EM, transverse section). (**B**) Adrenomyeloneuropathy. There are several narrow, more or less rectilinear inclusions in the cytoplasm of this myelinated Schwann cell (EM, transverse section). (**C**) Adrenomyeloneuropathy. At high magnification note the trilaminar structure of each inclusion. This appearance on ultrastructure seems to be specific for adrenoleucodystrophy or adrenomyeloneuropathy (EM, transverse section).

Pathology

Biopsy of peripheral nerve shows a reduced number of large myelinated fibers (Fig. 21.2A) and lamellar inclusions in Schwann cell cytoplasm (Fig. 21.2B,C) [16, 17].

Ataxia with vitamin deficiency (AVED)

Definition

Deficiency of vitamin E (a lipid-soluble and chain-breaking antioxidant in biological membranes) may result from fat malabsorption, deficient fat transport, or rarely, an isolated vitamin E deficiency [18]. Ataxia with vitamin E deficiency (AVED) is a rare autosomal recessive disorder phenotypically resembling Friedreich's ataxia (also called FAVED: Friedreich's ataxia phenotype with vitamin E deficiency) but due to a mutation of *TTPA* (alpha tocopherol transfer protein).

Clinical presentation

In AVED, early findings are hyporeflexia, decreased proprioception, distal muscle weakness, and night blindness (nyctalopia); later, patients develop truncal and limb ataxia, nystagmus, and diffuse muscle weakness. The neuropathy is a mild or moderate axonal sensory neuropathy [19].

Investigation

Plasma alpha tocopherol concentration is very low.

Pathology

Demyelinating neuropathy can be observed in isolated vitamin E deficiency: the sural nerve shows loss of large myelinated fibers with evidence of remyelination [18]. Compared with Friedreich's ataxia, myelinated fiber density is not as reduced, and signs of regeneration are prominent [19].

Treatment

High dose oral vitamin E supplementation halts disease progression and stabilizes the condition in most patients [20].

Neuroacanthocytosis (except beta-lipoprotein deficiency)

Acanthocytes are contracted red blood cells with a number of irregularly spaced thorny surface projections, often with terminal bulbs [21]. Acanthocytosis combined with a neurological disorder was first described in abetalipoproteinaemia, but the association also exists with McLeod syndrome and chorea-acanthocytosis [22].

Chorea-acanthocytosis

This is an autosomal recessive disorder, due to a mutation of the *ChAC* gene, characterized by progressive hyperkinetic movements and acanthocytosis without a lipid abnormality. Acanthocytosis is a hallmark of the disease, but there is variation in the efficacy of their detection, and they may appear only late in the course of the disease [22].

Most of the neurological manifestations are CNS disorders (chorea, dysphagia, dysarthria, repetitive motor tics, orofacial, and lingual movement abnormalities, Parkinsonism, cognitive impairment, and psychiatric symptoms), but in the PNS a predominantly distal motor axonal neuropathy can be found. Nerve conduction velocity is usually normal, with reduced sensory potentials in only half the patients [22].

Nerve biopsy shows depletion of large myelinated fibers, sometimes with signs of demyelination-remyelination [23], and rarely inflammatory signs [24]; on ultrastructural study, axonal swellings filled with accumulations of neurofilaments are found [25], suggesting slowed axonal transport as a possible mechanism for the axonal degeneration.

McLeod syndrome

This is a rare X-linked disorder (mutation of the *XK* gene) due to a lack of the Kx antigen (Kell system). Its phenotype is similar to that of chorea-acanthocytosis. There is a slowly progressive course with choreiform movements and associated peripheral neuropathy with generalized areflexia, myopathy with elevated serum creatine kinase level, and cardiomyopathy [22].

The PNS disorder is usually less important in McLeod syndrome than in chorea-acanthocytosis: electrophysiological study and nerve biopsy show axonal degeneration, sometimes with signs of demyelination [26]. Muscle biopsy can show type 2 fiber atrophy, increased variability in fiber size and central nucleation [27].

Porphyrias

Definition

Porphyrias are inherited or acquired metabolic disorders, affecting all ethnic groups; acquired porphyria is often the result of liver disease. The inherited forms result from a specific enzymatic alteration in the heme biosynthesis pathway leading to accumulation of porphyrins and porphyrin precursors [28]. Porphyrias can be divided into four forms of *acute hepatic porphyrias associated with neurological symptoms* (comprising acute intermittent porphyria, dehydratase deficiency porphyria, hereditary coproporphyria, and variegate porphyria) and four forms of *erythropoietic porphyrias with no neurological symptoms* (comprising congenital erythropoietic porphyria, erythropoietic protoporphyria, porphyria cutanea tarda, and the related hepatoerythropoietic porphyria). Many porphyrias are transmitted as autosomal dominant traits, but dehydratase deficiency porphyria and congenital erythropoietic porphyria are autosomal recessive and there is an X-linked dominant form of protoporphyria [28]. Sporadic forms account for 80% of porphyria cutanea tarda.

Clinical signs

The main signs of acute hepatic porphyrias are the triad of abdominal pain, neuropsychiatric symptoms, and neuropathy [29]. Porphyric neuropathy always occurs with other features of an acute attack of hepatic porphyria that may be precipitated or aggravated by many factors including medications [30]. Its incidence is unknown, and it is suggested that 10–40% of patients with porphyria develop a neuropathy. The neuropathy consists of both autonomic neuropathy (abdominal pain, decreased gastric motility, constipation, pseudo-obstruction, tachycardia, labile hypertension, or more rarely, symptomatic orthostatic hypotension, episodic diaphoresis, and urinary and rectal sphincter incontinence), and peripheral neuropathy. The peripheral neuropathy, usually an acute axonal motor neuropathy (sometimes mimicking Guillain–Barré syndrome), develops before the onset of abdominal pain, psychiatric abnormalities and other central nervous system manifestations: several forms have been described. The prognosis for an attack of porphyria is usually good, but the neuropathy recovers more slowly than other signs [30].

Investigations

Porphyrias can be diagnosed by quantifying the porphyrins and porphyrin precursors in urine and feces. Electrophysiological study confirms an axonal motor neuropathy without evidence of conduction block or marked conduction slowing: involvement is commonly proximal and affects the upper more than the lower limbs. The CSF may show pleocytosis and a high protein level [30].

Pathology

On nerve biopsy there is axonal loss with Wallerian degeneration associated with patchy areas of demyelination. Isolated demyelination is rare [31, 32].

Treatment

Treatment of porphyric neuropathy includes both aborting the acute attack and preventive therapies treating the underlying condition between attacks. Treatment for pain is also necessary [30].

PHARC syndrome

This is a progressive autosomal recessive neurodegenerative disease phenotypically resembling Refsum's disease, due to mutations of the *ABHD12* gene. PHARC is the acronym for Polyneuropathy, Hearing loss, Ataxia, Retinitis pigmentosa, and Cataract. The peripheral nerve disorder is a demyelinating polyneuropathy in most of cases [33].

DNA repair deficiencies

Human cells are constantly exposed to DNA damage from various endogenous sources: the four major pathways for repairing these damages are nucleotide excision repair, base excision repair, mismatch repair and double-strand break repair [34]. Deficiencies in DNA repair pathways can lead to an increase risk of cancer, and also to several hereditary DNA repair deficiency diseases.

Xeroderma pigmentosum

This rare autosomal recessive disease is due to a nucleotide excision repair deficiency, leading to short stature, microencephaly with bird-like face, cutaneous signs such as severe sunburn with blistering or persistent erythema after minimal sun exposure, poikiloderma, hyper- and hypo-pigmentation, skin atrophy, and later skin malignancies, ocular signs including photophobia, conjunctivitis, and later, malignant ocular tumors, as well as neurological symptoms.

The neurological symptoms appear before the age of 8 years with encephalopathy; patients then develop cerebellar disturbance, sensoneurial deafness, spastic tetraplegia, and moderate to marked axonal sensorimotor polyneuropathy [35].

Electron microscopy of the radial nerve shows increased interstitial collagen with reduced density of large and myelinated fibers, axonal atrophy, occasional regeneration clusters, and rare thinly myelinated fibers [36].

Cockayne syndrome

This is a rare autosomal recessive disease due to a nucleotide excision repair deficiency, characterized by progressive childhood neurological impairment resulting in growth failure, limited cognition, cachexia, premature aging, dementia, deteriorating vision and hearing, cutaneous photosensitivity (without a propensity to cancer), endocrinopathies, and neurological manifestations (progressive spasticity, ataxia, and sensorimotor peripheral neuropathy) [34, 37].

Peripheral nerve biopsy shows both axonal pathology and demyelination with remyelination [37]. Granular lysosomal inclusions can sometimes be observed on ultrastructural examination [38].

Spinocerebellar ataxia with axonal neuropathy (or SCAN1)

SCAN1 is a rare autosomal recessive neurodegenerative disease due to a single-stranded break repair deficiency caused by a mutation in the *DTP1* gene (encoding for tyrosyl-DNA phosphodiesterase 1) [34]. It is characterized by late-childhood-onset slowly progressive cerebellar ataxia followed by an axonal CMT-like polyneuropathy with distal weakness, marked muscular atrophy, pes cavus, and secondary sensory disturbances. Sural nerve biopsy shows a decrease in large myelinated fibers [39].

Ataxia-telangiectasia

This rare autosomal recessive disorder is characterized by ataxic movements and oculocutaneous telangiectasia resulting from mutations in the *ATM* (ataxia telangiectasia mutated) gene. It can rarely be associated with a neuropathy [34].

Ataxia with oculomotor apraxia type 1 (AOA1)

This is a rare autosomal recessive neurodegenerative disorder with progressive cerebellar atrophy, oculomotor apraxia, and late onset peripheral motor neuropathy.

Electrophysiological study shows an axonal motor neuropathy in all cases, and sural nerve biopsy shows loss of large myelinated fibers. In the spinal cord, the posterior columns are pale (more severe in the gracile than the cuneate fasciculus). Peripheral neuropathy in AOA1 is considered to be a sensory neuronopathy [40].

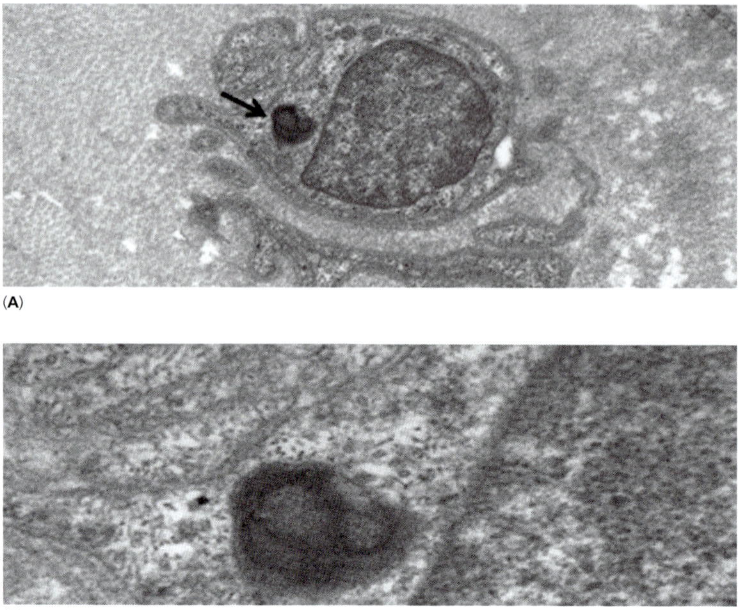

(A)

(B)

Figure 21.3 Chediak–Higashi syndrome. (**A**) Electron micrograph. Sural nerve (transverse section). The cytoplasm of an unmyelinated Schwann cell contains a lipofuscin-like inclusion. (**B**) At high magnification, the inclusion has a curvilinear and lamellar internal structure.

Ataxia with oculomotor apraxia type 2 (AOA2)

This rare autosomal recessive form of cerebellar ataxia (associated to oculomotor apraxia) is due to mutations in the *SETX* gene and is characterized by degeneration of the cerebellum, spinal cord, and peripheral nerves. Alpha-fetoprotein levels are elevated in patients' serum. Almost all patients with AOA2 have an axonal polyneuropathy. Peripheral nerve biopsy shows loss of large myelinated fibers without signs of regeneration [41].

Chediak–Higashi syndrome

Definition

Mutations in *LYST*, a gene encoding a putative lysosomal trafficking protein, cause Chediak–Higashi syndrome (CHS), an autosomal recessive multisystem disorder typically characterized by infantile-onset hemophagocytic syndrome, immunodeficiency, oculocutaneous albinism, and various neurologic problems.

Clinical presentation

Clinical neurological problems usually begin in early adulthood with cognitive decline, parkinsonism and features of spinocerebellar degeneration. Peripheral neuropathy is described in this disease, but is usually mild and manifests as isolated areflexia or moderate sensorimotor deficits.

Electrophysiology

Electrophysiological study indicates an "axonal" neuropathy.

Pathology

Nerve biopsy may demonstrate loss of myelinated nerve fibers, particularly those of larger size, and of unmyelinated axons [42]. In several published cases, there is a widespread infiltration of lymphohistiocytic cells, varying from fascicle to fascicle. Large anomalous granulations in circulating leukocytes and most tissue cells including the PNS and CNS are characteristic of CHS. They resemble lysosomes and lipofuscin granules, are PAS-positive and autofluorescent. In one personal unpublished case, abnormal infiltrates or nerve fiber abnormalities were not present on nerve biopsy, but many Schwann cells, axons, fibroblasts, capillary endothelial cells, pericytes, and a few macrophages showed numerous abnormal inclusions on electron microscopy (Fig. 21.3). Pathological changes in spinal motor neurons have been reported in a few autopsies and may possibly induce neurogenic atrophy in patients who have no involvement of peripheral nerves.

Treatment

Bone marrow transplant is effective in treating the hematologic and immune defects.

Animal models

The disease has been described in some animals such as mice, rats, cows, cats, mink, and whales [43].

References

1 Klein CJ, Duan X, Shy ME. (2013) Inherited neuropathies: clinical overview and update. *Muscle Nerve*; 48:604–622.

2 Irobi J, Dierick I, Jordanova A, Claeys KG, De Jonghe P, Timmerman V. (2006) Unraveling the genetics of distal hereditary motor neuronopathies. *Neuromol Med*;8: 131–146.

3 Ouvrier RA, McLeod JG, Conchin TE. (1982) Friedreich's ataxia. Early detection and progression of peripheral nerve abnormalities. *J Neurol Sci*;55:137–145.

4 Finsterer J, Löscher W, Quasthoff S, Wanschitz J, Auer-Grumbach M, Stevanin G. (2012) Hereditary spastic paraplegias with autosomal dominant, recessive, X-linked or maternal trait of inheritance. *J Neurol Sci*;318:1–18.

5 Timmermann V, Clowes VE, Eid E. (2013) Overlapping molecular pathological themes link Charcot–Marie–Tooth neuropathies and hereditary spastic paraplegia. *Exp Neurol*;246:14–25.

6 Schady W, Smith CM. (1994) Sensory neuropathy in hereditary spastic paraplegia. *J Neurol Neurosurg Psychiatry*; 57:693–698.

7 Mohamadynejad P, Ghaedi K, Shafeghati Y, *et al.* (2013) Identification of a novel missense mutation of PEX7 gene in an Iranian patient with rhizomelic chondrodysplasia punctata type 1. *Gene*;518:461–466.

8 Jansen GA, Waterham HR, Wanders RJ. (2004) Molecular basis of Refsum disease: sequence variations in phytanoyl-CoA hydroxylase (PHYH) and the PTS2 receptor (PEX7). *Hum Mutat*;23:209–218.

9 Thomas PK, Goebel HH. (2005) Inborn errors of metabolism with peripheral nerve involvement. Lysosomal and peroxysomal storage. In: Dyck PJ, Thomas PK (eds) *Peripheral Neuropathy*. Philadelphia: Elsevier Saunders: p. 2778.

10 Verny C, Prundean A, Nicolas G, *et al.* (2006) Refsum's disease may mimic familial Guillain Barre syndrome. *Neuromuscul Disord*;16:805–808.

11 Allen IV, Swallow M, Nevin NC, McCormick D. (1978) Clinicopathological study of Refsum's disease with particular reference to fatal complications. *J Neurol Neurosurg Psychiatry*;41:323–332.

12 Fardeau M, Engel WK. (1969) Ultrastructural study of a peripheral nerve biopsy in Refsum's disease. *J Neuropathol Exp Neurol*;28:278–294.

13 Zolotov D, Wagner S, Kalb K, Bunia J, Heibges A, Klingel R. (2012) Long-term strategies for the treatment of Refsum's disease using therapeutic apheresis. *J Clin Apher*;27:99–105.

14 Ferdinandusse S, Zomer AW, Komen JC, *et al.* (2008) Ataxia with loss of Purkinje cells in a mouse model for Refsum disease. *Proc Nat Acad Sci U S A*;105:17712–17717.

15 Ferrer I, Aubourg P, Pujol A. (2010) General aspects and neuropathology of X-linked adrenoleukodystrophy. *Brain Pathol*;20:817–830.

16 Tanaka K, Koyama A, Koike R, Ohno T, Atsumi T, Miyatake T. (1985) Adrenomyeloneuropathy: report of a family and electron microscopical findings in peripheral nerve. *J Neurol*;232:73–78.

17 Julien JJ, Vallat JM, Vital C, Lagueny A, Ferrer X, Darriet D. (1981) Adrenomyeloneuropathy: demonstration of inclusions at the level of the peripheral nerve. *Eur Neurol*;20: 367–373.

18 Puri V, Chaudhry N, Tatke M, Prakash V. (2005) Isolated vitamin E deficiency with demyelinating neuropathy. *Muscle Nerve*;32:230–235.

19 Zouari M, Feki M, Ben Hamida C, *et al.* (1998) Electrophysiology and nerve biopsy: comparative study in Friedreich's ataxia and Friedreich's ataxia phenotype with vitamin E deficiency. *Neuromuscul Disord*;8:416–425.

20 Mariotti C, Gellera C, Rimoldi M, *et al.* (2004) Ataxia with isolated vitamin E deficiency: neurological phenotype, clinical follow-up and novel mutations in TTPA gene in Italian families. *Neurol Sci*;25:130–137.

21 Brecher G, Bessis M. (1972) Present status of spiculed red cells and their relationship to the discocyte-echinocyte transformation: a critical review. *Blood*;40:333–344.

22 Rampoldi L, Danek A, Monaco AP. (2002) Clinical features and molecular bases of neuroacanthocytosis. *J Mol Med*;80:475–491.

23 Hardie RJ, Pullon HW, Harding AE, *et al.* (1991) Neuroacanthocytosis. A clinical, haematological and pathological study of 19 cases. *Brain*;114:13–49.

24 Lagreze HL, Kornguth SE, Brooks BR, Levine RL. (1988) Delayed immune response in chorea-amyotrophy with spherocytosis. *Neurology*;38:1642–1643.

25 Malandrini A, Fabrizi GM, Palmeri S, *et al.* (1993) Choreoacanthocytosis like phenotype without acanthocytes: clinicopathological case report. A contribution to the knowledge of the functional pathology of the caudate nucleus. *Acta Neuropathol*;86:651–658.

26 Danek A, Rubio JP, Rampoldi L, *et al.* (2001) McLeod neuroacanthocytosis: genotype and phenotype. *Ann Neurol*;50:755–764.

27 Dotti MT, Battisti C, Malandrini A, *et al.* (2000) McLeod syndrome and neuroacanthocytosis with a novel mutation in the XK gene. *Movement Disord*;15:1282–1284.

28 Puy H, Gouya L, Deybach JC. (2010) Porphyrias. *Lancet*;375:924–937.

29 Simon NG, Herkes GK. (2011) The neurologic manifestations of the acute porphyrias. *J Clin Neurosci*;18:1147–1153.

30 Albers JW, Fink JK. (2004) Porphyric neuropathy. *Muscle Nerve*;30:410–422.

31 Denny-Brown D, Sciarra D. (1945) Changes in the nervous system in acute porphyria. *Brain*;68:1–16.

32 Suarez JI, Cohen ML, Larkin J, Kernich CA, Hricik DE, Daroff RB. (1997) Acute intermittent porphyria: clinicopathologic correlation. Report of a case and review of the literature. *Neurology*;48:1678–1683.

33 Fiskerstrand C, H'Mida-Ben Brahim D, Johansson S, *et al.* (2010) Mutations in ABHD12 cause the neurodegenerative disease PHARC: an inborn error of endocannabinoid metabolism. *Am J Hum Genet*;87:410–417.

34 Jeppesen DK, Bohr VA, Stevnsner T. (2011) DNA repair deficiency in neurodegeneration. *Progr Neurobiol*; 94: 166–200.

35 Anttinen A, Koulu L, Nikoskelainen E, *et al.* (2008) Neurological symptoms and natural course of xeroderma pigmentosum. *Brain*;131:1979–1989.

36 Lai JP, Liu YC, Alimchandani M, *et al.* (2013) The influence of DNA repair on neurological degeneration, cachexia, skin cancer and internal neoplasms: autopsy report of four xeroderma pigmentosum patients (XP-A, XP-C and XP-D). *Acta Neuropathol Commun*;1:4.

37 Rapin I, Weidenheim K, Lindenbaum Y, *et al.* (2006) Cockayne syndrome in adults: review with clinical and pathologic study of a new case. *J Child Neurol*;21:991–1006.

38 Grunnet ML, Zimmerman AW, Lewis RA. (1983) Ultrastructure and electrodiagnosis of peripheral neuropathy in Cockayne's syndrome. *Neurology*;33:1606–1609.

39 Takashima H, Boerkoel CF, John J, *et al.* (2002) Mutation of TDP1, encoding a topoisomerase I-dependent DNA damage repair enzyme, in spinocerebellar ataxia with axonal neuropathy. *Nature Genet*;32:267–272.

40 Onodera O. (2006) Spinocerebellar ataxia with ocular motor apraxia and DNA repair. *Neuropathology*;26:361–367.

41 Tazir M, Ali-Pacha L, M'Zahem A, *et al.* (2009) Ataxia with oculomotor apraxia type 2: a clinical and genetic study of 19 patients. *J Neurol Sci*;278:77–81.

42 Misra VP, King RH, Harding AE, Muddle JR, Thomas PK. (1991) Peripheral neuropathy in the Chediak–Higashi syndrome. *Acta Neuropathol*;81:354–358.

43 Ward DM, Griffiths GM, Stinchcombe JC, Kaplan J. (2000) Analysis of the lysosomal storage disease Chediak–Higashi syndrome. *Traffic*;1:816–822.

CHAPTER 22

Adult polyglucosan body disease

Alexander Lossos,[1] Or Kakhlon,[1] and Dov Soffer[2]

[1] *Department of Neurology, Hadassah-Hebrew University Medical Centre, Jerusalem, Israel*

[2] *Department of Pathology, Hadassah-Hebrew University Medical Centre, Israel*

Definition of the disorder, major synonyms, and historical perspective

Adult polyglucosan body disease (APBD; OMIM 263570) is a late-onset slowly progressive disorder affecting the central and peripheral nervous systems [1]. Patients typically present in the fifth or early sixth decade with a variable combination of myelopathy, peripheral neuropathy, neurogenic bladder, and cognitive impairment. Pathologically, there is widespread accumulation of polyglucosan bodies (PBs) throughout the nervous system. These round intracellular inclusions are composed mostly of amylopectin-like polysaccharide and primarily involve neuronal and astrocytic processes [2].

Early reports of isolated [2, 3] and familial [4] cases in the 1970s were followed by a seminal study by Robitaille *et al.* [1] who categorized and named this disorder as a distinct clinico-pathological entity and outlined the main diagnostic criteria. In the 1990s, pathological similarities to glycogen storage disease type IV (GSD IV; OMIM 232500), also known as Andersen disease or amylopectinosis [1, 2, 5], led to the discovery of glycogen branching enzyme (GBE) deficiency in APBD patients of Ashkenazi Jewish origin [6] caused by recessively segregated mutations in the *GBE1* gene [7]. APBD is considered an allelic adult variant of GSD IV and adds to the list of hepatic and neuromuscular forms of perinatal, congenital or juvenile onset [8].

Epidemiology

Since the original description [1], approximately 100 cases of APBD with equal gender distribution have been reported but the true prevalence is unknown and many patients probably remain undiagnosed or misdiagnosed [9]. Although reported mostly in people of Ashkenazi Jewish background [7, 9], the disease is described in people from all over the world [9, 10]. APBD accounts for 1.6–10% of selected dementia autopsies [11, 12].

Clinical features and investigations

The disease usually begins around the age of 50 with symptoms of bladder dysfunction, followed slowly by paresthesia in the feet and by gait difficulties that progress over a decade when walking aids or wheelchair are required [9]. Clinically most patients manifest symmetric spastic paraparesis with bilateral extensor plantar response, brisk deep tendon reflexes, except for reduced ankle jerks, a gradient of distal more than proximal leg weakness, and distal superficial and vibration sensory deficits in the legs. The gait is unsteady and variably spastic. These findings suggest a combination of myelopathy with peripheral neuropathy. Mild cognitive impairment, saccadization of pursuit gaze, and late orthostatism and parkinsonian features can also occur.

Routine laboratory tests and CSF analysis are noncontributory, except for occasional elevation of serum creatine kinase [13]. Peripheral nerve conduction study demonstrates predominantly axonal sensorimotor peripheral neuropathy with reduced or absent compound motor action potentials and sensory nerve action potentials, often with an additional lumbosacral radicular involvement [9, 13]. Needle electromyography shows neurogenic changes in the legs and paraspinal muscles.

Cerebral and spinal MRI reveals progressive symmetric involvement of hemispheric and periventricular

Peripheral Nerve Disorders: Pathology and Genetics, First Edition. Edited by Jean-Michel Vallat, Joachim Weis, Francoise Gray, and Katy Keohane.

cerebral white matter, posterior limb of the internal capsule, the external capsule, cerebellar peduncles, and brainstem tracts with relative sparing of the subcortical U-fibers [9]. The lesions appear hyperintense on T2 and fluid-attenuated inversion recovery (FLAIR) sequences, and tend to be multifocal, symmetric, and confluent. Medullary and spinal cord atrophy are early invariable MRI findings, whereas cortical atrophy and a thin corpus callosum are seen later. MRS of the involved cerebral white matter may shows reduced NAA/Cr ratio and elevated lactate signal, reflecting the underlying processes involved in axonal loss and demyelination [14].

The diagnosis of APBD is suggested by the clinical and imaging findings but must be biochemically, genetically or pathologically confirmed to exclude differential diagnoses. These include a range of chronic progressive myelopathies and myeloneuropathies, complicated forms of hereditary spastic paraparesis, several late-onset leukoencephalopathies, including primary progressive multiple sclerosis, multiple system atrophy, and even prostatic enlargement in men with early urinary symptoms [9]. Definitive testing includes analysis of residual GBE activity in peripheral blood leukocytes or cultured skin fibroblasts [6] and *GBE1* genotyping [7]. If these tests are negative, inconclusive, or unavailable, PBs may be demonstrated in apocrine gland myoepithelial cells in axillary skin biopsy [15] or in sural nerve biopsy.

Pathology

Widespread accumulation of PBs throughout the nervous system is the pathological hallmark of APBD [1–4]. PBs also occur in liver, myocardium, and occasionally lungs, kidneys, gastrointestinal smooth muscle, in apocrine glands, and sometimes in skeletal muscle [15]. In the CNS, they occur in astrocytic and neuronal processes in all regions of the brain and spinal cord, but not in neuronal perikarya, allowing distinction from Lafora bodies [1]. Additional findings include cerebral demyelination and gliosis.

In the sural nerve, PBs are spherical, basophilic intra-axonal inclusions, sometimes concentrically laminated (Fig. 22.1A). Size varies from a few to 70 μm, but they are usually 10–15 μm in diameter and up to 100 μm in length. PBs are strongly PAS positive and diastase

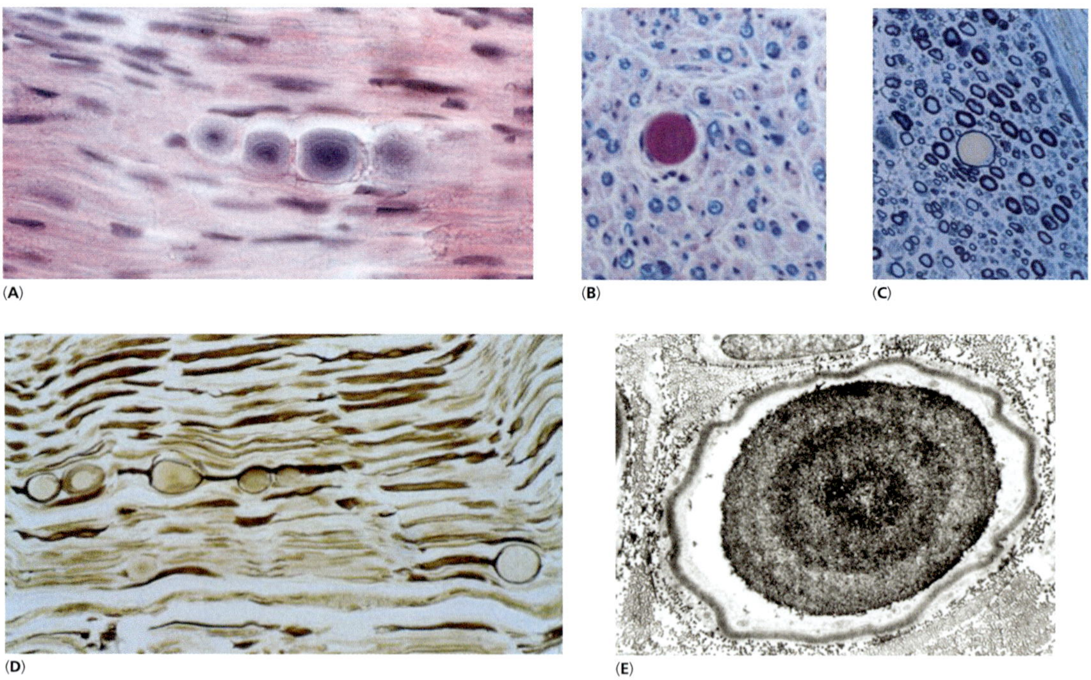

(A) (B) (C) (D) (E)

Figure 22.1 Sural nerve biopsy findings in APBD.(**A, D**) A string of intra-axonal PBs (**A**: H&E, ×400; **D**: Bielschowsky silver impregnation, ×400).(**B, C, E**) PB (**B**: luxol-fast blue – PAS, ×400; **C**: Semithin section stained with thionine and acridine orange, ×400; **E**: electron microscopy, ×12,500).

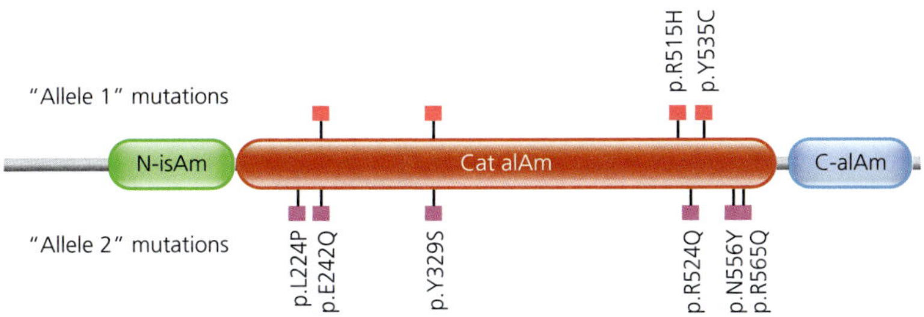

Figure 22.2 A schematic view of APBD-associated mutations in the *GBE1* gene (19)."Allele 1" mutations are shown above the protein sequence and "allele 2" mutations below. The p.R515H is observed in combination with the p.R524Q while other "allele 1" mutations are homozygous (p.E242Q and p.Y329S) or heterozygous (p.Y535C).The "allele 2" mutations are observed in combination with the p.Y329S in "allele 1", except for p.R524Q (with p.R515H in "allele 1"), p.N556Y (with pY329C in "allele 1") and the homozygous p.E242Q.The indicated protein domains are N-isAm for N-terminal isoamylase; Cat alAm for catalytic alpha amylase; C-alAm for C-terminal alpha amylase. The c.2003delA mutation (9) is not shown on this protein-based scheme.

resistant (Fig. 22.1B) and also stain with colloidal iron, Best's carmine, iodine, methenamine silver, and variably with alcian blue.

Ultrastructurally, they consist of a nonmembrane-bound compact mass of fine branching filaments, 5–8 nm in diameter, associated with granular and amorphous material (Fig. 22.1E). PBs are mainly seen in myelinated nerve fibers. If large, they distend axons causing thinning of myelin sheaths (Fig. 22.1C). They can be found in unmyelinated fibers and occasionally in Schwann cells. Some axons contain more than one PB (Fig. 22.1A,D). Other changes include mild loss of myelinated nerve fibers, occasional ovoids, regenerative clusters, mild endoneurial fibrosis, and rarely, poorly developed onion bulbs.

Nerve biopsy was originally required to confirm the diagnosis of APBD [1], but PBs are found as an age-dependent phenomenon in up to 8.5% of sural nerve biopsies from patients with unspecified polyneuropathies or rarely in other conditions, including normal aging [16]. Therefore biopsy findings must be interpreted in the appropriate clinical context. Intramuscular nerve twig PBs in adults are similarly nonspecific [17] (see also Fig. 7.14).

Genetics and pathogenesis

Most of the tested APBD patients show reduced GBE activity [7, 9, 10]. GBE is a widely expressed cytosolic enzyme of 702 amino acids encoded by the *GBE1* gene. Through its alpha amylase and glucosyl transferase (isoamylase) activities (Fig. 22.2), GBE enables branching of the growing glycogen molecule, which is essential for solubility. Excessive glycogen elongation unbalanced by adequate branching in GBE deficiency leads to the accumulation of amylopectin-like, poorly branched insoluble PBs in APBD. Because similar inclusions are observed as a result of overexpressed glycogen synthase [GS], it is the imbalance between GS-induced elongation to GBE-related branching that accounts for PB formation [18].

Of the multiple *GBE1* mutations associated with GSD IV [8, 19], only nine have been reported so far in APBD (Fig. 22.2). In contrast to early-onset forms of GSD IV, most mutations in APBD are "mild" missense substitutions [9] that presumably explain the relatively late onset and less severe clinical manifestations [19] and biochemical defect [4]. The p.Y329S mutation is found in 76% of patients, particularly of Ashkenazi Jewish ancestry [9]. Despite apparent autosomal recessive inheritance [6, 7], a proportion of APBD patients are p.Y329S heterozygotes [9, 14], yet are clinically and biochemically indistinguishable from homozygotes, suggesting additional genetic or environmental factors. Epidemiologically, one study showed this mutation to occur at a frequency of 1:34.5 in Ashkenazi Jewish population [20].

Using computational analysis (Fig. 22.3), the p.Y329S mutation is predicted to increase the conformational assembly of GBE leading to instability but not to complete unfolding. This is based on the Y329 location at a central cleft of the molecule and on its interaction with neighboring amino acids (Fig. 22.3).

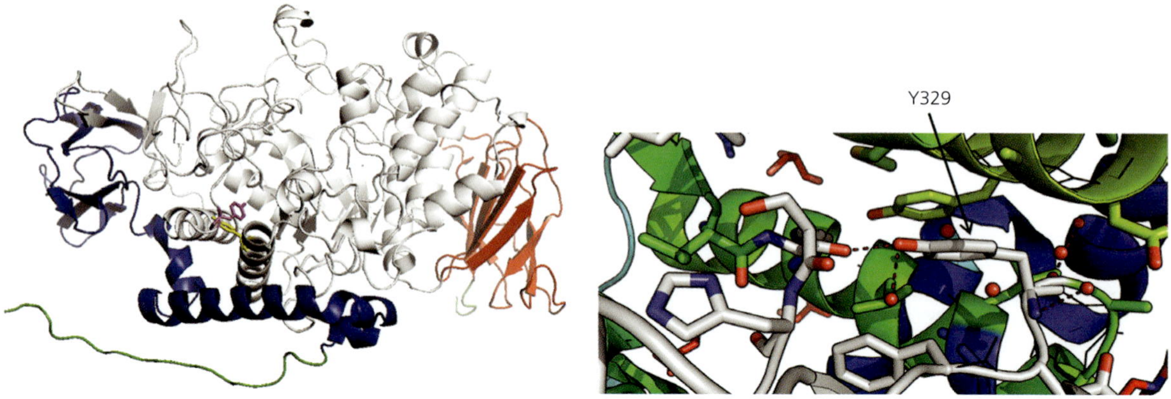

(A) (B)

Figure 22.3 A 3D model of the rice GBE close homolog (PDB ID: 3aml).(**A**) The different domains diagrammed in Fig. 20.2 are shown: blue and an unstructured N-terminal sequence in green refer to the N-terminal isoamylase, white to the catalytic alpha amylase, and red to the C-terminal alpha amylase. The most commonly mutated p.Y329 residue is shown in magenta in (**A**) and in white in (**B**) where its hydrogen bonds and pi-stacking interactions with another tyrosine in yellow (**A**) can be better appreciated. The specific inter-residue bonding and its location at a central cleft suggest how the p.Y329S mutation can destabilize the protein. Source: O. Furman. Reproduced with permission of O. Furman.

Animal models

In addition to several naturally occurring animal models of GSD IV, a mouse model with typical features of APBD was generated by *GBE1* manipulation [21].

Treatment

Currently there is no specific treatment for APBD. Symptomatic management of urodynamic, neurocognitive and autonomic disturbances, and intensive rehabilitation programs are important. Experimentally, the possibility of overcoming secondary energy metabolism impairment with anaplerotic diet therapy showed promising results [22].

References

1 Robitaille W, Carpenter S, Karpati G *et al.* (1980) A distinct form of adult polyglucosan body disease with massive involvement of central and peripheral neuronal processes and astrocytes. A report of four cases and review of the occurrence of polyglucosan bodies in other conditions such as Lafora's disease and normal ageing. *Brain* 103:315–336.

2 Peress NS, DiMauro S, Roxburgh VA (1979) Adult polysaccharidosis. Clinicopathological, ultrastructural, and biochemical features. *Arch Neurol* 36:840–845.

3 Suzuki K, David E, Kutschman B (1971) Presenile dementia with "Lafora-like" intraneuronal inclusions. *Arch Neurol* 25:69–80.

4 Carpenter S, Karpati G (1976) Intra-axonal polyglucosan bodies: an unusual lesion of peripheral nerves. *Neurology* 26:369.

5 McMaster KR, Powers JM, Hennigar GR *et al.* (1979) Nervous system involvement in type IV glycogenosis. *Arch Pathol Lab Med* 103:105–111.

6 Lossos A, Barash V, Soffer D *et al.* (1991) Hereditary branching enzyme dysfunction in adult polyglucosan body disease: a possible metabolic cause in two patients. *Ann Neurol* 30:655–662.

7 Lossos A, Meiner Z, Barash V *et al.* (1998) Adult polyglucosan body disease in Ashkenazi Jewish patients carrying the Tyr329Ser mutation in the glycogen branching enzyme gene. *Ann Neurol* 44:867–872.

8 Bao Y, Kishnani P, Wu J-Y, Chen Y-T (1996) Hepatic and neuromuscular forms of glycogen storage disease type IV caused by mutations in the same glycogen-branching enzyme gene. *J Clin Invest* 97:941–948.

9 Mochel F, Schiffmann R, Steenweg ME *et al.* (2012) Adult polyglucosan body disease: natural history and key magnetic resonance imaging findings. *Ann Neurol* 72: 433–441.

10 Bruno C, Servidei S, Shanske S *et al.* (1993) Glycogen branching enzyme deficiency in adult polyglucosan body disease. *Ann Neurol* 33:88–93.

11 Massoud F, Devi G, Moroney JT *et al.* (2000) The role of routine laboratory studies and neuroimaging in the diagnosis of dementia: a clinicopathological study. *J Am Geriatr Soc* 48:1204–1210.

12 Arnold SE, Franz BR, Trojanowski JQ (1994) Elderly patients with schizophrenia exhibit infrequent neurodegenerative lesions. *Neurobiol Aging* 15:299–303.

13 Klein CJ, Boes CJ, Chapin JE *et al.* (2004) Adult polyglucosan body disease: case description of an expanding genetic and clinical syndrome. *Muscle Nerve* 29:323–328.

14 Massa R, Bruno C, Martorana A *et al.* (2008) Adult polyglucosan body disease: proton magnetic resonance spectroscopy of the brain and novel mutation in the GBE1 gene. *Muscle Nerve* 37:530–536.

15 Busard HLSM, Gabreels-Festen AAWM, Renier WO *et al.* (1991) Adult polyglucosan body disease: The diagnostic value of axilla skin biopsy. *Ann Neurol* 29: 448–451.

16 Busard HLSM, Gabreels-Festen AAWM, van't Hof MA *et al.* (1990) Polyglucosan bodies in sural nerve biopsies. *Acta Neuropathol* 80:554–557.

17 Bernsen RAJAM, Busard HLSM, Ter Laak HJ *et al.* (1989) Polyglucosan bodies in intramuscular motor nerves. *Acta Neuropathol* 77: 629–633.

18 Raben N, Danon M, Lu N *et al.* (2001) Surprises of genetic engineering: a possible model of polyglucosan body disease. *Neurology* 56:1739–1745.

19 Magoulas PL, El-Hattab AW, Roy A *et al.* (2012) Diffuse reticuloendothelial system involvement in type IV glycogen storage disease with a novel GBE1 mutation: a case report and review. *Hum Pathol* 43:943–951.

20 Hussain A, Armistead J, Gushulak L *et al.* (2012) The adult polyglucosan body disease mutation GBE1 c.1076A>C occurs at high frequency in persons of Ashkenazi Jewish background. *Biochem Biophys Res Commun* 426: 286–288.

21 Akman HO, Sheiko T, Tay SK *et al.* (2011) Generation of a novel mouse model that recapitulates early and adult onset glycogenosis type IV. *Hum Mol Genet* 20:4430–4439.

22 Roe CR, Bottiglieri T, Wallace M *et al.* (2010) Adult polyglucosan body disease (APBD): anaplerotic diet therapy (triheptanoin) and demonstration of defective methylation pathways. *Molec Gen Metabol* 101:246–252.

Web references

APBDRF: Adult Polyglucosan Disease Research Foundation www.apbdrf.org/

OMIM: Online Mendelian Inheritance in Man www.ncbi.nlm.nih.gov/omim

GeneReviews ™: www.ncbi.nlm.nih.gov/books/NBK1116/

ORphanet: www.orpha.net/consor/www/cgi-bin/index.php?lng=EN

Clinicaltrials: clinicaltrials.gov/ct2/show/NCT00947960?term=adult+polyglucosan&rank=1

CHAPTER 23

Polyneuropathies associated with neurofibromatosis

Joachim Weis

Institute of Neuropathology, RWTH Aachen University Hospital and JARA Brain Translational Medicine, Aachen, Germany

Introduction

The neurofibromatoses are usually regarded as tumor syndromes that also feature maldevelopmental lesions. However, in neurofibromatosis 1, and quite frequently in neurofibromatosis 2, progressive, diffuse sensorimotor neuropathies can develop.

Neurofibromatosis 1 (*NF1*; MIM 162200)

Definition, genetics, and pathogenesis

Neurofibromatosis 1 is caused by autosomal dominant mutations of the *NF1* gene on chromosome 17q11.2, which encodes for the tumor suppressor protein neurofibromin 1. The spectrum of alterations includes neurofibromas and various other neoplasms such as gliomas, sarcomas and neuroendocrine tumors, osseous and vascular lesions, and café-au-spots. Neurofibromin 1 regulates the Ras/mitogen-activated protein kinase (MAPK) pathway and cyclic adenosine monophosphate (AMP) levels [1, 2].

Clinical presentation

Non-neoplastic nervous system disorders include macrocephaly, hydrocephalus due to aqueduct stenosis, epilepsy, and peripheral neuropathy. Neurofibromatous neuropathy affects 1–2% of neurofibromatosis 1 patients [1, 3]. These patients present with distal, predominantly sensory or sensorimotor symptoms that can show both demyelinating and axonal features electrophysiologically [4]. The nerves are often thickened and may show focal nodules [5]. Large root diffuse and other neurofibromas are particularly frequent in patients with neurofibromatous neuropathy; a much higher proportion of them develop malignant peripheral nerve sheath tumors (MPNST) than the whole population of NF1 patients [4].

Histopathology

In biopsied nerves, diffuse, variable neurofibromatous change is present, especially in the subperineurial zone [5] but also in the center of nerve fascicles [4]. The cells in these lesions may show schwannoid, fibroblast-like or perineurial differentiation [3, 5]. An abundant extracellular matrix containing many collagen fibers is deposited between these cells. Fibrous long-spaced collagen (FLC) can be found by electron microscopy [5]. The myelinated nerve fibers are reduced in density, with considerable focal variability and some myelin sheaths are thinned [3]. The perineurium may be disrupted focally and may be associated with hypercellularity of the epineurium [3].

Neurofibromatosis 2 (*NF2*; MIM 101000)

Definition and genetics

The spectrum of phenotypes in neurofibromatosis 2 comprises bilateral vestibular schwannomas, schwannomas of other nerves, meningiomas, gliomas and cerebral microhamartomas, meningioangiomatosis, and peripheral neuropathy [6, 7]. Neurofibromatosis 2 is caused by mutation of the *NF2* gene on chromosome

Peripheral Nerve Disorders: Pathology and Genetics, First Edition. Edited by Jean-Michel Vallat, Joachim Weis, Francoise Gray, and Katy Keohane.

22q12 that encodes for the tumor suppressor protein merlin (moesin-ezrin-radixin-like protein; synonym: schwannomin) [6]. Merlin regulates many cellular functions such as adhesion, cell motility, growth, proliferation, and survival by interacting with diverse pathways including receptor tyrosine kinases and integrins at the cell surface and ubiquitin E3 ligase activity in the nucleus [8].

Clinical presentation

Schwannomas and other tumors in *NF2* may cause isolated neurological deficits. However, *NF2* is more frequently associated with a diffuse, distally accentuated sensorimotor neuropathy than *NF1*.

Histopathology and pathogenesis

Reports on sural nerve biopsies [9–11] describe a predominantly axonal neuropathy, often associated with fibrosis and diffuse proliferation of Schwann cells, Schwann cell onion bulb formations with or without central myelinated axon and small endoneurial tumorlets of schwannomas (Fig. 23.1). Perineuriomas were found less frequently. The Ki-67 labeling index of endoneurial cells was mildly increased. Therefore, the axonopathy was thought to be caused by the space-occupying cell proliferations and a disturbed interaction between the altered Schwann cells and their axons.

An additional mechanism is suggested by recent results: Two alternatively spliced merlin isoforms were found to be expressed in the mammalian nervous system, only one of which, isoform 2, was found in axons [12]. Functional studies revealed that an isoform 2-dependent complex promotes activation of the GTPase RhoA, leading to neurofilament heavy chain phosphorylation [12]. Thus, impairment of intrinsic axonal functions of merlin might contribute to the neuropathy in *NF2*.

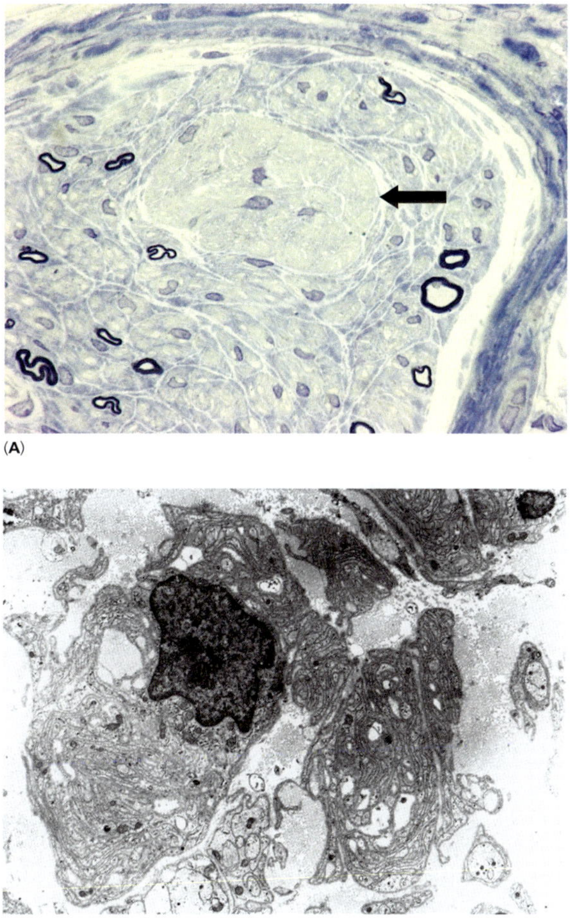

(A)

(B)

Figure 23.1 (**A**) Endoneurial cluster of abnormal schwannoid cells ("tumorlet", arrow) in a case of NF2-neuropathy. Sural nerve biopsy; semithin section, Toluidine blue. (**B**) EM of schwannoid cell of the same case. Note the numerous abnormal processes.

Schwannomatosis (MIM 162091)

Schwannomatosis is a prominent, diffuse endoneurial proliferation of Schwann cells without frank tumor formation, often occurring in the context of NF2 [7]. Familial schwannomatosis is characterized by multiple, often painful schwannomas at different sites, without vestibular schwannomas and other stigmata of neurofibromatosis [13]. The tumors can have a plexiform pattern and show a tendency to diffusely invade adjacent tissue [13]. Schwannomatosis is caused by mutation of *INI-1* (syn.: *SMARCB1, SWI/SNF-related, matrix-associated, actin-dependent regulator of chromatin, subfamily B, member 1*) [14]. Many tumors show additional *NF2* mutations [7].

References

1 Ferner RE, Gutmann DH (2013) Neurofibromatosis type 1 (NF1): diagnosis and management. *Handb Clin Neurol;* 115: 939–955.

2 Laycock-van Spyk S, Thomas N, Cooper DN, Upadhyaya M (2011) Neurofibromatosis type 1-associated tumors: their somatic mutational spectrum and pathogenesis. *Hum Genomics;*5:623–690.

3 Ferner RE, Hughes RA, Hall SM *et al.* (2004) Neurofibromatous neuropathy in neurofibromatosis 1 (NF1). *J Med Genet;* 41:837–841.

4 Drouet A, Wolkenstein P, Lefaucheur JP, Pinson S *et al.* (2004) Neurofibromatosis 1-associated neuropathies: a reappraisal. *Brain;*127:1993–2009.

5 Thomas PK, King RH, Chiang TR *et al.* (1990) Neurofibromatous neuropathy. *Muscle Nerve;*13:93–101.

6 Asthagiri AR, Parry DM, Butman JA *et al.* (2009) Neurofibromatosis type 2. *Lancet;*373:1974–1986.

7 Stemmer-Rachamimov AO, Wiestler OD, Louis DN (2007) Neurofibromatosis type 2. In: Louis DN, Ohgaki H, Wiestler OD, Cavenee WK (eds). *WHO Classification of Tumours of the Central Nervous System*. IVth edn. Lyon: IARC.

8 Zhou L, Hanemann CO. Merlin (2012) a multi-suppressor from cell membrane to the nucleus. *FEBS Lett;* 586(10):1403–1408.

9 Iwata A, Kunimoto M, Inoue K (1998) Schwann cell proliferation as the cause of peripheral neuropathy in neurofibromatosis-2. *J Neurol Sci;*156:201–204.

10 Sperfeld AD, Hein C, Schroder JM *et al.* (2002) Occurrence and characterization of peripheral nerve involvement in neurofibromatosis type 2. *Brain;*125:996–1004.

11 Hagel C, Lindenau M, Lamszus K *et al.* (2002) Polyneuropathy in neurofibromatosis 2: clinical findings, molecular genetics and neuropathological alterations in sural nerve biopsy specimens. *Acta Neuropathol;*104:179–187.

12 Schulz A, Baader SL, Niwa-Kawakita M *et al.* (2013) Merlin isoform 2 in neurofibromatosis type 2-associated polyneuropathy. *Nat Neurosci;*16:426–433.

13 MacCollin M, Woodfin W, Kronn D, Short MP (1996) Schwannomatosis: a clinical and pathologic study. *Neurology;* 46:1072–1079.

14 Hulsebos TJ, Plomp AS, Wolterman RA *et al.* (2007) Germline mutation of INI1/SMARCB1 in familial schwannomatosis. *Am J Hum Genet;*80:805–810.

CHAPTER 24
Vasculitides

Michael P. Collins[1] and P. James B. Dyck[2]
[1] *Department of Neurology, Medical College of Wisconsin, Wisconsin, USA*
[2] *Department of Neurology, Mayo Clinic, Rochester, USA*

Definition

The vasculitides are a clinically diverse spectrum of disorders that share the pathologic signature of inflammatory destruction of blood vessel walls, resulting in inflammatory and ischemic injury to the affected tissues [1]. They can result from direct infection of the vessel wall, but in most cases, the process involves autoimmune mechanisms. While immune-mediated vasculitides can be triggered by identifiable factors, such as drugs, infections, cancers, connective tissue diseases (CTDs), or other medical conditions, the underlying cause is usually unknown. The vasculitides have been the focus of ongoing investigation and serially updated definitional, diagnostic, and classification schemes since the original depiction of polyarteritis nodosa (PAN) by Kussmaul and Maier in 1866 [2].

When vasculitis affects vessels in the peripheral nervous system (PNS), a vasculitic neuropathy ensues. Peripheral nerve vasculitis is usually one of many clinical manifestations of a systemic disease, but vasculitis can be restricted to individual organs, including the PNS. Single-organ PNS vasculitis has most commonly been referred to as nonsystemic vasculitic neuropathy (NSVN) [3].

Epidemiology/classification

Classification of systemic vasculitides

Numerous classifications for the vasculitides have been proposed since the 1950s contingent on advances in our understanding of the etiology, mechanisms, clinical features, laboratory findings, and histological alterations of these disorders. Most have distinguished *primary* vasculitides, which lack an identified cause, from *secondary* vasculitides, which result from a known cause or predisposing condition. The most widely used classification criteria for the *primary* systemic vasculitides are those published by the American College of Rheumatology (ACR) in 1990 for PAN, Churg–Strauss syndrome, Wegener's granulomatosis, hypersensitivity vasculitis, Henoch–Schönlein purpura, giant cell arteritis (GCA), and Takayasu arteritis [4]. In 1994, the Chapel Hill Consensus Conference (CHCC 1994) defined 10 vasculitides based on size and pathology of involved vessels – GCA, Takayasu arteritis, PAN, Kawasaki disease, microscopic polyangiitis (MPA), Wegener's granulomatosis, Churg–Strauss syndrome, Henoch–Schönlein purpura, essential cryoglobulinemic vasculitis, and cutaneous leukocytoclastic angiitis [5].

The CHCC1994 and ACR systems have many limitations. They do not incorporate all of the primary systemic vasculitides or any of the secondary disorders. Apart from cutaneous leukocytoclastic angiitis, they do not address the "localized" or "single-organ" vasculitides [6]. When applied to the same cohort of patients, the criteria are often discordant [7]. Neither system functions well as diagnostic criteria for *de novo* patients. Equally important, neither system employs anti-neutrophil cytoplasmic antibodies (ANCAs). ANCAs are directed against cytoplasmic antigens in neutrophils and monocytes [8]. They are classified as perinuclear pANCAs or cytoplasmic cANCAs based on their immunofluorescent (IF) staining pattern on alcohol-fixed neutrophils. In vasculitis, cANCAs are usually directed

Peripheral Nerve Disorders: Pathology and Genetics, First Edition. Edited by Jean-Michel Vallat, Joachim Weis, Francoise Gray, and Katy Keohane.

against proteinase 3 (PR3) and pANCAs against myeloperoxidase (MPO). MPO/PR3-ANCAs are specific for systemic vasculitides affecting small-to-medium-sized vessels and exhibiting few vascular immune deposits. Indeed, ANCAs may participate in the pathogenesis of these small-vessel vasculitides [9]. The three ANCA-associated vasculitides (AAV) are Wegener's granulomatosis, MPA, and Churg–Strauss syndrome. PR3-ANCAs are strongly associated with Wegener's granulomatosis, while MPO-ANCAs occur most commonly in MPA and Churg–Strauss syndrome.

To address some of these failings, vasculitis experts developed new consensus methodology for classification of Wegener's granulomatosis, Churg–Strauss syndrome, MPA, and PAN in 2007 that utilized ACR criteria, CHCC1994 definitions, and ANCAs [10].

The 2012 Revised International CHCC (CHCC2012) convened to improve nomenclature for previously defined vasculitides and to add categories of vasculitis not included in CHCC1994 (Fig. 24.1) [11]. Eponyms were eliminated except for disorders with ill-defined pathogeneses. The nomenclature addresses only the noninfectious vasculitides, which are categorized by integrating knowledge about etiology, pathogenesis, pathology, demographics, and clinical markers. The first level of categorization is size of *predominantly* involved vessels. The "large-vessel vasculitides" are GCA and Takayasu arteritis. They sometimes also affect small- and medium-sized vessels. "Medium-vessel vasculitides" comprise PAN and Kawasaki disease. They affect small and medium-sized arteries but *not* the microvasculature. "Small-vessel vasculitides" primarily affect small arteries, arterioles, capillaries, and venules, but medium arteries and veins are also sometimes involved. In this nomenclature, large vessels are the aorta, vena cavae, and their major branches; medium vessels comprise the main visceral arteries and veins and their initial branches; and small vessels consist of the intraparenchymal vessels. The small-vessel vasculitides are divided into those associated with sparse versus prominent vascular wall deposits of immunoglobulin and complement. The "pauci-immune" disorders are the AAV with Wegener's granulomatosis renamed granulomatosis with polyangiitis (GPA) and Churg–Straus syndrome renamed eosinophilic granulomatosis with polyangitis (EGPA). Patients matching these definitions but lacking ANCAs are diagnosed with "ANCA-negative AAV." The "immune complex small-vessel vasculitides" exhibit "moderate-to-marked" immune deposits in small vessels. They include anti-glomerular basement disease (Goodpasture syndrome), cryoglobulinemic vasculitis, IgA vasculitis (Henoch–Schönlein purpura), and hypocomplementemic urticarial vasculitis (HUV). The "variable-vessel vasculitides" are Behçet disease and

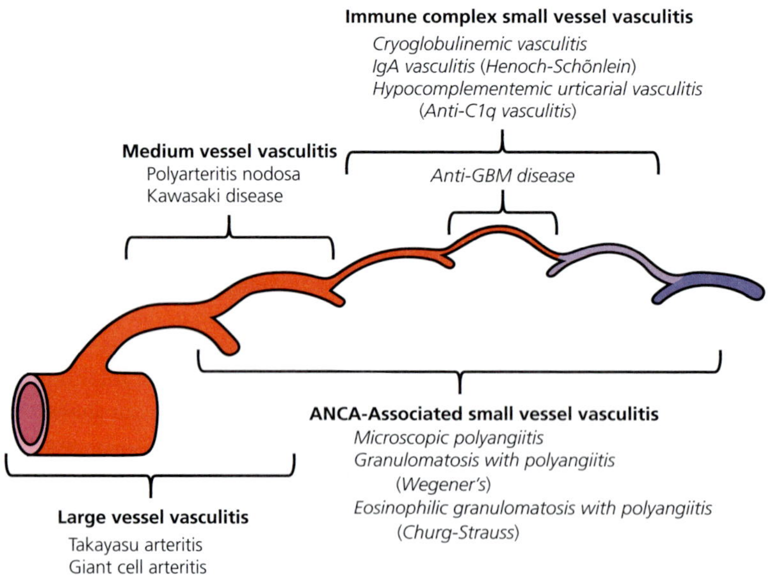

Figure 24.1 2012 Revised International Chapel Hill Consensus Conference Nomenclature of Vasculitides. Source: Jennette *et al.*, 2013. Reproduced with permission of Wiley.

Cogan syndrome. They affect vessels of all sizes and types non-preferentially. "Single-organ vasculitis" affects vessels of any type in a single organ/tissue with no signs of an underlying systemic vasculitis. NSVN should be categorized in this group. The many secondary causes of vasculitis are subsumed under "vasculitis associated with systemic disease" (e.g., rheumatoid arthritis, lupus) and "vasculitis associated with a probable etiology" (e.g., drug-associated, hepatitis B-associated PAN, hepatitis C-associated cryoglobulinemic vasculitis, and cancer-associated vasculitis).

Classification of vasculitides associated with neuropathy

Systemic vasculitic neuropathies (SVNs) occur most commonly in vasculitides affecting small arteries or large arterioles. Primary systemic vasculitides most likely to produce a neuropathy are EGPA, PAN, and MPA [12–14]. Of the secondary systemic vasculitides, nerves are most commonly affected in hepatitis B virus (HBV)-associated PAN, hepatitis C virus (HCV)-related cryoglobulinemic vasculitis, and rheumatoid vasculitis [13, 15, 16]. Neuropathies are uncommon in GCA, unreported in Takayasu arteritis and Kawasaki disease, and rare in Behçet disease, Cogan syndrome, and non-cryoglobulinemic immune complex small-vessel vasculitides. Based on these observations, a 2010 Peripheral Nerve Society task force derived a consensus classification for vasculitides associated with neuropathy (Table 24.1) [17].

Vasculitic neuropathies can also be divided into two groups based on the size of predominantly involved vessels: nerve large arteriole vasculitis and nerve microvasculitis [18]. All vessels in peripheral nerves are, by definition, "small vessels." Microvessels are venules, capillaries, and small arterioles (diameters <40 μm) [18]. Larger arterioles have diameters up to 100 μm. Arterial vessels with diameters >100 μm are referred to as small arteries. All endoneurial and perineurial vessels are microscopic, whereas most epineurial vessels are larger in size (50–300 μm) [19]. The nerve large arteriole vasculitides demonstrate primary involvement of small epineurial arteries/veins and large arterioles/venules combined with variable involvement of microvessels (Fig. 24.2). This group includes most of the SVNs [3, 19–23]. NSVN tends to involve smaller vessels (<100 μm) within this range but is not limited to microvessels [22, 24]. In accordance with CHCC2012, the systemic vasculitides causing nerve large arteriole vasculitis may be further divided into small vessel-predominant vasculitic neuropathy (e.g., MPA, EGPA), medium vessel-predominant vasculitic neuropathy (e.g., PAN), and large vessel-predominant vasculitic neuropathy (e.g., GCA), with the understanding that medium/large-vessel vasculitides can also affect small arteries and large arterioles.

The pathologic definition of "microvasculitis" varies between investigators. Some require only infiltration of microvessels by lymphocytic-predominant inflammatory cells without associated vascular damage ("lymphocytic" microvasculitis) [23, 25, 26]. However, PNS microvasculitis without vascular damage is a nonspecific alteration having only a weak association with clinicopathologic surrogates of vasculitic neuropathy [17]. It has been reported in such non-vasculitic disorders as chronic inflammatory demyelinating polyneuropathy, paraneoplastic, and Sjogren's-related sensory neuronopathy, motor neuron disease, Buerger's disease, diabetic polyneuropathy, infectious neuropathies, cholesterol emboli syndrome, coeliac disease, and multiple entrapments [17, 19, 25, 27]. For these reasons, the diagnosis of microvasculitis should be reserved for cases with vascular damage. To enhance identification of microvascular injury, nerve biopsies can be immunostained with antibodies against human smooth-muscle actin, assessing for fragmentation, loss, or destruction of vascular smooth muscle cells (Fig. 24.3) [18]. Nerve microvasculitis can occur in NSVN, Sjogren's syndrome, some virus-associated vasculitic neuropathies (e.g., HIV), diabetic radiculoplexus neuropathy (RPN), and non-diabetic RPN (clinical variant of NSVN) [18, 28, 29]. Nerve microvasculitis tends to correlate with nonsystemic or localized clinical features, whereas nerve large arteriole vasculitis associates more commonly with systemic vasculitides with other-organ involvement.

Epidemiology

Systemic vasculitides are uncommon diseases having an annual incidence of ~140 cases per million adults [30]. GCA and the predominantly cutaneous vasculitides are most common, followed by rheumatoid vasculitis, GPA, and MPA. For the primary vasculitides most routinely associated with neuropathy – MPA, PAN, EGPA, and GPA – the annual incidence rate is ~10–20 cases/million [31]. No study has determined the incidence or prevalence of any vasculitic neuropathy, but the *relative*

Table 24.1 Classification of vasculitides associated with neuropathy.

I Primary systemic vasculitides
1 Predominantly small vessel vasculitis
(a) Microscopic polyangiitis*
(b) Eosinophilic granulomatosis with polyangiitis (Churg–Strauss syndrome)*
(c) Granulomatosis with polyangiitis (Wegener's granulomatosis)*
(d) Essential mixed cryoglobulinemia (non-HCV)
(e) IgA vasculitis (Henoch–Schönlein purpura)
(f) Hypocomplementemic urticarial (anti-C1q) vasculitis
2 Predominantly medium vessel vasculitis
(a) Polyarteritis nodosa
3 Predominantly large vessel vasculitis
(a) Giant cell arteritis
II Secondary systemic vasculitides associated with one of the following
1 Connective tissue diseases
(a) Rheumatoid arthritis
(b) Systemic lupus erythematosus
(c) Sjogren's syndrome
(d) Systemic sclerosis
(e) Dermatomyositis
(f) Mixed connective tissue disease
2 Sarcoidosis
3 Behcet's disease
4 Cogan's syndrome
5 Infection (such as HBV, HCV, HIV, CMV, leprosy, Lyme disease, HTLV-I)
6 Drugs
7 Malignancy
8 Inflammatory bowel disease
III Nonsystemic/localized vasculitis
1 Nonsystemic vasculitic neuropathy
(a) Includes non-diabetic radiculoplexus neuropathy
(b) Includes some cases of Wartenberg's migrant sensory neuritis
2 Diabetic radiculoplexus neuropathy
3 Localized cutaneous/neuropathic vasculitis
(a) Cutaneous polyarteritis nodosa
(b) Others

*Anti-neutrophil cytoplasmic antibody (ANCA)-associated vasculitides

CMV = cytomegalovirus; HBV = hepatitis B virus; HCV = hepatitis C virus; HIV = human immunodeficiency virus; HTLV = human T-lymphotropic virus.

Source: Collins *et al.*, 2010. Reproduced with permission from Wiley.

frequency of these disorders can be derived from nerve biopsy series [26, 32]. The commonest vasculitic neuropathies in these series are NSVN and those associated with PAN, MPA, rheumatoid arthritis, and EGPA. In the primary small-to-medium-vessel systemic vasculitides, vasculitic neuropathy is not a risk factor for death or relapse, but it does reduce quality of life [33–35].

Vasculitic neuropathy can develop at any age but most commonly occurs in the sixth to eighth decades. The mean age at onset of a SVN ranges from 52–67 years in various series [3, 15, 21, 22, 36, 37]. For NSVN, age at diagnosis ranges from 13–88 years, with a mean of 59.5 and median of 63 years [26, 32, 37–39]. For systemic vasculitides, men are more frequently affected than women in PAN, MPA, rheumatoid vasculitis, and IgA vasculitis, while women are preferentially affected in GCA, lupus vasculitis, and cryoglobulinemic vasculitis. There is no significant association with gender for GPA and EGPA [1, 40]. For NSVN, reported women outnumber men by 5:4 [26, 32, 37–39].

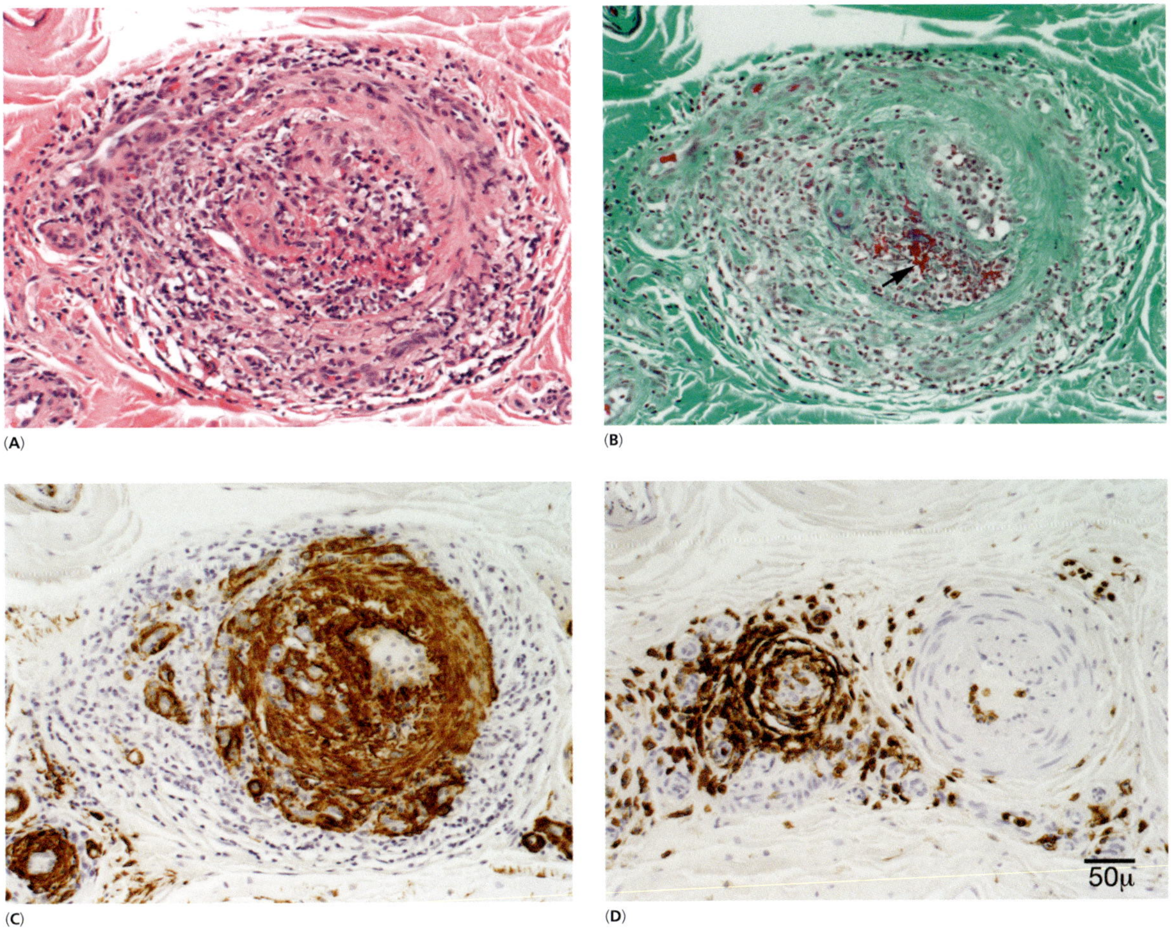

Figure 24.2 Serial paraffin-embedded cross sections of a sural nerve biopsy imaged at high power (original magnification 40×) in a patient with systemic vasculitis showing necrotizing vasculitis with fibrinoid necrosis (arrow) in a large arteriole/small artery. (**A**) is stained with H&E, (**B**) with Masson trichrome, (**C**) with anti-human smooth muscle actin primary antibodies, and (**D**) with anti-CD45 (leukocyte common antigen) primary antibodies.

Clinical features

Clinical presentation

The clinical presentation of PNS vasculitis depends on the distribution of affected nerves, disease severity, and spectrum of systemic involvement [3, 15, 17, 20–22, 26, 36–38, 41–46]. Signs and symptoms of multi-organ dysfunction are indicative of a systemic vasculitis or underlying CTD. Skin and mucous membranes are the most commonly affected non-PNS tissues in SVN [47]. By definition, NSVN is not accompanied by clinical evidence of extra-neurologic involvement. Constitutional symptoms such as fevers, weight loss, fatigue, and arthralgias occur in 70% of patients with SVN and 30% of NSVN [17].

Vasculitic neuropathy has a characteristic clinical picture whether occurring alone or as one feature of a systemic vasculitis, but SVNs tend to be more severe than NSVN [22]. While symptoms usually develop over several weeks to months, some patients present fulminantly, mimicking Guillain–Barre syndrome, and others follow an indolent course over several years prior to diagnosis [48, 49]. Median delay from onset to diagnosis ranges from 2–8 months in most series [21, 22, 37, 41–43]. Most patients experience one or more acute attacks, but one-third of them have a slowly progressive

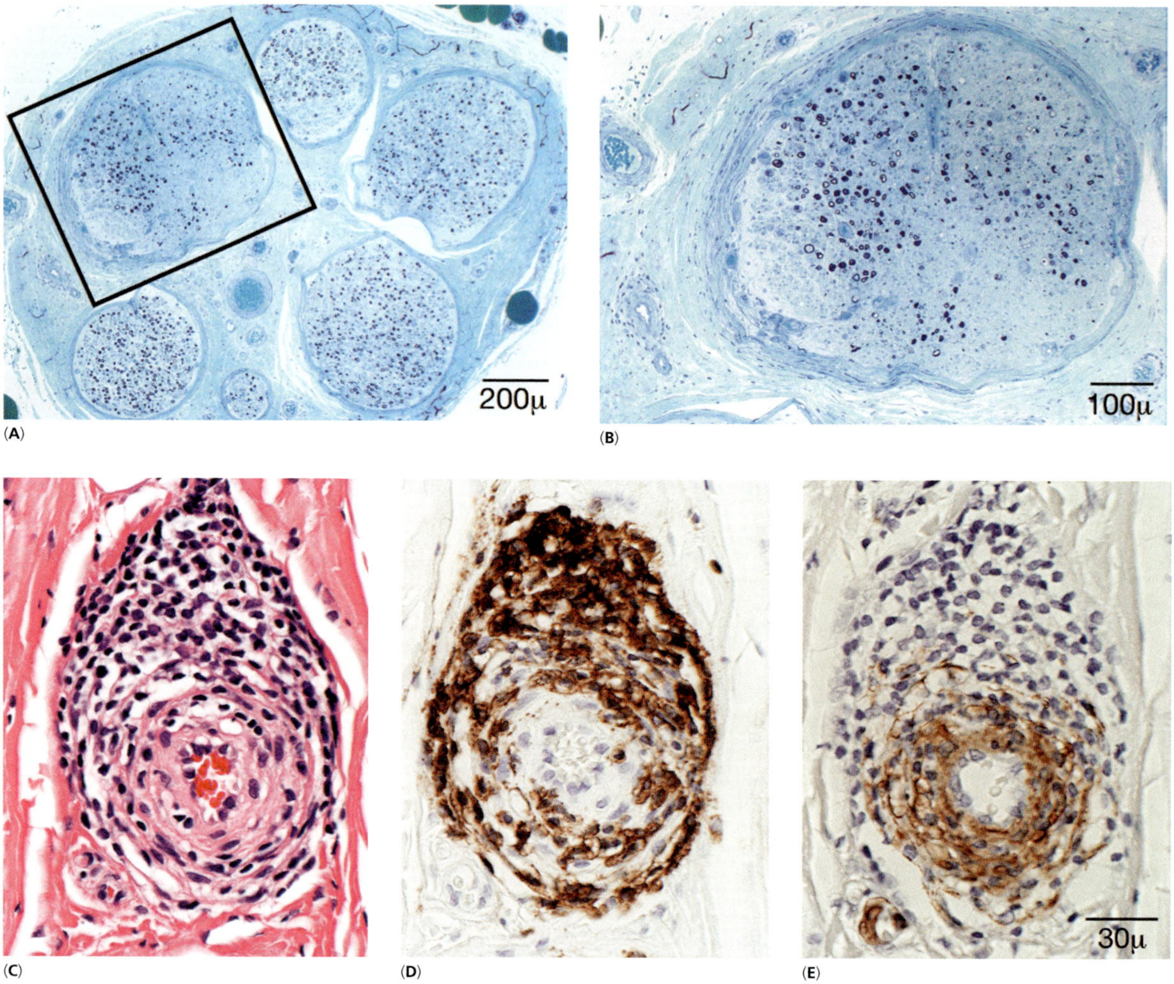

Figure 24.3 Sural nerve biopsy in patient with diabetic radiculoplexus neuropathy showing ischemic injury and definite microvasculitis. (**A**) is low power epoxy resin-embedded section stained with methylene blue demonstrating patchy/multifocal fiber loss. (**B**) is high power view of same process. (**C–E**) are serial paraffin-embedded cross sections imaged at high power showing microvasculitis (**C** is stained with H&E, **D** with anti-CD45 primary antibodies, and **E** with anti-human smooth muscle actin primary antibodies). Part (**E**) shows vessel wall fragmentation consistent with definite microvasculitis.

course from onset. PNS vasculitis exhibits three patterns of clinical involvement. The commonest (frequency 45%) and most distinctive is a *multiple mononeuropathy* (*multifocal neuropathy*), wherein patients develop pain, weakness, and/or sensory loss in the distribution of a single peripheral nerve, followed by stepwise involvement of other nerves. Although distinctive, this pattern is not pathognomonic for vasculitis. In other patients, individual mononeuropathies overlap, yielding an *asymmetric polyneuropathy* (frequency 35%). The least common and least specific pattern is a *distal, symmetric polyneuropathy* (frequency 20%). The symmetric phenotype is rare if minor asymmetries are not discounted [17]. Certain nerves are preferentially affected due to poor collateral or nutrient vessel supply. The most frequently affected individual nerve is the common peroneal or peroneal division of the distal sciatic nerve [3, 37, 43, 46]. In the arms, the ulnar nerve is most commonly involved. Neurological deficits are distally accentuated, but proximal involvement is not uncommon [43]. Cranial neuropathies occur in 10% of patients [22, 37, 43]. Most patients develop mixed sensory and motor deficits, but 15% have predominantly sensory symptoms [50]. Sensory dysfunction usually involves all modalities, but rare patients exhibit small fiber predominance [37]. Pure motor or autonomic presentations are exceptional. Eighty percent of vasculitic neuropathies are painful [17].

Laboratory evaluation

Evaluation of a patient with suspected vasculitic neuropathy requires laboratory tests, electrodiagnostic studies, and nerve or nerve/muscle biopsy in most cases. Laboratory workup assesses extra-neurologic involvement, markers of inflammation, and causes of multifocal or vasculitic neuropathy (Table 24.2). Laboratory studies predictive of biopsy-confirmed vasculitic neuropathy include decreased complement and elevated erythrocyte sedimentation rate (ESR), C-reactive protein, rheumatoid factor (RF), β2-microglobulin, MPO-ANCAs, and plasma vascular endothelial growth factor [17]. In NSVN, mildly to moderately elevated ESR occurs in 50% of patients, but severe elevation (≥100 mm/hour) suggests a systemic condition [17]. Other markers of inflammation or immune activation are less frequently abnormal: antinuclear antibodies (ANAs) 25%, anemia 20%, leukocytosis 15%, and RFs/hypocomplementemia < 10% [26, 32, 38]. ANCAs are rare and, if present, exclude the diagnosis [17]. In SVN, laboratory abnormalities are more common: elevated ESR 85%, leukocytosis 75%, anemia 45–50%, RFs 45%, hypocomplementemia 30%, and ANAs 30% [50]. CSF pleocytosis is uncommon (5%) in both SVN and NSVN. Mild to moderate CSF protein elevation occurs in only 30% of patients overall but is commoner in the proximal lower limb variant of NSVN, known as non-diabetic RPN [29, 50].

Electrodiagnostic studies are essential for identifying non-length-dependent features of the neuropathy, excluding a primary demyelinating disorder, and assisting with the selection of which nerve to biopsy [17, 51, 52]. Findings reflect the underlying pathology: multifocal axonal damage to motor and sensory fibers. Nerve conduction studies reveal low-amplitude or non-reproducible compound sensory nerve and muscle action potentials. Conduction velocities are normal or mildly reduced and distal latencies normal or mildly prolonged. H reflexes and F waves are often impersistent with normal or mildly prolonged latencies. "Pseudo" conduction blocks occur in some patients, resulting from acute Wallerian-like degeneration [53]. Needle EMG examination reveals fibrillation potentials in most patients, decreased recruitment in clinically weak muscles, and motor unit potential remodeling consistent with chronic reinnervation in those with sufficiently longstanding disease or pre-existing neurogenic disorders. A predominance of *demyelinating* features suggests an alternate diagnosis.

Types of vasculitic neuropathy

The *primary small-to-medium-vessel systemic vasculitides* are potentially life-threatening diseases characterized by vasculitic involvement of multiple organs [1, 11, 54]. They include PAN, MPA, EGPA, GPA, IgA vasculitis, anti-glomerular basement membrane disease, and HUV. Each disorder has distinguishing pathologic, laboratory, and clinical features (Table 24.3). AAV share a predilection for small vessels, paucity of immune deposits in vascular lesions, and potential for rapidly progressive glomerulonephritis and pulmonary capillaritis. Neuropathies occur in 60–70% of patients with PAN and EGPA [13, 14, 45, 55, 56]. The reported incidence of neuropathy in MPA is highly variable but averages ~45% in recent series [12, 57, 58]. In GPA, neuropathies are less common, occurring in 20–25% of patients [59–61], but cranial neuropathies are more common and develop in 15% [47, 58, 60]. Neuropathies are rare or unreported in IgA vasculitis, HUV, and anti-glomerular basement membrane disease.

The only *primary large-vessel vasculitis* associated with vasculitic neuropathy is GCA, a granulomatous vasculitis that primarily affects branches of the aortic arch and extracranial carotid arteries (Table 24.3) [62]. Focal/multifocal neuropathies suspicious for vasculitis occur in 6% of patients, most commonly involving the median nerve, C5/6 nerve roots, or upper brachial plexus [63–65].

Secondary systemic vasculitides are caused by infections, drugs, and diseases predisposing to autoimmune phenomena, such as CTDs, cryoglobulinemia, sarcoidosis, inflammatory bowel diseases, and cancers [11]. Vasculitic neuropathies are estimated to occur in ~10% of patients with rheumatoid arthritis, 3–4% of those with Sjogren's syndrome, 2–3% of patients with systemic lupus erythematosus, and <1% of patients with systemic sclerosis [50]. Virtually any infection can act as an antigenic stimulus to induce circulating immune complexes, immune responses directed against vascular autoantigens via

Table 24.2 Differential diagnosis of multifocal/asymmetric neuropathy.

A Ischemic neuropathies

1 Peripheral nerve vasculitis (see Table 24.1)
2 Livedoid vasculopathy
3 Sickle cell anemia
4 Cholesterol emboli syndrome
5 Atrial myxoma
6 Thrombophilic states

B Inflammatory/immune-mediated neuropathies

1 Sarcoidosis*
2 Multifocal acquired demyelinating motor and sensory neuropathy (Lewis–Sumner syndrome)
3 Multifocal motor neuropathy
4 Multifocal variants of Guillain–Barre syndrome
5 Neuralgic amyotrophy
6 Neuropathy with eosinophilic disorders*
7 Neuropathy with gastrointestinal disorders (Crohn's disease, ulcerative colitis, celiac sprue)*
8 Chronic graft versus host disease
9 Sensory perineuritis*

*C Infectious/toxic neuropathies**

1 Leprosy
2 Lyme disease
3 Viral (hepatitis C virus, hepatitis B virus, human immunodeficiency virus, human T cell lymphotropic virus type I, varicella zoster virus, cytomegalovirus, parvovirus B19, Epstein–Barr virus, West Nile virus, measles)
4 Other (infective endocarditis, leptospirosis, tuberculosis, sporotrichosis, meningococcus, group A β-hemolytic streptococcus, hepatitis A, *Mycoplasma pneumonia, Salmonella typhi, Pseudomonas aeruginosa*, trichinosis, ascaris, *Plasmodium falciparum*, scrub typhus, *Coxiella burnetii*, relapsing fever, *Trypanosoma cruzi*)

*D Drug-induced neuropathies**

1 Montelukast and other leukotriene receptor antagonists
2 Interferon-α
3 Tumor necrosis factor-α inhibitors
4 Antibiotics (penicillin, sulfonamides, minocycline)
5 Leflunomide
6 Drugs of abuse (amphetamines, cocaine, heroin)
7 Other (cromolyn, cimetidine, thiouracil, benzylthiouracil, allopurinol, amantidine, naproxen, piroxicam, valacyclovir, mesalazine, rituximab, masitinib, gasoline sniffing)

E Genetic neuropathies

1 Hereditary neuropathy with liability to pressure palsies
2 Hereditary neuralgic amyotrophy
3 Charcot–Marie–Tooth neuropathies (many)
4 Porphyria
5 Familial amyloid polyneuropathy
6 Tangier disease
7 Krabbe disease
8 Mitochondrial disorders

F Mechanical neuropathies

1 Multiple peripheral nerve injuries or burns
2 Multiple entrapment neuropathies
3 Wartenberg's migrant sensory neuritis (mechanical cases)

G Neuropathies related to neoplastic disease

1 Direct infiltration of nerves by tumor
2 Paraneoplastic (vasculitic and non-vasculitic)*
3 Multifocal peripheral nerve tumors with external/internal compression

(continued)

Table 24.2 *Continued*

4 Neurofibromatosis 2 (Schwann cell proliferation/dysfunction)
5 Lymphomatoid granulomatosis*
6 Intravascular large B cell lymphoma
7 Neoplastic meningitis
8 Primary AL amyloidosis
H *Intraneural hemorrhage*
1 Idiopathic thrombocytopenic purpura
2 Acute leukemia
3 Hemophilia
I *Degenerative disorders*
1 Motor neuron disease with sensory involvement

*Conditions occasionally or routinely associated with vasculitis

molecular mimicry, or altered immunoregulation with ensuing vasculitis [66, 67]. Organisms known to cause vasculitic neuropathy by direct infection of endothelial cells include cytomegalovirus (CMV) and varicella zoster virus [68, 69]. Viruses with persistent replication such as HBV, HCV, HIV, and parvovirus B19 have the strongest association with vasculitic neuropathies [66, 67, 70, 71]. In HBV-associated PAN, immune complex deposition appears to be the primary mechanism [66, 67]. Clinical features are similar to those in idiopathic PAN, but neuropathies occur in 85% of patients [13]. Chronic HCV infection can produce a cryoglobulinemic vasculitis [16, 72]. Mixed cryoglobulinemia occurs in 50% of patients with chronic HCV infection, but only 15% develop symptomatic disease [73]. The incidence of polyneuropathy in chronic hepatitis C is ~10%, but in patients with HCV-related cryoglobulinemic vasculitis, ~65% develop a clinically-defined neuropathy [73].

The only *single-organ vasculitides* involving the PNS are NSVN and diabetic RPN [3, 22, 24, 26, 28, 37, 41, 43]. A Peripheral Nerve Society guideline includes consensus diagnostic criteria for NSVN [17]. Patients are first required to have pathologically definite or clinically probable vasculitic neuropathy. Systemic features such as evidence of other-organ involvement, visceral aneurysms, ANCAs, ESR ≥ 100 mm/hour, cryoglobulins, pathologic evidence of vasculitis in non-neuromuscular tissues, or infection/medical condition/drug predisposing to vasculitis exclude the diagnosis. Constitutional symptoms, diabetes mellitus, and muscle vasculitis do not exclude NSVN.

Diabetic lumbosacral (LS) RPN is a unique syndrome that affects patients with type 2 diabetes mellitus in middle-to-old age, more commonly men than women [28]. The disorder bears no relationship to duration of diabetes, severity of glycemic dysregulation, or such diabetic complications as retinopathy and nephropathy. It usually starts with acute pain in the hip/thigh, and weakness emerges days to weeks later. Lower limb involvement is more commonly proximal than distal, but symptoms generally spread to other segments of the same limb. Clinical deficits tend to affect multiple leg, thigh, and pelvic nerves. Pain and weakness usually begin unilaterally and spread contralaterally in 80–90%. Most patients lose weight and develop autonomic symptoms. The syndrome is frequently accompanied by a thoracic radiculopathy (chest or abdominal wall pain and weakness). Upper limb involvement occurs in ~10%. Laboratory workup reveals elevated spinal fluid protein in 85%. Symptoms typically progress over several weeks/months and then slowly improve over 1–2 years, but 10–15% of patients relapse. Recovery is usually incomplete. Foot drop is the most common long-term sequel. Nerve biopsies reveal lymphocytic perivascular inflammation predominantly involving epineurial microvessels, occasional microvasculitis, and other changes suggestive of vasculitis (see next). An analogous syndrome is non-diabetic LSRPN, a proximally accentuated subtype of NSVN [29]. A painless form of diabetic RPN is also described characterized by slower progression, increased symmetry, greater upper limb involvement (75%), and distal predominance (55%) [74]. Upper limb involvement in painful LS diabetic RPN has been recognized for years, but a less common cervical variant of diabetic RPN manifesting with pure, predominant, or initial upper limb symptoms was recently highlighted [75]. All of the diabetic radiculoneuropathies appear to be microvasculitides [18].

Table 24.3 Clinical and pathologic features of primary vasculitides associated with neuropathy.

Disorder	Histopathology	Vessels affected	Other clinically involved organs (%)	Laboratory studies (%)	PNS, CNS changes
Polyarteritis nodosa	Necrotizing vasculitis; mixed infiltrate; sparse immune deposits	Small & medium arteries	Skin 55–60 Joints ~50 Kidneys 40–50 GI ~30 Testes 2–29 Heart 10–15 ENT – rare Lungs – rare	↑ESR ~85 ↑WBC ~70 ↓Hgb ~60 ↑Platelets ~60 RF ~30 Hep B 20–30 ↓Comp ~25 ANA ~15 Hep C 5–10 ANCA <10 Angio + 70 (aneurysm)	PNS 65–70 CrN <5 CNS ~5
Microscopic polyangiitis	Necrotizing vasculitis; mixed infiltrate; sparse immune deposits; LCV in skin	Arterioles, capillaries, venules, veins > small & medium arteries	Kidney 75–90 Joints 40–60 Skin 30–60 Lungs 35–50 GI 30–40 ENT 20–30 Heart 10–20 Testes – rare	↑ESR >90 ANCA 75–85 (MPO > PR3) RF 25–50 ANA 20–30 ↓Comp - rare Hep B/C (-) Angio - rare	PNS 40–50 CNS 10–15
Granulomatosis with polyangiitis (Wegener's granulomatosis)	Necrotizing vasculitis; granulomas; collagen necrosis; sparse immune deposits; LCV in skin	Small & medium arteries, arterioles, capillaries, venules, veins	ENT 90–95 Lungs 65–85 Kidney 60–75 Eyes 50–60 Skin 25–50 Joints 65–75 Heart 5–20 GI 5–10	ANCA 80–90 (PR3 > MPO) ↑ESR ~85 ↓Hgb ~75 ↑ Platelets 55 RF 50–60 ↑WBC ~35 ANA ~25	PNS 20–25 CNS 5–10 CrN 15
Eosinophilic granulomatosis with polyangiitis (Churg–Strauss syndrome)	Necrotizing vasculitis; mixed infiltrate with eosinophils; granulomas; sparse immune deposits; LCV in skin	Small & medium arteries, arterioles, capillaries, venules, veins	Lungs 100 (asthma) 40–75 (infiltrates) ENT (sinusitis, rhinitis) 60–80 Skin 50–70 GI 35–50 Joints 30–50 Heart 30–50 60 by MRI Kidney 15–30	↑Eos 100 ↑ESR ~85 ↑IgE ~75 ANCA 30–40 (MPO > PR3) RF 40–50 ANA ~10 ↓Comp – rare Hep B/C (-) Angio + 30	PNS 65 CrN <5 CNS 10–15

			GN ~40 children ~70 adults Testes ~15 Lungs – rare	↑ASO 20–50 Cryos 20–25 ↓Comp 10–20 ↓Hgb 5–15 RF ~5 ANA ~5 ANCA <5	
Cryoglobulinemic vasculitis	Necrotizing vasculitis; endoenurial microangiopathy; non-IgA immune deposits; LCV in skin	Small arteries, arterioles, capillaries, venules	Skin ~95 Joints 70–90 GN ~30 Salivary glands (sicca) ~30 Raynaud's 25–50 GI (pain) 10–20	Hep C 80–90 ↓Comp 70–90 RF 70–90 ↑ESR ~70 ↓Hgb ~70 ANA ~55 Hep B ~5 ANCA <5 Angio – infreq	PNS ~65 CNS - rare
Giant cell arteritis	Necrotizing vasculitis; mononuclear infiltrate; granulomas & giant cells ~50%	Medium-large arteries	PMR ~50 Liver ~30 (abnormal LFTs) Aorta 15–20 GN ~10 UE large vessel 6–8 LE large vessel 2–7	↑CRP 98–100 ↑ESR 85–100 ↓Hgb 55–60 ↑WBC 20–30 ANCA - rare RF (-) ANA (-)	Otologic 60–90 Optic nerve 15–20 PNS ~5 CNS ~5
Hypocomplementemic uricarial (C1q) vasculitis	LCV in skin and nerves; non-IgA immune deposits	Arterioles, capillaries, venules	Skin 100 Joints 50–75 Angioedema 50 Lungs 20–50 GN 10–50 Eyes 30 GI (pain) 20–30 Heart <5 Myositis – rare	C1q-Ab ~100 ↓ Comp ~100 ↑ESR 60–75 ANA ~50 RF ~10 dsDNA Ab<5 ANCA (-)	PNS - rare CNS - rare
Nonsystemic vasculitic neuropathy	Necrotizing vasculitis in epineurium/perineurium >>endoneurium; mononuclear infiltrate; immune deposits	Small arteries, arterioles, capillaries, venules	Muscle 25	↑ESR ~50 ANA ~25 ↓Hgb ~20 ↑WBC ~15 RF ~10 ↓Comp ~5	PNS 100 CNS 0

Ab = antibodies; ANCA = antineutrophil cytoplasmic antibodies; angio = abdominal angiographically-demonstrated microaneurysms; CNS = central nervous system; comp = circulating complement factors; CrN = cranial nerve involvement; cryos = cryoglobulins; dsDNA = double stranded DNA; ENT = upper respiratory tract involvement; GI = gastrointestinal involvement; GN = glomerulonephritis; Hep B = hepatitis B surface antigenemia; Hep C = hepatitis C antibodies cr RNA; Hgb = hemoglobin; LCV = leukocytoclastic vasculitis; LE large vessel = involvement of lower extremity large vessels (superficial femoral-popliteal); LFTs = liver function tests; MPO = myeloperoxidase; PMR = polymyalgia rheumatica; PNS = peripheral nervous system; PR3 = proteinase 3; RF = rheumatoid factor; UE large vessel = involvement of upper extremity large vessels (subclavian-axillary-brachia); WBC = white blood cell count

Pathology

Nerve pathologic findings

Almost all pathologic studies of SVN and NSVN have revealed changes indicative of a primary axonal process [19]. Axons are more vulnerable to ischemia than Schwann cells, fibroblasts, and perineurial cells. Affected fascicles show decreased myelinated nerve fiber density, prominent Wallerian-like degeneration, regenerating axonal clusters, and inconspicuous demyelination/remyelination. The mean percentage of teased nerve fibers undergoing axonal degeneration in vasculitic neuropathy series ranges from 60–80% (Fig. 24.4) [15, 21, 22, 36, 41, 76]. Segmental demyelination/remyelination tends to cluster on individual teased fibers, consistent with secondary demyelination induced by axonal atrophy [77]. These fibers predominate at margins of the ischemic core. Some studies have reported preferential involvement of larger myelinated nerve fibers [76], while others have not [22]. In fulminant vasculitis, all cellular elements are lost. Axon loss tends to be centrofascicular in proximal watershed areas (e.g., sciatic nerve bifurcation in distal thigh) but becomes multifocal in distal parts of the nerve due to intermingling of descending fibers (Fig. 24.5) [78–80].

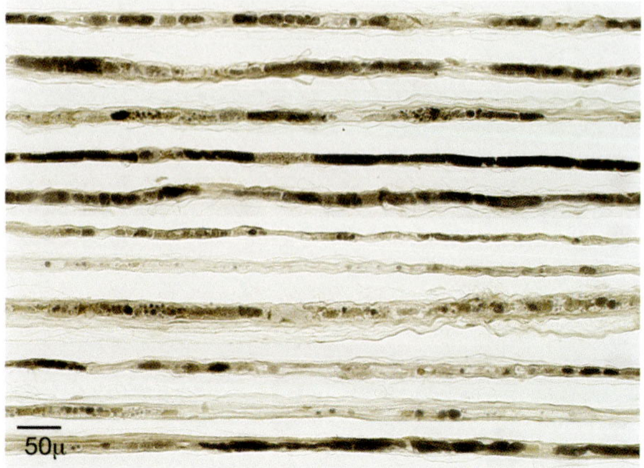

Figure 24.4 Teased nerve fibers showing abundant early axonal degeneration in vasculitic neuropathy (fixed in glutaraldehyde and osmicated).

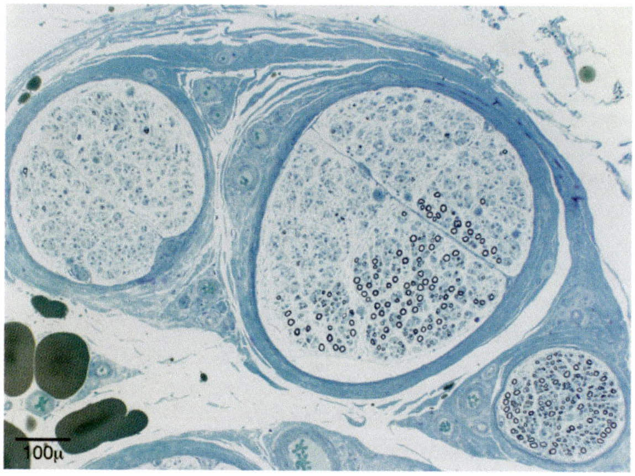

Figure 24.5 Low power view of epoxy resin-embedded cross section of sural nerve biopsy showing interfascicular and intrafascicular multifocal fiber loss (methylene blue stain).

Cellular infiltrates in cutaneous nerve biopsies in vasculitic neuropathy are perivascular and predominate in the epineurium. They consist primarily of T cells and macrophages, with T cells generally outnumbering macrophages by a factor of 2–3 [22, 36, 81, 82]. B cells are uncommon (2–3% of cells), and natural killer cells and polymorphonuclear leukocytes rare. Epineurial T cells are almost always CD4+ or CD8+ with varying CD4+/CD8+ ratios [22, 81, 83, 84]. There are no published immunohistochemical studies of plasma, dendritic, or T-regulatory cells. The vasculitic lesions are almost always located in the epineurium. Active vasculitic lesions are characterized by T cells and macrophages surrounding and invading vessel walls, with associated necrosis and other signs of vascular damage (Fig. 24.2). Direct IF shows deposits of IgM, fibrinogen, C3, and/or C5b-9 in epineurial vessel walls in up to 80% of patients (Fig. 24.6) [21, 41, 81, 85].

Endoneurial microvasculitis is rarely reported in EPGA, infections (e.g., HIV and CMV), CTDs (e.g., lupus and Sjogren's syndrome), cryoglobulinemic vasculitis, and diabetic RPN (Fig. 24.7) [19, 68, 73, 86, 87]. It might also occur in rare cases of MPA, GPA, IgA vasculitis, and paraneoplastic/drug-induced small-vessel vasculitis, but pathologic proof is lacking.

An investigation of the distribution of nerve pathology and vasculitis in sciatic/tibial and median nerves in autopsied cases of MPA-associated vasculitic neuropathy revealed no vasculitis in the spinal cord, lumbar dorsal root ganglia, lower thoracic sympathetic ganglia, and ventral/dorsal roots [80]. Instead, vasculitis was distributed in the epineurium throughout proximal and distal segments of the nerves. Medium-sized nutrient arteries were also affected. Myelinated fiber loss commenced in the middle nerve segments, corresponding to

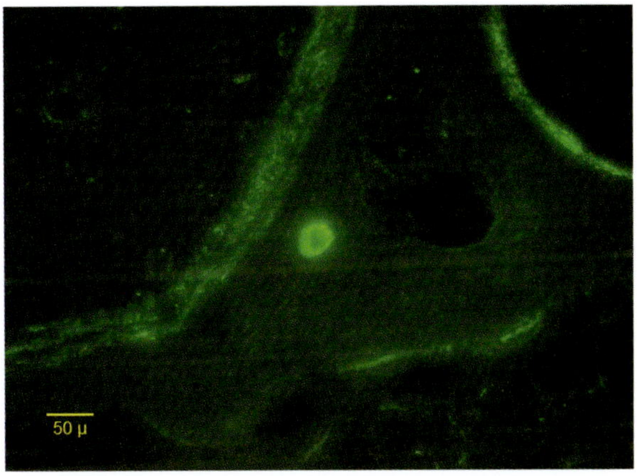

Figure 24.6 Fresh frozen cross section of superficial peroneal nerve in a patient with probable sarcoidosis-related vasculitic neuropathy showing intense deposition of complement terminal membrane attack complex in wall of a small epineurial vessel (indirect immunofluorescence with primary anti-C5b9 antibody, imaged with AlexaFluor488). The staining of the perineurium of three adjacent fascicles is a normal finding.

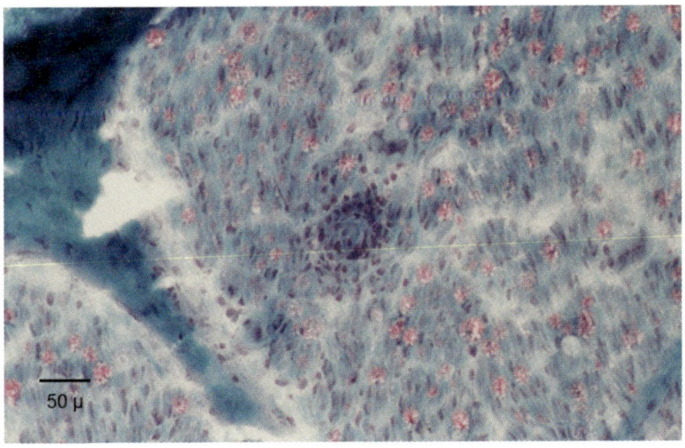

Figure 24.7 Fresh-frozen cross section of superficial peroneal nerve biopsy in patient with Sjogren's syndrome-related vasculitic neuropathy showing necrotizing vasculitis of an endoneurial microvessel (modified Gomori trichrome stain).

the distal arm and distal thigh. Likewise, the ischemic pattern of centrofascicular degeneration occurred only in proximal and middle nerve segments, while diffuse nerve loss predominated distally. In teased nerve fibers, axonal degeneration predominated in distal sections, while myelin wrinkling and mild demyelination/remyelination predominated proximally. These findings confirmed those in a prior autopsy study of rheumatoid vasculitis [79]. Systemic vasculitis tends to affect peripheral nerves diffusely but produces maximal damage in a borderzone vulnerable to ischemia in the proximal/middle portions of extremity nerves.

Diagnostic criteria

The Peripheral Nerve Society guideline on NSVN includes consensus diagnostic criteria for pathologically definite and probable vasculitic neuropathy (Tables 24.4, 24.5) [17]. A histologic diagnosis of *definite* vasculitic neuropathy requires inflammation within the vessel wall *and* signs of active or chronic vascular damage (Fig. 24.2). Perivascular or mural inflammation alone is nonspecific. Diagnostic criteria for pathologically *probable* vasculitic neuropathy require predominantly axonal alterations and either (1) perivascular inflammation combined with signs of active or chronic vascular damage, or (2) perivascular/vascular inflammation *without* vessel wall damage accompanied by one of five histologic predictors of vasculitic neuropathy: vascular deposits of IgM, complement, or fibrinogen by direct IF; hemosiderin deposits; asymmetric/multifocal nerve fiber loss; prominent axonal degeneration; or myofiber necrosis in peroneus brevis muscle (PBM) biopsy (Figs. 24.4–24.6, 24.8) [26, 42, 85, 88, 89]. Focal perineurial thickening/inflammation, injury neuroma with microfasciculation, neovascularization, endoneurial hemorrhage, and experimental axonal changes of acute ischemia might represent additional supportive features, but their specificity for vasculitis is not established (Fig. 24.9) [19, 23, 28, 78].

Biopsy

In the absence of a specific laboratory marker or clinical profile, nerve biopsy is required in all patients with suspected NSVN to confirm or refute the clinical diagnosis. In most patients with suspected SVN, nerve biopsy should also be performed, considering the many nonvasculitic causes of neuropathy in patients with systemic disease and the broad differential diagnosis of multifocal/asymmetric neuropathy (Table 24.2). Sural nerve is most commonly biopsied, but given reports of positive muscle biopsies in 50% of patients with PAN, combined nerve/muscle biopsies have become popular [90]. In one technique, superficial peroneal nerve (SPN) and PBM specimens are obtained through one incision in the distal leg (see Chapter 2) [20, 42]. Alternatively, sural nerve biopsy can be combined with soleus, gastrocnemius, quadriceps, or anterior tibialis muscle

Table 24.4 Diagnostic criteria for pathologically definite vasculitic neuropathy.

Active lesion: Nerve biopsy showing collection of inflammatory cells in vessel wall AND one or more signs of acute vascular damage:
1 Fibrinoid necrosis;
2 Loss/disruption of endothelium;
3 Loss/fragmentation of internal elastic lamina;
4 Loss/fragmentation of smooth muscle cells in media (can be highlighted with anti-smooth muscle actin staining);
5 Acute thrombosis;
6 Vascular/perivascular hemorrhage; OR
7 Leukocytoclasia.
Chronic lesion with signs of healing/repair: Nerve biopsy showing collection of mononuclear inflammatory cells in vessel wall AND one or more signs of chronic vascular damage with repair:
1 Intimal hyperplasia;
2 Fibrosis of media;
3 Adventitial/peri-adventitial fibrosis; OR
4 Chronic thrombosis with recanalization.
No evidence of another primary disease process that can mimic vasculitis pathologically, such as lymphoma, lymphomatoid granulomatosis, or amyloidosis.

*Presence of a chronic lesion does not exclude active vasculitis (vasculitides are usually segmental and multifocal, producing lesions of different ages in the same tissue or end-organ).
Source: Collins *et al.*, 2010. Reproduced with permission from Wiley.

Table 24.5 Diagnostic criteria for pathologically probable vasculitic neuropathy.

I Pathologically probable vasculitic neuropathy
1 Pathologic criteria for definite vasculitic neuropathy not satisfied (see Table 24.3); AND
2 Predominantly axonal changes; AND
3 Perivascular inflammation accompanied by signs of active or chronic vascular damage (as defined in Table 24.3); OR
Perivascular/vascular inflammation plus at least one additional class II or III *pathologic predictor* of definite vasculitic neuropathy:*
(a) Vascular deposition of complement, IgM, or fibrinogen by direct immunofluorescence;
(b) Hemosiderin deposits (Perls' stain for iron);
(c) Asymmetric nerve fiber loss or degeneration;
(d) Prominent active axonal degeneration; or
(e) Myofiber necrosis, regeneration, or infarcts in peroneus brevis muscle biopsy (not explained by underlying myopathy).
*Additional alterations used by some authorities as supportive of vasculitis but lacking in adequate evidence (more study required):
1 Neovascularization (Class II/III evidence suggests that this finding is probably not a predictor of vasculitis);
2 Endoneurial purpura (one negative class II study; one positive class III study);
3 Focal perineurial inflammation, degeneration, thickening (only class IV evidence);
4 Injury neuroma, microfasciculation (only class IV evidence); and
5 Swollen axons filled with organelles (one negative but non-convincing class II study) and other experimentally demonstrated axonal changes of acute ischemia, such as attenuated axons, flattened myelin profiles, tubular profiles, and axonal cytolysis.

Source: Collins *et al.*, 2010. Reproduced with permission from Wiley.

biopsy [37, 51, 91]. For patients in whom sural nerve or SPN are not clinically involved, the superficial radial, lateral antebrachial cutaneous, intermediate femoral cutaneous, or saphenous nerves can be biopsied. Others advocate fascicular biopsies of mixed proximal nerves in patients with abnormal MRIs of a proximal limb nerve, plexus, or root [92].

Although nerve is more commonly diagnostic than muscle in suspected vasculitic neuropathy, concomitant muscle biopsy may reveal vasculitis not found in the nerve due to sampling error. In patients diagnosed with vasculitic neuropathy, meta-analysis showed that concomitant muscle biopsy increased the yield for definite vasculitis by 15% [93]. However, in the

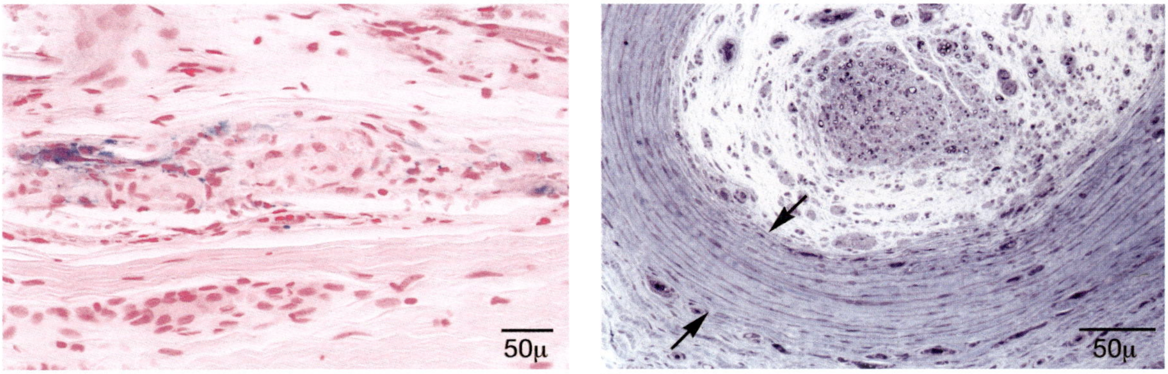

(A) (B)

Figure 24.8 (**A**) Longitudinal paraffin-embedded section of sural nerve biopsy at high power showing epineurial vessel with adjacent blue-staining hemosiderin deposits in patient with probable vasculitic neuropathy (Turnbull Blue stain). (**B**) Epoxy resin-embedded, high power cross section of sural nerve biopsy in patient with definite vasculitic neuropathy showing ischemic injury to one fascicle evidenced by complete loss of large myelinated fibers, reduced density of residual small myelinated fibers, and markedly thickened perineurium (arrows) (methylene blue stain).

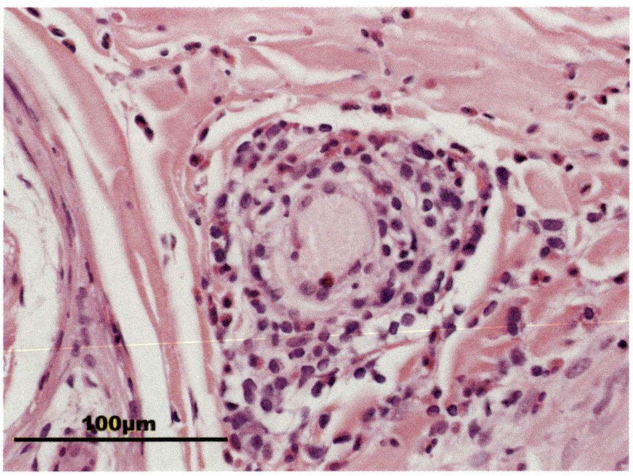

Figure 24.9 Paraffin-embedded cross section of sural nerve biopsy in patient with eosinophilic granulomatosis with polyangiitis (Churg–Strauss syndrome) presenting with vasculitic neuropathy showing epineurial large arteriolar vasculitis; the mixed cellular infiltrate disrupting the vessel wall includes many eosinophils (H&E).

only study in which a proximal muscle was biopsied (quadriceps), yield was not increased, suggesting that this conclusion pertains only to distal leg muscles [37]. In patients with NSVN, biopsies of distal leg muscles reveal definite vasculitis in 25% of patients [23, 26, 43, 44] (see also Chapter 2). Concomitant skin biopsy might enhance yield for vasculitis in patients with clinically suspected vasculitic neuropathy, but in two retrospective studies, distal leg skin biopsies in 23 patients with NSVN and three with SVN revealed no vasculitis [94, 95].

The true sensitivity of nerve or nerve/muscle biopsy for vasculitic neuropathy is unknowable in the absence of a reliable gold standard short of autopsy. However, in patients lacking nerve biopsy evidence of definite vasculitis, probable vasculitic neuropathy can be diagnosed by resorting to clinical and pathologic criteria. The Peripheral Nerve Society guideline on NSVN includes consensus diagnostic criteria for *clinically probable* vasculitic neuropathy [17]. Assuming these *probable* patients truly have vasculitic neuropathy, *estimated* diagnostic sensitivities can be derived. Pooling data from multiple studies, the estimated sensitivity of *definite* vasculitis in sural nerve biopsy is 50–55%, while that for combined SPN/PBM or sural nerve/distal muscle biopsy is 60% [96].

Two cohort studies of patients undergoing SPN/PBM biopsy for suspected vasculitic neuropathy determined diagnostic performance characteristics of "suspicious" biopsy features [26, 42]. In both studies, "suspicious" biopsies were defined as perivascular inflammation combined with at least one supportive pathologic alteration. Suspicious or positive biopsies had sensitivities of 85–86% and specificities of 80–85%, implying that ~15% of patients will still go undiagnosed when definite or probable diagnostic criteria are employed.

Differential diagnosis

The differential diagnosis of vasculitic neuropathy includes many other causes of sensorimotor or sensory asymmetric/multifocal neuropathy (Table 24.2). For patients diagnosed with definite or clinically probable vasculitic neuropathy, the differential diagnosis includes all conditions associated with PNS vasculitis (Table 24.1). Determination of the type of vasculitic neuropathy depends on clinical presentation, laboratory findings, and nerve pathology. Almost all vasculitides have the potential to involve vessels in a size range atypical for that disease. Because of this overlap, identification of the caliber and type of affected vessels does not indicate a specific disorder but may refine the differential diagnosis [21]. CHCC restricts PAN to small-medium-sized arteries, so microvascular or venular involvement excludes PAN [11]. Similarly, cellular content of vasculitic infiltrates does not, of itself, reliably distinguish between the vasculitides [21].

Pathologically, PAN is a necrotizing vasculitis of small-to-medium-sized arteries [97]. Granulomas and eosinophilic infiltrates are rarely observed. MPA is a necrotizing vasculitis primarily affecting arterioles, capillaries, and venules. In contrast to GPA and EGPA, there are no granulomas, and unlike IgA vasculitis, few immune deposits are seen [11, 98]. The three salient histopathological alterations of EGPA are eosinophilic tissue infiltration, extravascular granulomas, and small-vessel necrotizing vasculitis (Fig. 24.10) [11, 55, 99]. Although over 90% of

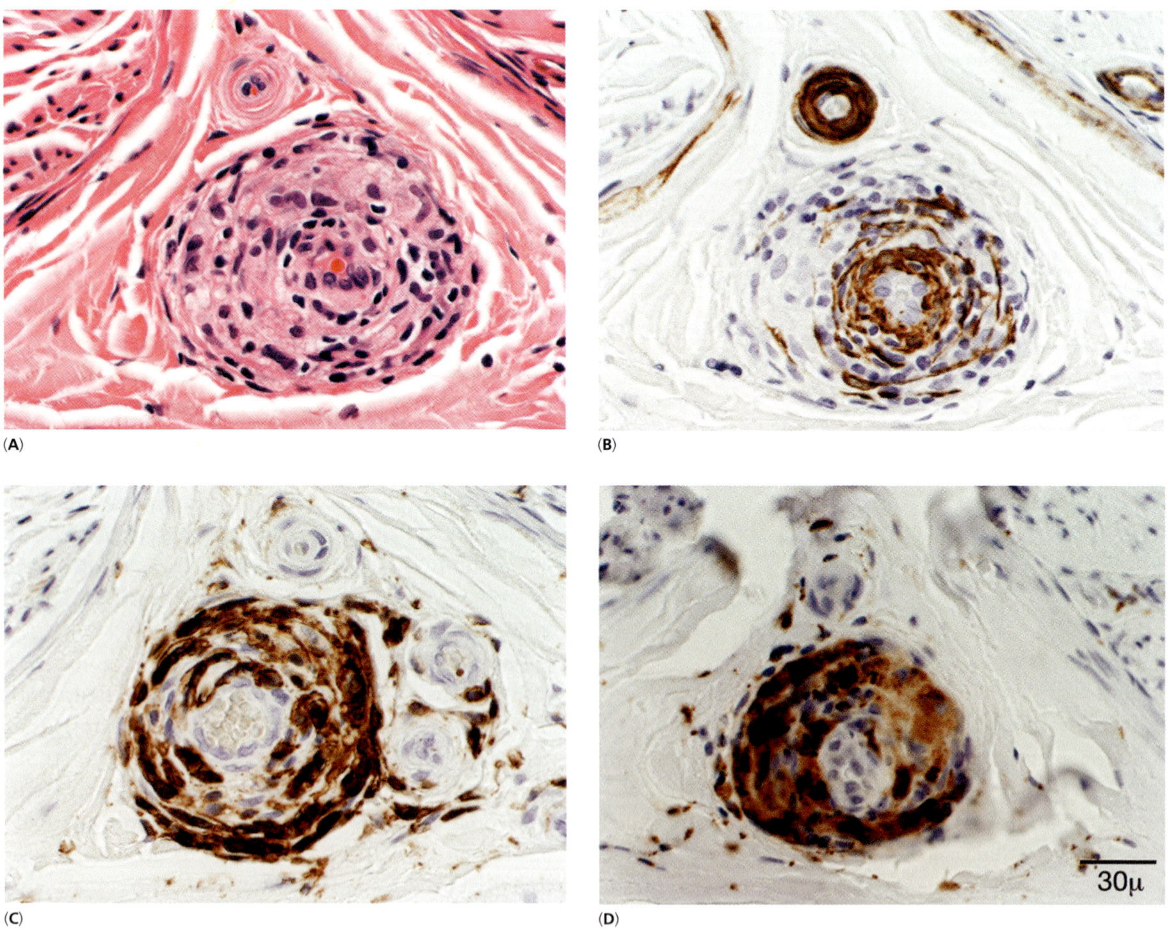

Figure 24.10 Serial low power cross sections of paraffin-embedded sural nerve biopsy in patient with granulomatosis with polyangiitis showing granulomatous vasculitis of an epineurial arteriole. (**A**) is stained with H&E, (**B**) with anti-human smooth muscle actin antibodies, (**C**) with anti-CD45 antibodies, and (**D**) with anti-CD68 antibodies (highlights macrophages and dendritic cells).

autopsies reveal vasculitis, only 40% show granulomas or eosinophilic infiltrates and only 24% contain all three lesions [55]. In four series reporting nerve biopsy findings, necrotizing vasculitis was observed in 30%, eosinophilic infiltrates in 35%, and granulomas in 10% [36, 100–102]. CD4+/CD8+ T cells are often the predominant cellular constituent in the vascular aggregates [36, 101]. GPA is defined by the pathological triad of granulomatous inflammation, necrosis, and vasculitis [103, 104]. The earliest pathologic alteration is fibrinoid degeneration of collagen with microabscess formation, which later evolves into palisading granulomas [105]. Vasculitis affects the microvasculature and small-to-medium-sized arteries and veins. Open lung biopsies are the most reliable method of diagnosis, yielding vasculitis, necrosis, and granulomas in 90% of specimens [106]. Information on nerve pathology is sparse (rare reports of granulomatous inflammation) [107]. NSVN exhibits nonspecific, non-granulomatous changes reminiscent of PAN or MPA, albeit with frequent vascular immune deposits.

GCA is a granulomatous vasculitis involving medium-to-large-sized arteries [108, 109]. Arterioles, capillaries, and veins are largely spared. Superficial temporal artery biopsy reveals granulomatous inflammation, infiltration of macrophages and T cells, and disruption of the internal elastic lamina. Multinucleated giant cells occur in less than 50% of biopsies. Vasculitic neuropathy is uncommon and generally results from nutrient artery vasculitis [63]. Of the few reported nerve biopsies, only one revealed healing epineurial vasculitis [110].

IgA vasculitis is characterized pathologically by leukocytoclastic vasculitis and IgA immune deposits in the walls of small vessels and glomeruli [11, 111]. Nerve pathology is not reported. HUV is another immune complex small-vessel vasculitis wherein lesional skin biopsies show leukocytoclastic vasculitis with complement and immunoglobulin (non-IgA) deposits in vessel walls [11]. In the rarely reported neuropathies associated with this condition, nerve biopsies have revealed leukocytoclastic vasculitis or probable vasculitis [112, 113].

In HCV-related cryoglobulinemic vasculitic neuropathy, nerve biopsies reveal (1) mononuclear-predominant perivascular inflammation in the epineurium; (2) epineurial vasculitis in 50%; and (3) endoneurial microangiopathy, characterized by endothelial cell swelling, luminal narrowing, and basal lamina reduplication, which might ensue from capillaritis, given infrequent reports of endoneurial hemorrhage and immunoglobulin/complement deposits in endoneurial vessels [73].

Nerve biopsies in CTD-related vasculitic neuropathies reveal alterations indistinguishable from those seen in other necrotizing vasculitides.

Pathogenesis

Whereas ANCAs appear important to the pathogenesis of AAV, they are unlikely to mediate vasculitic neuropathies. For example, nerve biopsies in patients with vasculitic neuropathies only rarely reveal neutrophils, the chief effector cells in AAV [22, 36, 81]. In addition, these biopsies commonly exhibit vascular immune deposits [85], contrasting with the "pauci-immune" nature of AAV. Moreover, in EGPA, an AAV closely associated with neuropathy, most patients with neuropathy are ANCA-negative [73]. Finally, in the most common vasculitic neuropathy, NSVN, ANCAs are rare [17].

Evidence suggests that NSVN and most SVNs are mediated primarily by cellular mechanisms (T cell cytotoxicity and chronic delayed-type hypersensitivity). First, DNA microarray and candidate-gene expression analyses of nerve biopsies in patients with SVNs have revealed upregulation of cytokines indicative of a Th1 response and many chemokine, chemokine receptor, and other genes involved in T cell and macrophage responses [114, 115]. Th1 cells activate macrophages, induce T cell proliferation, and promote T cell-mediated autoimmune diseases. Second, nerve biopsies in patients with vasculitic neuropathy demonstrate a predominance of CD4+ or CD8+ T cells and macrophages, with many of the T cells expressing markers of CTLs (cytotoxic T lymphocytes) [82, 116]. Third, antigen-presenting cells (APCs) are increased in the epineurium and endoneurium [81, 84, 117]. Fourth, co-stimulatory molecule ICOS (inducible costimulator), which is expressed preferentially by effector memory T cells, is upregulated on epineurial T cells, while ICOS-ligand is upregulated on epineurial macrophages, suggesting that macrophages act as APCs to re-stimulate activated T cells [118]. These and other observations support a pathogenic model wherein autoreactive T cells are recruited to the PNS, recognize self-glycolipid or peptide antigens presented by macrophages, Schwann cells, and/or endothelial cells, undergo activation, and then mature into or recruit CTLs that damage epineurial vessels.

Humoral mechanisms probably also contribute to PNS vasculitis pathogenesis. As noted previously, epineurial vessel walls often contain deposits of immunoglobulin and complement [85]. More compellingly, a DNA microarray analysis showed immunoglobulin genes exhibit maximally upregulated transcription, indicative of B cell selection and antigen recognition [115]. A C1q gene was also upregulated, suggesting concomitant activation of the classical complement pathway. Therefore, immune complex deposition or *in situ* formation followed by activation of complement and recruitment of phagocytes might also promote vascular damage in vasculitic neuropathy.

Conclusions and future perspectives

Vasculitis is an uncommon but treatable and thus important cause of neuropathy. Vasculitic neuropathy can occur in isolation (NSVN) but more frequently evolves in the setting of a primary or secondary systemic vasculitis. The nomenclature of the systemic vasculitides was updated by CHCC2012. PAN, AAV, rheumatoid vasculitis, and cryoglobulinemic vasculitis are the systemic disorders most commonly associated with neuropathy. Vasculitic neuropathy usually presents with a subacutely progressive, asymmetric/multifocal, painful, distal-predominant, axonal, sensor-imotor phenotype. Purely motor or primarily demyelinating presentations are rare. In patients lacking definite vasculitis in nerve biopsy, clinically probable vasculitic neuropathy can be diagnosed by resort to supportive clinicopathologic findings. Pathologic features such as caliber/type of affected vessels and content of inflammatory infiltrates are never pathognomonic for a specific disorder but can refine the diagnosis. Vasculitic neuropathies are more likely to be primarily mediated by cellular than humoral mechanisms. Serologic and pathologic markers of vasculitic neuropathy in patients with non-diagnostic biopsies and improved understanding of classification, natural history, pathogenic mechanisms, and optimal treatment of vasculitic neuropathies should be the focus of future investigations.

References

1 Langford CA, Fauci AS. (2012) The vasculitis syndromes. In: Longo DL, Fauci AS, Kasper DL, Hauser SL, Jameson JL, Loscalzo J, (eds) *Harrison's Principles of Internal Medicine*, 18th edn. McGraw-Hill, New York, www.accessmedicine.com/content.aspx?aID=9138083. Accessed April 3, 2014.

2 Kussmaul A, Maier R. (1866) Ueber eine bisher nicht beschriebene eigenthümliche Arterien-erkrankung (Periarteritis nodosa), die mit Morbus Brightii und rapid fortschreitender allgemeiner Muskellähmung einhergeht. *Deutsches Archiv fur Klinische Medizin* 1, 484–515.

3 Dyck PJ, Benstead TJ, Conn DL, Stevens JC, Windebank AJ, Low PA. (1987) Nonsystemic vasculitic neuropathy. *Brain* 110, 843–853.

4 Fries JF, Hunder GG, Bloch DA, *et al.* (1990) The American College of Rheumatology 1990 criteria for the classification of vasculitis. Summary. *Arthritis Rheum* 33, 1135–1136.

5 Jennette JC, Falk RJ, Andrassy K, *et al.* (1994) Nomenclature of systemic vasculitides. Proposal of an international consensus conference. *Arthritis Rheum* 37, 187–192.

6 Hernández-Rodríguez J, Hoffman GS. (2012) Updating single-organ vasculitis. *Curr Opin Rheumatol* 24, 38–45.

7 Bruce IN, Bell AL. (1997) A comparison of two nomenclature systems for primary systemic vasculitis. *Br J Rheumatol* 36, 453–458.

8 Wiik AS. (2010) Autoantibodies in ANCA-associated vasculitis. *Rheum Dis Clin North Am* 36, 479–489.

9 Jennette JC, Falk RJ, Hu P, Xiao H. (2013) Pathogenesis of antineutrophil cytoplasmic autoantibody-associated small-vessel vasculitis. *Annu Rev Pathol* 8, 139–60.

10 Watts R, Lane S, Hanslik T, *et al.* (2007) Development and validation of a consensus methodology for the classification of the ANCA-associated vasculitides and polyarteritis nodosa for epidemiological studies. *Ann Rheum Dis* 66, 222–227.

11 Jennette J, Falk R, Bacon P, *et al.* (2013) 2012 Revised International Chapel Hill Consensus Conference Nomenclature of Vasculitides. *Arthritis Rheum* 65, 1–11.

12 Guillevin L, Durand-Gasselin B, Cevallos R, *et al.* (1999) Microscopic polyangiitis: clinical and laboratory findings in eighty-five patients. *Arthritis Rheum* 42, 421–430.

13 Pagnoux C, Seror R, Henegar C, *et al.* (2010) Clinical features and outcomes in 348 patients with polyarteritis nodosa: a systematic retrospective study of patients diagnosed between 1963 and 2005 and entered into the French Vasculitis Study Group Database. *Arthritis Rheum* 62, 616–626.

14 Comarmond C, Pagnoux C, Khellaf M, *et al.* (2013) Eosinophilic granulomatosis with polyangiitis (Churg–Strauss syndrome) – clinical characteristics and long-term follow-up of the 383 patients enrolled in the FVSG cohort. *Arthritis Rheum* 65, 270–281.

15 Puéchal X, Said G, Hilliquin P, Coste J, *et al.* (1995) Peripheral neuropathy with necrotizing vasculitis in rheumatoid arthritis. A clinicopathologic and prognostic study of thirty-two patients. *Arthritis Rheum* 38, 1618–1629.

16 Terrier B, Cacoub P. (2013) Cryoglobulinemia vasculitis: an update. *Curr Opin Rheumatol* 25, 10–18.

17 Collins MP, Dyck PJ, Gronseth GS, *et al.* (2010) Peripheral Nerve Society Guideline on the classification, diagnosis, investigation, and immunosuppressive therapy of non-systemic vasculitic neuropathy: executive summary. *Peripher Nerv Syst* 15, 176–184.

18 Dyck PJB, Engelstad J, Dyck PJ. (2005) Microvasculitis. In: Dyck PJ, Thomas PK (eds) *Peripheral Neuropathy*, 4th edn, pp. 2405–2414. Elsevier Saunders, Philadelphia.
19 Said G, Lacroix-Ciaudo C, Fujimura H, *et al.* (1988) The peripheral neuropathy of necrotizing arteritis: a clinicopathological study. *Ann Neurol* 23, 461–465.
20 Hawke SH, Davies L, Pamphlett R, *et al.* (1991) Vasculitic neuropathy. A clinical and pathological study. *Brain* 114, 2175–2190.
21 Midroni G, Bilbao JM. (1995) *Biopsy Diagnosis of Peripheral Neuropathy*, pp. 105–117, 241–262. Butterworth-Heinemann, Boston.
22 Sugiura M, Koike H, Iijima M, *et al.* (2006) Clinicopathologic features of nonsystemic vasculitic neuropathy and microscopic polyangiitis-associated neuropathy: A comparative study. *J Neurol Sci* 241, 31–37.
23 Vital C, Vital A, Canron MH, *et al.* (2006) Combined nerve and muscle biopsy in the diagnosis of vasculitic neuropathy. A 16-year retrospective study of 202 cases. *J Peripher Nerv Syst* 11, 20–29.
24 Kararizou E, Davaki P, Karandreas N, *et al.* (2005) Nonsystemic vasculitic neuropathy: A clinicopathological study of 22 cases. *J Rheumatol* 32, 853–858.
25 Vincent D, Dubas F, Hauw JJ, *et al.* (1985) Nerve and muscle microvasculitis: 50 cases. *Rev Neurol* (Paris) 141, 440–446.
26 Agadi JB, Raghav G, Mahadevan A, *et al.* (2012) Usefulness of superficial peroneal nerve/peroneus brevis muscle biopsy in the diagnosis of vasculitic neuropathy. *J Clin Neurosci* 19, 1392–1396.
27 Leger JM, Bouche P, Chaunu MP, *et al.* (1988) Peripheral neuropathies with neural vasculitis. Clinical and electrophysiological aspects of 33 cases. *Presse Med* 17, 733–737.
28 Dyck PJ, Norell JE, Dyck PJ. (1999) Microvasculitis and ischemia in diabetic lumbosacral radiculoplexus neuropathy. *Neurology* 53, 2113–2121.
29 Dyck PJ, Norell JE, Dyck PJ. (2001) Non-diabetic lumbosacral radiculoplexus neuropathy: natural history, outcome and comparison with the diabetic variety. *Brain* 124, 1197–1207.
30 González-Gay MA, García-Porrúa C. (1999) Systemic vasculitis in adults in northwestern Spain, 1988–1997. Clinical and epidemiologic aspects. *Medicine* 78, 292–308.
31 Ntatsaki E, Watts RA, Scott DG. (2010) Epidemiology of ANCA-associated vasculitis. *Rheum Dis Clin North Am* 36, 447–461.
32 Collins MP, Periquet MI. (2008) Isolated vasculitis of the peripheral nervous system. *Clin Exp Rheumatol* 26, S118–130.
33 Guillevin L, Pagnoux C, Seror R, *et al.* (2011) French Vasculitis Study Group (FVSG). The Five-Factor Score revisited: assessment of prognoses of systemic necrotizing vasculitides based on the French Vasculitis Study Group (FVSG) cohort. *Medicine* 90, 19–27.
34 Walsh M, Flossmann O, Berden A, *et al.* (2012) Risk factors for relapse of antineutrophil cytoplasmic antibody-associated vasculitis. *Arthritis Rheum* 64, 542–548.
35 Walsh M, Mukhtyar C, Mahr A, *et al.* (2011) Health-related quality of life in patients with newly diagnosed antineutrophil cytoplasmic antibody-associated vasculitis. *Arthritis Care Res* 63, 1055–1061.
36 Hattori N, Ichimura M, Nagamatsu M, *et al.* (1999) Clinicopathological features of Churg–Strauss syndrome-associated neuropathy. *Brain* 122, 427–439.
37 Bennett DL, Groves M, Blake J, *et al.* (2008) The use of nerve and muscle biopsy in the diagnosis of vasculitis: a 5 year retrospective study. *J Neurol Neurosurg Psychiatry* 79, 1376–1381.
38 Restrepo JF, Rondón F, Matteson EL, *et al.* (2009) Necrotizing lymphocytic vasculitis limited to the peripheral nerves: report of six cases and review. *Int J Rheumatol* 2009, 368032.
39 Devigili G, Uçeyler N, Beck M, *et al.* (2011) Vasculitis-like neuropathy in amyotrophic lateral sclerosis unresponsive to treatment. *Acta Neuropathol* 22, 343–352.
40 González-Gay MA, García-Porrúa C. (2001) Epidemiology of the vasculitides. *Rheum Dis Clin North Am* 27, 729–749.
41 Davies L, Spies JM, Pollard JD, McLeod JG. (1996) Vasculitis confined to peripheral nerves. *Brain* 119, 1441–1448.
42 Collins MP, Mendell JR, Periquet MI, *et al.* (2000) Superficial peroneal nerve/peroneus brevis muscle biopsy in vasculitic neuropathy. *Neurology* 55, 636–643.
43 Collins MP, Periquet MI, Mendell JR, *et al.* (2003) Nonsystemic vasculitic neuropathy: Insights from a clinical cohort. *Neurology* 61, 623–630.
44 Seo JH, Ryan HF, Claussen GC, Thomas TD, *et al.* (2004) Sensory neuropathy in vasculitis: a clinical, pathologic, and electrophysiologic study. *Neurology* 63, 874–878.
45 Cattaneo L, Chierici E, Pavone L, *et al.* (2007) Peripheral neuropathy in Wegener's granulomatosis, Churg-Strauss syndrome and microscopic polyangiitis. *J Neurol Neurosurg Psychiatry* 78, 1119–1123.
46 Wolf J, Schmitt V, Palm F, *et al.* (2013) Peripheral neuropathy as initial manifestation of primary systemic vasculitides. *J Neurol* 260, 1061–1070.
47 Suppiah R, Hadden RD, Batra R, *et al.* (2011) Peripheral neuropathy in ANCA-associated vasculitis: outcomes from the European Vasculitis Study Group trials. *Rheumatology* 50, 2214–2222.
48 De Toni Franceschini L, Amadio S, Scarlato M, *et al.* (2011) A fatal case of Churg–Strauss syndrome presenting with acute polyneuropathy mimicking Guillain–Barré syndrome. *Neurol Sci* 32, 937–940.
49 Cassereau J, Baguenier-Desormeaux C, Letournel F, *et al.* (2012) Necrotizing vasculitis revealed in a case of multiple mononeuropathy after a 14-year course of spontaneous remissions and relapses. *Clin Neurol Neurosurg* 114, 290–293.
50 Collins MP, Kissel JT. (2014) Vasculitic neuropathies and neuropathies of connective tissue diseases. In: Katirji B, Kaminski HJ, Ruff RL, (eds) *Neuromuscular Disorders in Clinical Practice*. 2nd edn, pp. 733–785. Springer, New York.
51 Claussen GC, Thomas TD, Goyne C, *et al.* (2000) Diagnostic value of nerve and muscle biopsy in suspected vasculitis cases. *J Clin Neuromusc Dis* 1, 117–123.

52 Zivkovic SA, Ascherman D, Lacomis D. (2007) Vasculitic neuropathy – electrodiagnostic findings and association with malignancies. *Acta Neurol Scand* 115, 432–436.
53 McCluskey L, Feinberg D, Cantor C, Bird S. (1999) "Pseudo-conduction block" in vasculitic neuropathy. *Muscle Nerve* 22, 1361–1366.
54 Calabrese LH, Molloy ES, Duna G. (2009) Antineutrophil cytoplasmic antibody-associated vasculitis. In: Firestein GS, Budd RC, Harris ED, *et al.* (eds) *Kelley's Textbook of Rheumatology*, 8th edn, pp. 1429–1451. Saunders Elsevier, Philadelphia.
55 Lanham JG, Elkon KB, Pusey CD, *et al.* (1984) Systemic vasculitis with asthma and eosinophilia: a clinical approach to the Churg–Strauss syndrome. *Medicine* 63, 65–81.
56 Moosig F, Bremer JP, Hellmich B, *et al.* (2012) A vasculitis centre based management strategy leads to improved outcome in eosinophilic granulomatosis and polyangiitis (Churg–Strauss, EGPA): monocentric experiences in 150 patients. *Ann Rheum Dis* doi:10.1136/annrheumdis-2012–201531.
57 Cisternas M, Soto L, Jacobelli S, *et al.* (2005) Clinical features of Wegener granulomatosis and microscopic polyangiitis in Chilean patients. *Rev Med Chil* 133, 273–278.
58 Zhang W, Zhou G, Shi Q, *et al.* (2009) Clinical analysis of nervous system involvement in ANCA-associated systemic vasculitides. *Clin Exp Rheumatol* 27 (Suppl 52), S65–S69.
59 Hoffman GS, Kerr GS, Leavitt RY, *et al.* (1992) Wegener granulomatosis: an analysis of 158 patients. *Ann Intern Med* 116, 488–496.
60 Nishino H, Rubino FA, DeRemee RA, *et al.* (1993) Neurological involvement in Wegener's granulomatosis: an analysis of 324 consecutive patients at the Mayo Clinic. *Ann Neurol* 33. 4–9.
61 Holle JU, Gross WL, Latza U, *et al.* (2011) Improved outcome in 445 patients with Wegener's granulomatosis in a German vasculitis center over four decades. *Arthritis Rheum* 63, 257–266.
62 Borchers AT, Gershwin ME. (2012) Giant cell arteritis: A review of classification, pathophysiology, geoepidemiology and treatment. *Autoimmun Rev* 11, A544–A554.
63 Caselli RJ, Hunder GG, Whisnant JP. (1988) Neurologic disease in biopsy-proven giant cell (temporal) arteritis. *Neurology* 38, 352–359.
64 Nesher G. (2000) Neurologic manifestations of giant cell arteritis. *Clin Exp Rheumatol* (Suppl 20) 18, S24–S26.
65 Pfadenhauer K, Roesler A, Golling A. (2007) The involvement of the peripheral nervous system in biopsy proven active giant cell arteritis. *J Neurol* 254, 751–755.
66 Pagnoux C, Cohen P, Guillevin L. (2006) Vasculitides secondary to infections. *Clin Exp Rheumatol* 24 (2 Suppl 41), S71–S81.
67 Lidar M, Lipschitz N, Langevitz P, *et al.* (2009) The infectious etiology of vasculitis. *Autoimmunity* 42, 432–438.
68 Said G, Lacroix C, Chemouilli P, *et al.* (1991) Cytomegalovirus neuropathy in acquired immunodeficiency syndrome: a clinical and pathological study. *Ann Neurol* 29, 139–146.
69 Chretien F, Gray F, Lescs MC, *et al.* (1993) Acute varicella-zoster virus ventriculitis and meningo-myelo-radiculitis in acquired immunodeficiency syndrome. *Acta Neuropathol* 86, 659–665.
70 Lenglet T, Haroche J, Schnuriger A, *et al.* (2011) Mononeuropathy multiplex associated with acute parvovirus B19 infection: characteristics, treatment and outcome. *J Neurol* 258, 1321–1326.
71 Patel N, Patel N, Khan T, Patel N, *et al.* (2011) HIV infection and clinical spectrum of associated vasculitides. *Curr Rheumatol Rep* 13, 506–512.
72 Ramos-Casals M, Stone JH, Cid MC, Bosch X. (2012) The cryoglobulinaemias. *Lancet* 379, 348–360.
73 Collins MP. (2012) The vasculitic neuropathies: an update. *Curr Opin Neurol* 25, 573–585.
74 Garces-Sanchez M, Laughlin RS, Dyck PJ, *et al.* (2011) Painless diabetic motor neuropathy: a variant of diabetic lumbosacral radiculoplexus neuropathy? *Ann Neurol* 69, 1043–1054.
75 Massie R, Mauermann ML, Staff NP, *et al.* (2012) Diabetic cervical radiculoplexus neuropathy: a distinct syndrome expanding the spectrum of diabetic radiculoplexus neuropathies. *Brain* 135, 3074–3088.
76 Fujimura H, Lacroix C, Said G. (1991) Vulnerability of nerve fibres to ischaemia. A quantitative light and electron microscope study. *Brain* 114, 1929–1942.
77 Dyck PJ, Johnson WJ, Lambert EH, *et al.* (1971) Segmental demyelination secondary to axonal degeneration in uremic neuropathy. *Mayo Clin Proc* 46, 400–431.
78 Nukada H, Dyck PJ. (1984) Microsphere embolization of nerve capillaries and fibre degeneration. *Am J Pathol* 115, 275–287.
79 Dyck PJ, Conn DL, Okazaki H. (1972) Necrotizing angiopathic neuropathy. Three-dimensional morphology of fibre degeneration related to sites of occluded vessels. *Mayo Clin Proc* 47, 461–475.
80 Morozumi S, Koike H, Tomita M, *et al.* (2011) Spatial distribution of nerve fibre pathology and vasculitis in microscopic polyangiitis-associated neuropathy. *J Neuropathol Exp Neurol* 70, 340–348.
81 Kissel JT, Riethman JL, Omerza J, *et al.* (1989) Peripheral nerve vasculitis: Immune characterization of the vascular lesions. *Ann Neurol* 25, 291–297.
82 Satoi H, Oka N, Kawasaki T, *et al.* (1998) Mechanisms of tissue injury in vasculitic neuropathies. *Neurology* 50, 492–496.
83 Engelhardt A, Lorler H, Neundorfer B. (1993) Immunohistochemical findings in vasculitic neuropathies. *Acta Neurol Scand* 87, 318–321.
84 Khalili-Shirazi A, Gregson NA, Londei M, *et al.* (1998) The distribution of CD1 molecules in inflammatory neuropathy. *J Neurol Sci* 158, 154–163.
85 Collins MP, Periquet-Collins I, Sahenk Z, *et al.* (2010) Direct immunofluoresence in vasculitic neuropathy: specificity of vascular immune deposits. *Muscle Nerve* 42, 62–69.

86 Midroni G, Cohen SM, Bilbao JM. (2000) Endoneurial vasculitis and tubuloreticular inclusions in peripheral nerve biopsy. *Clin Neuropathol* 19, 70–76.

87 Said G, Lacroix C, Lozeron P, *et al.* (2003) Inflammatory vasculopathy in multifocal diabetic neuropathy. *Brain* 126, 376–385.

88 Adams CW, Buk SJ, Hughes RA, *et al.* (1989) Perls' ferrocyanide test for iron in the diagnosis of vasculitic neuropathy. *Neuropathol Appl Neurobiol* 15, 433–439.

89 Vrancken AFJE, Notermans NC, Jansen GH, *et al.* (2004) Progressive idiopathic axonal neuropathy – a comparative clinical and histopathological study with vasculitic neuropathy. *J Neurol* 251, 269–278.

90 Fort JG, Griffin R, Tahmoush A, *et al.* (1994) Muscle involvement in polyarteritis nodosa: report of a patient presenting clinically as polymyositis and review of the literature. *J Rheumatol* 21, 945–948.

91 Sanchez J, Coll-Canti J, Ariza A, *et al.* (2001) Neuropathy due to necrotizing vasculitis: a study of the clinical anatomy, neurophysiological characteristics, and clinical course of the disorder in 27 patients. *Rev Neurol* 33, 1033–1036.

92 Dyck PJB, Spinner RJ, Amrami KK, Klein CJ, Englestad JK, Dyck PJ. (2010) MRI-targeted fascicular nerve biopsies of proximal nerves: historic reports and illustrative case reports. In: Dyck PJ, Dyck PJB, Klein CJ, Low P, Amrami KK, Englestad JK, (eds) *Companion to Peripheral Neuropathy*, pp. 3–14. Saunders Elsevier, Philadelphia.

93 Vrancken AF, Gathier CS, Cats EA, *et al.* (2011) The additional yield of combined nerve/muscle biopsy in vasculitic neuropathy. *Eur J Neurol* 18, 49–58.

94 Lee JE, Shun CT, Hsieh SC, *et al.* (2005) Skin denervation in vasculitic neuropathy. *Arch Neurol* 62, 1570–1573.

95 Uçeyler N, Devigili G, Toyka KV, *et al.* (2010) Skin biopsy as an additional diagnostic tool in non-systemic vasculitic neuropathy. *Acta Neuropathol* 120, 109–116.

96 Collins MP, Arnold WD, Kissel JT. (2013) The neuropathies of vasculitis. *Neurol Clin* 31, 557–595.

97 Bonsib SM. (2001) Polyarteritis nodosa. *Semin Diagn Pathol* 18, 14–23.

98 Jennette JC, Thomas DB, Falk RJ. (2001) Microscopic polyangiitis (microscopic polyarteritis). *Semin Diagn Pathol* 18, 3–13.

99 Churg J, Strauss L. (1951) Allergic granulomatosis, allergic angiitis, and periarteritis nodosa. *Am J Pathol* 27, 277–301.

100 Vital A, Vital C, Viallard JF, *et al.* (2006) Neuro-muscular biopsy in Churg–Strauss syndrome: 24 cases. *J Neuropathol Exp Neurol* 65, 1871–92.

101 Oka N, Kawasaki T, Matsui M, *et al.* (2011) Two subtypes of Churg–Strauss syndrome with neuropathy: the roles of eosinophils and ANCA. *Mod Rheumatol* 21, 290–295.

102 Shimoi T, Shojima K, Murota A, *et al.* (2012) Clinical and pathological features of Churg–Strauss syndrome among a Japanese population: a case series of 18 patients. *Asian Pac J Allergy Immunol* 30, 61–70.

103 Godman GC, Churg J. (1954) Wegener's granulomatosis: pathology and review of the literature. *AMA Arch Pathol* 58, 533–553.

104 Yi ES, Colby TV. (2001) Wegener's granulomatosis. *Semin Diagn Pathol* 18, 34–46.

105 Mark EJ, Matsubara O, Tan-Liu NS, *et al.* (1988) The pulmonary biopsy in the early diagnosis of Wegener's (pathergic) granulomatosis: a study based on 35 open lung biopsies. *Hum Pathol* 19, 1065–1071.

106 Travis WD, Hoffman GS, Leavitt RY, *et al.* (1991) Surgical pathology of the lung in Wegener's granulomatosis. Review of 87 open lung biopsies from 67 patients. *Am J Surg Pathol* 15, 315–333.

107 Finkelman R, Munsat T, Mandell H, *et al.* (1993) Neuromuscular manifestations of Wegener's granulomatosis: a case report. *Neurology* 43, 617–618.

108 Lie JT. (1996) Temporal artery biopsy diagnosis of giant cell arteritis: lessons from 1109 biopsies. *Anat Pathol* 1, 69–97.

109 Weidner N. (2001) Giant-cell vasculitides. *Semin Diagn Pathol* 18, 24–33.

110 Bridges AJ, Porter J, England D. (1989) Lower extremity peripheral neuropathy and ischemic ulcers associated with giant cell arteritis. *J Rheumatol* 16, 1366–1369.

111 Poterucha TJ, Wetter DA, Gibson LE, *et al.* (2012) Correlates of systemic disease in adult Henoch–Schönlein purpura: a retrospective study of direct immunofluorescence and skin lesion distribution in 87 patients at Mayo Clinic. *J Am Acad Dermatol* 67, 612–616.

112 Zeiss CR, Burch FX, Marder RJ, *et al.* (1980) A hypocomplementemic vasculitic urticarial syndrome. Report of four new cases and definition of the disease. *Am J Med* 68, 867–875.

113 Filosto M, Cavallaro T, Pasolini G, *et al.* (2009) Idiopathic hypocomplementemic urticarial vasculitis-linked neuropathy. *J Neurol Sci* 284, 179–181.

114 Saadoun D, Bieche I, Maisonobe T, *et al.* (2005) Involvement of chemokines and type 1 cytokines in the pathogenesis of hepatitis C virus-associated mixed cryoglobulinemia vasculitis neuropathy. *Arthritis Rheum* 52, 2917–2925.

115 Kinter J, Broglio L, Steck AJ, *et al.* (2010) Gene expression profiling in nerve biopsy of vasculitic neuropathy. *J Neuroimmunol* 225, 184–189.

116 Heuss D, Probst-Cousin S, Kayser C, *et al.* (2000) Cell death in vasculitic neuropathy. *Muscle Nerve* 23, 999–1004.

117 Van Rhijn I, Van den Berg LH, Bosboom WM, *et al.* (2000) Expression of accessory molecules for T-cell activation in peripheral nerve of patients with CIDP and vasculitic neuropathy. *Brain* 123, 2020–2029.

118 Hu W, Janke A, Ortler S, *et al.* (2007) Expression of CD28-related costimulatory molecule and its ligand in inflammatory neuropathies. *Neurology* 68, 277–282.

CHAPTER 25

Infectious and tropical neuropathies

Leila Chimelli[1] and Jean-Michel Vallat[2]

[1] *Department of Pathology, University Hospital, Federal University of Rio de Janeiro, Rio de Janeiro, Brazil*

[2] *Neurology Laboratory, National Referral Center for Rare Peripheral Neuropathies, University Hospital, Limoges, France*

Introduction

Infectious diseases are important in the differential diagnosis of peripheral nerve disorders because they are amongst the most treatable. Diagnosis may be challenging because of variability in the pattern of deficits, geographic distribution of pathogens, interval from the time of infection to the development of neuropathy, and mechanism of nerve injury. The important points are that these neuropathies are treatable and often preventable [1, 2].

Infectious neuropathy affects a large number of people worldwide. It may be due to direct invasion of nerves by the agent, including viruses, especially retroviruses, parasites, and bacilli (Table 25.1), or to the patient's immune reaction, or secondary to drug toxicity associated with treatment [3].

Infectious neuropathies primarily involve the interstitial supporting tissue of the nerve and vessels, secondarily damaging nerve fibers. Vasculitis (cf. Chapter 24), which is a frequent cause of interstitial neuropathy, may also be related to infections.

Bacterial neuropathies

Leprosy

Definition and pathogenesis

Leprosy or Hansen's disease is due to infection by *Mycobacterium leprae* or Hansen's bacilli (HB). A wide variety of peripheral neuropathies and peripheral nerve lesions are found in all forms of leprosy. HB has a predilection for Schwann cells, where the organism multiplies unimpeded by organism-specific host immunity, resulting in destruction of myelin, secondary inflammatory changes, and destruction of the nerve architecture [4, 5].

The disease course and the clinical features are determined by the degree of host immune response. The lepromatous (Virchowian) form is associated with a low level immune response and hematogenous spread of organisms (multibacillary forms). The tuberculoid form is associated with a high level immune response, limiting the proliferation and spread of bacilli, which are sparse (paucibacillary forms). In the individual patient, the type of leprosy is determined by the clinical manifestations, histologic response to bacilli, and number of bacilli [4]. Leprosy reactions may increase nerve damage and neurological complications. Leprosy reactions include: Type 1 (Reversal reactions) and Type 2 (Erythema Nodosum Leprosum) in which arteritic leprosy lesions involving epineurial vessels may cause additional nerve damage.

Inflammation within and around the nerve is a feature common to all types and is induced by mediators such as cytokines and chemokines. Apart from the bacillus, the nerve may be damaged by increased pressure due to endoneurial edema and inflammatory cell infiltration (especially in leprosy reactions) and by vascular lesions including necrosis and granulomatous reaction [5–7].

Epidemiology

Leprosy is one of the most common causes of nontraumatic peripheral neuropathy in the developing world including Asia, Africa, and South America. Although

Peripheral Nerve Disorders: Pathology and Genetics, First Edition. Edited by Jean-Michel Vallat, Joachim Weis, Francoise Gray, and Katy Keohane.

Table 25.1 Main causes of infectious neuropathies.

Infectious Neuropathies		
Bacterial	Leprosy	
	Lyme	
	Diphtheria	
Viral	Herpes virus	Simplex
		Varicella Zoster
		Epstein–Barr virus
		Cytomegalovirus
	HVC	
	HIV	
	HTLV-1	
	Arbovirus	
Parasitic	*T cruzi*	
	Schistosomiasis	
	Strongyloidiasis	
	Malaria	
	Toxoplasmosis	
	Cyclosporidiosis	
	Giardiasis	
	Leishmaniasis	
	Cysticercosis,	
	Dracunculosis	
	Coenurosis	
	Onchocerciasis	
	Hydatidosis	

considered exotic and rare, leprous neuropathy occurs in developed countries, due to worldwide travel and immigration [8] and should be considered in the differential diagnosis of neuropathies. Despite widespread implementation of effective multidrug therapy, leprosy has not been eradicated and continues to be a global challenge to health. About 250,000 new cases are detected annually [6]. The mode of transmission is human to human but the incubation period is not known and may be very prolonged. Damage to nerves may occur before, during, and after treatment, resulting in disabilities and long-term disfigurement, which is associated with stigma. Early diagnosis is important to alleviate patient suffering and prevent and reverse nerve damage. Recent reports of co-infected patients with *M. leprae* and HIV are described next.

Clinical features including appropriate investigations

The cardinal diagnostic features of leprosy are anesthetic skin lesions, neuropathy, and positive skin smears demonstrating the bacilli. Uncommonly, pure neuritic leprosy without skin lesions occurs [9] so leprosy must be considered in the differential diagnosis of a peripheral neuropathy, even without skin lesions, especially in a patient from an endemic country [3, 4].

The lepromatous (Virchowian) form usually presents as a symmetric polyneuropathy with sensory loss, initially for pain and temperature. The tuberculoid form is a well-localized, asymmetrical disease process with mono- or polyneuropathies. The borderline type is most unstable, and deteriorates towards the lepromatous form in the absence of treatment, or improves towards the tuberculoid form with treatment. Intermediate leprosy is a transitional form of the early infection with subtle clinical manifestations and usually consists of a solitary hypopigmented macule with impaired sensation. In leprosy late-onset neuropathy (LLON), patients have a painful neuropathy (PN) with no concurrent cause apart from a past history of successfully treated leprosy [10]. A delayed immune reaction could explain the late onset. A painful multiplex neuritis and polyneuropathy, respectively, were reported in two cases.

In addition to clinical examination, neurophysiological investigations can be helpful. Early in the disease there may be demyelinating features but as the disease progresses secondary axonal damage commonly ensues. In leprosy patients, motor weakness in the muscles innervated by the ulnar nerve correlates with both ultrasound evidence of ulnar nerve thickening and slowing of ulnar nerve motor conduction. Ultrasound provides additional information of an altered echogenic signal in the involved nerve and of the location of nerve enlargement [11].

Morphological aspects

Nerve biopsy is an important means of diagnosing leprosy in neural forms where skin lesions are not clinically or histologically definitive [7, 12]. Additionally, PCR on nerve biopsy tissue and enzyme-linked immunosorbent assay (ELISA) to detect anti-phenolic glycolipid 1 IgM antibodies may be helpful [13]. Biopsy is also useful to assess the efficacy of treatment, since cutaneous lesions regress but neurological manifestations persist in some cases and viable bacilli may be present in the nerve. The sural nerve, superficial radial or dorsal cutaneous branch of the ulnar (DCBU), the normal morphology and morphometry of which have been described [14], are most commonly biopsied.

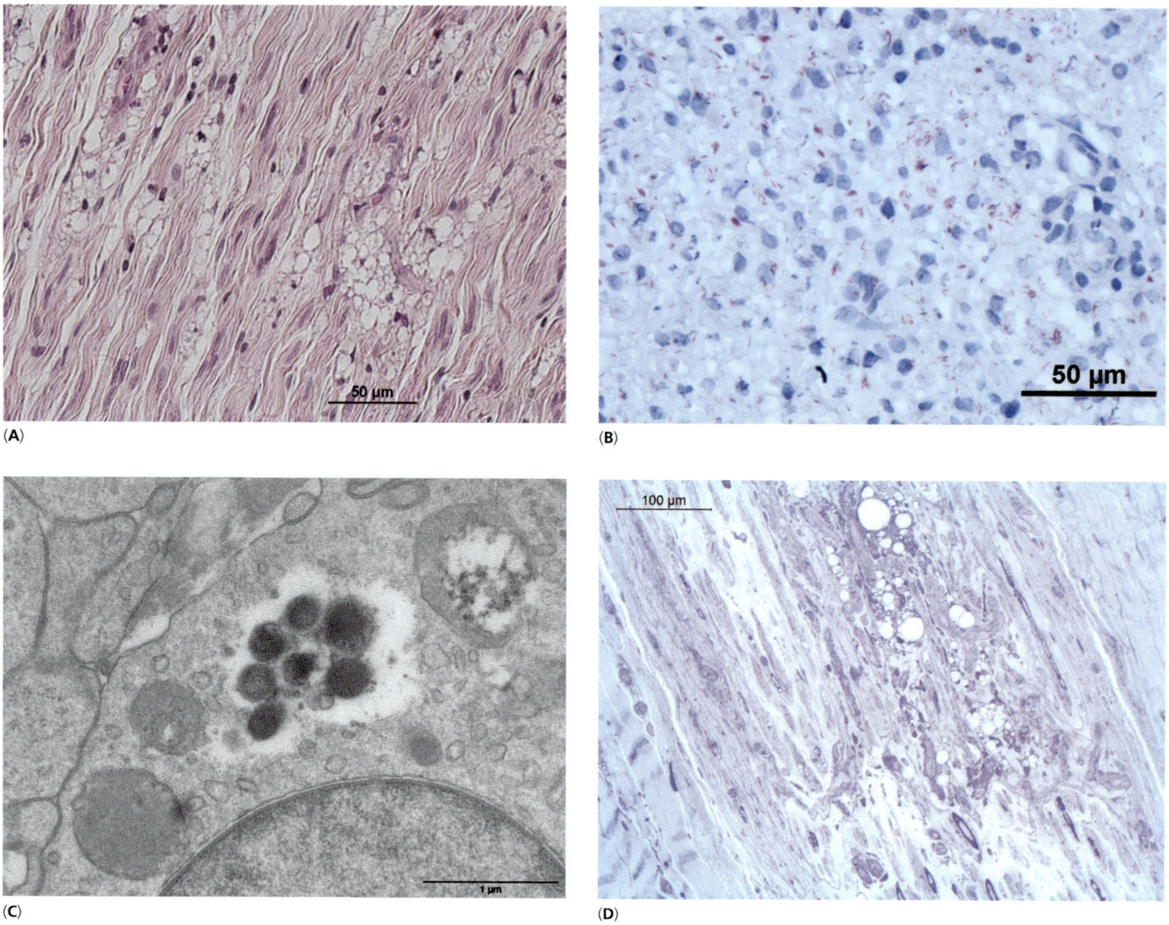

Figure 25.1 Lepromatous leprosy. (**A**) Numerous Virchow's cells in lepromatous leprosy (H&E, ×50). (**B**) Ziehl method for AFB, shows numerous Hansen's bacilli in Virchow's cells × 500). (**C**) Ultrastructural image of numerous bacilli in a Virchow cell. (**D**) Chronic treated case: Empty vacuoles that previously contained bacilli are seen on a semi-thin (1 µm) section (toluidine blue, ×250).

In *Virchowian (multibacillary, lepromatous) leprosy*, there is nearly always widespread cutaneous sensory nerve involvement even in patients with no clinical signs of neuropathy. Most cases show moderate inflammation with widespread infiltration of the endoneurium, perineurium, and epineurium by numerous macrophages (Fig. 25.1A). The macrophage cytoplasm is filled with acid-fast bacilli (AFB) (Fig. 25.1B), sometimes arranged in large aggregates (globi). The bacilli are abundant, especially in the cytoplasm of Remak cells. On ultrastructural examination, they predominate in macrophages and Schwann cells, but may also be seen in axons and in endothelial cell cytoplasm. Individual or groups of bacteria are surrounded by a clear electron-lucent halo (Fig. 25.1C). There is demyelination and axonal loss, predominantly involving small myelinated and unmyelinated fibers. In chronic treated cases, there may be empty vacuoles that previously contained bacilli (Fig. 25.1D).

In *tuberculoid (pauci bacillary) leprosy*, bacilli are either absent or extremely rare on light microscopic examination resulting in a well-localized, asymmetrical disease process. Granulomatous infiltrates predominate, consisting of T-lymphocytes with some B cells, plasma cells, Langhans giant cells, and histiocytes (Fig. 25.2A). Caseous necrosis may occur, producing abscesses. There is marked distortion of the walls of capillaries and small vessels due to inflammation (Fig. 25.2B). Axons, Schwann cells, and myelin are lost, and there is perineurial and endoneurial fibrosis (Fig. 25.2C); the nerves adjacent to granulomatous

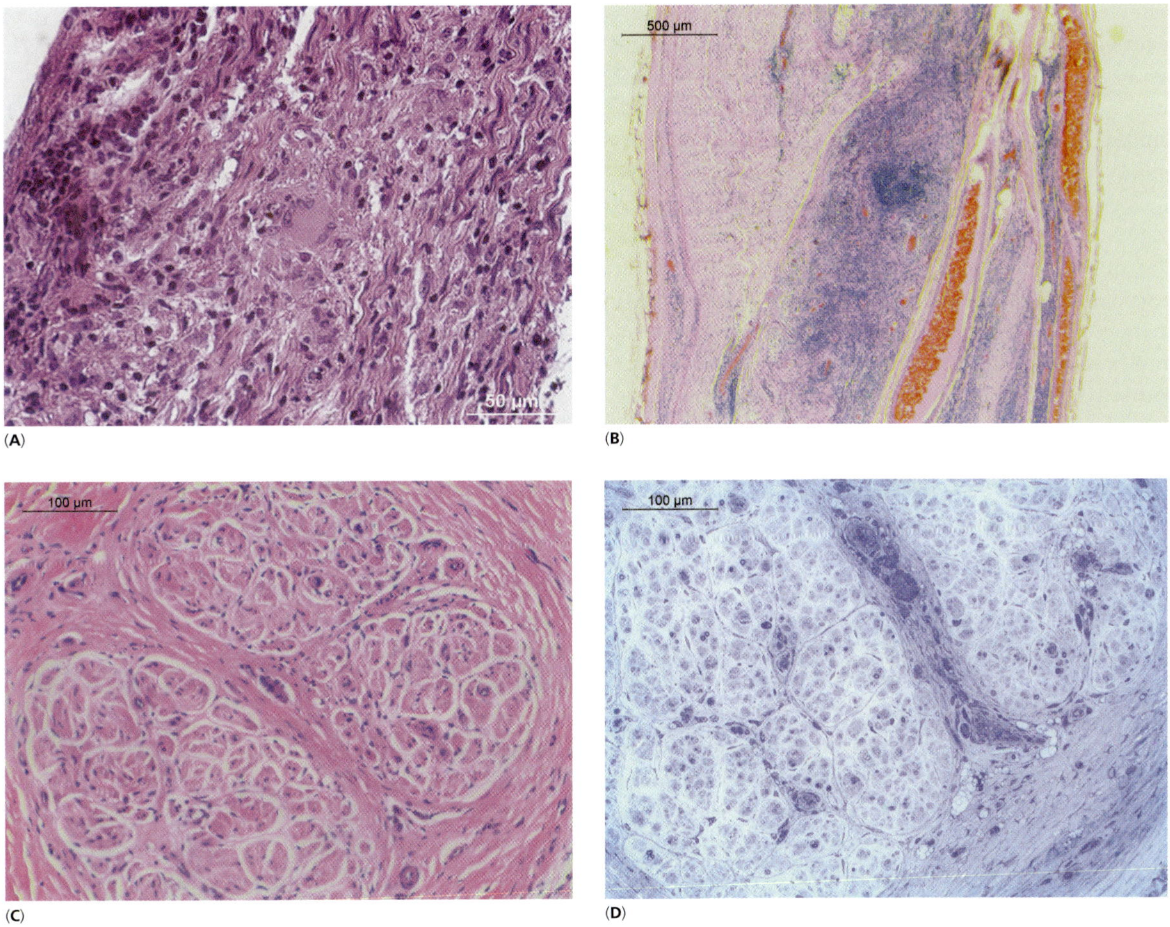

Figure 25.2 Leprosy. (**A**) Granulomatous infiltration in the endoneurium consisting of lymphocytes, plasma cells, Langhans giant cells, and histiocytes (H&E). (**B**) Dense inflammatory infiltrate in one fascicle distorting endoneurial vessels (H&E, ×25). (**C**) Epineurial and endoneurial fibrosis. Microfasciculation of the endoneurium can also be seen in this paraffin embedded tissue (H&E, ×200). (**D**) Microfasciculation of the endoneurium in a semithin (1 µm) section (Toluidine Blue, ×250).

foci of inflammation are partially or completely destroyed and replaced by fibrous tissue and become abnormally firm with nodular thickenings.

Borderline leprosy is characterized by variable combinations of the changes in lepromatous and tuberculoid forms and is responsible for pure neural leprosy.

In the *indeterminate form*, nerve trunks are usually not affected. There is mild inflammatory infiltration in cutaneous nerves and a small number of bacilli. Skin biopsies are also useful to detect early changes in dermal and epidermal nerves.

Microfasciculation is a perineurial response in leprosy neuropathies and is strongly associated with perineurial damage and a multibacillary inflammatory process in the nerves, particularly in the perineurium [15]. Microfascicles are composed predominantly of unmyelinated fibers and denervated Schwann cells surrounded by fibroblast-perineurial cells (Fig. 25.2D) and were found more frequently in actively inflamed leprosy nerves with AFB and perineurial damage.

In *LLON* microvasculitis was seen on nerve biopsy with no bacilli.

Secondary amyloidosis may occur.

Genetics

Genomics have provided insight into the biology and drug resistance of HB. *M. leprae* has undergone reductive evolution and pseudogenes now occupy half of its genome. Comparative genomics of four different strains revealed remarkable conservation of the genome (99.995% identity) yet uncovered 215 polymorphic sites, mainly single nucleotide polymorphisms, and a handful of new pseudogenes. Mapping these polymorphisms in a large panel of strains defined 16 single nucleotide polymorphism-subtypes with strong geographical associations, which helped retrace the evolution of *M. leprae*. Host genetics are also important in susceptibility to leprosy. The results of genome-wide analyses (linkage and association) and candidate gene studies suggest an independent genetic control over both susceptibility to leprosy per se and development of clinical subtype [16].

Treatment and future perspectives

Immune responses and mechanisms involved in nerve damage are not clearly understood. There is no test for predicting the extent of nerve damage and no good evidence on the best treatment [6]. A third of newly diagnosed patients has nerve damage and is at risk of disability. Several factors, including the level of self-care, influence the risk.

Research on diagnosis, treatment, and prevention, such as further use of molecular analysis of the *Mycobacterium leprae* genome, implementation of BCG vaccination, and chemoprophylaxis for household contacts are recommended. The development of tools for early diagnosis and detection of infection and nerve damage, and strategies to manage the chronic complications of leprosy, such as immune-mediated reactions and neuropathy, are also necessary.

Advances in understanding the pathogenesis, mapping the genome, and other developments in molecular biology may result in better preventive and therapeutic measures, and the goal of eradicating leprosy as a global problem may yet be realized.

At the present time, in early cases, standard therapy recommended by WHO includes rifampicin, dapsone, and clofaimine for 6–12 months, depending on the form of the disease.

Diphtheria

Diphtheria is due to an infection by a Gram positive *Corynebacterium diphtheriae* causing sore throat and upper respiratory or skin infection transmitted by aerosols. It is rare nowadays since its occurrence is entirely preventable by immunization, but small epidemics continue to occur [17]. Ten percent of patients develop a neuropathy that represents the prototypic demyelinating neuropathy.

Neuropathic symptoms first appear 2–7 weeks after onset of the infection and include numbness of the tongue and face and dysphonia, impaired swallowing and respiratory function, and oculomotor disturbance. Motor and sensory deficits occur in limbs when the cranial nerve deficits have begun to abate.

Nerve biopsy is very rarely undertaken in diphtheria. Neuropathological changes are confined to the PNS, have a patchy distribution and consist of segmental demyelinating changes extending from the paranodes. There is minimal inflammation and axonal degeneration is rare.

Molecular pathogenesis and pathophysiology are explained by a toxic protein secreted by *C. diphtheriae*, encoded by the *tox* bacteriophage gene.

Borreliosis, or Lyme disease (tick-bite meningoradiculoneuritis)

Definition

Lyme disease (LD) is caused by infection with several genospecies from the spirochete *Borrelia burgdorferi* (B.b) sensu lato complex and is transmitted by bites of infected ixodoid ticks. It is a multisystem infectious disease affecting individuals exposed professionally as well as individuals resident in or visiting an endemic area.

Epidemiology

LD is the most common tick-borne infectious disease in North America and in European and Asian countries with moderate climates. About 10–15% of infected patients develop a neuropathy, in Germany the figure is about 5% [18].

Clinical features

At the earliest stage, a few days or weeks after a tick bite, a skin lesion (erythema migrans) appears at the site of inoculation and disappears in several weeks. Symptoms and signs of PNS involvement appear at the second stage, a few weeks or months later, and may be associated with involvement of the meninges, the heart, and the joints. Acute, sensory-motor painful radiculopathy, plexopathy, multiplex neuropathy, or polyneuropathy can occur; cranial nerves are also often involved. ENMG usually shows anomalies suggesting an axonal neuropathy; CSF study reveals pleocytosis and elevated protein.

In late LD, which is quite rare, peripheral nerve involvement (axonal) is more or less latent, often associated with acrodermatitis chronica atrophicans (ACA). CSF is normal.

At every stage, the diagnosis is suspected on clinical signs and confirmed by a specific serology.

Pathology

Signs of acute axonal involvement are found in nerve biopsies in the secondary stage; nerve roots, dorsal root ganglia, and distal nerve segments are involved. There is a strong inflammatory mononuclear reaction around blood vessels in the endoneurium, perineurium, and epineurium (Fig. 25.3). Lymphocytes appear mainly of the B-type. In our experience, demyelinating lesions or infiltrating inflammatory cells with dissociation of myelin lamellae like that seen in GBS did not occur, and there was no necrosis of vessel walls [19]. Schafers *et al.* have studied various types of cytokines in the nerves of several patients [18].

A few authors have reported neuropathies associated with ACA in the tertiary stage; the lesions were axonal without inflammatory cells. In one case, PCR confirmed B.b DNA in the sural nerve demonstrating that the spirochete was still localized in the PNS; complement membrane around small vessels confirmed an associated immune process.

Nerve biopsy is not used to diagnose LD in the second stage but should be considered in neuropathy of undetermined cause with a combination of axonal involvement and signs of inflammation.

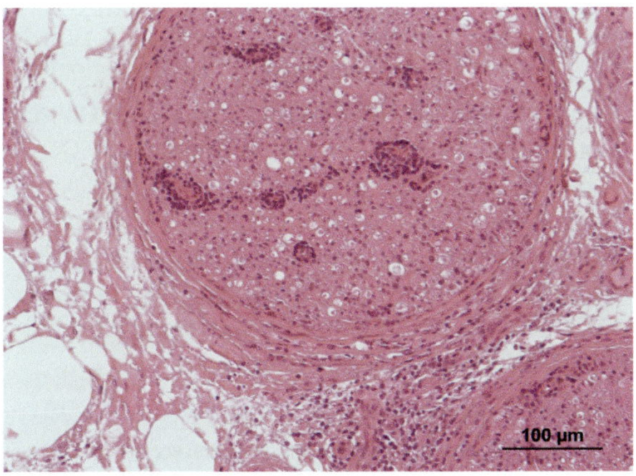

Figure 25.3 Lyme disease. Paraffin embedded transverse section of a sural nerve (H&E). Numerous mononuclear cells. around all vessels of the endoneurium and in the perineurium and epineurium. The vessel walls are not necrotic.

Pathogenesis and animal models

The pathogenesis of peripheral nerve lesions is unknown. The efficacy of antibiotics suggests direct infiltration by the organisms although they have never been seen within nerves in humans. The infection may also induce post-infectious autoimmune reactions perhaps due to molecular mimicry. Primates inoculated with a strain of B.b develop infection of multiple tissues including CNS and PNS; the spirochete has a tropism for meninges and connective tissues. Several innate immune defects modulating disease development have been observed in human and experimental infections, and significant heterogeneity exists between B.b spirochetes. These factors could explain why the infection induces a significant variety of disorders.

Treatment

Antibiotics are beneficial for all clinical manifestations of LD. In the second stage, parenteral therapy with ceftriaxone or doxycycline or penicillin G should be used for 3 weeks.

Viral infections

A number of viruses may infect the PNS and cause peripheral neuropathies. However, in some cases, neuropathy is not observed. As an example, rabies virus invades PNS axons thereby spreading to the CNS, but it does not induce any peripheral neuropathy.

Herpes viruses

Neuropathies may be produced by five types of human herpes viruses (HHV) (Table 25.2) [20].

Herpes simplex virus (HSV) 1 and 2

Neurologic disease usually occurs after reactivation of the latent virus. Primary HSV infection typically involves the oropharynx and genitals. Most infections are subclinical and are followed by latent infection in ganglionic neurons.

Neurologic complications include encephalitis (usually with HSV-1) or aseptic meningitis and recurrent radiculopathy (usually with HSV-2). Extension of virus into the meninges may produce aseptic meningitis,

Table 25.2 Neuropathies associated with human herpes viruses infections.

HSV-1	HSV-2	VZV	EBV	CMV
Bell's palsy	Radiculopathy	Zoster (radicular pain with rash)	Cranial neuropathies	Polyradiculopathy
		Zoster sine herpete	Radiculopathy with or without myelitis and encephalitis	Retinopathy
		(radicular pain without rash)	Acute autonomic neuropathy	Guillain–Barré syndrome
		Postherpetic neuralgia		Mononeuritis multiplex

often recurrent. The same mechanism probably accounts for isolated cases of HSV radiculitis, but peripheral nerves are not involved by HSV.

Varicella zoster virus (VZV)

VZV is a neurotropic human herpes virus that, after causing chickenpox (varicella), becomes latent in cranial nerve, dorsal root, and autonomic nervous system ganglia. Reactivation produces shingles (zoster), characterized by pain and a rash usually restricted to one to three dermatomes. There is increased incidence in elderly and immune-compromised individuals. Post herpetic neural pain may persist for months or years and may reflect a chronic VZV ganglionitis. VZV DNA is latent in ganglia of over 90% of normal adults.

Epstein–Barr virus (EBV)

EBV is the cause of infectious mononucleosis and is latent in most adult humans. It may cause aseptic meningitis, cerebellar ataxia, encephalitis, myelitis, neuritis, or overlapping myeloneuritis. Biological signs of EBV infection may be found in some patients presenting a Guillain–Barré or a Miller–Fisher syndrome. The pathology corresponds to these syndromes and may be quite inflammatory.

Cytomegalovirus (CMV)

CMV is the most common opportunistic pathogen in immune compromised individuals, in whom reactivation leads to infection in multiple organs including the CNS and PNS.

Myeloradiculopathy usually occurs in HIV-infected patients, but has decreased since the introduction of highly active antiretroviral therapy (HAART). Pathological changes include a prominent polymorphonuclear and mononuclear cell infiltrate involving the sacral spinal cord, cauda equina, and lumbosacral nerve roots associated with both demyelination and axonal destruction. CMV antigens and sometimes inclusion bodies (Fig. 25.4A) are present in Schwann cells and endothelial cells of involved roots.

Mononeuritis multiplex in AIDS patients is due to infarction of cranial and peripheral nerves. Nerve biopsies show polymorphonuclear cells associated with multifocal necrotic endoneurial lesions and frank necrotizing arteritis with fibrinoid necrosis. CMV inclusions may be seen in infiltrating inflammatory cells, Schwann cells, and endothelial cells of the vasa nervorum.

CMV infection may precede GBS in both immune-competent and immune-compromised individuals; the mechanism is probably via molecular mimicry. Anti-GM2 antibodies have been detected in sera from approximately 40% of GB patients with recent CMV infection

Human T cell lymphotropic virus 1 (HTLV-1)

Most cases of HTLV-1 infection of the nervous system have been associated with tropical spastic paraparesis (TSP). There are some poorly-documented instances of peripheral nerve involvement that may reflect lesions induced by vasculitis involving the *vasa nervorum* (Fig. 25.4B). A few patients show muscle atrophy indicative of anterior horn cell involvement [21].

Peripheral neuropathies associated with human immunodeficiency (HIV) infection

Peripheral neuropathy has become the chief neurological syndrome in individuals infected with HIV-1 [22]. Between 5 and 40% of these patients have some clinical

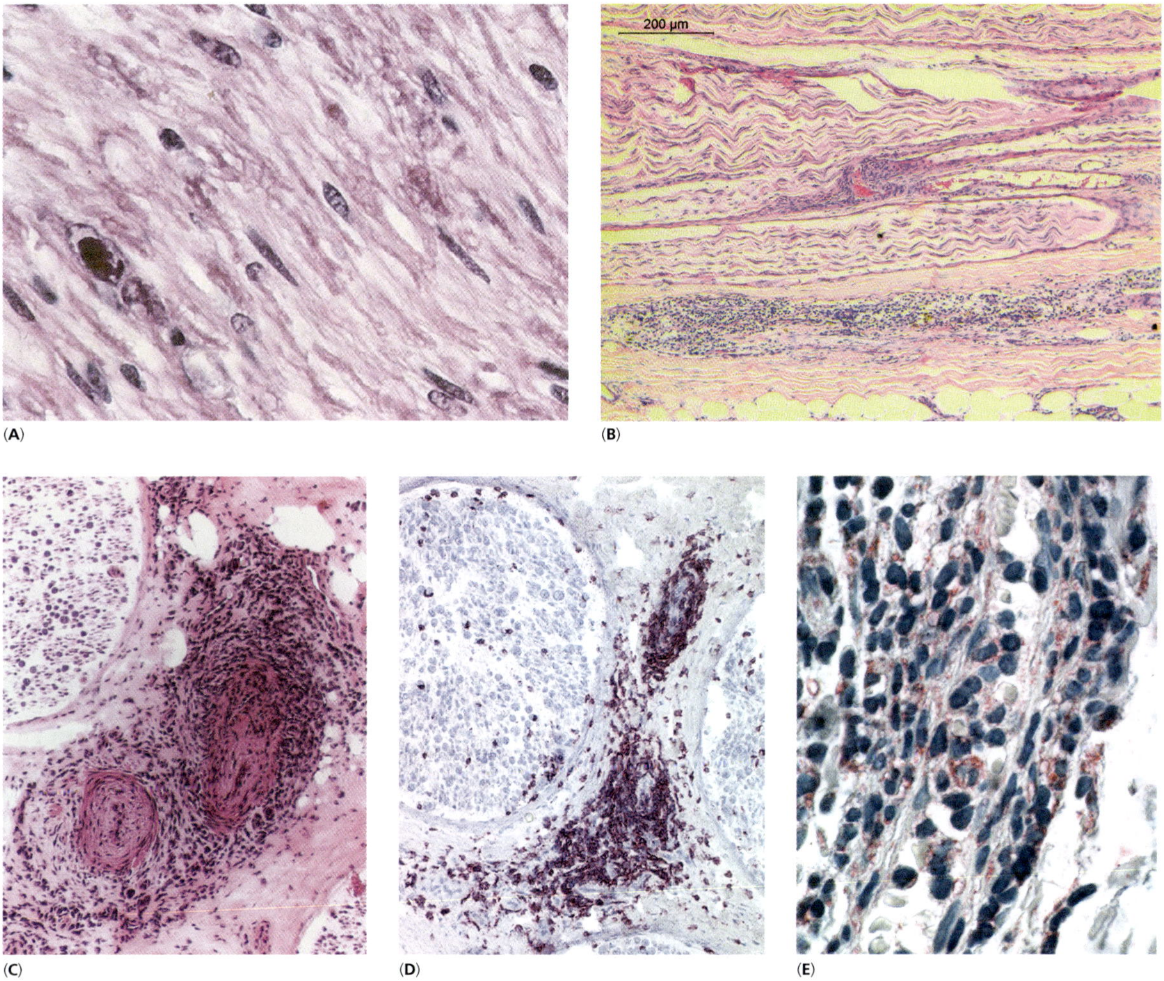

Figure 25.4 Viral neuropathies. (**A**) CMV cytomegalic cell with a characteristic intranuclear inclusion body in a case of CMV myeloradiculitis in an AIDS patient (H&E, ×500). (**B**) Lymphocytic infitrate and vasculitis in vasa nervorum of neuropathy associated with HTLV-1 infection (H&E, ×40). (**C, D, E**) DILS (courtesy of Fabrice Chrétien). (**C**) Massive perivascular lymphocytic infiltration of the epineurium (H&E, ×100). (**D**) CD8 Immunostaining shows that most lymphocytes in the epineurium are CD8+ lymphocytes; CD8+ lymphocytes are also present in the endoneurium (×100). (**E**) Immunostaining for HIV protein p24 shows abundant viral load in perivascular macrophages (×400).

evidence of peripheral neuropathy; those due to antiretroviral therapies, which are increasingly frequent, may be clinically indistinguishable from those caused by HIV or by cytomegalovirus (cf. Section on Cytomegalovirus). A number of HIV-associated neuropathies have been described that do not seem to be the direct result of viral infection; however, *in situ* hybridization and immunocytochemistry have detected viral antigen in mononuclear endoneurial cells.

Different types of neuropathies related to HIV infection

Different types of neuropathies related to HIV infection have been described (Table 25.3).

DSP, the most common subtype of HIV-associated neuropathy is characterized by axonal and distal dying back degeneration of long axons, unmyelinated fiber loss and varying degrees of macrophage infiltration. Its pathogenesis is unclear. HIV has been

Table 25.3 Neuropathies associated with human immunodeficiency virus infection.

Inflammatory demyelinating polyradiculoneuropathies (GBS, CIDP)	Occur mainly in the early stages of the disease Frequently associated with pleocytosis in CSF
Distal symmetric predominantly sensory neuropathy (DSP)	
Acute or subacute mononeuritis multiplex	Due to vasculitis or necrotizing vasculitis Some related to CMV opportunistic infection Rare lymphomatous neuropathies which can present as a lumbosacral radiculoplexus neuropathy and tend to be asymmetrical [29]
Autonomic neuropathy	
Diffuse infiltrative lymphocytic syndrome (DILS)	

identified in DSP nerve biopsies; however, viral replication is limited to a small percentage of macrophages. It seems likely that nerve damage can be mediated by macrophage activation and the effects of pro-inflammatory cytokines similar to the proposed mechanism in the CNS. However, *in situ* end-labeling detected DNA strand breaks in DRG neurons of AIDS patients with axonal polyneuropathy suggesting that apoptosis of DRG neurons may play a role in the pathogenesis of DSP [23].

Autonomic dysfunction is common in HIV and associated with distal symmetric polyneuropathy [24]. Post-mortem examination of sensory and autonomic ganglia may show lymphocytes, activated macrophages, and loss of ganglion cells [25]. HIV p24 antigen was detected by PCR or *in situ* hybridization in the absence of sensory neuropathy, or autonomic disorder indicating that infection occurs early before the development of neuropathy in some patients.

Diffuse infiltrative lymphocytosis syndrome (DILS) is a rarer form of neuropathy associated with HIV due to a systemic host-determined antigen response to HIV. It is characterized by persistent CD8 hyperlymphocytosis and a Sjögren-like syndrome with multivisceral CD8 T cell infiltration associated with expression of HIV protein and HIV genome [26, 27]. Nerve biopsy in DILS shows marked angiocentric CD8 infiltrate without mural necrosis (Fig. 25.4C,D) and abundant expression of HIV p24 protein in macrophages (Fig. 25.4E). Localized DILS predominantly affecting the PNS (lumbosacral roots, plexus, and lower limb nerves) have been described [28] and may resemble a lymphomatous neuropathy [29].

Toxic neuropathies

Toxic neuropathies, caused by the *dideoxinucleosides* (ddI, ddC, and d4T) are dose-dependent and neurotoxicity is usually the dose-limiting factor in antiretroviral therapy. Clinically, they resemble DSP and have mainly sensory manifestations that occur in later stages of HIV infection. Interference in DNA synthesis and mitochondrial abnormalities produced by nucleoside antiretrovirals are considered to be factors involved in toxic neuropathies.

Sural nerve biopsies in patients with ddC neuropathy show intense axonal destruction, especially of unmyelinated fibers, abnormal mitochondria with broken ridges in axons, increased lactate production, and accumulation of fat in the affected cells.

Skin biopsies

Skin biopsies have become useful in the evaluation of HIV-associated neuropathies. Reduced fiber density, increased frequency of varicosities, and fragmentation of fibers are common findings [30] (cf. Chapter 3).

HIV neuropathies in the HAART era

Following the introduction of HAART, the prevalence of DSP decreased significantly. Also opportunistic infections and DILS declined, but the prevalence of toxic neuropathies increased, probably related to antiretroviral nucleoside analogues. A classification based on the stage and CD4 cell count [22] has been proposed (Table 25.4).

Co-infection of HIV and leprosy

Early in the HIV epidemic, it was predicted that HIV infection would worsen leprosy outcomes. However, epidemiologic and clinical studies suggest that the

Table 25.4 Classification of HIV-associated neuropathies in the HAART era.

Early HIV disease CD4 cell count >500 cells/μl	Seroconversion neuropathies (facial nerve palsy) GBS
Moderately advanced HIV disease CD4 cell count 200–500 cells/μl	Vasculitis CIDP Superimposed infections (Hepatitis C, HTLV-1, *Varicella Zoster*) Diffuse infiltrative lymphocytic syndrome (DILS)
Advanced HIV disease CD4 cell count <200 cells/μl	DSP CMV-related neuropathy
Antiretroviral drug related neuropathies *Autonomic neuropathy*	

course of leprosy in co-infected patients has not been greatly altered by HIV infection. In contrast, initiation of antiretroviral treatment has been associated with activation of subclinical *Mycobacterium leprae* infection and exacerbation of existing leprosy lesions [31], including leprosy-associated immune reconstitution inflammatory syndrome (IRIS).

Co-infection of HIV and hepatitis C

Co-infection of HIV and hepatitis C has become increasingly prevalent [32]. It is a major source of morbidity in HIV-infected populations. The symptoms and signs of HIV and hepatitis C neuropathy overlap.

Neuropathies associated with hepatitis virus infection

Hepatitis C (HCV)

In several cases, cryoglobulinemia (CG) (mainly mixed: type II and III) elicit inflammation and occlusion of small and medium sized blood vessels and induce vasculitis or necrotizing arteritis. In cases without CG, immune complexes or HCV-induced autoimmune mechanisms cause vascular and perivascular inflammation. In these cases, nerve lesions are axonal; clinically the patients present with mononeuropathy or mononeuritis multiplex.

Pure symmetrical sensory neuropathies are the most common type. They are considered as probably secondary to ganglioneuritis. Chronic demyelinating inflammatory neuropathies (CIDP, Lewis–Sumner syndrome) can also occur; in a few cases, treatment with interferon alpha has been performed.

Hepatitis B

Hepatitis B infection can cause neuropathy either due to vasculitis associated with polyarteritis nodosa or immune-mediated neural damage.

Chikungunya virus (CHIKV)

Chikungunya is a relatively rare and benign arboviral infection caused by a RNA-virus belonging to genus *Alphavirus* of *Togaviridae* family. It is transmitted from primates to humans by *Aedes aegypti* mosquito causing an acute symptomatic illness with fever, skin rash, and incapacitating arthralgia. The risk of importation and spreading disease has increased given the global distribution of the vectors [33]. In this context, peripheral nerve involvement presents as a typical GBS.

Parasitic infections of the peripheral nervous system

Only a few parasites damage the peripheral nervous system, either by direct invasion, with concurrent tissue damage, or by indirectly affecting host tissues and organs through metabolic disturbances, pressure effects, aberrant migration, toxins, and immunologic mechanisms [34].

American T rypanosomiasis or Chagas' disease

American Trypanosomiasis or Chagas' disease is one of the most prevalent and important parasitic infections affecting the peripheral nervous system. Chagas' disease is caused by the protozoan *Trypanosoma cruzi* and is widespread throughout Latin America, particularly in rural areas, despite a substantial reduction in its incidence. It is transmitted mainly by the insect vector hematophagous triatomine bugs (80–90%), but also by blood transfusion (5–20%), congenital routes (0.5–8%), organ transplants, and accidental laboratory infection. Trypomastigotes is the form responsible for the dissemination of the infection through the blood or lymphatic circulation and infects autonomic ganglia, nerve fibers of the heart and the enteric plexuses of Meissner and Auerbach.

During the acute phase, about 10% of the patients, especially children, develop a severe acute illness with encephalitis and myocarditis. Scanty parasitized cells persist as a latent infection, within inflammatory foci in cardiac and extra-cardiac tissues. CNS lesions are not prominent in the absence of immunosuppression, but peripheral nerves, particularly the autonomic nerves are frequently involved in the chronic phase. The conduction systems of the heart and autonomic plexus in the wall of the esophagus and gut are particularly affected leading to dysfunction in peristalsis, which culminates in the development of megaesophagus and/or megacolon. Peripheral somatosensory neuropathies including involvement of dorsal root ganglia, anterior horn neurons, and peripheral sensory and motor nerve fibers are less frequent. Both axonal and demyelinating neuropathies have been diagnosed and may result from several autoimmune mechanisms.

Hypervariable nuclear markers such as microsatellites are now used to investigate the genetics of *Trypanosoma cruzi* and determine the clinical course of Chagas' disease [35].

Schistosoma

Early and late lesions of *Schistosomal neuritis* have been described involving the terminal ramifications of the median nerve in the forearm and nerves of the ureter, characterized by perineuritis in which the schistosomal ova penetrated the nerve sheath and, along with the granulomatous reaction, strangled the nerve bundles [36].

Other parasitic infections involving peripheral nerves

Facial and abducens nerves are occasionally affected in *angiostrongyliasis*. There may be inflammation caused by migration of living larvae or dead and degenerated parasites in the neural tissue [34].

Peripheral neuropathy has also been described in *trichinosis*, characterized by foot drop and facial palsy due to a peripheral neuritis.

In *giardiasis* denervation of distal muscles has been described but may be caused by malabsortion, which is common in this disease.

Isolated cases of *cysticerci* causing peripheral neuropathy due to mechanical and inflammatory effects of larva adherent to nerve have also been described and were characterized by dense inflammatory tissue surrounding a gelatinous material identified as the parasite *Cysticercus cellulosae*.

Cranial nerves can be involved in *Coenurosis*. Symptoms are due to a single cyst resulting in space-occupying lesion.

Rarely, footdrop and peripheral neuropathy caused by mechanical compression by intrapelvic *hydatid cysts* have been reported. Distal paresthesias and weakness are possibly immunoallergic.

Entrapment neuropathy of the median nerve resulting in carpel tunnel syndrome may occur in *dracunculiasis* or guinea worm disease.

Compression of the median nerve has been observed in *onchocerciasis* and is characterized by an adult *O. volvulos* worm surrounded by a granulomatous reaction and eosinophilic infiltration.

In cutaneous and visceral forms of *leishmaniasis*, nerves may be infiltrated with lymphohistiocytic cells and occasionally parasites.

Other parasitic diseases such as *malaria and toxoplasmosis* may be associated with GBS.

Genetic approaches for investigation of parasitic diseases

Genetic markers are now accessible for all organisms, including parasites. Amplified fragment length polymorphism (AFLP), a PCR-based marker, is an advanced type of genetic marker for the rapid screening of genetic diversity and intraspecific variation [37, 38].

Tropical neuropathies

Definition, historical perspective, and epidemiology

Tropical neuropathies are known for more than a century, since the first report by Strachan [39]. They constitute a heterogeneous group of neuromyelopathies of obscure etiology that occurs in geographical isolates, in tropical regions of Africa, Asia, and Latin America [40, 41] and thus may represent an important differential diagnosis for a number of infectious neuropathies. Usually most of the patients come from a rural background.

Clinical

Tropical neuropathies are broadly categorized into tropical ataxic neuropathy (TAN) with prominent sensory ataxia and symmetrical sensory polyneuropathy (most of the patients are complaining of "burning feet"), sensory-motor polyneuropathy and tropical spastic paraparesis (TSP) with prominent spastic gait disturbance with minimal sensory deficit. In addition, deafness and optic atrophy are not uncommonly encountered [41]. A majority of patients have gradual onset of symptoms, while acute or subacute onset rarely occurs. Overt causes of neuropathies such as diabetes mellitus, nutritional deficiency, toxin exposure, porphyria, paraneoplastic syndrome, and vasculitis have to be excluded [42].

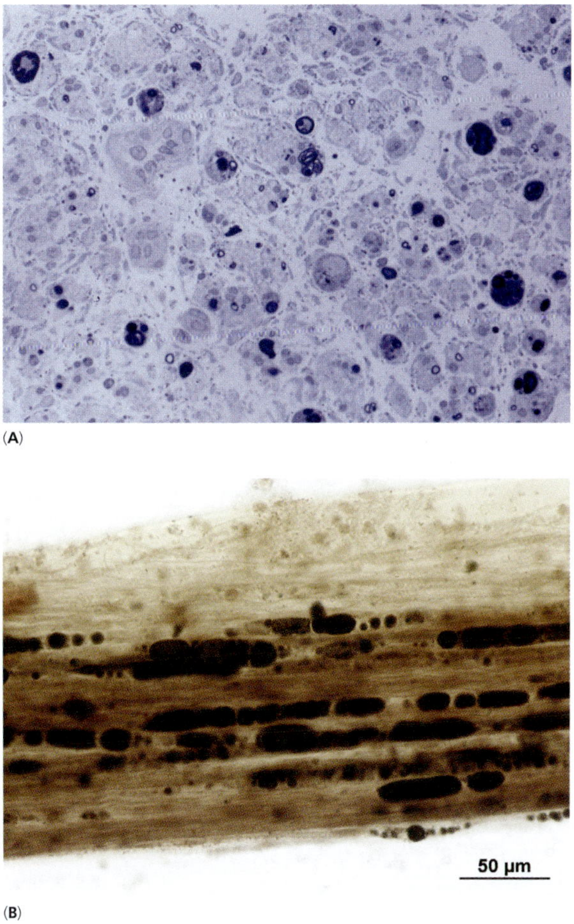

Figure 25.5 Tropical neuropathy. (**A**) Semithin transverse section: Toluidine blue. There are no normal myelinated fibers; there are numerous "ovoids" typical of acute axonal lesions. (**B**) Incomplete teasing. The rows of "ovoids" replace normal myelinated fibers that have completely disappeared.

Pathology

Pathological studies are quite rare in the literature [43]. Microscopic signs consist of severe axonal involvement affecting both unmyelinated and myelinated fibers. In the latter group, the larger fibers are usually most affected. Very few signs of regeneration are seen.

It is possible to discriminate acute, subacute, and chronic stages. At the acute stage, there are many ovoids attesting the severity of the lesions of the myelinated fibers (Figs 25.5A,B), while the destruction of the unmyelinated fibers are clearly detected by electron microscopy. At the chronic stage, there is a severe rarefaction of both myelinated and unmyelinated fibers, but after a few years, nerve fibers may regenerate. There are no inflammatory cells in the interstitial tissue, but numerous macrophages are present at the acute stage.

No histological signs can be found that might give a clue to the possible etiology of this disorder.

Pathogenesis and genetics

It is uncertain whether the clinical heterogeneity of tropical myeloneuropathies is related to differences in the etiopathogenesis, to genetic predispositions, or to a combination of these factors. The early descriptions attributed tropical neuromyelopathies to a nutritional deficiency resulting from combined poor dietary intake and malabsorption, later reports incriminated cassava neurotoxicity [42]. There is no history of diarrhea, malabsorption, or other intercurrent diseases prior to onset of symptoms. In a few females, the onset of symptoms correlated with the post-partum period of breast feeding.

Some cases of TSP and Tropical neuropathies have been associated with HTLVI infection with some poorly-documented instances of peripheral nerve involvement, possibly due to an underlying process such as vasculitis. Also, some cases of co-infection by HIV viruses have been observed.

References

1 Robinson-Papp J (2012) Infectious neuropathies. *Continuum (Minneap Minn)* 18: 126–138.
2 Said G (2007) Infectious neuropathies. *Neurol Clin* 25: 115–137.
3 de Freitas MR (2007) Infectious neuropathy. *Curr Opin Neurol* 20: 548–552.
4 Ooi WW, Srinivasan J (2004) Leprosy and the peripheral nervous system: basic and clinical aspects. *Muscle Nerve* 30: 393–409.
5 Scollard DM (2008) The biology of nerve injury in leprosy. *Lepr Rev* 79: 242–253.
6 Rodrigues LC, Lockwood DN (2011) Leprosy now: epidemiology, progress, challenges, and research gaps. *Lancet Infect Dis* 11: 464–470.
7 Chimelli L, Freitas M, Nascimento O (1997) Value of nerve biopsy in the diagnosis and follow-up of leprosy: the role of vascular lesions and usefulness of nerve studies in the detection of persistent bacilli. *J Neurol* 244: 318–323.
8 Koike H, Hashimoto R, Tomita M *et al.*(2011) The wide range of clinical manifestations in leprous neuropathy: two case reports. *Intern Med* 50: 2223–2226.
9 Nascimento OJ, Freitas MR, Escada T *et al.*(2012) Leprosy late-onset neuropathy: an uncommon presentation of leprosy. *Arq Neuropsiquiatr* 70: 404–406.
10 Bathala L, Kumar K, Pathapati R *et al.*(2012) Ulnar neuropathy in Hansen disease: clinical, high-resolution ultrasound and electrophysiologic correlations. *J Clin Neurophysiol* 29: 190–193.
11 Wen Y, Xing Y, Yuan LC *et al.*(2013) Whole-blood nested-PCR amplification of M. leprae-specific DNA for early diagnosis of leprosy. *Am J Trop Med Hyg* 88: 918–922.
12 Vallat J-M, Anthony D, De Girolami U (2004) *Peripheral Nerve Diseases*. In: Gray F, De Girolami U, Poirier J (eds) *Escourolle & Poirier Manual of Basic Neuropathology* 4th edn, pp. 315–343. Butterworth-Heinemann, Philadelphia.
13 Antunes SL, Chimelli L, Jardim MR *et al.* (2012). Histopathological examination of nerve samples from pure neural leprosy patients: obtaining maximum information to improve diagnostic efficiency. *Mem Inst Oswaldo Cruz* 107: 246–253.
14 Oliveira AL, Fazan VP, Marques W Jr *et al.* (2011) Dorsal cutaneous branch of the ulnar nerve: a light and electron microscopy histometric study. *J Peripher Nerv Syst* 16: 98–101.
15 Antunes SL, Medeiros MF, Corte-Real S (2011) Microfasciculation: a morphological pattern in leprosy nerve damage. *Histopathology* 58: 304–311.
16 Eiglmeier K, Simon S, Garnier T *et al.* (2001) The integrated genome map of Mycobacterium leprae. *Lepr Rev* 72: 462–469.
17 Pleasure D, Messing A (2005) Diphtheric Polyneuropathy. In: Dyck PJ and Thomas PK (eds) *Peripheral Neuropathy*, 4th edn, pp. 2147–2151. Elsevier Saunders, Philadelphia.
18 Schafers M, Neurkichen S, Toyka KV *et al.* (2008) Diagnostic value of sural nerve biposy in patients with suspected Borrelia neuropathy. *J Periph Nerv Syst* 13: 81–91.
19 Vallat JM, Hugon J, Lubeau M *et al.* (1987) Tick-bite meningo-radiculoneuritis. *Neurology* 37: 749–753.
20 Gilden DH, Tyler KL (2005). Herpes Infection and Peripheral Neuropathy. In: Dyck PJ and Thomas PK (eds) *Peripheral Neuropathy*, 4th edn, pp. 2117–2127. Elsevier Saunders, Philadelphia.
21 Leite AC, Silva MT, Alamy AH *et al.* (2004) Peripheral neuropathy in HTLV-I infected individuals without tropical spastic paraparesis/HTLV-I-associated myelopathy. *J Neurol* 251: 877–881.
22 Brew BJ (2003) The peripheral nerve complications of human immunodeficiency virus (HIV) infection. *Muscle Nerve* 28:542–552.
23 Adle-Biassette H, Bell JE, Creange A *et al.* (1998) DNA breaks detected by in situ end-labelling in dorsal root ganglia of patients with AIDS. *Neuropathol Appl Neurobiol* 24: 373–380.
24 Robinson-Papp J, Sharma S, Simpson DM *et al.* (2013) Autonomic dysfunction is common in HIV and associated with distal symmetric polyneuropathy. *J Neurovirol* 19: 172–180.
25 Chimelli L, Martins AR (2002) Degenerative and inflammatory lesions in sympathetic ganglia: further morphological evidence for an autonomic neuropathy in AIDS. *J NeuroAIDS* 2: 67–82.
26 Moulignier A, Authier FJ, Baudrimont M, *et al.* (1997) Peripheral neuropathy in human immunodeficiency virus-infected patients with the diffuse infiltrative lymphocytosis syndrome. *Ann Neurol* 41: 438–445.
27 Gherardi RK, Chretien F, Delfau-Larue MH, *et al.* (1998) Neuropathy in diffuse infiltrative lymphocytosis syndrome: an HIV neuropathy, not a lymphoma. *Neurology* 50: 1041–1044.
28 Chahin N, Temesgen Z, Kurtin PJ *et al.* (2010) HIV lumbosacral radiculoplexus neuropathy mimicking lymphoma: Diffuse Infiltrative Lymphocytosis Syndrome (DILS) restricted to Nerve? *Muscle Nerve* 41: 276–282.
29 Gold JE, Jimenez E, Zalusky R (1988) Human immunodeficiency virus-related lymphoreticular malignancies and peripheral neurologic disease. A report of four cases. *Cancer* 61: 2318–2324.
30 Mellgren SI, Nolano M, Sommer C (2013) The cutaneous nerve biopsy: technical aspects, indications, and contribution. *Handb Clin Neurol* 115: 171–188.
31 Pavie J, De Castro N, Molina JM *et al.* (2010) Severe peripheral neuropathy following HAART initiation in an HIV-infected patient with leprosy. *J Int Assoc Physicians AIDS Care (Chic)* 9: 232–235.
32 Estanislao LB, Morgello S, Simpson DM (2005) Peripheral neuropathies associated with HIV and hepatitis C co-infection: a review. *AIDS* 19 Suppl 3: S135–139.

33 Das T, Jaffar-Bandjee MC, Hoarau JJ (2010) Chikungunya fever: CNS infection and pathologies of a re-emerging arbovirus. *Prog Neurobiol* 91: 121–129.
34 Pottumarthy S, Fritsche TR. (2005) Parasitic infections of the Peripheral nervous system. In: Dyck PJ and Thomas PK (eds) *Peripheral Neuropathy*, 4th edn, pp. 2153–2176. Elsevier Saunders, Philadelphia.
35 Valadares HM, Pimenta JR, de Freitas JM (2008) Genetic profiling of Trypanosoma cruzi directly in infected tissues using nested PCR of polymorphic microsatellites. *Int J Parasitol* 38: 839–850.
36 Gentile R, Oliveira G (2008) Brazilian studies on the genetics of *Schistosoma mansoni*. *Acta Trop* 108: 175–178.
37 Biron DG, Loxdale HD (2013). Host-parasite molecular cross-talk during the manipulative process of a host by its parasite. *J Exp Biol* 216: 148–160.
38 Kumar A, Misra P, Dube A (2013) Amplified fragment length polymorphism: an adept technique for genome mapping, genetic differentiation, and intraspecific variation in protozoan parasites. *Parasitol Res* 112: 457–466.
39 Strachan H (1897) On a form of multiple neuritis prevalent in the West Indies. *Practitioner* 59: 477–484
40 Osuntokun BO (1968) An ataxic neuropathy in Nigeria: a clinical, biochemical and electrophysioloigical study. *Brain* 91: 215–248.
41 Román GC, Spencer PS, Schoenberg BS (1985) Tropical myeloneuropathies: the hidden endemias. *Neurology* 35: 1158–1170.
42 Oluwole OSA, Onabolu AO, Cotgreave IA, Rosling H, Persson A, Link H (2003) Incidence of endemic ataxic polyneuropathy and its relation to exposure to cyanide in a Nigerian community. *J Neurol Neurosurg Psychiatry* 74: 1417–1422.
43 Vallat JM, Dumas M, Giordano C, Piquemal M, Sonan Th (1987) Histologic study of peripheral nerve biopsies from 20 patients with tropical ataxic neuropathy. *Neurology* 37 (Suppl 1): 255.

CHAPTER 26
Sarcoid neuropathy

Anne Vital
Department of Pathology-Neuropathology, Hôpital Pellegrin, Bordeaux, France

Definition

Sarcoidosis is a multisystem disorder of unknown origin characterized histologically by non-caseating epithelioid cell granulomas mainly in lymph nodes, lung, eyes, and skin. The liver, spleen, heart, muscle, nervous system, and other organs may also be involved [1, 2].

Epidemiology

Sarcoidosis affects all races, both sexes, and all ages with a predilection for young and middle-aged adults. Swedes, Danes, and African Americans appear to have the highest prevalence rates in the world [1]. Neurosarcoidosis is relatively rare and may involve cranial nerves, brain parenchyma, leptomeninges, dura, and peripheral nerves [3]. Neurological symptoms are observed in 5–13% of sarcoidosis, but are often attributable to another cause [4–6]. Cranial neuropathies, particularly facial palsy, and optic neuritis, are the most common manifestations of neurosarcoidosis whereas peripheral nervous system involvement is less common and its prevalence varies depending on diagnosis criteria [4–6].

Clinical features

Clinical features of peripheral nervous system involvement vary, but most cases present with a chronic sensorimotor axonal polyneuropathy or mononeuropathy multiplex, or less frequently an inflammatory demyelinating polyneuropathy [7, 8]. The differential diagnosis of sarcoid neuropathy is wide, including vasculitis, leprosy, amyloidosis, acute or chronic inflammatory demyelinating polyneuropathy and lymphomatous neuropathy. Peripheral neuropathy secondary to glucose intolerance may also develop in patients with sarcoidosis undergoing steroid therapy. Chronic pain is a common complaint among patients with sarcoidosis and small fiber neuropathy is regarded as the cause [9, 10].

Sarcoid neuropathy may occur at different stages of sarcoidosis, either isolated to nerves or associated with other organ involvement. When isolated, the diagnosis is often not suspected before nerve biopsy [7]. A subsequent search for extraneural locations is necessary, and the proportion of chest involvement in sarcoid peripheral neuropathy is similar to that found in neurosarcoidosis (78%) [7, 11]. In a report of 30 patients with neurosarcoidosis, five had peripheral nervous system involvement and none of these had associated central nervous system signs [5].

Serum angiotensin-converting enzyme (ACE) levels are of limited value in neurosarcoidosis [1]. Typical CSF finding include elevated protein levels and a lymphocytosis, but normal results do not exclude neurosarcoidosis. The value of CSF ACE is controversial, but an elevated level can provide supportive evidence for the diagnosis [6]. Nerve conduction studies and electromyography should be performed in patients with suspected peripheral neuropathy; and MRI has become useful to demonstrate enlarged segments of roots or nerve [12, 13].

Peripheral Nerve Disorders: Pathology and Genetics, First Edition. Edited by Jean-Michel Vallat, Joachim Weis, Francoise Gray, and Katy Keohane.

The risk of progression in sarcoid neuropathy is low, in contrast to CNS sarcoidosis, which is associated with a poor prognosis [6]. Neurosarcoidosis usually does not spontaneously remit, with the exception of facial nerve palsy, and patients with sarcoid peripheral neuropathy usually respond well to high-dose corticosteroid therapy although no standard treatment has been established. Patients refractory to treatment or with complications of corticosteroids may require second-line treatments with immunosuppressants or cytotoxic agents [6].

Pathology

As most cases of sarcoid neuropathy are improved by steroid therapy, a definite diagnosis based on characteristic histopathological features is mandatory. In practice, the diagnosis is often made indirectly by histologic confirmation in extraneural sites coupled with clinical symptoms of peripheral neuropathy, but it is likely that symptoms are not always due to sarcoidosis in the nerve.

Sarcoid granulomas are randomly distributed in nerve and muscle (Fig. 26.1), and *combined nerve and muscle*

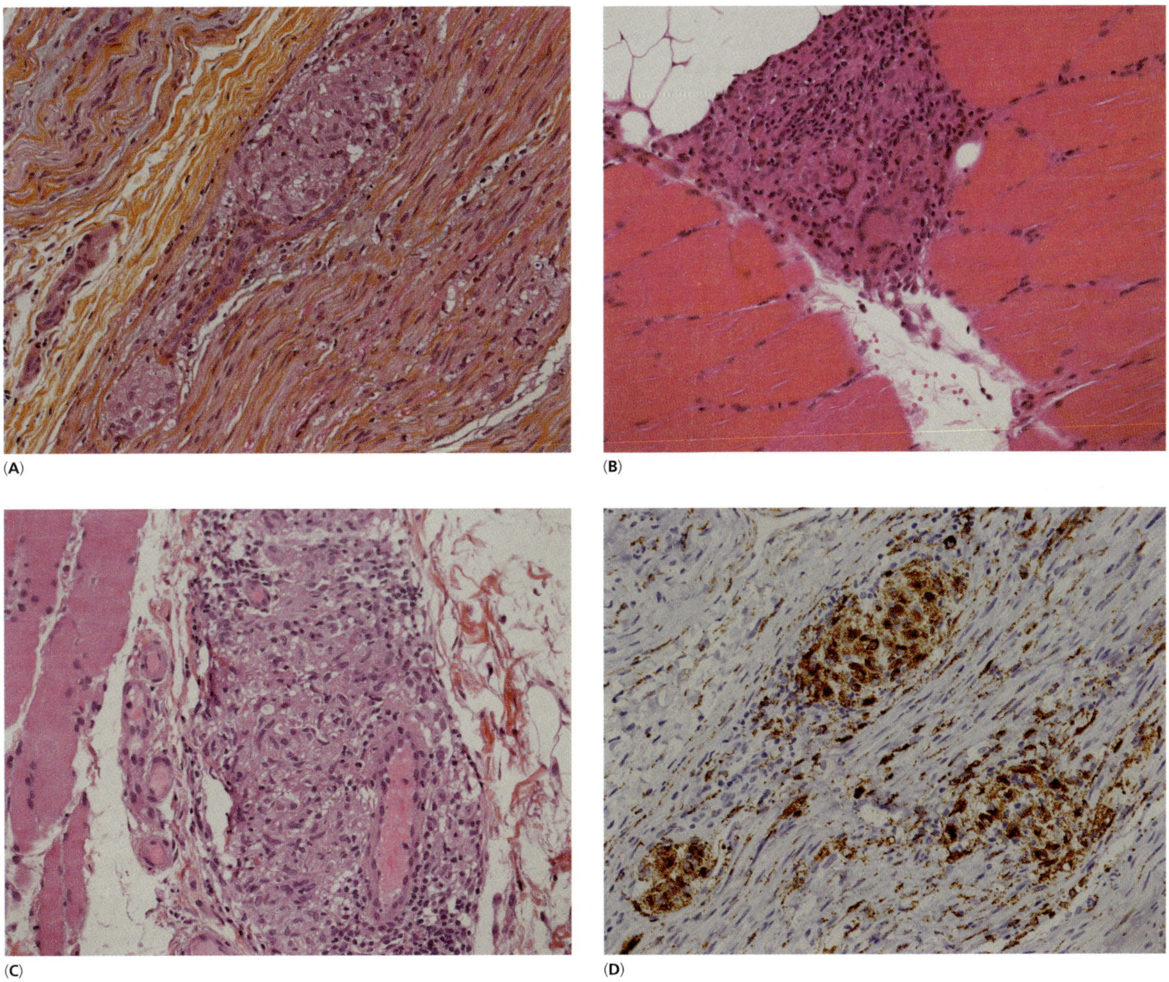

Figure 26.1 (**A**) A subperineurial non-caseating sarcoid granuloma. (**B**) Giant cells are visible within a large granuloma in the vicinity of muscle fibers. (**C**) This sarcoid granuloma involves a small vessel in a muscle specimen. (**D**) Anti-CD68 immunohistochemistry highlights small sarcoid granulomas within the endoneurium.

biopsy is the most useful tool for diagnosis because muscle involvement is frequent (cf. Chapter 2). Non-caseating granulomas are well developed between muscle fibers, whereas they are frequently smaller within epineurium or endoneurium. Granulomas in muscle also help differentiate sarcoidosis from tuberculoid leprosy. Punch skin biopsy is useful to confirm small fiber neuropathy in patients with pain and/or autonomic dysfunction, without visible sarcoid granulomas in the superficial dermis [9].

Sarcoid granulomas are mainly composed of tightly aggregated epithelioid cells mixed with a few multinucleated giant cells. A few lymphocytes, predominantly CD4 T helper cells may be present mainly at the periphery of granulomas, similar to sarcoid granulomas in other locations [7]. A collagenous reaction around granulomas is sometimes visible. Focal necrosis is very rare in neurosarcoidosis and has never been reported in the PNS.

Immunohistochemistry is not absolutely necessary for diagnosis, but anti-CD68 helps to detect small epithelioid granulomas. On ultrastructural examination, epithelioid cells have long intermingled cytoplasmic processes, their cytoplasm contains numerous mitochondria, Golgi complexes, and segments of rough endoplasmic reticulum [8].

In 2008, a well-illustrated review of 38 nerve biopsies with description of microscopic lesions was published [8]. Three additional cases have been reported with chronic sensory neuropathy [14], acute inflammatory demyelinating polyneuropathy [15], and chronic sensory motor neuropathy [16]. A case presenting as acute inflammatory demyelinating polyneuropathy with pleocytosis in the CSF prompted a search for systemic disease and sarcoid granulomas were found in nerve and muscle specimens [15]. Vascular involvement is not uncommon in sarcoid neuropathy and may manifest as necrotizing vasculitis or microvasculitis with sarcoid granulomas encroaching on or abutting a vessel wall [8, 14, 16]. A recent severe vasculitic neuropathy was attributed to sarcoidosis, subsequently confirmed by mediastinal lymph node biopsy [16].

Genetics

Intriguing spatial clustering of sarcoidosis suggests a common environmental exposure, infectious agent or genetic predisposition with an abnormal immune response [1]. The human leukocyte antigen (HLA) allele HLA-DRB1*0 is associated with sarcoidosis and HLA-DRB1*0301/DQB1*0201 genotype is associated with a good prognosis in Löfgren syndrome, the triad of erythema nodosum, bilateral hilar lymphadenopathy and arthralgia. Genome scans in African Americans show linkage to Chr 5 and the Butyrophilin-Like 2 (MHC Class II associated) BTNL2 gene on Chr 6 has been associated with sarcoidosis, but not specifically with neurosarcoidosis [17].

Experimental models and pathogenesis

The spectrum of sarcoid neuropathies is wide and authors have tried to assess the respective roles of mechanical compression, vasculitis, or local action of cytokines and immune factors. Sarcoid neuropathies in the form of chronic sensory motor polyneuropathy or mononeuropathy multiplex are mainly due to axonal degeneration, probably due to direct compression of nerve fibers by endoneurial sarcoid granulomas. However, vascular insufficiency may also play a role, particularly when axonal lesions are well limited to an area of the endoneurium [7, 8]. Primary myelin pathology is rarely observed, but isolated remyelinating fibers can occur, and fascicular demyelination was observed in a unique case reminiscent of experimental hypoperfusion models [8, 18].

Sarcoidosis is regarded as a T cell-mediated inflammation, in which memory T cells recruit and activate macrophages. These become epithelioid cells, may fuse to multinucleated giant cells, and release noxious secretory products that can induce axonal degeneration or demyelination of neighboring nerve fibers, or fibrinoid necrosis of the vessel walls [7, 19].

The mechanism responsible for the development of small fiber neuropathy in sarcoidosis is unclear [20].

Future directions and conclusions

Sarcoid neuropathy is a rare manifestation of sarcoidosis that may occur in isolation without other organ involvement. The diagnosis should not be missed since it is treatable. Diagnosis of isolated sarcoid neuropathy is often problematic, but is improved by *combined nerve and muscle biopsy* demonstrating characteristic granulomas, indicating that clinical symptoms are related to sarcoidosis. Treatment has not been subjected to rigorous study, but high-dose corticosteroid therapy typically produces substantial benefit.

References

1 Statement on sarcoidosis. Joint statement of the American Thoracic Society (ATS), the European Respiratory Society (ERS), and the World Association of Sarcoidosis and Other Granulomatous Disorders (WASOG) adopted by the ATS Board of Directors and by the ERS Executive Committee (1999). *Am J Respir Crit Care Med* 160, 736–755.

2 Judson MA. (2008) Sarcoidosis: clinical presentation, diagnosis, and approach to treatment. Am J Med Sci 335, 26–33.

3 Judson MA, Baughman RP, Teirstein AS et al. (1999) Defining organ involvement in sarcoidosis: the ACCESS proposed instrument. ACCESS Research Group. A Case Control Etiologic Study of Sarcoidosis. Sarcoidosis Vasc Diffuse Lung Dis 16, 75–86.

4 Lacomis D. (2011) Neurosarcoidosis. Curr Neuropharmacol 9, 429–436.

5 Gascon-Bayarri J, Mana J, Martinez-Yelamos S et al. (2011) Neurosarcoidosis: report of 30 cases and literature survey. Eur J Intern Med 22, e125–132.

6 Nozaki K, Judson MA. (2012) Neurosarcoidosis: clinical manifestations, diagnosis and treatment. Presse Med 41, e331–348.

7 Said G, Lacroix C, Plante-Bordeneuve V et al. (2002) Nerve granulomas and vasculitis in sarcoid peripheral neuropathy. A clinicopathological study of 11 patients. Brain 125, 264–275.

8 Vital A, Lagueny A, Ferrer X et al. (2008) Sarcoid neuropathy: clinico-pathological study of 4 new cases and review of the literature. *Clin Neuropathol* 27, 96–105.

9 Hoitsma E, Marziniak M, Faber CG *et al.* (2002) Small fibre neuropathy in sarcoidosis. *Lancet* 359, 2085–2086.

10 Bakkers M, Faber CG, Drent M *et al.* (2010) Pain and autonomic dysfunction in patients with sarcoidosis and small fibre neuropathy. *J Neurol* 257, 2086–2090.

11 Sharma OP. (1997) Neurosarcoidosis. A personal perspective based on the study of 37 patients. *Chest* 112, 220–228.

12 Moore FG, Andermann F, Richardson J *et al.* (2001) The role of MRI and nerve root biopsy in the diagnosis of neurosarcoidosis. *Can J Neurol Sci* 28, 349–353.

13 Burns TM, Dyck PJ, Aksamit AJ *et al.* (2006) The natural history and long-term outcome of 57 limb sarcoidosis neuropathy cases. *J Neurol Sci* 244, 77–87.

14 Zivkovic SA, Lacomis D. (2004) Sarcoid neuropathy. Case report and review of the literature. *J Clin Neuromusc Dis* 5, 184–189.

15 Vital C, Bonnin A, Dumas P *et al.* (2009) Acute sarcoid neuropathy developed 4 months after the occurrence of a gastrointestinal stromal tumor (GIST). *Sarcoidosis Vasc Diffuse Lung Dis* 26, 69–72.

16 Souayah N, Chodos A, Krivitskaya N *et al.* (2008) Isolated severe vasculitic neuropathy revealing sarcoidosis. *Lancet Neurol* 7, 756–760.

17 Iannuzzi MC. (2007) Genetics of Sarcoidosis. *Semin Respir Crit Care Med.* 1, 15–21.

18 Myers RR, Heckman HM, Galbraith JA *et al.* (1991) Subperineurial demyelination associated with reduced nerve blood flow and oxygen tension after epineurial vascular stripping. *Lab Invest* 65, 41–50.

19 Said G, Hontebeyrie-Joskowicz M. (1992) Nerve lesions induced by macrophage activation. *Res Immunol* 143, 589–599.

20 Judson MA. (2011). Small fibre neuropathy in sarcoidosis: something beneath the surface. *Respir Med* 105, 1–2.

CHAPTER 27

Guillain–Barré syndromes and chronic inflammatory demyelinating polyradiculoneuropathy

Laurent Magy

Neurology Laboratory, National Referral Center for Rare Peripheral Neuropathies, University Hospital, Limoges, France

The Guillain–Barré syndromes

Definition of the disorder, major synonyms, and historical perspective

The Guillain–Barré syndrome (GBS) is an acute inflammatory disorder of the peripheral nervous system, described in 1916 by Guillain, Barré, and Strohl although previous reports of patients with the same disorder existed [1]. GBS is characterized by an acute flaccid paralysis with elevated protein and normal cell count in the cerebrospinal fluid (CSF). In its classical form, GBS is also called Acute Inflammatory Demyelinating Polyradiculoneuropathy (AIDP), its pathological hallmark being inflammatory-mediated demyelination. Since its first description, several variants have been described including the Miller–Fisher syndrome (characterized by the association of ophthalmoplegia, ataxia, and areflexia), Acute Motor Axonal Neuropathy (AMAN) and Acute Motor and Sensory Axonal Neuropathy (AMSAN).

Epidemiology: Incidence and prevalence, sex, age, geographical distribution, risk factors

The incidence of GBS is presumably variable among countries. In the Western world, it ranges from 0.89–1.89 cases (median, 1.11) per 100,000 person-years according to a recent review [2]. The disease can start at any age but increases by 20% every decade after the first decade [3]. The sex ratio is 1.78 (95% confidence interval, 1.36 to 2.33) [2]. Most patients who develop GBS have a preceding diarrhea or upper respiratory tract infection. About one third of patients have a *Campylobacter Jejuni* infection; other microorganisms such as *Cytomegalovirus*, *Epstein Barr virus*, and *Mycoplasma Pneumoniae* have been linked to GBS.

Clinical features including appropriate investigations and important differential diagnosis

Most patients with GBS have paresthesia and numbness that progress from the extremities to proximal areas, and are rapidly followed by weakness in a matter of days [4]. Low back and limb pain may precede or accompany the other symptoms, sometimes in a nerve root distribution [5]. The condition typically worsens over less than four weeks (usually about 10 days) to reach a plateau phase. Bulbar weakness and other cranial nerve palsies may occur as well as respiratory distress due to diaphragm weakness [6]. Tendon jerks are usually decreased or absent although they may be brisk in variant forms of the disease [7].

Nerve conduction studies may be normal at the very beginning but usually show signs of a demyelinating neuropathy with variable degrees of axonal involvement in the demyelinating form of the disorder, which may be called acute inflammatory demyelinating polyneuropathy AIDP [8].

Lumbar puncture is usually performed in suspected GBS and typically shows albuminocytologic dissociation, defined by a raised protein content without an elevated cell count, in about 50–75% of patients.

Peripheral Nerve Disorders: Pathology and Genetics, First Edition. Edited by Jean-Michel Vallat, Joachim Weis, Francoise Gray, and Katy Keohane.

Recovery is usually slow over weeks to months and may be quickened by intravenous immunoglobulin or plasma exchange. About 20% of adult patients with GBS have persistent disability, but 90% of children have a complete recovery in the long term [9].

Axonal forms of GBS have been described and seem more prevalent in Asian countries [10]. The electrodiagnostic findings are consistent with primary axonal involvement in motor nerves (AMAN) [11] or in motor and sensory nerves (ASMAN) [12]. Recently, the definitions of axonal forms have been refined and cases with acute conduction blocks that may be rapidly reversible or lead to secondary axon loss have been described [13]. The Miller–Fisher syndrome is a sensory variant of the disease, which is more common in eastern countries. It is clinically characterized by the association of sensory ataxia, areflexia, and ophthalmoplegia [14].

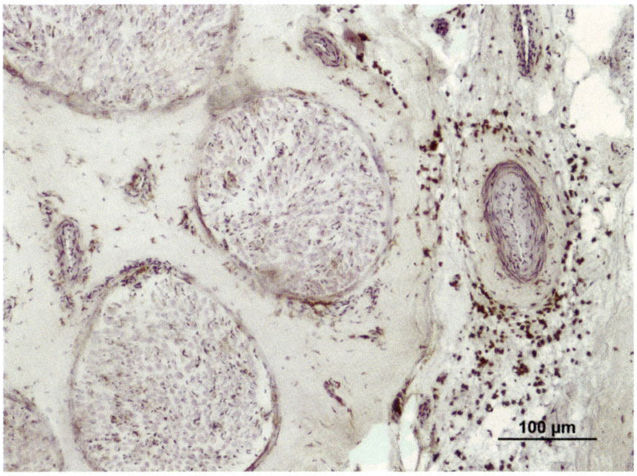

Figure 27.1 An epineurial blood vessel is surrounded by numerous T lymphocytes labeled with anti-CD45 antibody, in a patient with Guillain–Barré syndrome. Sural nerve biopsy: Frozen transverse section.

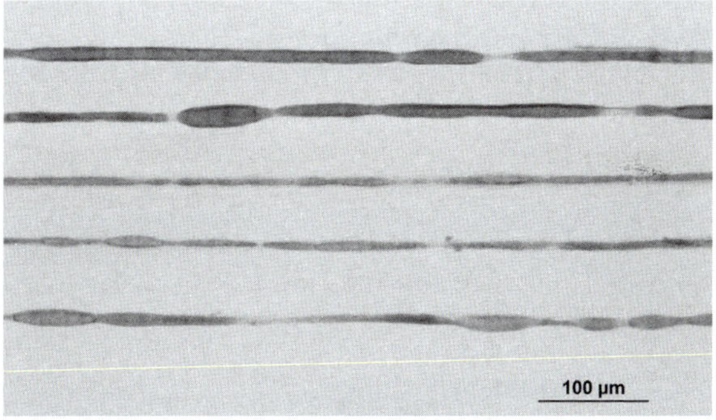

Figure 27.2 Teased fibers of the same patient as in Fig. 27.1 show a mixture of myelin swelling (reflecting the very early stage of the disease) and occasional segmental demyelination.

Pathology, including histopathology, electron microscopy, immunocytochemistry

Pathological examination is not required to diagnose GBS, but it may be performed in atypical cases or for research purposes. Up to now, probably <5% of patients die from GBS in developed countries [15] and many hallmarks of pathology that have been described years ago are based on autopsy findings [16]. It must be emphasized that nerve lesions may predominate in proximal sites including nerve roots and plexuses, and that changes are unevenly distributed along nerve trunks [17]. In AIDP, inflammation, demyelination, and variable degrees of axon loss are key features.

As a consequence of blood-nerve barrier breakdown, lymphocytic infiltration is frequent and often appears as perivascular cuffs in the endoneurium or epineurium (Fig. 27.1). Occasionally there are diffuse endoneurial infiltrates, sometimes near areas where axons are demyelinated. Lymphocytic infiltration is an early event in the course of the disease but may remain prominent long after the active phase [16].

Demyelination, the second key feature of AIDP, can be seen on light or electron microscopy. On semithin sections, demyelinated and partially remyelinated fibers may be observed. Teased fibers are more suitable to assess the longitudinal extent of these changes (Fig. 27.2). A few internodes are usually demyelinated in single fibers. Neighboring axons may be normal, suggesting a patchy and random pattern of demyelination within and between fascicles. Nerve fiber edema is an early but rarely mentioned feature [18], particularly seen in myelin structures (Fig. 27.2). Ultrastructural examination in AIDP may usually show at least two different patterns of demyelination. In one, macrophages are often seen stripping myelin lamellae after penetrating the basal lamina of Schwann cells surrounding axons that look otherwise normal (Fig. 27.3) [19]. In the other, naked axons surrounded by macrophages filled with myelin debris forming vesicular or bubble-like formations are seen (Fig. 27.4). Early vesicular changes are thought to be caused by complement and immunoglobulin deposition, followed by macrophages entering the fibers to clear myelin debris [20]. Axonal degeneration

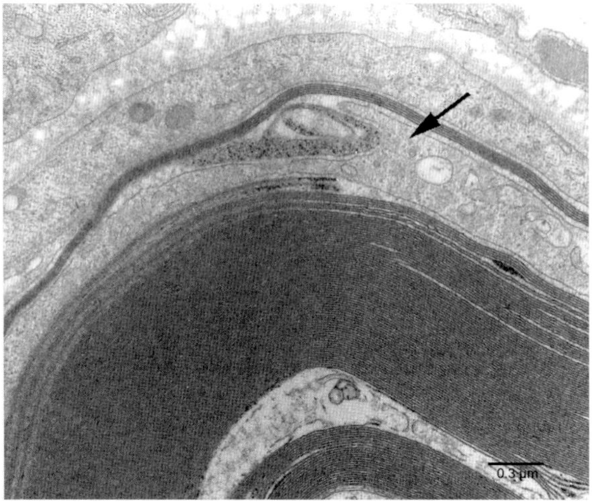

Figure 27.3 In this patient suffering from GBS, a macrophage has penetrated the myelin sheath and can be seen splitting the myelin lamellae. The axon is intact. Sural nerve biopsy. Electron micrograph, transverse section. Source: Jean-Michel Vallat, CHU de Limoges, France. Reproduced with permission of Jean-Michel Vallat.

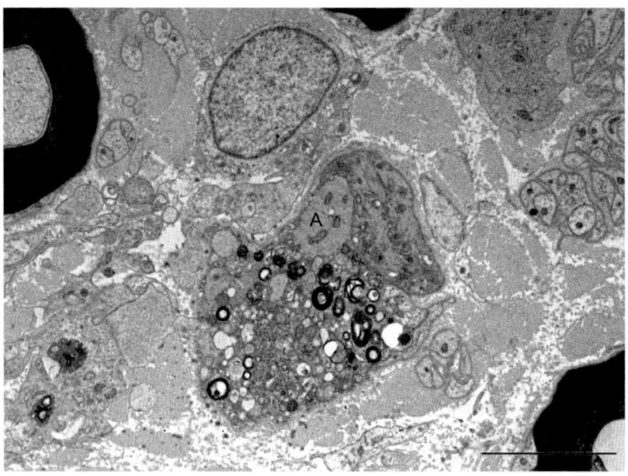

Figure 27.4 A macrophage full of myelin debris is in close contact with an axon (A), in a patient with Guillain–Barré syndrome. Sural nerve biopsy. Electron micrograph, transverse section.

secondary to demyelination is a constant feature in AIDP although it is highly variable among patients. There is currently no reasonable explanation for this variability although one may speculate that it correlates with the degree of early inflammation in nerve.

The concept of an axonal form of GBS was introduced by Feasby and coworkers in 1986, based on the description of five patients who developed a flaccid paralysis with inexcitable motor nerves, one of whom had extensive Wallerian-like degeneration without overt inflammation in the nerves and roots at autopsy [21]. The pattern of nerve damage in AMAN and AMSAN is quite different from that of AIDP. The pathology in AMAN is restricted to motor fibers, and pathological studies mainly come from autopsy cases in Chinese patients in the mid-1990s [22]. In AMAN, sensory nerves are essentially preserved although subtle changes may be found in some cases. Usually, ventral roots and motor nerves undergo Wallerian-like degeneration, highly variable in extent. Segmental demyelination seems very rare, although nodal lengthening has been demonstrated in teased nerve fiber studies. Lymphocytic infiltration seems to be rare and self-limited. In motor nerve fibers macrophages are prominent and are located in the periaxonal space, without disruption of the myelin sheath. Interestingly, in the case series reported by Griffin and co-workers, several patients had minimal changes in ventral roots and motor nerves, which seemed disproportional to the extent of paralysis that led to the patient's death [22]. Changes in these minimal cases mostly consisted of small numbers of degenerating fibers and mild paranodal changes with occasional nodal swelling. These important findings suggested functional changes causing flaccid paralysis, which could revert to normal in a few days or lead to axonal damage, a concept that has since been extensively discussed [23–26].

The pathology of AMSAN mostly consists of axon loss with signs of acute Wallerian-like degeneration. As in AMAN, these cases are also characterized by the paucity of inflammatory infiltrates and by the presence of macrophages in the adaxonal space. Finally, the only clear pathological difference between AMAN and AMSAN seems to be the involvement of sensory fibers in the latter [27].

Although GBS is considered a PNS-specific disorder, pathological changes in the CNS of patients with GBS are described. Some features such as posterior column and anterior horn cell degeneration may be secondary to PNS pathology, but inflammatory infiltrates have also been shown mainly in the gray matter of the spinal cord [28, 29]. This questions whether GBS is truly a PNS-specific disease and may suggest that antigenic targets in the CNS may be involved.

Pathogenesis

In AIDP, early changes in the nerve include antibody binding and complement deposition on Schwann cell surface and myelin, followed by invasion of T cells and macrophages [20]. The target of the pathological process is believed to be on myelin itself and not on Schwann cells, as macrophages are usually seen invading the myelin sheath, leaving the remaining Schwann cell cytoplasm largely intact in the early phases of the disease [17].

In AMAN, IgG and complement deposition occur at the axolemma of nodes of Ranvier of motor fibers [23]. Thereafter, nodal lengthening and axonal degeneration seem to be mainly caused by the membrane attack complex, and Wallerian-like degeneration occurs from ventral roots to motor nerves. Macrophages may be found overlying nodes or within the internodal periaxonal space, separating the axon from the adaxonal Schwann cell and myelin sheath. Experimental models of AMAN using animals sensitized by the ganglioside GM1 create very similar lesions to the human disorder and have helped to understand its pathogenesis [30].

The pathogenesis of GBS is likely to involve molecular mimicry between some surface components (lipooligosaccharides) of various microorganisms and peripheral nerve gangliosides. This has only been convincingly demonstrated in patients previously infected by *Campylobacter jejuni* [31].

The search for genetic factors associated with an increased risk of GBS has been the subject of many publications. In a recent review, there is no convincing evidence to draw firm conclusions favoring one or several factors in sufficiently large studies to date [32].

Animal models

Experimental autoimmune neuritis (EAN), an animal model of AIDP can be induced by immunization with peripheral nerve myelin [33]. More precisely EAN can be provoked in susceptible animals by active immunization using peripheral nerve homogenate, whole myelin, myelin proteins P0 and P2 (or peptides issued from these proteins), and galactocerebroside. Alternatively, EAN can be elicited by passive transfer of T cells previously immunized against proteins of peripheral nerve myelin. Pathologic examination of animals affected by EAN clearly shows invasion by lymphocytes and macrophages, and multifocal demyelination associated with variable degrees of axon loss. This animal model nicely reproduces clinical and pathological features of GBS and has given much information on its pathogenesis. Other models that mimic sensory ataxic neuropathy linked to antibodies against peripheral nerve gangliosides have allowed therapeutic strategies to be tested [34].

Treatment, future perspective, conclusions

The first line of treatment for patients with GBS is supportive. The improvement in nursing care and the development of mechanical ventilation in patients with diaphragm weakness, have greatly improved the prognosis of GBS. Immunomodulatory treatment must be started as soon as possible, the two options being plasma exchange [35] and IVIg [36]. To date, no other pharmacological intervention has proved beneficial in patients with Guillain–Barré syndrome, emphasizing the need for new treatment options in this disabling disorder [37].

Although nerve biopsy is no longer performed in the diagnosis of GBS and its variants, in the last few decades pathology has provided a better understanding of its pathogenesis. The development of biomarkers for these disorders, whether derived from blood samples, CSF, or nerve tissue, should help in further understanding of their mechanisms and in development of appropriate therapies.

Chronic inflammatory demyelinating polyradiculoneuropathy

Definition of the disorder, major synonyms, and historical perspective

Chronic Inflammatory Demyelinating Polyradiculoneuropathy (CIDP) is a chronic, assumed immune-mediated neuropathy that may be considered as the chronic counterpart of GBS [38]. It usually consists of a grossly symmetrical sensory and motor neuropathy with diffuse areflexia. Nerve conduction studies show features of a heterogeneously distributed demyelinating neuropathy with frequent conduction block and/or temporal dispersion. CSF protein is usually elevated and the pathological hallmark of the disease is inflammatory-mediated demyelination [39]. The disorder had been described for decades and was given different names [40–42] until it was termed chronic inflammatory polyradiculoneuropathy [39] and then chronic inflammatory demyelinating polyradiculoneuropathy [43].

Epidemiology: Incidence and prevalence, sex, age, geographical distribution, risk factors

Persons of any age may develop CIDP but little is known about its global epidemiology. Its prevalence could be between 1 and 10 in 100,000 and its geographical distribution is mostly unknown although it has been described in the US, Europe, and eastern countries. For example, the incidence of CIDP in Olmsted County, Minnesota has been reported to be 1.6/100,000/year and its prevalence 8.9/100,000 persons [44]. The crude prevalence of CIDP in southeast England has been recently reported to be 2.84/100,000 with men being more affected than women [45]. The lowest prevalence of CIDP has been reported in Japan, where it is 1.61/100,000 in the total population; 2.01 in males and 1.23 in females [46]. Approximately one third of patients develop the disorder following an infectious disease although the direct relationship between the two disorders has not been yet elucidated, and CIDP has been associated with various other autoimmune diseases and hematological disorders. Interestingly, a CIDP-like illness has been reported in people exposed to aerosolized porcine brain tissue in a working environment, suggesting that autoantigens are present in nerve tissue [47].

Clinical features including appropriate investigations (biochemistry, electrophysiology, imaging, etc.) and important differential diagnosis

The clinical presentation of CIDP is relatively heterogeneous. Patients suffering from the classic form usually present with a sensory and motor polyneuropathy developing over eight weeks or longer, involving both proximal and distal segments of limbs. A subacute form of CIDP (subacute inflammatory demyelinating polyneuropathy SIDP) has been described, where symptoms and signs progress over 4–8 weeks and have a fairly good prognosis with complete recovery in most patients [48]. Areflexia is usually diffuse and some patients may have cranial nerve involvement. Nerve conduction studies reveal a diffuse polyneuropathy involving all four limbs with features suggesting patchy demyelination, the hallmark of which is conduction block and temporal dispersion.

With improving electrodiagnostic techniques, nerve conduction parameters have greatly improved the diagnostic accuracy of CIDP without requiring pathological confirmation [49–53]. As in GBS, CSF examination may reveal an elevated protein level without elevation of cell count in patients with CIDP. In occasional cases, magnetic resonance imaging shows nerve root or plexus hypertrophy and/or contrast enhancement [54]. The workup for patients with suspected CIDP includes different investigations to confirm its diagnosis and rule out other conditions that may mimic the disorder [55].

The differential diagnosis includes polyneuropathies such as POEMS syndrome (Polyneuropathy, Organomegaly, Endocrinopathy, M protein, and Skin changes), which has a completely different management to CIDP [56]. Prominent axonal features in the lower limbs on electrodiagnostic studies [57–59] and raised vascular endothelial growth factor (VEGF) level [60] are key features of POEMS along with a lambda light chain monoclonal gammopathy. Amyloidosis can also mimic CIDP [61, 62]. Lastly, hereditary demyelinating neuropathy in sporadic cases may be mistaken for CIDP.

Besides its core clinical presentation, there are some clinical variants of CIDP. Sensory forms are usually characterized by a sensory ataxic neuropathy, although nerve conduction studies frequently also display motor nerve involvement in these patients [63]. Distal forms sometimes referred to as DADS (distal acquired demyelinating symmetrical neuropathy) present with bilateral foot drop and sensory loss in a stocking distribution [53]. Multifocal forms may be called MADSAM (multifocal acquired demyelinating sensory and motor neuropathy) or the Lewis–Sumner syndrome [53]. They are characterized by a multifocal sensory and motor involvement of individual nerves with conduction block [64].

In children, a subacute onset and a relapsing course seem more frequent than in adults and the prognosis is favorable with complete remission and recovery after a few months in many cases [9, 65].

Pathology, including histopathology, electron microscopy, immunocytochemistry

Nerve biopsy must be performed in an affected nerve and may provide supportive evidence of CIDP in patients with an unusual course or presentation [51]. Pathological findings may help confirm the diagnosis if there is unequivocal evidence of inflammatory-mediated demyelination in patients with various presentations [66]. It must be remembered that nerve lesions in CIDP are segmental and multifocal, so that

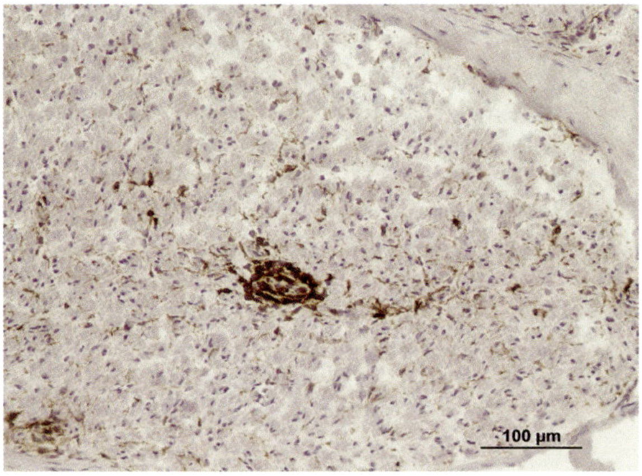

Figure 27.5 A cluster of T cells labeled with anti-CD45 antibody is seen in the endoneurium of this sural nerve of a patient with CIDP. Sural nerve biopsy. Transverse frozen section.

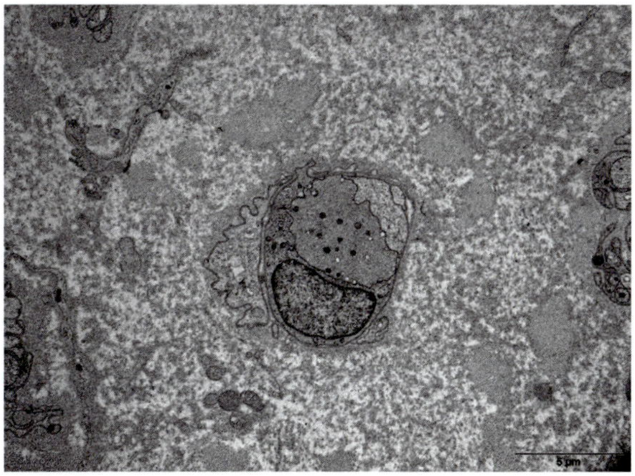

Figure 27.6 A completely demyelinated mid-diameter axon can be seen in a patient with CIDP. Sural nerve biopsy. Electron micrograph, transverse section.

neuropathological findings may differ between patients. It is important to study an affected nerve in order to find the characteristic lesions, which is sometimes difficult when the proximal segments of nerve are mainly or exclusively involved [67]. CIDP is an acquired demyelinating neuropathy, so its hallmark is inflammatory mediated segmental demyelination and remyelination with various degrees of axon loss associated with axonal sprouting. The prevalence of inflammatory infiltrates in nerve samples from patients with CIDP is highly variable, probably depending on the disease itself (which is quite heterogeneous) and also on the timing of nerve biopsy in the course of the disease. T cell infiltrates may be seen in the epineurium and/or endoneurium (Fig. 27.5), sometimes in close vicinity to demyelinating lesions. In the endoneurium, macrophages are frequently associated with axons undergoing demyelination and may be seen as small clusters around endoneurial blood vessels [68]. Demyelinated axons may be seen on transverse Toluidine blue-stained semi-thin sections, although they are easier to see by electron microscopy (Fig. 27.6). On teased nerve fiber preparation, segmental demyelination and remyelination is visible and may be associated with some degree of axonal degeneration. Attempted remyelination in CIDP frequently gives rise to onion bulbs that are occasionally very prominent. Axons surrounded by onion bulb formations are readily seen on semi-thin sections (Fig. 27.7). Although onion bulb-like formations are frequently prominent in CIDP, they have not been

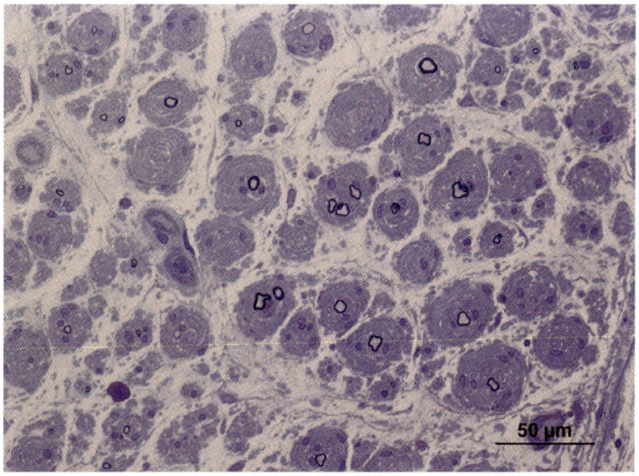

Figure 27.7 Virtually all small and large diameter axons in this field are surrounded by large onion bulb formations. Sural nerve biopsy of a patient with CIDP. Epon embedded tissue. Transverse semi-thin section stained with Toluidine blue.

reported in 15 patients with SIDP, its subacute form [69]. One of the key characteristics of CIDP is the distribution of anomalies is typically heterogeneous within or between fascicles (Fig. 27.8). This patchy distribution may be useful in differentiating CIDP from Charcot–Marie–Tooth disease. There are differences in onion bulb structures between patients with CIDP and patients with CMT. In patients with CIDP, the interspaces of onion bulbs are usually packed with collagen whereas these interspaces are open in patients with CMT1A. Additionally, onion bulbs are strongly immunoreactive for extracellular matrix protein like Tenascin-C in CIDP

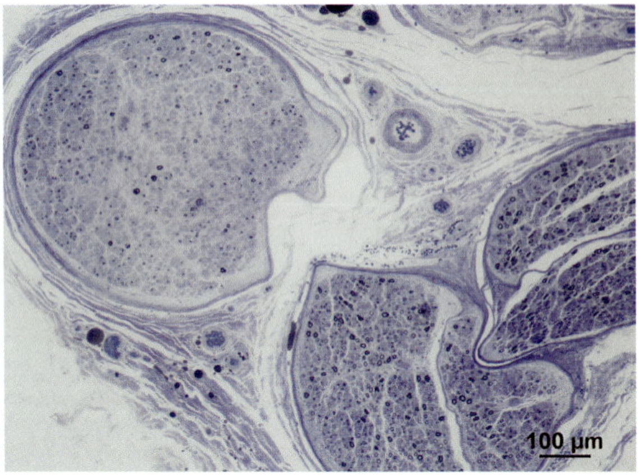

Figure 27.8 This photograph displays the heterogeneity of nerve involvement in a patient with CIDP. In the top left fascicle, there is a loss of large myelinated fibers and many remaining fibers are demyelinated (not visible at this magnification). In the bottom right fascicles, axon loss is less obvious and many axons appear remyelinated, with a thin-for-diameter myelin sheath. Sural nerve biopsy. Transverse semi-thin section stained with Toluidine blue.

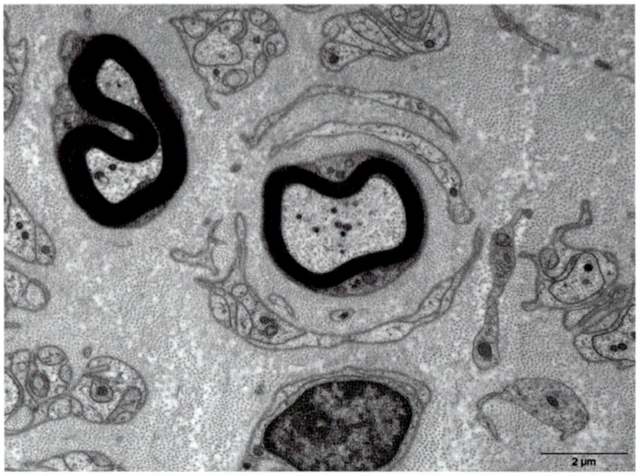

Figure 27.9 A mid-diameter axon is surrounded by an incipient onion bulb-like formation. Sural nerve biopsy of a patient with CIDP. Electron micrograph, transverse section.

nerve samples whilst immunoreactivity is rare in CMT1A [69]. Another classical feature of CIDP is endoneurial edema, defined by the increase of interstitial tissue within fascicles. Although endoneurial edema is sometimes readily visible, it is not readily quantifiable and there are no strict defining criteria. Macrophage-mediated demyelination is typically seen on electron microscopic examination in patients with CIDP and is probably the most specific tissue lesion [70]. Similar to GBS, macrophages may be seen splitting the myelin lamellae of large diameter axons. In other instances, macrophages full of myelin debris are seen around naked but intact axons. Onion bulb-like formations that are often visible on semi-thin sections are sometimes easier to see by electron microscopy when they are composed of just a few Schwann cell layers (Fig. 27.9).

Pathological data on childhood CIDP are scarce in the literature. In a Japanese series, sural nerve biopsy was undertaken in nine children with CIDP [71]. Subperineurial edema was a prominent feature, whereas onion bulb-like formations were found in only two cases. The paucity of onion bulbs in this series is likely to reflect the course of the disease, as six out of nine patients had a subacute onset. The density of myelinated fibers was always reduced and cellular infiltration was seen in six cases. Teased fiber preparation was useful as it showed signs of demyelination/remyelination in 6.3–34% of fibers [71].

Pathogenesis

CIDP is considered and inflammatory autoimmune disorder, based on CSF and pathological findings, and on its favorable response to immunotherapy. Several findings at the cellular and humoral level suggest that T lymphocytes and their partners play a crucial role and that damage of the blood/nerve barrier is a key event in the cascade of factors leading to nerve damage [72]. It is tempting to postulate that peripheral blood T cells become activated at some point against an autoantigen of peripheral myelin and/or axons. However, although several components of peripheral nerve have been considered as putative autoantibodies in CIDP, there is no convincing evidence of a specific target to date.

Some works have focused on genetic susceptibility to CIDP, but due to its rarity, studies have not been large enough to provide clear evidence of variants that have a clear influence on its development [73].

Animal models

Although the classical model of EAN consists of an acute inflammatory neuropathy with a monophasic course, grossly mimicking GBS, other models of inflammatory neuropathies have been developed that have a chronic course resembling CIDP [74]. Although these models have shed light on the cellular and molecular events that occur in the early phases of autoimmune neuropathies, triggering events, and autoantigens in CIDP are still largely not understood.

Treatment, future perspective, conclusions

Therapeutic options for CIDP include corticosteroids [75], IVIg [76], and plasma exchange [77]. The first choice is usually corticosteroids or IVIg, depending on potential contraindications and patients' associated conditions. Steroids are usually started at a dose of 60 mg of prednisone or prednisolone with subsequent tapering [43], but pulse doses of oral dexamethasone [78, 79] and intravenous methylprednisolone [80] have recently been used. Regardless of the first choice of treatment, the long-term management of patients with CIDP who have not remitted usually requires individual dose adjustment and prolonged maintenance therapy [81]. In these patients, alternative therapy is needed to minimize discomfort and side effects of current treatment, but is not yet available [82].

CIDP is a chronic, sometimes devastating immune-mediated neuropathy, whose pathogenesis is still not completely known. Progress has been achieved in both the diagnosis and treatment. Numerous studies have shown that nerve biopsy is still useful in this disorder when the clinical/neurophysiological presentation is atypical or unusual. Moreover, nerve tissue provides a unique opportunity to understand its pathogenesis and help develop new therapeutic strategies for the patients who do not respond to standard treatment.

References

1 Guillain G, Barré JA, Strohl A (1916) Sur un syndrome de radiculonévrite avec hyperalbuminose du liquide céphalo-rachidien sans réaction cellulaire: remarques sur les caractères cliniques et graphiques des réflexes tendineux. *Bull Soc Med Hop Paris;*40:1962.

2 Yuki N, Hartung HP (2012) Guillain–Barre syndrome. *N Engl J Med;*366:2294–2304.

3 Sejvar JJ, Baughman AL, Wise M, Morgan OW (2011) Population incidence of Guillain-Barre syndrome: a systematic review and meta-analysis. *Neuroepidemiology;*36:123–133.

4 Hahn AF (1998) Guillain–Barre syndrome. *Lancet;*352:635–641.

5 Ruts L, van Doorn PA, Lombardi R, *et al.* (2012) Unmyelinated and myelinated skin nerve damage inGuillain–Barre syndrome: correlation with pain and recovery. *Pain;*153:399–409.

6 Durand MC, Porcher R, Orlikowski D, *et al.* (2006) Clinical and electrophysiological predictors of respiratory failure in Guillain–Barre syndrome: a prospective study. *Lancet Neurol;*2006;5:1021–1028.

7 Yuki N, Kokubun N, Kuwabara S, *et al.* (2012) Guillain–Barre syndrome associated with normal or exaggerated tendon reflexes. *J Neurol;*259:1181–1190.

8 Albers JW, Kelly JJ, Jr (1989) Acquired inflammatory demyelinating polyneuropathies: clinical and electrodiagnostic features. *Muscle Nerve;*12:435–451.

9 Rabie M, Nevo Y (2009) Childhood acute and chronic immune-mediated polyradiculoneuropathies. *Eur J Paediatr Neurol;*13:209–218.

10 Yuki N, Yoshino H, Sato S, Miyatake T (1990) Acute axonal polyneuropathy associated with anti-GM1 antibodies following Campylobacter enteritis. *Neurology;*40: 1900–1902.

11 McKhann GM, Cornblath DR, Griffin JW, *et al.* (1993) Acute motor axonal neuropathy: a frequent cause of acute flaccid paralysis in China. *Ann Neurol;*33:333–342.

12 Capasso M, Notturno F, Manzoli C, Uncini A (2011) Involvement of sensory fibres in axonal subtypes of Guillain-Barre syndrome. *J Neurol Neurosurg Psychiatry;* 82:664–670.

13 Uncini A, Kuwabara S (2012) Electrodiagnostic criteria for Guillain–Barre syndrome: a critical revision and the need for an update. *Clin Neurophysiol;*123:1487–1495.

14 Yuki N (2009) Fisher syndrome and Bickerstaff brainstem encephalitis (Fisher–Bickerstaff syndrome). *J Neuroimmunol;* 215:1–9.

15 Walgaard C, Lingsma HF, Ruts L *et al.* (2011) Early recognition of poor prognosis in Guillain–Barre syndrome. *Neurology;*76:968–975.

16 Asbury AK, Arnason BG, Adams RD (1969) The inflammatory lesion in idiopathic polyneuritis. Its role in pathogenesis. *Medicine (Baltimore);*48:173–215.

17 Prineas JW (1981) Pathology of the Guillain–Barre syndrome. *Ann Neurol;*9 Suppl:6–19.

18 Haymaker WE, Kernohan JW (1949) The Landry–Guillain–Barre syndrome; a clinicopathologic report of 50 fatal cases and a critique of the literature. *Medicine (Baltimore);* 28:59–141.

19 Prineas JW (1972) Acute idiopathic polyneuritis. An electron microscope study. *Lab Invest;*26:133–147.

20 Hafer-Macko CE, Sheikh KA, Li CY, *et al.* (1996) Immune attack on the Schwann cell surface in acute inflammatory demyelinating polyneuropathy. *Ann Neurol;*39: 625–635.

21 Feasby TE, Gilbert JJ, Brown WF, *et al.* (1986) An acute axonal form of Guillain–Barre polyneuropathy. *Brain;*109 (Pt 6):1115–1126.

22 Griffin JW, Li CY, Ho TW, *et al.* (1995) Guillain–Barre syndrome in northern China. The spectrum of neuropathological changes in clinically defined cases. *Brain;*118 (Pt 3): 577–595.

23 Hafer-Macko C, Hsieh ST, Li CY, *et al.* (1996) Acute motor axonal neuropathy: an antibody-mediated attack on axolemma. *Ann Neurol*;40:635–644.
24 Kokubun N, Nishibayashi M, Uncini A *et al.* (2010) Conduction block in acute motor axonal neuropathy. *Brain*;133:2897–2908.
25 Uncini A, Yuki N (2009) Electrophysiologic and immunopathologic correlates in Guillain–Barre syndrome subtypes. *Expert Rev Neurother*;9:869–884.
26 Yuki N, Kuwabara S (2007) Axonal Guillain–Barre syndrome: carbohydrate mimicry and pathophysiology. *J Peripher Nerv Syst*;12:238–249.
27 Griffin JW, Li CY, Ho TW, *et al.* (1996) Pathology of the motor-sensory axonal Guillain–Barre syndrome. *Ann Neurol*;39:17–28.
28 Maier H, Schmidbauer M, Pfausler B *et al.* (1997) Central nervous system pathology in patients with the Guillain–Barre syndrome. *Brain*;120 (Pt 3):451–464.
29 Muller HD, Beckmann A, Schroder JM (2003) Inflammatory infiltrates in the spinal cord of patients with Guillain–Barre syndrome. *Acta Neuropathol*;106:509–517.
30 Susuki K, Rasband MN, Tohyama K, *et al.* (2007) Anti-GM1 antibodies cause complement-mediated disruption of sodium channel clusters in peripheral motor nerve fibres. *J Neurosci*;27:3956–3967.
31 Yuki N, Taki T, Inagaki F, *et al.* (1993) A bacterium lipopolysaccharide that elicits Guillain–Barre syndrome has a GM1 ganglioside-like structure. *J Exp Med*;178:1771–1775.
32 Wu LY, Zhou Y, Qin C, Hu BL (2012) The effect of TNF-alpha, FcgammaR and CD1 polymorphisms on Guillain–Barre syndrome risk: evidences from a meta-analysis. *J Neuroimmunol*;243:18–24.
33 Waksman BH, Adams RD (1955) Allergic neuritis: an experimental disease of rabbits induced by the injection of peripheral nervous tissue and adjuvants. *J Exp Med*;102:213–236.
34 Kusunoki S, Shimizu J, Chiba A *et al.* (1996) Experimental sensory neuropathy induced by sensitization with ganglioside GD1b. *Ann Neurol*;39:424–431.
35 Raphael JC, Chevret S, Hughes RA, Annane D (2012) Plasma exchange for Guillain–Barre syndrome. *Cochrane Database Syst Rev*;7:CD001798.
36 Hughes RA, Swan AV, van Doorn PA (2012) Intravenous immunoglobulin for Guillain–Barre syndrome. *Cochrane Database Syst Rev*;7:CD002063.
37 Hughes RA, Pritchard J, Hadden R (2013). Pharmacological treatment other than corticosteroids, intravenous immunoglobulin and plasma exchange for Guillain–Barre syndrome. *Cochrane Database Syst Rev*;2:CD008630.
38 Hinman RC, Magee KR (1967) Guillain–Barre syndrome with slow progressive onset and persistent elevation of spinal fluid protein. *Ann Intern Med*;67:1007–1012.
39 Dyck PJ, Lais AC, Ohta M *et al.* (1975) Chronic inflammatory polyradiculoneuropathy. *Mayo Clin Proc*;50:621–637.
40 Austin JH (1958) Recurrent polyneuropathies and their corticosteroid treatment; with five-year observations of a placebo-controlled case treated with corticotrophin, cortisone, and prednisone. *Brain*;81:157–192.
41 Dolman CL, Allan BM (1973) Relapsing hypertrophic neuritis. *Arch Neurol*;28:351–353.
42 Thomas PK, Lascelles RG, Hallpike JF, Hewer RL (1969) Recurrent and chronic relapsing Guillain–Barre polyneuritis. *Brain*;92:589–606.
43 Dyck PJ, O'Brien PC, Oviatt KF, *et al.* (1982) Prednisone improves chronic inflammatory demyelinating polyradiculoneuropathy more than no treatment. *Ann Neurol*;11:136–141.
44 Laughlin RS, Dyck PJ, Melton LJ, *et al.* (2009) Incidence and prevalence of CIDP and the association of diabetes mellitus. *Neurology*;73:39–45.
45 Mahdi-Rogers M, Hughes RA (2013) Epidemiology of chronic inflammatory neuropathies in south-east England. *Eur J Neurol*;21:28–33.
46 Iijima M, Koike H, Hattori N, *et al.* (2008) Prevalence and incidence rates of chronic inflammatory demyelinating polyneuropathy in the Japanese population. *J Neurol Neurosurg Psychiatry*;79:1040–1043.
47 Tracy JA, Dyck PJ (2011) Auto-immune polyradiculoneuropathy and a novel IgG biomarker in workers exposed to aerosolized porcine brain. *J Peripher Nerv Syst*;16 Suppl 1:34–37.
48 Oh SJ, Kurokawa K, De Almeida DF *et al.* (2003) Subacute inflammatory demyelinating polyneuropathy. *Neurology*;61:1507–1512.
49 Research criteria for diagnosis of chronic inflammatory demyelinating polyneuropathy (CIDP). Report from an ad hoc subcommittee of the American Academy of Neurology AIDS Task Force. (1991) *Neurology*;41:617–618.
50 Bromberg MB (2011) Review of the evolution of electrodiagnostic criteria for chronic inflammatory demyelinating polyradicoloneuropathy. *Muscle Nerve*;43:780–794.
51 Joint Task Force of the EFNS and the PNS. European Federation of Neurological Societies/Peripheral Nerve Society Guideline on management of chronic inflammatory demyelinating polyradiculoneuropathy: report of a joint task force of the European Federation of Neurological Societies and the Peripheral Nerve Society – First Revision. (2010) *J Peripher Nerv Syst*;15:1–9.
52 Nicolas G, Maisonobe T, Le Forestier N *et al.* (2002) Proposed revised electrophysiological criteria for chronic inflammatory demyelinating polyradiculoneuropathy. *Muscle Nerve*;25:26–30.
53 Saperstein DS, Katz JS, Amato AA, Barohn RJ (2001) Clinical spectrum of chronic acquired demyelinating polyneuropathies. *Muscle Nerve*;24:311–324.
54 Tazawa K, Matsuda M, Yoshida T, *et al.* (2008) Spinal nerve root hypertrophy on MRI: clinical significance in the diagnosis of chronic inflammatory demyelinating polyradiculoneuropathy. *Intern Med*;47:2019–2024.

55 French CIDP Study Group (2008) Recommendations on diagnostic strategies for chronic inflammatory demyelinating polyradiculoneuropathy *J Neurol Neurosurg Psychiatry;*79:115–118.

56 Dispenzieri A (2012) POEMS syndrome: update on diagnosis, risk-stratification, and management. *Am J Hematol;*87:804–814.

57 Cui RT, Huang XS, Liu JX *et al.* (2012) Electrophysiological characteristics of polyneuropathy in POEMS syndrome: comparison with CIDP. *J Clin Neurophysiol;*29:345–348.

58 Mauermann ML, Sorenson EJ, Dispenzieri A *et al.* (2012) Uniform demyelination and more severe axonal loss distinguish POEMS syndrome from CIDP. *J Neurol Neurosurg Psychiatry;*83:480–486.

59 Nasu S, Misawa S, Sekiguchi Y *et al.* (2012) Different neurological and physiological profiles in POEMS syndrome and chronic inflammatory demyelinating polyneuropathy. *J Neurol Neurosurg Psychiatry;*83:476–479.

60 Nobile-Orazio E, Terenghi F, Giannotta C *et al.* (2009) Serum VEGF levels in POEMS syndrome and in immune-mediated neuropathies. *Neurology;*72:1024–1026.

61 Mathis S, Magy L, Diallo L *et al.* (2012) Amyloid neuropathy mimicking chronic inflammatory demyelinating polyneuropathy. *Muscle Nerve;*45:26–31.

62 Plante-Bordeneuve V, Ferreira A, Lalu T, *et al.* (2007) Diagnostic pitfalls in sporadic transthyretin familial amyloid polyneuropathy (TTR-FAP). *Neurology;*69:693–698.

63 Oh SJ, Joy JL, Kuruoglu R (1992) "Chronic sensory demyelinating neuropathy": chronic inflammatory demyelinating polyneuropathy presenting as a pure sensory neuropathy. *J Neurol Neurosurg Psychiatry;*55:677–680.

64 Saperstein DS, Amato AA, Wolfe GI *et al.* (1999) Multifocal acquired demyelinating sensory and motor neuropathy: the Lewis–Sumner syndrome. *Muscle Nerve;*22:560–566.

65 McMillan HJ, Kang PB, Jones HR, Darras BT (2013) Childhood chronic inflammatory demyelinating polyradiculoneuropathy: combined analysis of a large cohort and eleven published series. *Neuromuscul Disord;*23:103–111.

66 Vallat JM, Tabaraud F, Magy L *et al.* (2003) Diagnostic value of nerve biopsy for atypical chronic inflammatory demyelinating polyneuropathy: evaluation of eight cases. *Muscle Nerve;*27:478–485.

67 Midroni G, Dyck PJ (1996) Chronic inflammatory demyelinating polyradiculoneuropathy: unusual clinical features and therapeutic responses. *Neurology;*46:1206–1212.

68 Sommer C, Koch S, Lammens M *et al.* (2005) Macrophage clustering as a diagnostic marker in sural nerve biopsies of patients with CIDP. *Neurology;*65:1924–1929.

69 Oka N, Kawasaki T, Unuma T *et al.* (2013) Different profiles of onion bulb in CIDP and CMT1A in relation to extracellular matrix. *Clin Neuropathol;*32(5):402–412.

70 Vital C, Vital A, Lagueny A, *et al.* (2000) Chronic inflammatory demyelinating polyneuropathy: immunopathological and ultrastructural study of peripheral nerve biopsy in 42 cases. *Ultrastruct Pathol;*24:363–369.

71 Hattori N, Ichimura M, Aoki S *et al.*(1998) Clinicopathological features of chronic inflammatory demyelinating polyradiculoneuropathy in childhood. *J Neurol Sci;*154:66–71.

72 Vallat JM, Sommer C, Magy L (2010) Chronic inflammatory demyelinating polyradiculoneuropathy: diagnostic and therapeutic challenges for a treatable condition. *Lancet Neurol;*9:402–412.

73 Notturno F, Pace M, De Angelis MV *et al.* (2008) Susceptibility to chronic inflammatory demyelinating polyradiculoneuropathy is associated to polymorphic GA repeat in the SH2D2A gene. *J Neuroimmunol;*197:124–127.

74 Soliven B (2012) Autoimmune neuropathies: insights from animal models. *J Peripher Nerv Syst;*17 Suppl 2:28–33.

75 Hughes RA, Mehndiratta MM (2012) Corticosteroids for chronic inflammatory demyelinating polyradiculoneuropathy. *Cochrane Database Syst Rev;*8:CD002062.

76 Eftimov F, Winer JB, Vermeulen M *et al.* Intravenous immunoglobulin for chronic inflammatory demyelinating polyradiculoneuropathy. *Cochrane Database Syst Rev;9:*CD001797.

77 Mehndiratta MM, Hughes RA (2012) Plasma exchange for chronic inflammatory demyelinating polyradiculoneuropathy. *Cochrane Database Syst Rev;*9:CD003906.

78 Eftimov F, Vermeulen M, van Doorn PA *et al.*(2012) Predict. Long-term remission of CIDP after pulsed dexamethasone or short-term prednisolone treatment. *Neurology;*78:1079–1084.

79 van Schaik IN, Eftimov F, van Doorn PA, *et al.* (2010) Pulsed high-dose dexamethasone versus standard prednisolone treatment for chronic inflammatory demyelinating polyradiculoneuropathy (PREDICT study): a double-blind, randomised, controlled trial. *Lancet Neurol;*9:245–253.

80 Nobile-Orazio E, Cocito D, Jann S, *et al.* (2012) Intravenous immunoglobulin versus intravenous methylprednisolone for chronic inflammatory demyelinating polyradiculoneuropathy: a randomised controlled trial. *Lancet Neurol;*11:493–502.

81 Hughes RA, Donofrio P, Bril V *et al.* (2008) Intravenous immune globulin (10% caprylate-chromatography purified) for the treatment of chronic inflammatory demyelinating polyradiculoneuropathy (ICE study): a randomised placebo-controlled trial. *Lancet Neurol;*7:136–144.

82 Mahdi-Rogers M, van Doorn PA, Hughes RA. (2013) Immunomodulatory treatment other than corticosteroids, immunoglobulin and plasma exchange for chronic inflammatory demyelinating polyradiculoneuropathy. *Cochrane Database Syst Rev;*6:CD003280.

CHAPTER 28
Diabetic neuropathies

Robert E. Schmidt
Department of Pathology and Immunology, Division of Neuropathology, Washington University School of Medicine, St. Louis, USA

Introduction

Diabetes is a near-epidemic disease causing a number of different neuropathic presentations, most typically involving the sensory and autonomic nervous systems. Some diabetic patients have other superimposed neuropathic processes, requiring careful neurologic, laboratory, and metabolic workup. Neuropathy may be the presenting symptom of patients with unrecognized but established diabetes leading to a first-time diagnosis, while others only have impaired glucose tolerance and whether their neuropathy is diabetic is less certain. Many pathogenetic mechanisms have been proposed and tested in animal models. It is considered likely that diabetic neuropathies have different pathogenetic mechanisms and possibly require different therapies.

Epidemiology

As diabetes becomes an epidemic (WHO estimates >400 million worldwide), diabetic neuropathy (DNP) is increasing and is now the commonest neuropathy in the world. The prevalence of neuropathy in adult diabetics is approximately 30%. Over 50% develop neuropathy at some time during their disease, although numbers range from 10–90% depending on selection criteria and analytic methods. Risk factors include the presence of retinopathy and nephropathy, duration of diabetes, age, hypertension, smoking (in type 1 diabetes), patient height, alcohol consumption, and worsening degree of glycemic control. Diabetic sensory and autonomic neuropathy increases the risk for lower limb amputation, sudden death and, in 10–20% of the diabetic population, chronic debilitating pain. Neuropathy may lead to the initial recognition of already established but unsuspected diabetes, represent progressive disease in known long-term diabetics, or accompany incipient (pre)diabetes. Both types 1 and 2 diabetes may be complicated by DNP at any time during their course. Although the Diabetes Control and Complications Trial (DCCT) established a 60% reduction in the incidence of sensory DNP in type 1 diabetic patients receiving enhanced glucose control, multiple studies support only a modest reduction in neuropathy in strictly-controlled type 2 diabetic patients [1], suggesting different mechanisms. Curiously, protection against cardiac autonomic neuropathy persisted years after the close out of the DCCT study, despite deterioration of overall glycemic control.

Forms of diabetic neuropathy

Diabetic neuropathy is not a single entity; rather, it is a complex spectrum of neuropathies (Table 28.1), including symmetrical sensorimotor, asymmetrical (involving cranial and somatic nerves) and autonomic neuropathies [2, 3]. Patients may present with sensory loss, often accentuated in the distal limbs and occasionally complicated by disabling neuropathic pain, autonomic insufficiency involving many modalities and distributions, or asymmetric pain and weakness in the distribution of individual peripheral or cranial nerves. Not all patients with diabetes and neuropathy have DNP; some have an undiagnosed, unsuspected or superimposed

Peripheral Nerve Disorders: Pathology and Genetics, First Edition. Edited by Jean-Michel Vallat, Joachim Weis, Francoise Gray, and Katy Keohane.

Table 28.1 Forms of diabetic neuropathy.

Impaired glucose tolerance and hyperglycemic neuropathy
Generalized (symmetrical) neuropathies
Sensorimotor
Small fiber predominant (acute painful, including treatment-induced)
Autonomic
Acute motor
Focal and multifocal neuropathies (including mononeuritis multiplex)
Cranial
Thoracolumbar
Lumbosacral radioplexus (Bruns–Garland syndrome)
Other forms
Carpal & Cubital Tunnel
Meralgia Paraesthetica
Superimposed chronic inflammatory demyelinating neuropathy (CIDP) (debated)
Hypoglycemic neuropathy

Source: Llewelyn *et al.*, 2005 [3]. Adapted with permission of Elsevier.

secondary process (e.g., paraneoplastic, vasculitic, compressive, CIDP). Patients with typical patterns of DNP are infrequently biopsied, those presenting with severe sensory loss (particularly large fiber joint and vibration sense) out of proportion to the severity of their diabetes, asymmetric involvement, dominant motor symptoms, or an acute rapidly worsening course may be biopsied.

Neuropathy with impaired glucose tolerance

Some patients present with an idiopathic, typically painful neuropathy that develops in the absence of elevated HbA1c or fasting hyperglycemia, and are only found to have impaired glucose tolerance [4]. There is a predilection for small axons, particularly epidermal, which may be the earliest detectable sign of neuropathy in glucose dysmetabolism [5].

Hyperglycemic neuropathy

A syndrome of paresthesias and pain in newly diagnosed diabetes ("hyperglycemic neuropathy," [6]) may be particularly sensitive to normalization of blood glucose values.

Treatment-induced neuropathy ("insulin neuritis")

Diabetic patients with newly instituted, sometimes over-aggressive insulin therapy may develop acute pain or autonomic symptoms. This is commonest in type 1 diabetics, and is usually transient. Patients who intentionally withhold insulin for weight loss ("diabetic anorexia") may be at particularly high risk. Irrespective of its old name, "insulin neuritis," there is no solid evidence that it is an inflammatory condition [7].

Symmetrical sensorimotor polyneuropathy

Clinical

The best known of the neuropathies of diabetes [2, 3], symmetrical sensorimotor polyneuropathy, ranges from subclinical electrophysiological alterations to distal "stocking-glove" anesthesia. Loss of sensation may be accompanied by paresthesias, Charcot joints, loss of reflexes, increased incidence of amputation, and trophic changes in skin.

Pathology

There is loss of myelinated and unmyelinated axons, variable in severity from fascicle to fascicle (Fig. 28.1A) particularly distally in the lower limbs. Often fascicles show evidence of regeneration forming axon clusters (white arrows, Fig. 28.1B), regenerated axons with myelin sheaths that are too-thin-for-axon-caliber (red arrows, Fig. 28.1B) and relatively normal axons (black arrows, Fig. 28.1B). Active axonal degeneration (blue arrows, Fig. 28.1C) may occur on a background of residual axonal and myelin debris, numerous bands of Büngner, regenerative axonal clusters (red arrow, Fig. 28.1C), and regenerated axons (black arrow, Fig. 28.1C) [8]. In severely affected nerves or late in the course of DNP, few axons remain, and even Schwann cell processes may be lost. Pathological findings are frequently patchy but summate to a diffuse symmetrical fascicular involvement distally. Axonal degeneration and regeneration occasionally produce a mini-neuroma with interruption of the perineurium. Some patients with chronic involvement or mild symptoms show primary and secondary demyelination, remyelination, and scattered onion bulbs. The apparent increase in CIDP in diabetics may contribute to this pathologic appearance, although the presence of distinctive macrophage-mediated demyelination favors coexistent CIDP rather than diabetes alone. Without teased fiber analysis it may be difficult to distinguish thinly myelinated regenerated axons from true demyelination; however, the presence of active axonal degeneration, numerous aggregates of Schwann processes (bands of Büngner) and regenerative axonal clusters suggests that most thinly-myelinated-for-axon-caliber axons

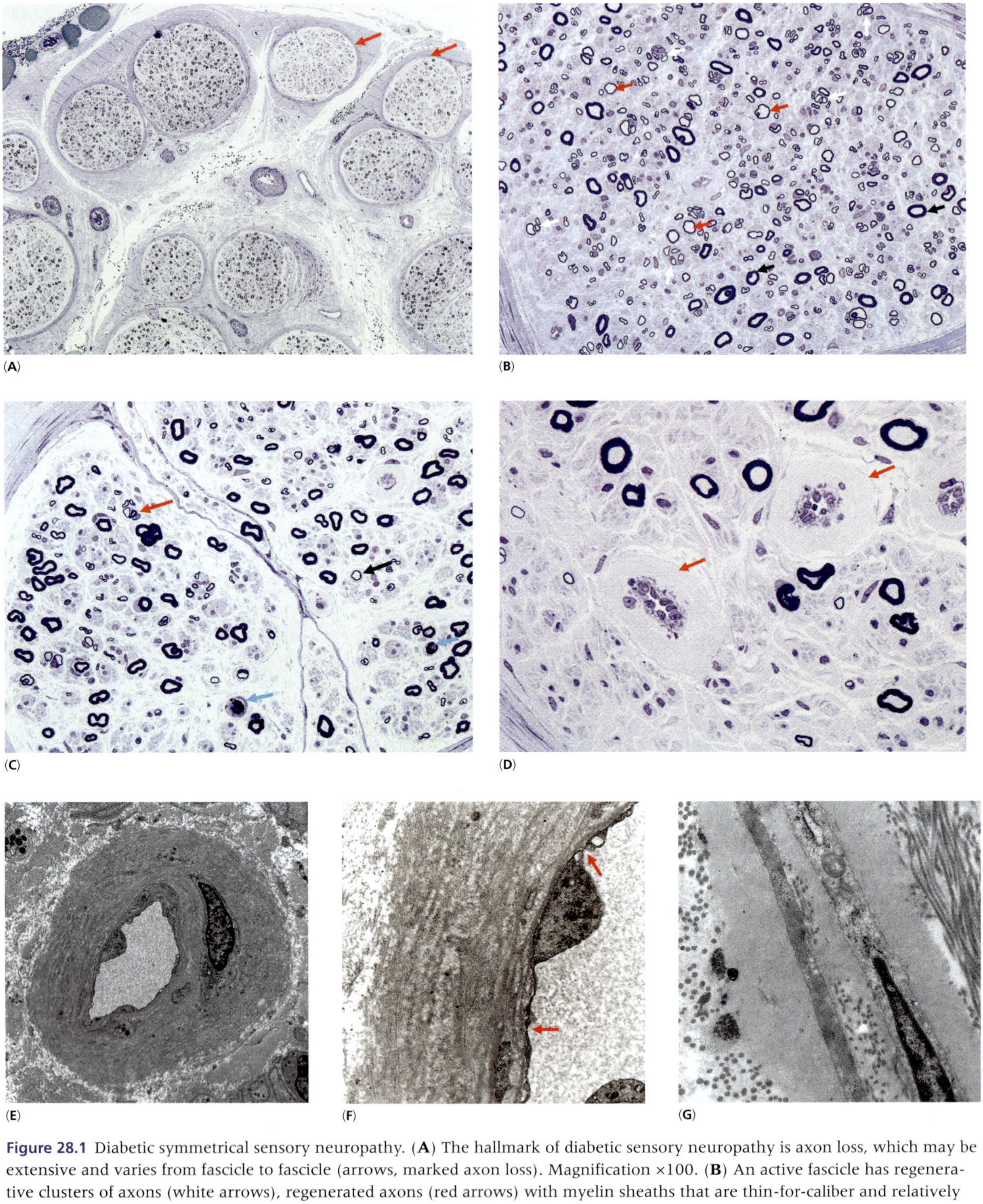

Figure 28.1 Diabetic symmetrical sensory neuropathy. (**A**) The hallmark of diabetic sensory neuropathy is axon loss, which may be extensive and varies from fascicle to fascicle (arrows, marked axon loss). Magnification ×100. (**B**) An active fascicle has regenerative clusters of axons (white arrows), regenerated axons (red arrows) with myelin sheaths that are thin-for-caliber and relatively normal axons (black arrows). Magnification ×400. (**C**) A fascicle that has lost significant numbers of axons shows ongoing degeneration/debris (blue arrows), regenerative clusters (red arrow) and axons that have thinned myelin (black arrow). Magnification ×600. (**D**) Markedly thickened microvasculature (red arrows) may mimic amyloid deposition, although symmetrical. Magnification ×1000. (**E, F**) Marked thickening of endoneurial venules and capillaries is produced by accumulation of concentric multilamellar collections of basal laminae, seen at higher magnification in **F**. Notice fenestrations (**F**, arrows). Magnification: **E**, ×5000; **F**, ×15,000. (**G**) Diabetic perineurium shows marked thickening of basement membranes. Magnification ×30,000.

originate as part of axonal degeneration/regeneration (Fig. 28.1A–C). Nonetheless, studies of early diabetic neuropathy have reported paranodal abnormalities, segmental demyelination and remyelination in the absence of myelinated axon degeneration [9]. Axonal atrophy has not been demonstrated consistently in human diabetic neuropathy. Endoneurial microvasculature shows marked thickening (Fig. 28.1D) that results from accumulation of layers of thickened basement membranes (Fig. 28.1E,F). These probably reflect deficient turnover of glycated basement membrane, and are prominent in endoneurial microvasculature [10], Schwann and perineurial cells (Fig. 28.1G) but are not pathognomonic of DNP.

Both type 1 and 2 diabetics develop sensory DNP; type 1 patients are reported to develop fewer degenerating axons and more myelinopathy than type 2, in whom axonal degeneration is most prominent. Axoglial dysjunction, an unusual and debated ultrastructural and molecular alteration of the perinodal junctional apparatus, has been described to explain paranodal demyelination and conduction defects, especially in type 1 diabetes in rats and humans [11].

Skin biopsies in diabetic peripheral neuropathy

Skin biopsies have recently been used to assess diabetic symmetrical sensory polyneuropathy and autonomic neuropathy [12–14] (see Chapter 3). Intra-epidermal nerve fibers (IENF) are unmyelinated unsheathed sensory fibers expressing the transient receptor potential vanilloid type 1 (TRPV1) receptor, also known as the capsaicin receptor. Distal sensory unmyelinated axon loss in skin biopsies may occur in the absence of more proximal sural axon loss in diabetic sensory neuropathy. The absolute IENFD values from distal leg are lower in early type 2 diabetes and prediabetic patients compared to controls and may improve with appropriate intervention [15]. Small thinly myelinated Aδ (A-delta) axons, innervating cutaneous mechanoreceptors and thermal receptors, can also be demonstrated using skin biopsies. Skin biopsies can be used to indicate incipient neuropathy at a very early, treatable stage by demonstrating an 80% slower rate of IENF regeneration in diabetics than controls after capsaicin-induced sensory skin denervation. Distal preterminal nerve-fiber swellings in diabetes may represent a "pre-degenerative" change but are also seen in control patients. Skin biopsies also enable assessment of sudomotor innervation [14].

Painful neuropathy

Definition, clinical, and pathogenesis

Painful neuropathy [16] is a major debilitating symptom of diabetic neuropathy. Numerous studies confirm the role of diabetes in small fiber neuropathy as defined by IENFD. A near majority of patients with IGT or diabetes have small fiber neuropathy, the prototype of painful neuropathy, with burning feet, accompanied by thermal-evoked pain and/or allodynia. Ectopic discharges related to pain perception arise from DRG neurons and axons and accompany changes in sensory neuron sodium channels [17, 18]. The NaV1.7 sodium channel accumulates at nerve fiber endings and amplifies small sub-threshold depolarizations, regulating excitability. In large studies of type 2 diabetics, SCN9A mutations resulted in a gain of function in the sodium channel Nav1.7 in 28% of patients with biopsy-confirmed small fiber neuropathy [17, 18]. Loss-of function mutations in SCN9A are associated with congenital insensitivity to pain and gain-of-function mutations have been linked to spontaneous pain in several rare disorders. Antisense knockdown of Nav1.7 attenuates Freund's adjuvant-induced thermal hyperalgesia and diabetic pain. The transient receptor potential ankyrin 1 (TRPA1) ion channel on primary afferent nerve fibers also appears involved in painful diabetic neuropathy, due to sustained activation by reactive compounds generated in diabetes [19]. Alterations in DRG Ca(v)3.2T-type and TRPV1 channel function may also contribute to the variety of pain syndromes induced by type 1 diabetes [20]. In diabetes, up-regulation of cutaneous NGF may overstimulate surviving axons, which may participate in the genesis of painful diabetic neuropathy. Injured small caliber peripheral nerve fibers may cause localized imbalance of sensory inputs between small and large caliber injured and uninjured nerve fibers producing aberrant painful sensations. Diabetic patients may also have altered CNS pain perception processing causing input from mechanoreceptive A fibers to be perceived as pain. Changes in purinergic signaling by microglia responding to nociceptive transmission in neurons may also contribute to neuropathic pain in humans.

Corneal confocal microscopy

Non-invasive *in vivo* confocal microscopic measurements of corneal nerve fiber length correlate well with the severity of DNP, the degree of IENF loss, the presence of painful DNP, and improvement following combined pancreas/kidney transplantation [21].

Asymmetrical diabetic neuropathies

This category includes diabetic lumbosacral radiculoplexus neuropathy (DLRPN; also known as "diabetic amyotrophy," "Bruns–Garland syndrome," "femoral neuropathy of diabetes," and "proximal diabetic neuropathy"), cervical radiculoplexus neuropathy (DCRPN), truncal radiculopathy, upper limb mononeuropathy, and cranial nerve palsies (usually cranial nerves III, IV, and VI) [22].

Clinical

Occasionally, especially early in type 2 diabetes, patients develop sudden or subacute motor dysfunction following institution of insulin therapy, not obviously related to glycemic control or associated with significant weight loss. Onset with deep aching or burning tingling severe unilateral thigh pain is followed by progressive atrophy, weakness, and muscle wasting, involving the distribution of large nerves to the lower limbs or cranial nerves. The symptoms typically spread throughout the limb and eventually involve the contralateral side. Rarely, upper limb involvement occurs as part of the recently described entity DCRPN, often following an immune trigger such as immunization, viral syndrome, trauma, or surgery [23].

Pathology

Pathological findings in this group of neuropathies include an inflammatory microvasculitis (Fig. 28.2A), dominated by T cell infiltrates but typically lacking angionecrosis, involving the epineurial vasa nervorum often with endoneurial and perineurial hemosiderin deposition. Vascular changes are accompanied by perineuritis (Fig. 28.2A), perineurial thickening with macrophage infiltration (Fig. 28.2B) and axonopathy, ranging from multifocal degenerating axons to neuroma formation [24]. Loss of intra-epidermal nerve fibers is described in biopsies from symptomatic areas [13]. These findings in diabetic LRPN are identical to those in patients with non-diabetic LRPN; some of the latter have abnormal glucose tolerance, indicating a pre-diabetic condition. The usual course results in spontaneous recovery over several months. Although DLRPN may represent an autoimmune vasculopathy, it is resistant to immunotherapy. Pathology of the rarer cranial nerve palsies is assumed to be similar since occasionally cranial nerve palsies accompany DLRPN.

Diabetic autonomic neuropathy (DANP)

Clinical

Diabetic patients can develop a myriad of autonomic symptoms, targeted individually or in functional groups [25]. Cardiovascular complications include abnormal R-R interval, loss of cardiac reflexes, silent myocardial

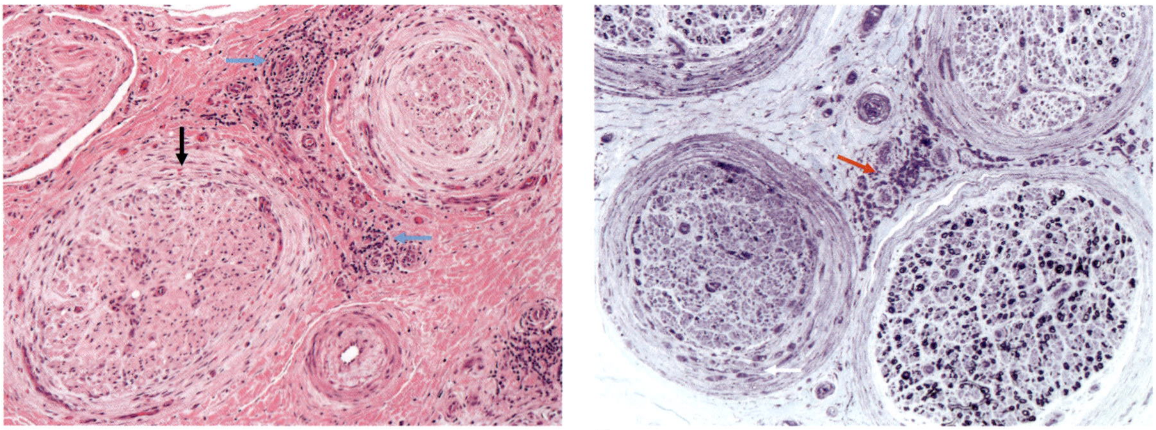

(A) (B)

Figure 28.2 Diabetic lumbosacral radiculoplexus neuropathy. (**A**) Characteristic pathological findings include perivascular inflammation involving the epineurial vessels (blue arrows) and proliferation of perineurial cells (black arrow). Magnification ×200. (**B**) The inflammatory infiltrate is clustered around small epineurial vessels (red arrow) and is accompanied by perineuritis and macrophage infiltration (white arrow). Magnification ×200.

infarction (sensory fibers), and often late orthostatic hypotension. Other symptoms include gastrointestinal dysfunction, such as esophageal dysmotility, gastroparesis, and chronic diarrhea or constipation; bladder distension and infection; erectile deficiency, and pupillomotor or sweating abnormalities. Symptomatic DANP increases morbidity and mortality several fold, possibly autonomic imbalance between sympathetic and parasympathetic nervous systems results in cardiac arrhythmias, nephropathy, stroke, or increased perioperative mortality [3, 26]. Diabetic gastrointestinal dysfunction also involves the enteric nervous system itself, the non-adrenergic non-cholinergic pathway in the pylorus, and the visceral sensory nervous system, particularly for urinary bladder function. Autonomic and peripheral somatic neuropathies may be divergent in diabetic patients, suggesting different underlying pathophysiological processes or separately targeted subpopulations of autonomic neurons/axons.

Pathology

Both sympathetic and parasympathetic dysfunction occurs in diabetes and may be accompanied and exaggerated by superimposed enteric or visceral sensory dysfunction. Examination of sweat gland, arrector pili, and arteriolar innervation in skin biopsies allows analysis of autonomic nerves and different neurotransmitters in DANP [14]. Skin biopsy correlates sweat gland nerve fiber density with neuropathic symptoms, neurological deficits, and sweat production in diabetic patients. Systematic autopsy studies of diabetic patients have demonstrated markedly swollen neurofilament-laden axons and synapses, that is, neuroaxonal dystrophy (Fig. 28.3) in the relative absence of neuron loss in diabetic prevertebral sympathetic autonomic ganglia that serve the bowel and viscera [27]. Lymphocytic infiltrates in sympathetic ganglia of diabetic patients have been interpreted as evidence for its possible autoimmune pathogenesis, although lymphocytic infiltration was neither more frequent nor of greater intensity in diabetic subjects than controls in one large autopsy series. Significant loss of preganglionic myelinated axons in the greater splanchnic and abdominal vagus nerves in diabetic gastroparesis has also been described. Studies of parasympathetic ganglia and projections suggest the selective loss of nitrergic innervation of the stomach and penis of diabetic rodents, which shows a biphasic degenerative response: initially insulin-reversible loss of

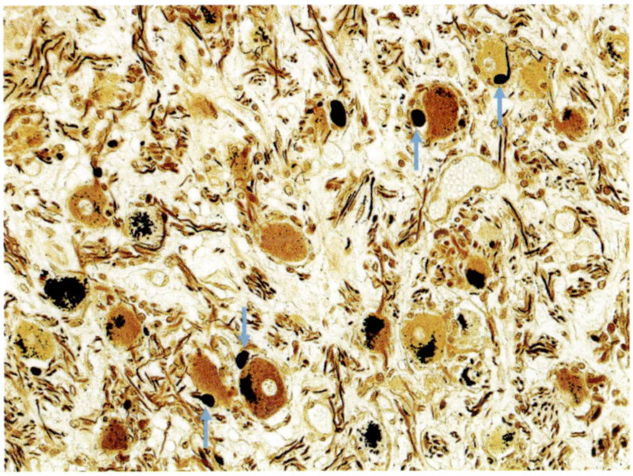

Figure 28.3 Diabetic autonomic neuropathy. Numerous dystrophic swellings (arrows) involve terminal axons and synapses in diabetic prevertebral sympathetic ganglion. Bielschowsky stain, 600×.

axonal nitric oxide synthase (NOS) and later irreversible neuron loss [28]. In other diabetic animal models, subpopulations of autonomic fibers within the gut, bladder, penis, and other end organs may show preferential damage [29].

Hypoglycemic neuropathy

A predominantly motor and upper extremity sensorimotor hypoglycemic neuropathy has been described as part of insulinoma-induced maintained hypoglycemia. However, in diabetes-related neuropathy a role for hypoglycemia is not clearly established [3].

Animal models

Genetic (Biobreeding Wor: BBW and Zucker Diabetic Fatty: ZDF rats, non-obese diabetic: NOD, db/db, Akita mice), spontaneous and pancreatic beta cell toxin (alloxan, streptozotocin)-induced rodent models of types 1 and 2 diabetes have been developed and used in DNP research over the last 50 years. No model accurately reproduces the entire range of distribution and histologic features of diabetic symmetrical sensorimotor neuropathy, particularly regarding the degree and distribution of somatic axon loss; however, individual features of the neuropathy (nerve conduction and biochemical changes, skin denervation, etc.) have been modeled. Animal models of DANP are more faithful models of dystrophic changes but significant differences to patients do exist.

Proposed pathogenetic mechanisms of diabetic neuropathy

The pathogenesis of diabetic neuropathy is unknown. Several mechanisms [3, 30, 31] have been proposed and tested in experimental animal models including oxidative stress [32–34] mitochondrial dysfunction [35–39] and deficiencies or surpluses in the amount or regulation of neurotrophic substances (e.g., NGF [40], BDNF [41], CNTF [42], NT-3, IGF-I, insulin [43], C-peptide [44], erythropoietin [45]). There is currently no consensus regarding which of several mechanisms operate, and multiple mechanisms may interact and account for differences in diabetic neuropathies.

The relevance of ischemia in the pathogenesis of diabetic neuropathy has been debated [46, 47]. Some have argued that while nerve ischemia is associated with neuropathy, it may not be its primary or major cause, only accelerating the process [3].

The substantially reduced incidence of sensory neuropathy in type 1 diabetic patients subjected to intensive glucose control contrasts with a modest reduction in type 2 diabetics [1], and suggests different mechanisms. Epidemiologic studies show that obesity, levels of high density lipoproteins/hyperlipidemia, and hypertension are all independently associated with the development of DNP. Microarray analysis of nerves from type 2 diabetic mice with polyneuropathy reveals that genes associated with lipid metabolism and immune response are highly dysregulated, similar to man. Variation of the severity of diabetic complications in comparable diabetic patients is not understood, however, there is likely a genetic component to diabetic neuropathy that is being actively investigated [48].

Differences in types 1 and 2 diabetes include: C-peptide levels, differences in levels of insulin/IGF-I serving as neurotrophic substances, neuronal insulin resistance [49] with altered downstream phosphatidylinositol 3-kinase (PI3K)/pAkt/GSK-3b signaling pathways, mitochondrial biogenesis and dysfunction, multiple sources of oxidative stress and 12/15 lipoxygenase activation [50] with attendant increased oxidative-nitrosative stress and levels of free fatty acids. Type 2 diabetes induces significant and persistent increase of Nav1.6 expression in the DRG, which may participate in diabetic neuropathic pain.

Somatic neuropathy in type 1 diabetic BB/Wor rats is characterized by severe nerve conduction defects, axonal atrophy, node of Ranvier-based pathology with molecular alterations of nodal proteins, defects in axonal regeneration and, eventually, significant loss of myelinated axons [11]. In comparison, diabetic somatic neuropathy in type 2 diabetic BBZDR/Wor rats is associated with only mild atrophy of myelinated axons, minimal nodal pathology with no molecular changes, segmental demyelination, and active Wallerian degeneration in the absence of axon loss, which may reflect increased axonal regeneration [11].

References

1 Callaghan BC, Cheng HT, Stables CL, *et al.* (2012) Diabetic neuropathy: clinical manifestations and current treatments. *Lancet Neurol* 11, 521–534.

2 Smith AG, Singleton JR. (2012) Diabetic neuropathy. *Continuum Lifelong Learning Neurol* 18, 60–84.

3 Llewelyn J, Tomlinson D, Thomas P. (2005) Diabetic neuropathies. In: Dyck P and Thomas P (eds) *Peripheral Neuropathy*, pp. 1951–1991. Elsevier-Saunders, Philadelphia.

4 Novella SP, Inzucchi SE, Goldstein JM. (2001) The frequency of undiagnosed diabetes and impaired glucose tolerance in patients with idiopathic sensory neuropathy. *Muscle Nerve* 24, 1229–1231.

5 Smith AG, Ramachandran P, Tripp S, *et al.* (2001) Epidermal nerve innervation in impaired glucose tolerance and diabetes-associated neuropathy. *Neurology* 57, 1701–1704.

6 Watkins PJ, Thomas PK. (1998) Diabetes mellitus and the nervous system. *J Neurol Neurosurg Psychiatry* 65, 620–632.

7 Ellenberg M. (1974). Diabetic neuropathic cachexia. *Diabetes* 23, 418–423.

8 Midroni G, Bilbao JM. (1995) *Biopsy Diagnosis of Peripheral Neuropathy*, pp. 313–321. Butterworth-Heinemann, Boston.

9 Malik RA, Tesfaye S, Newrick PG, *et al.* (2005) Sural nerve pathology in diabetic patients with minimal but progressive neuropathy. *Diabetologia* 48, 578–585.

10 King RH, Llewelyn JG, Thomas PK, *et al.* (1989) Diabetic neuropathy: abnormalities of Schwann cell and perineurial basal laminae. Implications for diabetic vasculopathy. *Neuropathol Appl Neurobiol* 15, 339–355.

11 Sima AA, Zhang W, Xu G, *et al.* (2000) A comparison of diabetic polyneuropathy in type II diabetic BBZDR/Wor rats and in type I diabetic BB/Wor rats. *Diabetologia* 43, 786–793.

12 Malik RA, Veves A, Tesfaye S *et al.* (2011) Small fibre neuropathy: role in the diagnosis of diabetic sensorimotor polyneuropathy *Diab Metab Res Rev* 27, 678–684.

13 Lauria G, McArthur JC, Hauer PE, *et al.* (1998) Neuropathological alterations in diabetic truncal neuropathy: evaluation by skin biopsy. *J Neurol Neurosurg Psychiatry* 65, 762–766.

14 Luo KR, Chao CC, Chen YT, *et al.* (2011) Quantitation of sudomotor innervation in skin biopsies of patients with diabetic neuropathy. *J Neuropathol Exp Neurol* 70, 930–938.
15 Divisova S, Vlckova E, Hnojcikova M, *et al.* (2012) Prediabetes/early diabetes-associated neuropathy predominantly involves sensory small fibres. *J Periph Nerv Syst* 17, 341–350.
16 von Hehn CA, Baron R, Woolf CJ. (2012) Deconstructing the neuropathic pain phenotype to reveal neural mechanisms. *Neuron* 73, 638–652.
17 Sung J-Y, Park SB, Liu Y-T, *et al.* (2012) Progressive axonal dysfunction precedes development of neuropathy in type 2 diabetes. *Diabetes* 61, 1592–1598.
18 Faber CG, Hoeijmakers JG, Ahn HS, *et al.* (2012) Gain of function Nav1.7 mutations in idiopathic small fiber neuropathy. *Ann Neurol* 71, 26–39.
19 Koivisto A, Hukkanen M, Saarnilehto M, *et al.* (2012) Inhibiting TRPA1 ion channel reduces loss of cutaneous nerve fiber function in diabetic animals: Sustained activation of the TRPA1 channel contributes to the pathogenesis of peripheral diabetic neuropathy. *Pharmacol Res* 65, 149–158.
20 Khomula EV, Viatchenko-Karpinski VY, Borisyuk AL, *et al.* (2013) Specific functioning of Cav3.2 T-type calcium and TRPV1 channels under different types of STZ-diabetic neuropathy. *Biochim Biophys Acta doi:* 10.1016/j.bbadis.2013.01.017.
21 Tavakoli M, Mitu-Pretorian M, Petropoulos IN, *et al.* (2013) Corneal confocal microscopy detects early nerve regeneration in diabetic neuropathy after simultaneous pancreas and kidney transplantation. *Diabetes* 62, 254–260.
22 Younger DS. (2011) Diabetic lumbosacral radiculoplexus neuropathy: a postmortem studied patients and review of the literature. *J Neurol* 258, 1364–1367.
23 Massie R, Mauermann ML, Staff NP, *et al.* (2012) Diabetic cervical radiculoplexus neuropathy: a distinct syndrome expanding the spectrum of diabetic radiculoplexus neuropathies. *Brain* 135, 3074–3088.
24 Llewelyn JG, Thomas PK, King RH. (1998) Epineurial microvasculitis in proximal diabetic neuropathy. *J Neurol* 245, 159–165.
25 Rundles R. (1945) Diabetic neuropathy: general review with report of 125 cases. *Medicine* 24, 111–160.
26 Ewing DJ, Campbell IW, Clarke BF. (1980) The natural history of diabetic autonomic neuropathy. *Quart J Med* 49, 95–108.
27 Schmidt RE. (2002) Neuropathology and pathogenesis of diabetic autonomic neuropathy. *Int Rev Neurobiol* 50, 267–292.
28 Cellek S, Foxwell NA, Moncada S. (2003) Two phases of nitrergic neuropathy in streptozotocin-induced diabetic rats. *Diabetes* 52, 2353–2362.
29 Schmidt RE. Autonomic Neuropathy in Experimental Models of Diabetes Mellitus. *In* Zochodne D and Malik R, (eds). *Handbook of Clinical Neurology*, in press.
30 Obrosova IG. (2009) Diabetes and the peripheral nerve. *Biochim Biophys Acta* 1792, 931–940.
31 Vincent AM, Callaghan BC, Smith AL, *et al.* (2011) Diabetic neuropathy: cellular mechanisms as therapeutic targets. *Nat Rev Neurol* 7, 573–583.
32 Obrosova IG. (2002) How does glucose generate oxidative stress in peripheral nerve? *Int Rev Neurobiol* 50, 3–35.
33 Campanucci V, Krishnaswamy A, Cooper E. (2010) Diabetes depresses synaptic transmission in sympathetic ganglia by inactivating nAChRs through a conserved intracellular cysteine residue. *Neuron* 66, 827–834.
34 Zherebitskaya E, Akude E, Smith DR, *et al.* (2009) Development of selective axonopathy in adult sensory neurons isolated from diabetic rats: role of glucose-induced oxidative stress. *Diabetes* 58, 1356–1364.
35 Brownlee M. (2001) Biochemistry and molecular cell biology of diabetic complications. *Nature* 414, 813–820.
36 Chowdhury SKR, Dobrowsky RT, Fernyhough P. (2011) Nutrient excess and altered mitochondrial proteome and function contribute to neurodegeneration in diabetes. *Mitochondrion* 11, 845–854.
37 Chowdhury SKR, Zherebitskaya E, Smith DR, *et al.* (2010) Mitochondrial respiratory chain dysfunction in dorsal root ganglia of streptozotocin-induced diabetic rats and its correction by insulin treatment. *Diabetes* 59, 1082–1091.
38 Chowdhury SKR, Smith DR, Saleh A, *et al.* (2012) Impaired adenosine monophosphate-activated protein kinase signaling in dorsal root ganglia neurons is linked to mitochondrial dysfunction and peripheral neuropathy in diabetes. *Brain* 135, 1751–1766.
39 Chowdhury SK, Smith DR, Fernyhough P. (2013) The role of aberrant mitochondrial bioenergetics in diabetic neuropathy. *Neurobiol Dis* 51, 56–65.
40 Diemel LT, Brewster WJ, Fernyhough P, *et al.* (1994) Expression of neuropeptides in experimental diabetes: effects of treatment with nerve growth factor or brain-derived neurotrophic factor. *Brain Res Mol Brain Res* 21, 171–175.
41 Schmidt RE, Dorsey DA, Beaudet LN, *et al.* (1999) Insulin-like growth factor I reverses experimental diabetic autonomic neuropathy. *Am J Pathol* 155, 1651–1660.
42 Saleh A, Roy Chowdhury SK, Smith DR, *et al.* (2013) Ciliary neurotrophic factor activates NF-kappaB to enhance mitochondrial bioenergetics and prevent neuropathy in sensory neurons of streptozotocin-induced diabetic rodents. *Neuropharmacol* 65, 65–73.
43 Singhal A, Cheng C, Sun H, *et al.* (1997) Near nerve local insulin prevents conduction slowing in experimental diabetes. *Brain Res* 763, 209–214.
44 Ekberg K, Brismar T, Johansson BL, *et al.* (2003) Amelioration of sensory nerve dysfunction by C-peptide in patients with type 1 diabetes. *Diabetes* 52, 536–541.
45 Bianchi R, Buyukakilli B, Brines M, *et al.* (2004) Erythropoietin both protects from and reverses experimental diabetic neuropathy. *Proc Natl Acad Sci USA*, 101, 823–828.

46 Zochodne DW. (2002) Nerve and ganglion blood flow in diabetes: an appraisal. *Int Rev Neurobiol* 50, 161–202.
47 Theriault M, Dort J, Sutherland G, *et al.* (1997) Local human sural nerve blood flow in diabetic and other polyneuropathies. *Brain* 120, 1131–1138.
48 Hur J, Sullivan KA, Pande M, *et al.* (2011) The identification of gene expression profiles associated with progression of human diabetic neuropathy. *Brain* 134:3222–3235.
49 Kim B, Feldman EL. (2012) Insulin resistance in the nervous system. *Trends Endo Metab* 23, 133–141.
50 Stavniichuk R, Drel VR, Shevalye H, *et al.* (2010) Role of 12/15-lipoxygenase in nitrosative stress and peripheral prediabetic and diabetic neuropathies. *Free Rad Biol Med* 49, 1036–1045.

CHAPTER 29

Neuropathies in metabolic diseases other than diabetes mellitus

Martin Lammens

Department of Pathology, Antwerp University Hospital, Edegem, and University of Antwerp, Antwerp, Belgium

Introduction

Diabetes mellitus is the most prevalent acquired metabolic disorder that causes peripheral neuropathy. Other conditions such as hypothyroidism, hyperthyroidism, chronic kidney, liver and lung diseases, and hyperuricemia are associated with several forms of peripheral neuropathy. The causes of these disease states may be quite diverse and, especially in advanced liver and kidney diseases, there are often several associated pathologies that make it difficult to determine the primary pathological basis of the neuropathy. This chapter reviews the neuropathies associated with thyroid, renal, hepatic, and lung disorders.

Peripheral neuropathies in diseases of the thyroid gland

Both hypothyroidism and hyperthyroidism may lead to disorders of the peripheral nerves. In a clinical and electrophysiological prospective study on newly diagnosed thyroid disorders, 42% of hypothyroid patients had signs of sensorimotor axonal neuropathy, and 29% had carpal tunnel syndrome; 19% of hyperthyroid patients had sensorimotor axonal neuropathy but none had carpal tunnel syndrome [1]. This is in line with earlier mostly retrospective studies [2, 3] in patients with hypothyroidism. Recently, studies of intra-epidermal nerve fibers (IENF) found small fiber neuropathy in up to 60% of patients with overt hypothyroidism and in up to 25% of cases with subclinical hypothyroidism [4].

Hypothyroidism

In patients with hypothyroidism sensory symptoms prevail [5]. Carpal tunnel syndrome is a major issue, starting with numbness and tingling in the distribution area of the median nerve, mostly bilateral [1, 2]. In patients with polyneuropathy, distal paresthesias commonly occur, and others complain of lancinating pains. The patients present with unsteady gait and have loss of vibration and position sense more than small-fiber modalities. In more severe cases, the distal muscles of the lower limbs are weak [6] and there is loss of deep tendon reflexes at the ankles.

Most neurophysiological studies in hypothyroid polyneuropathy describe axonal changes with mild conduction velocity slowing and reduced amplitudes but in severe cases, sensory action potentials may be absent. In some studies conduction velocities typical for demyelinating neuropathy are found. The neurophysiological changes precede the clinical symptoms in hypothyroidism.

Sural nerve biopsies in hypothyroid polyneuropathy show a combination of axonal and demyelinating features. There is a reduction in the number of myelinated fibers, especially of large diameter fibers. Distinct aggregates of glycogen in Schwann cell cytoplasm and more diffuse glycogen in myelinated and unmyelinated axons are found on electron microscopy [6]. More recently several studies of skin biopsies for IENF confirmed the loss of small unmyelinated fibers with a length-dependent distribution [4].

The assumption that carpal tunnel syndrome in hypothyroidism is due to deposition of acid mucopolysaccharide protein complexes in nerves could not be confirmed.

Peripheral Nerve Disorders: Pathology and Genetics, First Edition. Edited by Jean-Michel Vallat, Joachim Weis, Francoise Gray, and Katy Keohane.

It is probably due to synovial and tendon thickening by deposition of these acid mucopolysaccharides [7].

The symptoms of carpal tunnel syndrome normally resolve with thyroid replacement therapy. The polyneuropathy also responds well to the treatment of hypothyroidism.

Hyperthyroidism

In the study of Duyff *et al.* [1], 4 of 21 thyrotoxic patients had signs of peripheral neuropathy, including depressed deep tendon reflexes and symmetric distal sensory disturbances, confirmed by electrophysiological evidence of peripheral neuropathy in 24% of patients. Other patients have been described with carpal tunnel syndrome or a mononeuropathy [8–10]. In most cases the neuropathy has been deemed due to thyrotoxicosis, largely because the two conditions are apparently simultaneous and the neuropathy resolves after correction of the thyrotoxicosis.

There are a few descriptions of acute or subacute weakness of the lower limbs (Basedow's paraplegia) in patients with hyperthyroid thyrotoxicosis [11, 12]. The patients usually present with severe proximal and distal lower limb weakness and decreased tendon reflexes, or areflexia. Sphincters are not involved and there is minimal or no sensory disturbance. Electrophysiological studies reveal a mixed axonal and demyelinating sensorimotor neuropathy. Although rare, this peripheral neuropathy may be an initial clinical feature of hyperthyroidism [13]. Symptoms and signs in such acute cases usually resolve with restoration to a euthyroid state.

Thyrotoxic periodic paralysis is the most frequent form of periodic paralysis in Asian people and is classically due to the associated hypokalemia. There are a few cases described with thyrotoxic normokalemic periodic paralysis [14], clinically and electrophysiologically resembling Guillain–Barré syndrome, but responding very well to control of the hyperthyroidism.

Uremic neuropathy

It has been long known that chronic renal failure is accompanied by polyneuropathy. It is often difficult to determine what is due to the underlying disorder, what is due to renal failure, and what is due to therapy such as hemodialysis. Jebsen *et al.* [15] proved that decreased motor nerve velocity could be improved by hemodialysis, and it became clear that uremia was the cause of the neuropathy, which was later confirmed by numerous other studies.

Neuropathy in renal failure occurs irrespective of the underlying disorder, although concomitant diseases such as diabetes increase the susceptibility for uremia. Clinical or neurophysiological evidence of neuropathy is found in 65–80% of patients with chronic renal failure [16–18], with a glomerular filtration rate of less than 10–12 ml/min or plasma creatinine level of more than 5–6 mg/dl. It is more frequent in males than in females.

Patients typically present with a distal sensorimotor polyneuropathy, starting in the distal lower limbs with tingling, paresthesias, tenderness, or burning sensations of the feet. Restless legs are a very common complication of uremia. Sensory loss is followed by motor weakness of the distal lower limbs, especially of toe and ankle dorsiflexors, with loss of deep tendon reflexes at the ankles. There is loss of vibration and position sense with relative sparing of pinprick and thermal sensibility. Nowadays dialysis is widely available and renal transplantation is often performed, so that extreme motor involvement with upper limb weakness or loss of ambulation is rarely seen. Autonomic neuropathy is also present with sexual, bladder and bowel dysfunction, bloating, and orthostatic hypotension.

Rarely a motor neuropathy resembling acquired inflammatory polyradiculopathy with flaccid quadriplegia may occur [19].

In renal failure mononeuropathies may be found as complications of hemodialysis [20, 21]. Carpal tunnel syndrome may be due to accumulation of Beta2-microglobulin-associated amyloid in the nerve and in the flexor tendon ligament, secondary to using cuprophan membranes [21]. Ischemic forearm neuropathy may be associated with the placement of arteriovenous shunts for dialysis [20].

Sural nerve biopsies revealed axonal degeneration with secondary segmental demyelination, and axonal atrophy with loss of fibers of all sizes most pronounced distally [22–24]. These changes are typical for a length-dependent distal axonopathy, but are non-specific (Figs 29.1 and 29.2). Nerve biopsy is not indicated in typical cases of uremic neuropathy.

For decades, many possible toxins can be filtered during hemodialysis, but no single uremic toxin has been found to be responsible for the polyneuropathy [25].

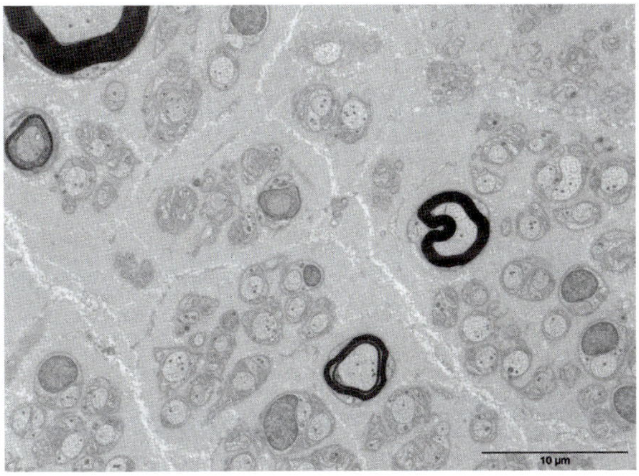

Figure 29.1 Uremic neuropathy: Electron micrograph, transverse section. Sural nerve. Severe reduction of myelinated and unmyelinated fibers corresponding to an axonal neuropathy. Source: Jean-Michel Vallat, CHU de Limoges, France. Reproduced with permission of Jean-Michel Vallat.

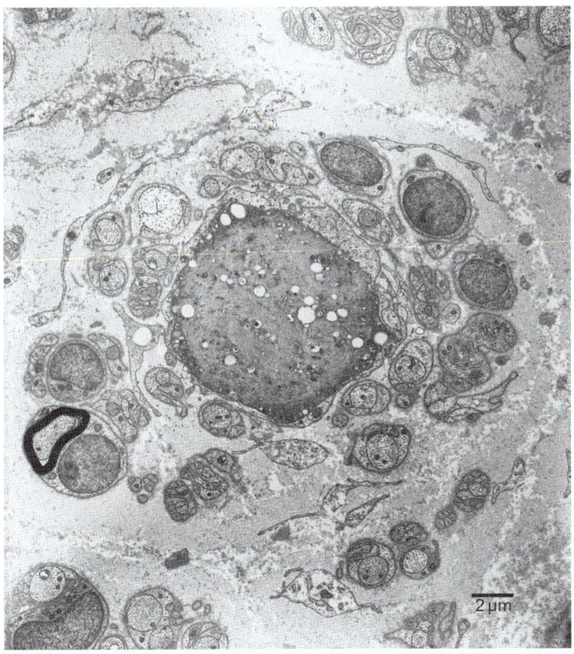

Figure 29.2 Uremic neuropathy: Electron micrograph, transverse section. Sural nerve. Large dilated degenerating unmyelinated axon; the axoplasm is filled with vacuoles, dense bodies, filaments, mitochondria. These findings are non-specific and, although few in this case, correspond to a severe axonal neuropathy. Source: Jean-Michel Vallat, CHU de Limoges, France. Reproduced with permission of Jean-Michel Vallat.

The hypothesis that incomplete clearance of molecules in the range of 0.5–500 kDa in size are the cause of neurotoxicity in renal failure could not be proven because of conflicting results when techniques to improve the clearance of these molecules changed. The pathogenesis probably involves a sequence of metabolic abnormalities leading to impairment of energy supplies, axonal transport, or both [25].

Uremic neuropathy is completely reversible with renal transplantation. The motor and sensory functions improve after a few months, continuing for 12 months or more [26]. During dialysis uremic neuropathy considerable improves, but a complete recovery is rare in the more severe cases [25].

Neuropathy and liver failure

In a study of 83 patients awaiting liver transplantation tested for the presence of peripheral and autonomic neuropathy, 65% had evidence of neuropathy [27]. Many liver diseases such as alcoholic cirrhosis, hepatic porphyria, fat and vitamin E malabsorption, hepatitis C infection with vasculitis and cryoglobulinemia, infections leading to Guillain–Barré syndrome, and others, are accompanied by peripheral neuropathy. In patients with liver failure there are often other concomitant diseases such as diabetes mellitus or renal failure that can also cause a peripheral neuropathy, as can a hepatorenal syndrome. This makes it difficult to define a neuropathy that is primarily due to the metabolic dysfunction of liver failure. The study of Cocito *et al.* [27] found a correlation between the prevalence of neuropathy and the severity of liver disease, suggesting that liver dysfunction might be the primary cause of neuropathy.

Symptoms are predominantly sensory with distal paresthesias and numbness. In more severe cases motor symptoms also occur with weakness especially in the lower limbs. On clinical examination there is loss of sensation, especially vibration sense and loss of deep tendon reflexes of the knees and ankles. Impaired cardiovagal function [28, 29] is an important sign of autonomic neuropathy and may have a more serious prognosis in advanced hepatic disease [28]. This was found in 36.8% of end-stage liver patients in the study of Cocito *et al.* [27].

Neurophysiological studies [27, 30–32] are abnormal in 35–60% of patients. Nerve conduction studies reveal a length-dependent neuropathy with sensory and motor potentials of reduced amplitude and slightly reduced conduction velocity.

Nerve biopsies are consistent with an axonal neuropathy with secondary demyelination [33].

A study of Chopra *et al.* [34] suggested that portosystemic shunting and hepatocellular damage were the two most important factors in the pathogenesis of hepatic neuropathy. However, other studies found that undergoing a portocaval shunt made no difference in patients with cirrhosis [35]. Furthermore, experimental portocaval anastomosis in rats [36] also favored hepatocellular failure as the principal pathophysiological mechanism in neuropathy. One study showed a mild depolarization of the resting axonal membrane potential [37]. Many patients with hepatic neuropathy reported cramps, probably due to intramuscular nerve axonal hyperexcitability [37]. Ischaemia of vasa nervorum and changes in the axonal membrane excitability due to changes in metabolites and toxins could be the primary pathogenetic mechanism of nerve dysfunction [37]. Such depolarization is likely to result from poor nerve perfusion. The hypothesis of a nerve ischemia is supported by histopathological studies [33].

Neuropathy in other acquired metabolic diseases

Chronic pulmonary disease

An association of neuropathy with primary chronic pulmonary disease has been described in several studies [38–40], and the presence of polyneuropathy correlated with the degree of hypoxemia. In the study of Pfeiffer *et al.* [41], 8% of 151 patients with chronic obstructive pulmonary disease (COPD) had clinical polyneuropathy. A neurophysiological study performed in 49 COPD patients, found a subclinical neuropathy in 45% of the patients [42].

Patients complain of distal numbness and paresthesias, there is a mild distal sensory loss and reduced ankle reflexes. Muscle strength is usually normal. Neurophysiologic studies reveal length-dependent axonal neuropathy with reduced sensory and motor amplitudes and normal or slightly reduced nerve conduction velocities. Stoebner *et al.* found signs of axonal degeneration, secondary demyelination and endoneurial vessels with thickened basal lamina in superficial peroneal nerve biopsies of COPD patients [43].

Hyperuricemia

There are several reports of compression neuropathy, especially carpal tunnel neuropathy, due to hyperuricemia (gout) in which tophaceous deposits were found at surgery [44]. In a large population study of one million Taiwani people, an association of gout and carpal tunnel syndrome was found with a ratio of 2.29 [45]. Symptoms of neuropathy improved and relapsed in one patient in accordance with uricemia [46]. It must be kept in mind that colchicine, used in the therapy of gout, especially in transplantation patients, is toxic for peripheral nerves and may lead to an acute myopathy with neuropathy [47].

References

1 Duyff RF, Van den Bosch J, Laman DM *et al.* (2000) Neuromuscular findings in thyroid dysfunction: a prospective clinical and electrodiagnostic study. *J Neurol Neurosurg Psychiatry*. 68:750–755.

2 Murray IP, Simpson JA (1958) Acroparaesthesia in myxoedema; a clinical and electromyographic study. *Lancet*. 1: 1360–1363.

3 Rao SN, Katiyar BC, Nair KR, Misra S (1980) Neuromuscular status in hypothyroidism. *Acta Neurol Scand*. 61:167–177.

4 Magri F, Oliviero A, Rotondi M, Chiovato L (2010) Comments on "aspects of peripheral nerve involvement in patients with treated hypothyroidism." *Eur J Neurol*. 17:e13.

5 Nickel SN, Frame B, Bebin J *et al.* (1961). Myxedema neuropathy and myopathy. A clinical and pathologic study. *Neurology*. 11:125–137.

6 Dyck PJ, Lambert EH (1970) Polyneuropathy associated with hypothyroidism. *J Neuropathol Exp Neurol*. 29:631–658.

7 Gelberman RH, Aronson D, Weisman MH (1980) Carpal-tunnel syndrome. Results of a prospective trial of steroid injection and splinting. *J Bone Joint Surg Am*. 62:1181–1184.

8 Ijichi S, Niina K, Tara M *et al* (1990) Mononeuropathy associated with hyperthyroidism. *J Neurol Neurosurg Psychiatry*. 53:1109–1110.

9 Roquer J, Cano JF (1993) Carpal tunnel syndrome and hyperthyroidism. A prospective study. *Acta Neurol Scand*. 88:149–152.

10 Beard L, Kumar A, Estep HL (1985) Bilateral carpal tunnel syndrome caused by Graves' disease. *Arch Intern Med*. 145: 345–346.

11 Feibel JH, Campa JF (1976) Thyrotoxic neuropathy (Basedow's paraplegia). *J Neurol Neurosurg Psychiatry*. 39:491–497.

12 Sahni V, Gupta N, Anuradha S *et al.* (2007) Thyrotoxic neuropathy – an under diagnosed condition. *Med J Malaysia* 62:76–77.

13 Kung AW (2007) Neuromuscular complications of thyrotoxicosis. *Clin Endocrinol (Oxf)*. 67:645–650.

14 Wu CC, Chau T, Chang CJ, Lin SH (2003) An unrecognized cause of paralysis in ED: thyrotoxic normokalemic periodic paralysis. *Am J Emerg Med.* 21:71–73.
15 Jebsen RH, Tenckhoff H, Honet JC (1967) Natural history of uremic polyneuropathy and effects of dialysis. *N Engl J Med.* 277:327–333.
16 Bazzi C, Pagani C, Sorgato G *et al.* (1991) Uremic polyneuropathy: a clinical and electrophysiological study in 135 short- and long-term hemodialyzed patients. *Clin Nephrol.* 35176–35181.
17 Raskin NH, Fishman RA (1976 A) Neurologic disorders in renal failure (first of two parts). *N Engl J Med.* 294: 143–148.
18 Raskin NH, Fishman RA (1976 B) Neurologic disorders in renal failure (second of two parts). *N Engl J Med.* 294: 204–210.
19 Ropper AH (1993) Accelerated neuropathy of renal failure. *Arch Neurol.* 50:536–539.
20 Harding AE, Le Fanu J (1977) Carpal tunnel syndrome related to antebrachial Cimino-Brescia fistula. *J Neurol Neurosurg Psychiatry.* 40:511–513.
21 Charra B, Calemard E, Uzan M *et al.* (1985) Carpal tunnel syndrome, shoulder pain and amyloid deposits in long-term haemodialysis patients. *Proc Eur Dial Transplant Assoc Eur Ren Assoc.* 21:291–295.
22 Dyck PJ, Johnson WJ, Lambert EH, O'Brien PC (1971) Segmental demyelination secondary to axonal degeneration in uremic neuropathy. *Mayo Clin Proc.* 46:400–431.
23 Said G, Boudier L, Selva J *et al.* (1983) Different patterns of uremic polyneuropathy: clinicopathologic study. *Neurology.* 33:567–574.
24 Ahonen RE (1981) Peripheral neuropathy in uremic patients and in renal transplant recipients. *Acta Neuropathol.* 54:43–53.
25 De Deyn PP, Saxena VK, Abts H *et al.* (1992) Clinical and pathophysiological aspects of neurological complications in renal failure. *Acta Neurol Belg.* 92:191–206.
26 Nielsen VK (1974) The peripheral nerve function in chronic renal failure. IX. Recovery after renal transplantation. Electrophysiological aspects (sensory and motor nerve conduction). *Acta Med Scand.* 195:171–180.
27 Cocito D, Maule S, Paolasso I *et al.* (2010) High prevalence of neuropathies in patients with end-stage liver disease. *Acta Neurol Scand.* 122:36–40.
28 Hendrickse MT, Thuluvath PJ, Triger DR (1992) Natural history of autonomic neuropathy in chronic liver disease. *Lancet.* 339:1462–1464.
29 Hendrickse MT, Triger DR (1993) Autonomic dysfunction in chronic liver disease. *Clin Auton Res.* 3:227–231.
30 Knill-Jones RP, Goodwill CJ, Dayan AD, Williams R (1972) Peripheral neuropathy in chronic liver disease: clinical, electrodiagnostic, and nerve biopsy findings. *J Neurol Neurosurg Psychiatry.* 35:22–30.
31 Kardel T, Nielsen VK (1974) Hepatic neuropathy. A clinical and electrophysiological study. *Acta Neurol Scand.* 50:513–526.
32 Fierro B, Modica A, D'Arpa A *et al.* (1986) The F-wave in uremic neuropathy. *Acta Neurol (Napoli).* 8:404–411.
33 Chari VR, Katiyar BC, Rastogi BL, Bhattacharya SK (1977) Neuropathy in hepatic disorders. A clinical, electrophysiological and histopathological appraisal. *J Neurol Sci.* 31:93–111.
34 Chopra JS, Samanta AK, Murthy JM *et al.* (1980) Role of porta systemic shunt and hepatocellular damage in the genesis of hepatic neuropathy. *Clin Neurol Neurosurg.* 82:37–44.
35 Kardel T, Nielsen VK (1974) Hepatic neuropathy. A clinical and electrophysiological study. *Acta Neurol Scand.* 50:513–526.
36 Hindfelt B, Holmin T (1980) Experimental porta-caval anastomosis and motor nerve conduction velocity in the rat. *J Neurol.* 223:171–15.
37 Ng K, Lin CS, Murray NM *et al.* (2007) Conduction and excitability properties of peripheral nerves in end-stage liver disease. *Muscle Nerve.* 35:730–738.
38 Appenzeller O, Parks RD, MacGee J (1968) Peripheral neuropathy in chronic disease of the respiratory tract. *Am J Med.* 44:873–880.
39 Faden A, Mendoza E, Flynn F (1981) Subclinical neuropathy associated with chronic obstructive pulmonary disease: possible pathophysiologic role of smoking. *Arch Neurol.* 38:639–642.
40 Jarratt JA, Morgan CN, Twomey JA *et al.* (1992) Neuropathy in chronic obstructive pulmonary disease: a multicentre electrophysiological and clinical study. *Eur Respir J.* 5:517–524.
41 Pfeiffer G, Kunze K, Brüch M *et al.* (1990) Polyneuropathy associated with chronic hypoxaemia: prevalence in patients with chronic obstructive pulmonary disease. *J Neurol.* 237:230–233.
42 Ozge A, Atiş S, Sevim S (2001) Subclinical peripheral neuropathy associated with chronic obstructive pulmonary disease. *Electromyogr Clin Neurophysiol.* 41:185–191.
43 Stoebner P, Mezin P, Vila A *et al.* (1989) Microangiopathy of endoneurial vessels in hypoxemic chronic obstructive pulmonary disease (COPD). A quantitative ultrastructural study. *Acta Neuropathol.* 78:388–395.
44 Fitzgerald BT, Setty A, Mudgal CS (2007) Gout affecting the hand and wrist. *J Am Acad Orthop Surg.* 15:625–635.
45 Tseng CH, Liao CC, Kuo CM *et al.* (2012) Medical and nonmedical correlates of carpal tunnel syndrome in a Taiwan cohort of one million. *Eur J Neurol.* 19:91–97.
46 Delaney P (1983) Gouty neuropathy. *Arch Neurol.* 40: 823–824.
47 Lai IC, Cheng CY, Chen HH *et al.* (2006) Colchicine myoneuropathy in chronic renal failure patients with gout. *Nephrology (Carlton).* 11:147–150.

CHAPTER 30

Toxic neuropathies

Sebastian Brandner

Division of Neuropathology and Department of Neurodegenerative Disease, National Hospital for Neurology and Neurosurgery, and UCL Institute of Neurology, London, UK

Definition of the disorder and historical perspective

Peripheral neuropathies caused by occupational or environmental exposure, by medication or nutrition can be classified under the umbrella term *toxic neuropathies*. This chapter specifically excludes all forms of toxic optic neuropathies and neuropathies due to malnutrition or nutritional-toxic causes, such as alcoholic neuropathies (see Chapter 33). Depending on the etiology, toxic neuropathies have also been designated drug-related, medication-induced, nutritional, nutritional-toxic, alcohol-induced, and so on. Removal of the offending agent may alleviate or reverse some or all of the symptoms.

Historical reports of toxic neuropathies highlight the impact of occupational surveillance: the most commonly reported occupational and environmental toxins in industrialized countries used to be lead, arsenic, mercury, thallium, acrylamide, organophosphates, trichlorethylene, DDT, tetrachlorethane, and pentachlorophenol [1]. Many of these toxins have now been phased out in western industrialized countries (such as the European Union and the United States) due to stricter control on their usage and exposure, but are on the rise in emerging economies where environmental pollution and occupational exposure are poorly controlled. Medication-induced neuropathies have long been known for well-established drugs such as Amiodarone [2] (Fig. 30.1A–D) or Chloroquine [3] (Fig. 30.1G,H) but have recently become more prevalent, due to the development and availability of a multitude of increasingly sophisticated drugs, which have added to the spectrum of offending agents [4, 5]. The increasing use of recreational drugs such as nitric oxide [6] has also led to unexpected complications, including toxic neuropathies. It is important to recognize the causes of toxic neuropathies because they are treatable and preventable.

Epidemiology

Individuals with toxic neuropathies will have had either an environmental, occupational or iatrogenic exposure to an offending toxin.

Iatrogenic toxic neuropathy, unavoidable in the context of chemotherapy, is usually controlled by adjusting the medication.

Occupational or environmental toxic neuropathies may be acute, subacute, or chronic due to exposure to metals, solvents, pesticides, as a result of war (e.g., chemical warfare), environmental disasters (oil spills, accidents in the chemical industry), and other contaminants [7–9]. Genetic, physiological, and environmental factors determine an individual's metabolic make-up, and may influence differences in the sensitivity of exposed individuals.

Chemotherapy-induced toxic peripheral neuropathies (CIPN) are an increasingly frequent problem [4, 10, 11]. Neurotoxicity is usually dependent on the cumulative dose where the severity of the neuropathy increases with duration of treatment. Cessation or completion of the treatment usually stops progression of CIPN, except for platinum compounds where symptoms progress or at least persist for several months. Often, only symptomatic

Peripheral Nerve Disorders: Pathology and Genetics, First Edition. Edited by Jean-Michel Vallat, Joachim Weis, Francoise Gray, and Katy Keohane.

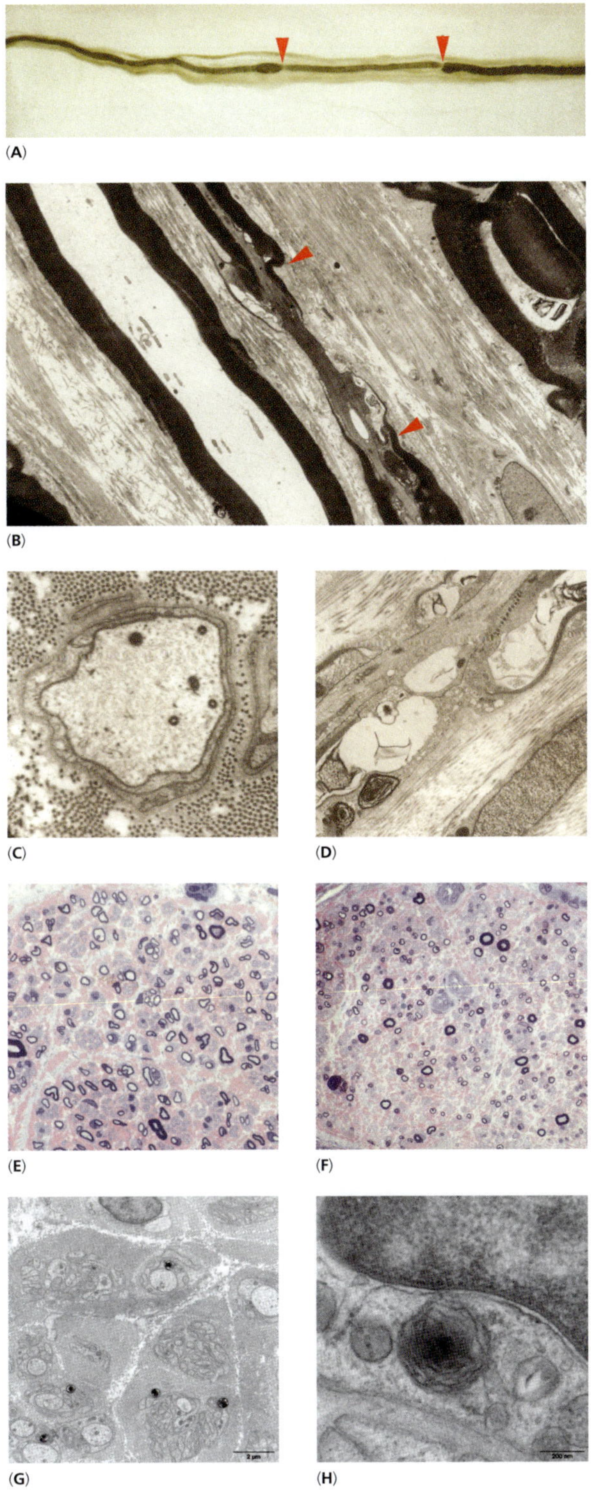

Figure 30.1 Examples of microscopic and ultrastructural (EM) findings in toxic neuropathies: **(A–D)** Amiodarone-induced toxic neuropathy with demyelination. (**A**) teased fiber preparation with segmental demyelination, (**B**) ultrastructural examination shows demyelination in the nodal region, next to an unaffected myelinated axon, (**C**) transverse section of demyelinated fiber, and (**D**) longitudinal section with nodal changes. **(E)** Widespread regeneration in a sural nerve of a patient surviving a suicide attempt with podophyllin, a once commonly used tincture against HPV-induced warts. **(F)** Thalidomide toxicity with widespread rarefaction of large and small myelinated fibers due to axonal neuropathy. **(G, H)** Chloroquine-induced neuropathy: Note the lamellar inclusions in Schwann cells. Source: Michael Groves, National Hospital for Neurology and Neurosurgery, UK (parts A–F) and Jean-Michel Vallat, CHU de Limoges, France (parts G–H); Reproduced with permission of Michael Groves and Jean-Michel Vallat.

treatment is available so neurotoxicity poses a major dose-limiting factor. Rarely, prophylaxis or specific treatments are available. The epidemiology of CIPN is still unclear, and several drug-dependent pathogenetic mechanisms exist (see section on pathogenesis). Patients with pre-existing neuropathies, such as subclinical HSMN have a greater risk of developing CIPN [12].

Clinical features including appropriate investigations and important differential diagnosis

The clinical presentation resulting from the exposure to toxins can mimic hereditary, autoimmune, or metabolic (e.g., diabetic) neuropathies. The classification can be based on (1) etiology, (2) clinical picture, or (3) the pathological-anatomical involvement (Table 30.1). Symptoms correspond to sensory, motor, or autonomic involvement [9], and have to be validated by electrical studies, to assess large fiber neuropathies.

CIPNs are predominantly sensory, length-dependent neuropathies that develop after a typical cumulative dose. CIPN generally appear in a dose-dependent manner, although with oxaliplatin and taxanes, immediate toxic effects can occur. The most frequent substances causing CIPN are platin compounds, vinca alkaloids, taxanes, bortezomib, and thalidomide (Table 30.1 and Fig. 30.1 F). The role of synergistic neurotoxicity caused by previously given or concomitant chemotherapies and the role of a pre-existent neuropathy on the development of a CIPN is likely to vary from case to case.

The commonest type of axonal neuropathy in the context of exposure to toxins is usually a dying back type axonal neuropathy (Wallerian degeneration) and will result in reduced sensory amplitudes [8, 9]. Demyelinating neuropathies are less common, and result in a conduction block [9, 13, 14].

The strengths of electrophysiology are (1) it is non-invasive, (2) it allows multiple assessments to map natural history, (3) it gives detailed analysis of the somatosensory evoked potentials to map conduction along the peripheral nerves, roots, spinal cord, brainstem, and brain [15]. Its limitations are that (1) it is generally sensitive, but non-specific and (2) it represents a summary of the activity of all fibers so that damage in a small number of neurons can remain undetected in the averaged response [5, 7, 16]. Electrophysiology is not synonymous with nerve function; most measures reflect activity in only a subset of neurons, and for a restricted set of functions.

As more long-term cancer patients survive, a new focus emerges on the long-term effects of chemotherapy-induced neuropathies, and rehabilitation is required to improve patients' functions and quality of life.

Pathology

Histopathological assessment of peripheral nerves is rightfully considered the gold standard of peripheral nerve analysis, including the examination of toxic neuropathies [7]. It can provide an accurate view of the natural history ranging from initial changes to end-stage processes, such as Wallerian degeneration.

Histological and ultrastructural analysis of nerve biopsies can identify the anatomical target of the toxin. These comprise alterations of axons (associated with axonal swellings similar to those in giant axonal neuropathy, axonal degeneration, axonal loss with reduced fiber density and clusters of regenerating nerve fibers) and alterations of Schwann cells (leading to abnormal Schwann cell morphology, demyelination and remyelination). Moreover, alterations of the interstitium and of blood vessels as well as inflammatory infiltrates are detected [8].

The analysis can be aided by morphometry to determine the g-ratio, numbers of large and small fibers, and the ratio between unmyelinated, small and large myelinated fibers. As for all neuropathies, the limitation of a biopsy is the restriction of sampling, which provides a "regional snapshot." Microscopically observable nerve regeneration and clinical improvement may follow cessation of exposure.

The morphological features of relevant, paradigmatic toxic neuropathies are summarized in Table 30.1 and typical examples are given in Fig. 30.1.

Genetics and pathogenesis

Cells of the peripheral nervous system are sensitive to toxins due to their particular unique anatomical location and environment. Sensory neurons, located within ganglia, are not protected by the blood brain barrier, but are supplied by capillaries that allow free exchange of molecules between the circulation and the interstitium of ganglia. Peripheral nervous system axons are

References	Histopathology B = Biopsy on patients E = Experimental	Target or mechanism of action	Type and involvement of neuropathy	Etiology E = Environ O = Occup M = Medical	Type, use, or occurrence of toxin	Toxin
[35]	Sciatic nerve Schwann cells and myelin; DRG and axonal degeneration (E)	Mitochondrial and endoplasmic reticulum damage	Axonal, small-fiber sensory, distal, and highly length dependent; rare motor	M	Polycyclic derivative of boronic acid, proteasome inhibitor	Bortezomib
[36]	Severe DRG damage in rodents (E)	Microtubule stabilization (fast axonal transport)	Axonal, sensory distal neuropathy	M	Semisynthetic analogue of the natural product epothilone B	Ixabepilone
[33]	Focal axonal (Wallerian) degeneration (E)	Structural change of DNA	Large fiber neuropathy	M	Platinum compounds	Cisplatin, Carboplatin
[37]		Structural change of DNA	Cold hypersensitivity, limb paresthesia	M	Organo-platinum compound	Oxaliplatin
[32]	Injury of vasa nervorum (Axonal neuropathy (E, B)	Angiogenesis inhibition	Paresthesia, sensation, pain in the feet and hands. proprioceptive sensory loss	M	Paclitaxel (taxol) and docetaxel (taxotere) a	Taxanes
[13, 32] (Fig. 30.1 F)	Reduction of vasa nervorum (E)	Antiangiogenesis	Predominantly sensory; can be irreversible; less commonly demyelinating polyneuropathy (more severe but reversible)	M	VEGF inhibitor	Thalidomide
[3] (Fig. 30.1G,H)	Biopsy: Segmental demyelination and axonopathy with myeloid bodies. Ultrastructure: myelin figures in Schwann cell cytoplasm surrounding myelinated and unmyelinated axons	Antimalarial drugs accumulate in lysosomes and raise the intralysosomal pH	Peripheral neuropathy	M	Antimalaria drug (CQ) Antirehumatic drug (HCQ)	Chloroquin (CQ), Hydroxychloroquin (HCQ)
[10]		Mitotic spindle inhibitors	Dose-related sensorimotor neuropathy	M	Anti-mitotic and anti-microtubule agents	Vinca alkaloids
[38]	Wallerian degeneration; De- and remyelination	Uncoupling G protein from receptor	Chronic: mild distal axonal neuropathy; Acute: polyradiculoneuropathy, demyelination	M	Polysulfonated naphthylurea	Suramin
[2] (Fig. 30.1A–D)	Severe acute motor axon degeneration; delayed complete regeneration (E) Induction of heterogeneous osmiophilic, lipidic intra lysosomal inclusions	Antiarrhythmic drug	Peripheral neuropathy (NOS)	M	Inhibitory effect on lysosomal phospholipases A1 and A2, (formation of lysosomal phospholipid-containing inclusions in many cell types).	Amiodarone

(Continued)

Table 30.1 (*Continued*)

References	Histopathology B = Biopsy on patients E = Experimental	Target or mechanism of action	Type and involvement of neuropathy	Etiology E = Environ O = Occup M = Medical	Type, use, or occurrence of toxin	Toxin
[39]		Inhibits bacterial synthesis of dihydrofolic acid	Peripheral neuropathy (NOS)	M	Diamino-diphenyl sulfone, antimycotic, (m. leprae)	Dapsone
[40]	De- and remyelination >>axonal degeneration (E)	Prodrug, activated by a bacterial peroxidase prevention and treatment of tuberculosis	Peripheral neuropathy (NOS)	M	Inhibition of the activity of vitamin B6. Reversal by pyridoxine administration	Isoniazid
[41]	Axonal degeneration	Medication particularly for anaerobic bacteria and protozoa	Length-dependent painful neuropathy	M	Nitroimidazole antibiotic	Metronidazole
[34]	Axonal degeneration	Disruption neuronal mitochondrial DNA synthesis	Glove and stocking, epidermal, and sweat gland innervation	M	Stavudine, zalcitabine didanosine	Nucleoside reverse transcriptase inhibitors (NRTI) ddI, ddC, d4T
[9]	Distal axon degeneration (E)	Axoplasmic Na-K ATPase, Presynaptic toxicity on nerve terminals; kinesin-based fast axonal transport	Distal axon degeneration	O	Mining and tunneling, polymers, paper and fabric industry, dyes, adhesives, waste treatment	Acrylamide
[9, 24]	Axonal degeneration	Inhibits glutathione reductase and diminishes intracellular reduced glutathione cell cycle arrest at G0/G1 phase, induction of apoptosis	Axonal large fiber sensorimotor neuropathy	O, E	Pesticides, pigments, seafood, wood preservative, tanning, pharmaceuticals, glass	Arsenic
[9, 42]	Axonal degeneration	Disruption of neurofilaments homeostasis (E). Decrease of microtubules	Polyneuropathy, ascending from distal to proximal.	O	Viscose Rayon, electroplating, cellophane, plywood and pesticides, rubber vulcanization, explosives	Carbon disulfide
[43]	Axonal degeneration	Mitochondria	Sensorimotor polyneuropathy	O	Heavy metal prosthetic material, such as hip replacement	Cobalt
[9, 44, 45]	Axonal degeneration	Dysregulation of serine/threonine protein phosphatases Ca++ mimetic action.	Paresthesia and pain or impaired sensation	O, E	Solderers, insecticides, batteries, smelters, pipes, paint	Lead

[9, 46]	Axonal degeneration	Cytoskeletal reorganization of structural proteins (E) Disruption of membrane structure	Peripheral neuropathy with distal latency sensory slowing, and motor slowing for long-term exposures	O, E	Organic: agricultural and industrial poisons: elemental and inorganic: electronics, paint, metal and textile production, chemical catalyst, pharmaceuticals, dental amalgams, gold mining, photography, felt making, consumption of fish	Mercury
[9, 47, 48]	Multifocal loss of myelinated fibers, segmental de-and remyelination. Axon degeneration.	Free radical generator forming a methyl radical, a highly reactive species	Chronic peripheral sensorimotor neuropathy	O, E	Fumigant, fire retardant, refrigerant, insecticide	Methyl bromide
[9, 14]	Reduced number of small and medium sized unmyelinated fibers. Regeneration. Focal fusiform axon enlargement. Masses of 9–10-nm filaments in enlarged axons.	Impaired neurofilament transport along the length of the axon.	Focal, partial conduction block	O, E	Paints, lacquers, adhesives, solvents, component of naphtha	N-hexane
[9, 49]	Axonal swelling, segmental demyelination (E) Axonal degeneration and regeneration, demyelination (B)	Irreversible AChE inhibition	Distal numbness and paresthesia, followed by progressive weakness	O, E	Agricultural pesticide	Organophosphates
[9, 23, 50]	Degenerating axons, disruption of myelin. Ultrastructurally, disturbance of neurofilament structure and fragmentation. Degeneration of unmyelinated axons.	Oxidative stress, Lipid peroxidation	Paresthesia, dysesthesia, severe pain	O, E	Glass and alloys, rodenticides	Thallium
[9, 25, 51]	Intramyelin oedema induced by triethyl-tin, and neuronal necrosis caused by trimethyl-tin.		Peripheral neuropathy with paresthesia and slowed sensory nerve conduction	O, E	Plastic polymers and catalysts in polyurethane, silicone and epoxy curing. Biocidal, repellent and wood and textile preservation, disinfectants, antifungal agents	Tin

Key: E = Environmental, O = Occupational, M = Medical/Iatrogenic; NOS = not otherwise specified generally susceptible to any substances interfering with energy metabolism or axonal transport. Drugs disrupting microtubules in the mitotic spindle (e.g., Vinca alkaloids, podophyllin, Fig. 30.1E) inevitably also disrupt microtubule-based axonal transport (Table 30.1). Agents targeting the increased mitochondrial activity of cancer cells may impair axonal transport. Finally, neurons have programmed cell death pathways that are particularly sensitive to DNA damage induced by chemotherapeutic agents. Genetic variability (polymorphisms) influence the susceptibility to toxins; an example is the δ-Aminolaevulinic acid dehydratase genotype, which modulates susceptibility to lead-induced neuropathies [17].

Animal models and pathogenesis

Experimental models of neurotoxicity, usually in rodents, have identified a number of molecular and cellular targets of some compounds, at both histological and biochemical levels. Although specific molecular targets have been identified for a number of environmental/occupational and therapeutic agents, it is speculated that these targets may ultimately prove to involve a mechanism at the single cell level, for example, cell division [18, 19]. The direct targets of a toxin may be a presumed single molecular or receptor target or a toxin can affect multiple targets. Cell and animal models have aided the understanding of the mechanisms of toxicity of occupational or environmental agents, such as acrylamide [20], 2,5 Hexanedione [21, 22], Thallium [23], Arsenic [24], Tin [25], or of medication-induced neuropathies such as Taxol [26], 5-lipoxygenase inhibitors (used in asthma, rheumatoid arthritis, and psoriasis) [27], Amiodarone [28], isoniazid [29], nuclear reverse transcriptase inhibitors [30, 31], Thalidomide [32].

Treatment, future perspective, conclusions

The effective use of many anti-cancer drugs can be limited by a dose-dependent peripheral neuropathy. To identify the mechanisms of toxicity, generation and validation of animal models (see previously) is essential to reproduce pathology, identify the molecular targets and then determine a mechanism by which the side effects can be controlled [10, 19]. Several models exist: Apfel *et al.* (26) established an animal model to analyze Taxol-mediated neuropathies and then demonstrated that treatment with nerve growth factor significantly ameliorates the toxicity. Cisplatin has anti-angiogenic effects, and VEGF treatment is beneficial to reduce neuropathy [33]. Clinical studies of successful treatment include the inhibition of Taxol and Thalidomide toxicity by VEGF-mediated antiangiogenesis [32], or L-Carnitine to reduce antiretroviral toxic neuropathies [34]. An overview of the most commonly used chemotherapy agents and their treatment is given in [10].

References

1 Barnes JM (1969) Toxic chemicals and peripheral neuropathy: experimental studies. *Proc R Soc Med*;62:205–208.
2 Orr CF, Ahlskog JE (2009) Frequency, characteristics, and risk factors for amiodarone neurotoxicity. *Arch Neurol*;66: 865–869.
3 Estes ML, Ewing-Wilson D, Chou SM *et al.* (1987) Clinical and pathologic perspective. *Am J Med*;82:447–455.
4 Manji H (2011) Toxic neuropathy. *Curr Opin Neurol*;24: 484–490.
5 Weimer LH, Sachdev N (2009) Update on medication-induced peripheral neuropathy. *Curr Neurol Neurosci Rep*;9:69–75.
6 Cheng HM, Park JH, Hernstadt D (2013) Subacute combined degeneration of the spinal cord following recreational nitrous oxide use. *BMJ Case Rep*;2013.
7 Arezzo JC, Litwak MS, Zotova EG (2011) Correlation and dissociation of electrophysiology and histopathology in the assessment of toxic neuropathy. *Toxicol Pathol*;39:46–51.
8 Scelsi R, Candura SM (2012) Occupational toxic neuropathies: morphology in peripheral nerve biopsies. *G Ital Med Lav Ergon*;34:410–419.
9 Rutchik J (2009) Occupational medicine physician's guide to neuropathy in the workplace, part 2: electromyography and cryptogenic and toxic neuropathy. *J Occup Environ Med*;51:622–625.
10 Grisold W, Cavaletti G, Windebank AJ (2012) Peripheral neuropathies from chemotherapeutics and targeted agents: diagnosis, treatment, and prevention. *Neuro Oncol*;14 Suppl 4:45–54.
11 Windebank AJ, Grisold W (2008) Chemotherapy-induced neuropathy. *J Peripher Nerv Syst*;13:27–46.
12 Chaudhry V, Chaudhry M, Crawford TO *et al.* (2008) Toxic neuropathy in patients with pre-existing neuropathy. *Neurology*;60:337–340.
13 Chaudhry V, Cornblath DR, Polydefkis M *et al.* (2008) Characteristics of bortezomib- and thalidomide-induced peripheral neuropathy. *J Peripher Nerv Syst*;13:275–282.

14 Chang AP, England JD, Garcia CA, Sumner AJ (1998) Focal conduction block in n-hexane polyneuropathy. *Muscle Nerve*;21:964–969.

15 Arezzo JC, Schaumburg HH, Spencer PS (1982) Structure and function of the somatosensory system: a neurotoxicological perspective. *Environ Health Perspect*;44:23–30.

16 Arezzo JC, Zotova E (2002) Electrophysiologic measures of diabetic neuropathy: mechanism and meaning. *Int Rev Neurobiol*;50:229–255.

17 Zheng G, Tian L, Liang Y *et al.* (2011) delta-Aminolevulinic acid dehydratase genotype predicts toxic effects of lead on workers' peripheral nervous system. *Neurotoxicology*; 32:374–382.

18 Xiao WH, Bennett GJ (2012) Effects of mitochondrial poisons on the neuropathic pain produced by the chemotherapeutic agents, paclitaxel and oxaliplatin. *Pain*;153:704–709.

19 Zheng H, Xiao WH, Bennett GJ (2012) Mitotoxicity and bortezomib-induced chronic painful peripheral neuropathy. *Exp Neurol*;238:225–234.

20 Sickles DW, Stone JD, Friedman MA (2002) Fast axonal transport: a site of acrylamide neurotoxicity? *Neurotoxicology*; 23:223–251.

21 Sterman AB, Delannoy MR (1985) Cell body responses to axonal injury: traumatic axotomy versus toxic neuropathy. *Exp Neurol*;89:408–419.

22 Zhao L, Liu Q, Chen H *et al.* (2011) The effect of 2,5-hexanedione on myelin protein zero expression, and its mitigation using Ginkgo biloba extract. *Biomed Environ Sci*;24:374–382.

23 Galvan-Arzate S, Martinez A, Medina E *et al.* (2000) Subchronic administration of sublethal doses of thallium to rats: effects on distribution and lipid peroxidation in brain regions. *Toxicol Lett*;116:37–43.

24 Banerjee N, Banerjee M, Ganguly S *et al.* (2008) Arsenic-induced mitochondrial instability leading to programmed cell death in the exposed individuals. *Toxicology*;246: 101–111.

25 Trabucco A, Di Pietro P, Nori SL *et al.* (2009) Methylated tin toxicity a reappraisal using rodents models. *Arch Ital Biol*;147:141–153.

26 Apfel SC, Lipton RB, Arezzo JC, Kessler JA (1991) Nerve growth factor prevents toxic neuropathy in mice. *Ann Neurol*;29:87–90.

27 Gunson DE, Sahota PS, Iverson WO *et al.* (1992) Toxic peripheral neuropathy with demyelination in Sprague–Dawley rats given CGS 21595 – a 5-lipoxygenase inhibitor. *Vet Pathol*;29:145–151.

28 Santoro L, Barbieri F, Nucciotti R *et al.* (1992) Amiodarone-induced experimental acute neuropathy in rats. *Muscle Nerve*;15:788–795.

29 Naba I, Yoshikawa H, Sakoda S *et al.* (2000) Successful generation of peripheral neuropathy with onion-bulb formation in the macrophage scavenger receptor classA knockout mouse treated with isoniazid. *Neurosci Lett*;290:5–8.

30 Keswani SC, Chander B, Hasan C *et al.*(2003) FK506 is neuroprotective in a model of antiretroviral toxic neuropathy. *Ann Neurol*;53:57–64.

31 Youle M (2007) Acetyl-L-carnitine in HIV-associated antiretroviral toxic neuropathy. *CNS Drugs*;21 Suppl 1:25–30; discussion 45–46.

32 Kirchmair R, Tietz AB, Panagiotou E *et al.* (2007) Therapeutic angiogenesis inhibits or rescues chemotherapy-induced peripheral neuropathy: taxol- and thalidomide-induced injury of vasa nervorum is ameliorated by VEGF. *Mol Ther*;15:69–75.

33 Kirchmair R, Walter DH, Ii M *et al.* (2005) Antiangiogenesis mediates cisplatin-induced peripheral neuropathy: attenuation or reversal by local vascular endothelial growth factor gene therapy without augmenting tumor growth. *Circulation*;111:2662–2670.

34 Youle M, Osio M (2007) A double-blind, parallel-group, placebo-controlled, multicentre study of acetyl L-carnitine in the symptomatic treatment of antiretroviral toxic neuropathy in patients with HIV-1 infection. *HIV Med*; 8:241–250.

35 Argyriou AA, Iconomou G, Kalofonos HP (2008) Bortezomib-induced peripheral neuropathy in multiple myeloma: a comprehensive review of the literature. *Blood*;112:1593–1599.

36 Argyriou AA, Marmiroli P, Cavaletti G, Kalofonos HP (2011) Epothilone-induced peripheral neuropathy: a review of current knowledge. *J Pain Symptom Manage*;42:931–940.

37 Lehky TJ, Leonard GD, Wilson RH *et al.* (2004) Oxaliplatin-induced neurotoxicity: acute hyperexcitability and chronic neuropathy. *Muscle Nerve*;29:387–392.

38 Chaudhry V, Eisenberger MA, Sinibaldi VJ *et al.* (1996) A prospective study of suramin-induced peripheral neuropathy. *Brain*;119 (Pt 6):2039–2052.

39 Mery L, Dega H, Prost C, Dubertret L (2003) Dapsone-induced sensory peripheral neuropathy. *Ann Dermatol Venereol*;130:447–449.

40 Kass JS, Shandera WX (2010) Nervous system effects of antituberculosis therapy. *CNS Drugs*;24:655–667.

41 Tan CH, Chen YF, Chen CC *et al.* (2011) Painful neuropathy due to skin denervation after metronidazole-induced neurotoxicity. *J Neurol Neurosurg Psychiatry*;82:462–465.

42 Song F, Zhang C, Wang Q *et al.* (2009) Alterations in neurofilaments content and calpains activity of sciatic nerve of carbon disulfide-treated rats. *Arch Toxicol*;83:587–594.

43 Catalani S, Rizzetti MC, Padovani A, Apostoli P (2012) Neurotoxicity of cobalt. *Hum Exp Toxicol*;31:421–437.

44 Rubens O, Logina I, Kravale I *et al.* (2001) Peripheral neuropathy in chronic occupational inorganic lead exposure: a clinical and electrophysiological study. *J Neurol Neurosurg Psychiatry*;71:200–204.

45 Rahman A, Brew BJ, Guillemin GJ (2011) Lead dysregulates serine/threonine protein phosphatases in human neurons. *Neurochem Res*;36:195–204.

46 Choi WS, Kim SJ, Kim JS (2011) Inorganic lead (Pb)- and mercury (Hg)-induced neuronal cell death involves cytoskeletal reorganization. *Lab Anim Res*;27:219–225.

47 Cavalleri F, Galassi G, Ferrari S *et al.*(1995) Methyl bromide induced neuropathy: a clinical, neurophysiological, and morphological study. *J Neurol Neurosurg Psychiatry*;58:383.

48 Shaw I (2010) Motor neurone disease – a methyl bromide exposure cluster points to a causal mechanism. *Hum Exp Toxicol*;29:241–242.

49 Vasilescu C, Alexianu M, Dan A (1984) Delayed neuropathy after organophosphorus insecticide (Dipterex) poisoning: a clinical, electrophysiological and nerve biopsy study. *J Neurol Neurosurg Psychiatry*;47:543–548.

50 Kuo HC, Huang CC, Tsai YT *et al.* (2005) Acute painful neuropathy in thallium poisoning. *Neurology*;65:302–304.

51 Dopp E, von Recklinghausen U, Hippler J *et al.* Toxicity of volatile methylated species of bismuth, arsenic, tin, and mercury in mammalian cells in vitro. *J Toxicol*;2011:503576.

CHAPTER 31

Polyneuropathy associated with a monoclonal gammopathy

Yuichi Kawagashira,[1] Haruki Koike,[1] Jean-Michel Vallat,[2] and Gen Sobue[1]

[1] *Department of Neurology, Nagoya University Graduate School of Medicine, Nagoya, Japan*

[2] *Neurology Laboratory, National Referral Center for Rare Peripheral Neuropathies, University Hospital, Limoges, France*

Introduction

There are no large prospective studies of the prevalence of neuropathies in patients with monoclonal gammopathy (MG); however, polyneuropathies (PN) can occur in any type of benign or malignant MG and are a frequent complication of plasma-cell dyscrasias such as "monoclonal gammopathy of undetermined significance" (MGUS), multiple myeloma, Waldenström's disease, POEMS (polyneuropathy, organomegaly, endocrinopathy, monoclonal gammopathy, and skin changes) syndrome, Castleman's disease, and light-chain amyloidosis. These clinically diverse peripheral neuropathies can occur before or after discovery of the gammopathy.

Nerve biopsy can be particularly useful in patients undergoing potentially neurotoxic chemotherapy. Clinical and electrophysiological findings alone cannot discriminate between drug-induced PN and other causes. Depending on the nerve biopsy findings, aggressive chemotherapy and/or a bone marrow transplant may be indicated.

Endoneurial immunoglobulin deposits

Intramyelin infiltration

IgM

Of the many complications of monoclonal gammopathies [1–5], IgM is the most common M protein to cause neuropathy; it commonly causes demyelinating neuropathy [5, 6]. IgM causes several forms of neuropathy, possibly reflecting different pathogenic mechanisms and is associated with Waldenstrom's disease or MGUS. [7–10, 11–15]. Although various antibodies against sulfatides, chondroitin sulfate C, cytoskeletal proteins, and several gangliosides have been detected in the serum of these patients, the best defined and most frequent are anti-MAG antibodies [16–18]. Anti-MAG neuropathy has distinctive clinical, electrophysiological and pathological features that may help to distinguish it from other demyelinating chronic neuropathies [13–15, 19].

Clinical manifestations, anti- MAG antibodies and electrophysiological findings

Approximately 80–90% of the patients are men. In most patients, symptoms appear late in life: typically in the sixth or seventh decade, and occasionally after the age of 80 [13, 14, 16].

Almost all patients have symmetrical sensory symptoms in the distal legs, often associated with a sensory ataxia [16]. Mild to moderate distal muscle weakness, first noted in the toe extensors, develops over the course of years [13, 14, 16]. Some patients present with sensorimotor neuropathy, which has predominant muscle weakness and wasting [14, 20]. A postural tremor in the upper limbs is present at onset in a number of patients [16]. After onset, the vast majority of patients progress slowly with symmetric, predominantly distal impairment affecting the lower limbs more severely than the upper limbs.

MAG is the most extensively studied antigen, it is highly specific, and is recognized as the antigen responsible for many cases of IgM monoclonal gammopathy. In approximately half the patients with IgM monoclonal gammopathy, the monoclonal antibody reacts with

Peripheral Nerve Disorders: Pathology and Genetics, First Edition. Edited by Jean-Michel Vallat, Joachim Weis, Francoise Gray, and Katy Keohane.

MAG [16, 21]. The IgM reactivity against MAG is usually demonstrated by Western blot using purified MAG or myelin proteins from autopsied human brain, or by ELISA that appears to be more useful in detecting anti-MAG IgM antibodies [22].

Electrophysiological studies show a widespread symmetrical, predominantly distal, reduction of conduction velocities, which is more severe in sensory than in motor nerves, usually without conduction block [23]. Nerve fiber endings are particularly affected, as shown by a disproportionate prolongation of distal latencies [24]. This finding can help distinguish anti-MAG neuropathy from other chronic acquired or inherited demyelinating polyneuropathies. [24–27].

Pathology

Light microscopy: Morphological studies on nerve biopsy tissue in patients with anti-MAG neuropathy do not show significant abnormalities on paraffin sections. On semithin cross sections a variable loss of myelinated fibers, especially of large myelinated fibers is usually observed, [28, 29]. Vasculitis, infiltration of inflammatory cells, and amyloid deposits in the endoneurium are not generally detected. Changes due to demyelination, including naked axons, thinly myelinated fibers, and regenerating clusters of axons are commonly seen (Fig. 31.1A). Redundant myelin loops, typical of hypermyelination are not uncommon. Hypermyelination is inappropriately thickened myelin sheaths relative to the size of the axon. Onion bulb formations are occasionally observed. Teased fiber studies commonly show coexistence of segmental demyelination, remyelination, hypermyelination, and axonal degeneration (Fig. 31.1B). Segmental de/remyelination is extensive, whereas severe axonal lesions are rarely found [29, 30].

Electron microscopy: On transverse sections, many demyelinating axons, remyelinating fibers with very thin myelin sheaths and fibers with a tomaculous appearance are identified (Fig. 31.2A). The ultrastructural

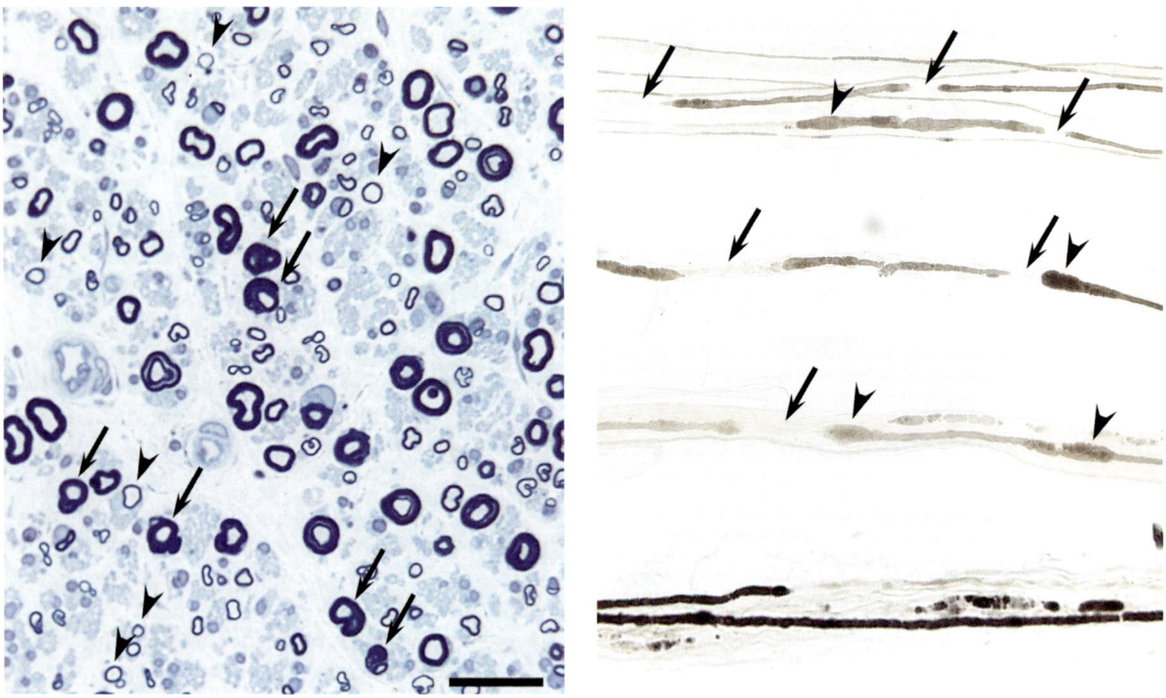

(A) (B)

Figure 31.1 (**A**) Transverse section of a sural nerve specimen from anti-MAG neuropathy. There is moderate loss of myelinated fibers, especially large myelinated fibers. Some fibers show myelin abnormalities, such as thin myelin (arrowheads) and focal myelin thickenings (arrows). (**B**) Teased-fiber preparations. Segmental demyelination (arrows), and tomaculous appearances (arrowheads) are shown. The lowest panel shows fibers undergoing degeneration. Scale bar = (A) 20 μm.

hallmark of anti-MAG neuropathy is the presence of fibers with widely spaced myelin (WSM) (Fig. 31.2B) in which the distance between neighboring intraperiod lines is increased [31, 32] (Fig. 31.2C). WSM is found in over 90% of patients with anti-MAG neuropathy [28, 29] and is preferentially located in the outer layers of the myelin sheath. Some fibers show more severe WSM involving the entire myelin thickness. While the typical appearance of WSM consists of several consecutive layers of separated intraperiod lines, sometimes only the outermost layer is separated. In many fibers, the length of the outer mesaxon, which is the external surface of the fiber in the space between the Schwann cell plasma membrane and the basement membrane, is also extended (Fig. 31.2D). There are redundant myelin loops with a tomaculous appearance consisting of an infolding (Fig. 31.2A) and an outfolding (Fig. 31.2E) of the myelin sheaths. Almost all fibers with a tomaculous appearance also have WSM of the outermost or outer few layers of the myelin sheath. The frequency of WSM varies from case to case, correlates positively with the frequency of demyelination and tomacula on teased fiber study, and correlates negatively with the total myelinated fiber density. These findings indicate that

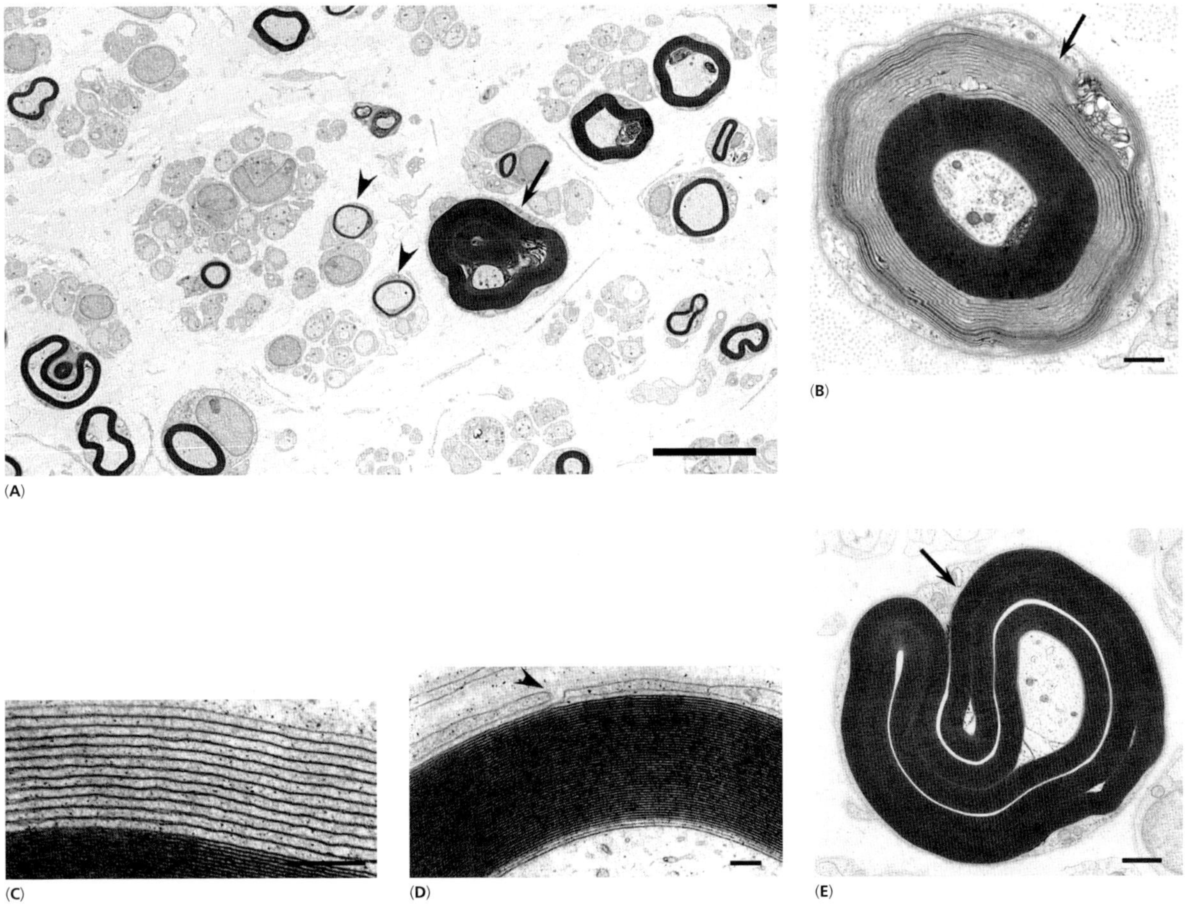

Figure 31.2 Electron micrograph of a transverse section. (**A**) Tomaculous appearance with axonal atrophy (arrow) and thin myelination (arrowheads) are shown. Unmyelinated nerve fibers are well preserved. (**B**) Typical widening of the outer myelin lamellae (arrow). (**C**) WSM is caused by separation of the intraperiod line. (**D**) Electron micrograph showing widening of external mesaxon (arrowhead). (**E**) Redundant myelin loops, such as myelin infolding and outfolding (arrow), are thought to be related to tomacula in teased-fiber preparations. Scale bars = (A) 5 μm; (B) 1 μm; (C) 0.1 μm; (D) 0.1 μm; (E) 1 μm.

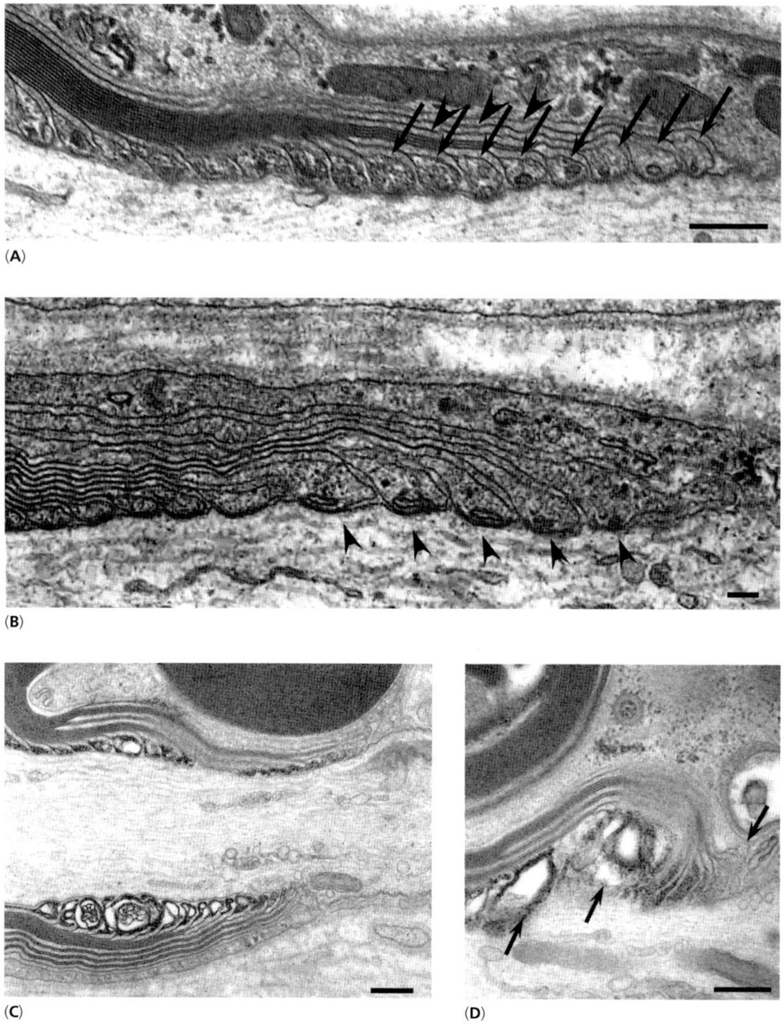

Figure 31.3 Electron micrographs of longitudinal sections of the paranodal region in anti-MAG neuropathy. (**A**) Widening of spaces between terminal myelin loops (arrows) is observed. There is WSM in some outer layers (arrowheads). (**B**) High-power detail of terminal myelin loops adjacent to the node of Ranvier. The spaces between terminal myelin loops are widened, and the outer terminal myelin loops are apparently swollen (arrowheads). (**C**) WSM, which is consecutive with a paranodal region, is frequently observed in demyelinating fibers. (**D**) Terminal myelin loops are dissociated from the paranodal axolemma (arrows). Scale bars = (**A**, **C**, **D**) 0.5 μm; (**B**) 0.1 μm.

WSM induces demyelination and tomacula formation in anti-MAG neuropathy [29]. In contrast to myelinated fibers, unmyelinated fibers are relatively preserved. Ballooning of axons, accumulation of specific organelles, and other morphologic abnormalities suggestive of axonal damage are not apparent in unmyelinated fibers (Fig. 31.2A).

On longitudinal sections, WSM is found in association with the paranodal regions and Schmidt–Lanterman incisures [29]. As observed in transverse sections WSM is preferentially located in the outer layers of myelin sheaths [29]. In the paranodal regions, the spaces between the terminal myelin loops are widened, especially adjacent to the nodes of Ranvier (Fig. 31.3A). Some terminal myelin loops, especially those adjacent to nodes of Ranvier, show concomitant apparent swelling in the processes during the time in which myelin is altered (Fig. 31.3B). The widened spaces between terminal myelin loops continue into the juxtaparanodal regions (Fig. 31.3C). In demyelinating fibers, detachment of terminal myelin loops from the paranodal axolemma is observed [29] (Fig. 31.3D). In addition to the association of paranodal terminal myelin loops with WSM, WSM is also observed frequently in Schmidt–Lanterman incisures, but demyelination is not.

Tomacula are found in both paranodal and internodal regions on longitudinal sections. Almost all fibers with tomacula have WSM, especially in the outer layers of the myelin sheath [29]. Large tomacula with complex redundant myelin loops in juxtaparanodal regions are accompanied by widened nodes of Ranvier.

In anti-MAG neuropathy longitudinal sections show a significantly increased neurofilament density in axons is in all regions, including the paranode, juxtaparanode, and internode, compared with controls [29]. The density is most prominent in the paranodal regions.

Immunofluorescence and immunohistochemistry: Immunofluorescence and immunohistochemical studies of anti-MAG neuropathy demonstrate that anti-MAG IgM antibodies play an important pathogenic role in this neuropathy [28, 29, 33, 34].

To assess antimyelin activity, patients' serum is tested on normal frozen human peripheral nerve by indirect immunofluorescence. In positive cases, all myelin sheaths react to the immune serum IgM. Direct immunofluorescence on frozen sections of patients' nerve biopsies is performed to search for IGM that binds to myelin sheaths, and visualized on both cross and longitudinal sections. Specific antisera for IgG, IgA, IgM, lambda and kappa light chains, and C3d conjugated to fluorescein are used to reveal IgM deposits on myelin sheaths.

Many reports have confirmed monoclonal proteins localized in the myelin sheaths [28, 31–34, 35]. Immunohistochemical analysis of sural nerve cross-sections reveals anti-MAG IgM antibody deposits on both large and small myelinated nerve fibers derived from patients with anti-MAG neuropathy (Fig. 31.4A). The IgM antibody deposits appear as either a thin line on the outside of myelinated fibers or as thick rings that extend into the inner layer of the myelin sheath (Fig. 31.4B), confirmed on longitudinal sections. Longitudinal sections also reveal that IgM antibody deposits are continuous along the outermost layer of the myelin sheaths and are concentrated at both the paranodal regions and Schmidt–Lanterman incisures (Fig. 31.4C). These findings are consistent with the location of WSM. IgM antibodies are not seen on the periaxonal membrane of longitudinal sections. Confocal microscopy reveals colocalization of anti-IgM antibodies and complement C3d, possibly activated by the complement pathway [34].

Pathogenesis and animal models

Animal studies also support a direct causal link between anti-MAG antibodies and neuropathy. Experimental demyelination of nerve involving activation of the complement pathway is induced in animals by intraneural or systemic injection of serum containing anti-MAG antibodies [36–40].

Significant titers of anti-MAG antibodies (above 1/5000 by ELISA) are reliably associated with a demyelinating symmetric polyneuropathy. Anti-MAG antibodies are occasionally found in asymptomatic patients, but most of these patients have a subclinical neuropathy that later becomes clinically manifest [41, 42]. In contrast, the lack of correlation between anti-MAG antibody titers and the severity of neuropathy in different individuals argue against a possible pathogenic role of anti-MAG antibodies [43]. However, such discrepancies are not unusual in autoimmune diseases and may reflect differences in antibody specificities or affinities [44, 45].

Anti-MAG IgM antibodies and complement are both deposited on myelinated fibers, suggesting that the activated complement pathway may be necessary to induce demyelination. The deposits correlate with sites of MAG localization: regions of noncompacted myelin, including periaxonal membranes, Schmidt–Lanterman incisures, paranodal loops, and the outer mesaxon [46]. This binding alters the adhesion properties of MAG, which eventually leads to abnormal myelin spacing [47–50]. The WSM visible on longitudinal sections suggests that early myelin changes occur in the myelin terminals of paranodal regions, and impaired adhesion between terminal myelin loops and paranodal axolemma results in extensive demyelination and subsequent axonal damage in anti-MAG neuropathy [29].

Neurofilament spacing in the axons of demyelinated fibers is altered in the sural nerves of patients with anti-MAG neuropathy [39]. This supports the observation in MAG knockout mice that MAG may be implicated in the signaling cascade controlling neurofilament phosphorylation and spacing [51, 52]. On electron

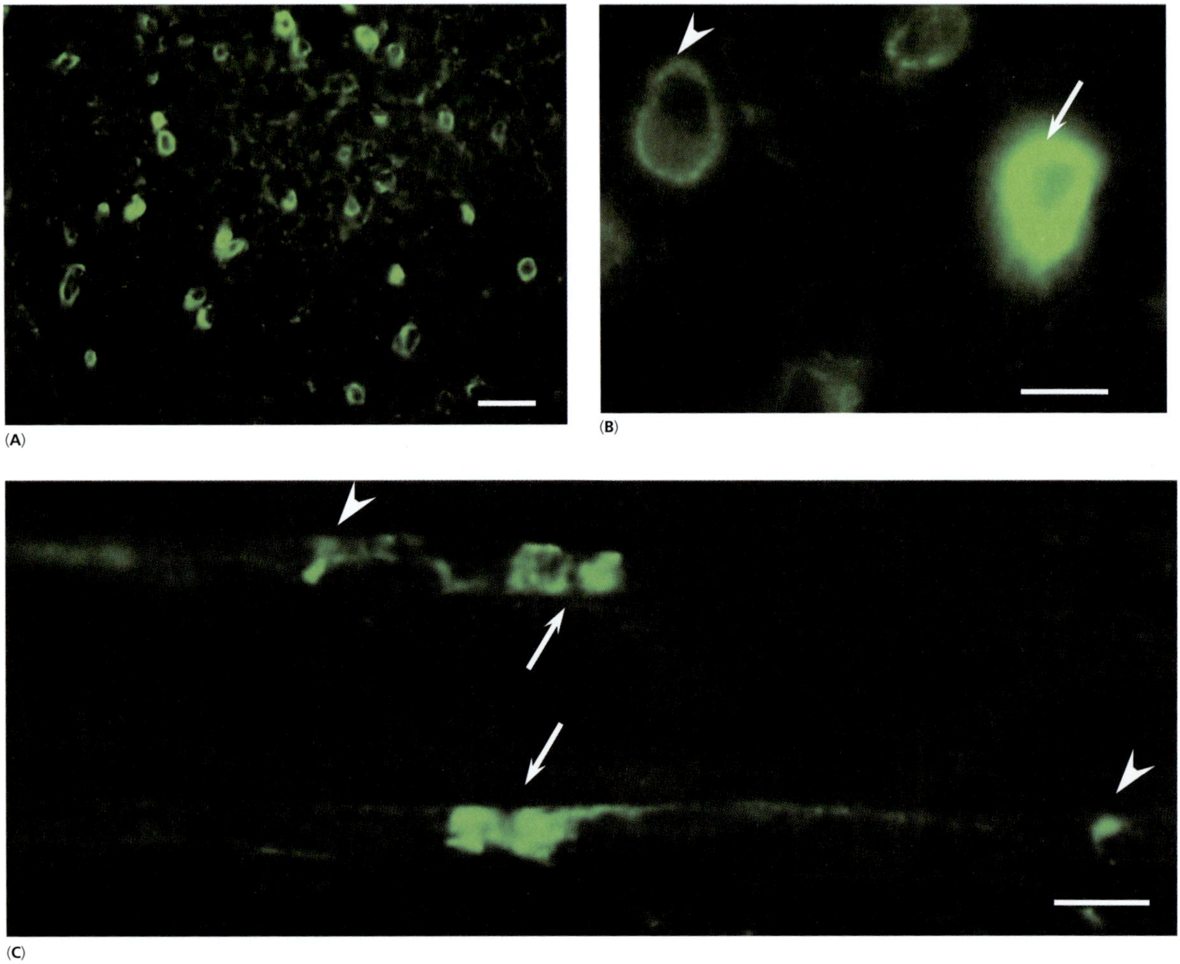

Figure 31.4 Immunofluorescence with IgM antibody on cross sections and longitudinal sections. (**A**) IgM antibody deposits are present on both large and small myelinated nerve fibers. (**B**) Detail of IgM antibody deposits. IgM antibodies appear as either a thin line at the periphery of myelinated fibers (arrowhead) or as thick rings extending into the inner layer of the myelin sheath (arrow). (**C**) Immune reactions with IgM antibodies are concentrated in both the paranodal regions (arrows) and Schmidt–Lanterman incisures (arrowheads). Scale bars = (**A**) 10 μm; (**B**) 5 μm; (**C**) 5 μm.

microscopy, longitudinal sections show that neurofilament density is significantly increased in all domains of myelinated fibers [29]. The presence of MAG in unmyelinated fibers has not been assessed, but since unmyelinated fibers are preserved, in contrast to myelinated fibers, it is likely that demyelination is the primary cause of axonal damage in this neuropathy.

Conclusion

Pathological studies reveal that morphological changes in terminal myelin loops, formation of WSM at the paranodes, and subsequent dissociation from paranodal axolemma, possibly caused by activation of the complement pathway, may play an important role in demyelination. Loosening of compact myelin due to WSM in various sites seems to contribute to the formation of tomacula. As the neurofilament density is high in the paranodes, demyelination initiated from the paranodal regions may be attributable to axonal damage in anti-MAG neuropathy.

If anti-MAG antibodies are significantly elevated, nerve biopsy is usually not done. Nevertheless, in a few reported cases, biopsy has revealed other lesions associated with WSM, such as malignant cells and amyloid deposits [53].

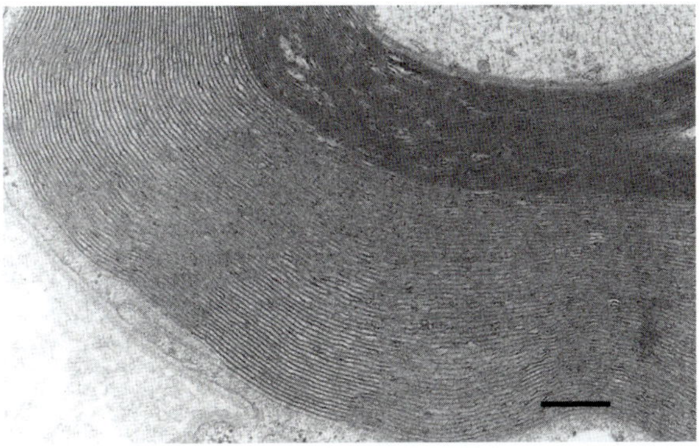

Figure 31.5 Electron microscopy, transverse section. Polyneuropathy associated with IgA monoclonal gammopathy. In this myelin sheath, there are numerous and regular widenings due to the intramyelinic infiltration of IgA (see Fig. 31.6).

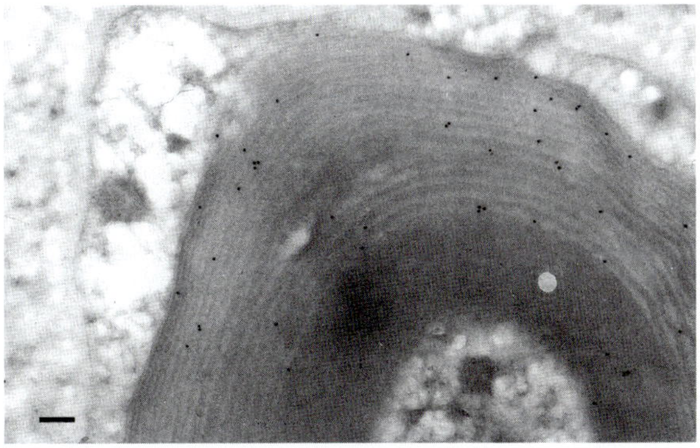

Figure 31.6 Immunoelectron microscopy, transverse section. IgA specifically labeled by gold particles, is seen at the level of widenings of the myelin lamellae.

IgG; IgA

In these patients the antigens are unknown, there is no anti-MAG activity. In a few cases, immunofluorescence using specific antibodies on frozen nerve sections demonstrates annular binding to numerous myelin sheaths corresponding to widened myelin lamellae comparable to those described in IgM-anti MAG neuropathies (Figs 31.5 and 31.6). Sometimes these lesions may be associated with immunoglobulin deposits in endoneurial interstitial tissue (see the next section on immunoglobulins, supporting the view that the MG causes the neuropathy [48, 54].

Deposits in the interstitial tissue

Immunoglobulins

Immunoglobulin deposits of any kind: IgG, IgA or IgM or light chains can only be proven by nerve biopsy [55, 56]. These monoclonal dysglobulinemias are usually malignant (multiple myeloma, Waldenstrom's disease or non-Hodgkin's lymphoma). They must not be confused with amyloidosis on routine stains and are best identified by immunocytochemistry on frozen sections and by EM [57]. Depending on their size, they can be detected either by immunofluorescence on frozen sections or only by EM. Ultrastructurally, they can have a characteristic appearance as digitiform, fibrillar, or tubular structures but if these are not present immunoEM using anti-immunoglobulin antibodies has to be done to confirm their specificity (Fig. 31.7). If immunoglobulin deposits are found, a cryoprotein should be looked for

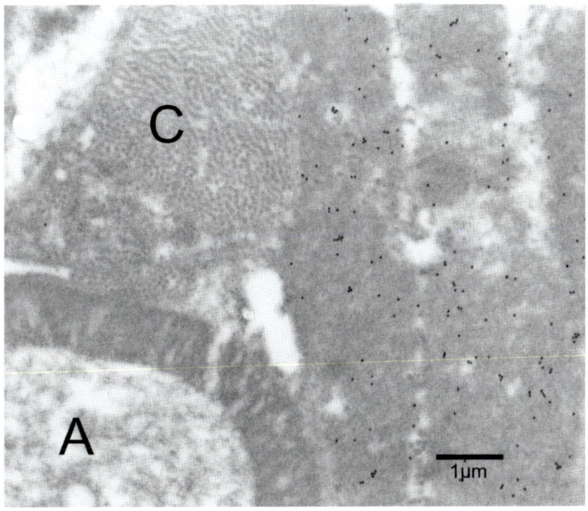

Figure 31.7 Immunoelectron microscopy, transverse section. Gray deposits infiltrate the interstitial tissue and surround Schwann cell cytoplasm (A = axon). These IgM deposits are specifically labeled by gold particles, but collagen fibers (C) are not. As there was no frozen sample available, immunofluorescence was not performed.

carefully; if present, we recommend fixing it and comparing its ultrastructure with that of the endoneurial deposits; if ultrastructurally similar, it confirms abnormal immunoglobulin in the nerve [58].

Amyloid deposits

Amyloid deposits are multifocal, so they are not seen on all sections of the NB and can be missed. They are quite rare and are induced by myeloma or Waldenstrom's disease. A negative examination does not exclude an amyloid neuropathy. The sensitivity of nerve biopsy for the diagnosis of systemic amyloidosis is said to be around 85% [59].

On paraffin-embedded sections, amyloid deposits appear round, are scattered in the endoneurium and sometimes attached to thickened capillary walls [60]. AL amyloidosis results from the transformation of an immunoglobulin light chain, which may be identified on frozen specimens with a specific antibody. These deposits are stained by Congo red and thioflavine. On EM, amyloid deposits are extracellular and composed of characteristic bundles of unbranched, 7–10 nm-wide fibrils in an irregular matted form; they are sometimes seen in intimate contact with the basement membranes of endothelial cells and Schwann cells. Severe lesions of myelinated and unmyelinated fibers are common in amyloidosis, whether of genetic or dysimmune origin.

It is recommended to test for a transthyretin (TTR) mutation, even when amyloid neuropathy is associated with monoclonal IgG, since the association could be coincidental [61]. Immuno-EM can help differentiate light chain amyloidosis from TTR amyloidosis, which has important genetic consequences.

POEMS (polyneuropathy, organomegaly, endocrinopathy, M protein, skin lesions) syndrome (Crow– Fukase syndrome)

Usually, the diagnosis is clinical and is confirmed by increased levels of vascular endothelial growth factor (VEGF) in the serum. Nerve biopsy is performed when clinical signs are not typical. The M protein is almost always an IgG or less often an IgA heavy chain, associated with a lambda light chain, and with these dysglobulinemias there is usually an underlying solitary osteosclerotic plasma cell tumor.

EM may show uncompacted myelin lamellae (UML) (Fig. 31.8) that are characteristic of this condition and are visible in 1–7% of the myelinated fibers [62]. The myelin changes correspond to portions of the mesaxon that are neither flattened nor compacted and are visible around at least one semi-circumference of the axon on three or more consecutive lamellae so there is an abnormally widened space between major dense lines. Fragments of cytoplasm are often seen between these lamellae. These unusual lesions are found in the inner and middle layers of the myelin sheaths, but may involve the outer layer. They must be differentiated from widened myelin lamellae, seen in IgM-antiMAG positive patients. Numerous UML on a nerve biopsy can help distinguish POEMS from CIDP and other demyelinating peripheral nerve disorders, especially in the early phase. The significance of UML in the pathogenesis of POEMS is still unknown.

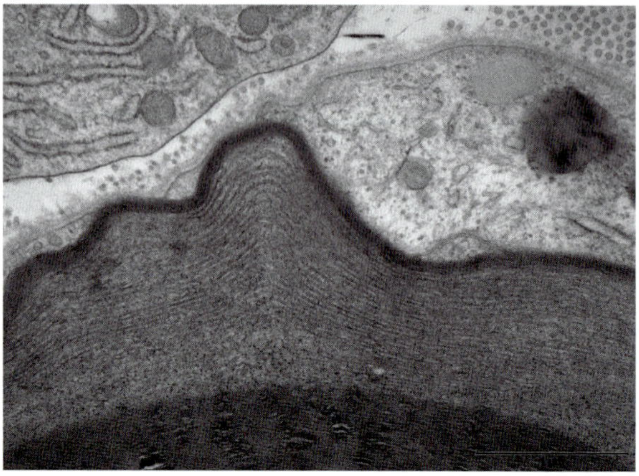

Figure 31.8 Electron microscopy, transverse section. POEMS syndrome. Typical appearance of uncompacted myelin lamellae in the myelin sheath.

Immunocytochemistry using specific immunoglobulin antibodies are negative.

Other nerve fiber lesions are usually a mixture of segmental demyelination and axonal degeneration. In some cases pure axonal lesions are present [63]. There may be sparse inflammatory infiltration of the endoneurium and, occasionally, the epineurium; in addition prominent vascular proliferation is sometimes described, possibly a consequence of the high levels of VEGF in these patients [64].

Malignant cells

Infiltration by B or T cell lymphoma in the peripheral nerve parenchyma, usually in the epineurium, can only be shown by nerve biopsy; the malignant cells are detected on routine paraffin embedded sections (Fig. 31.9) and their phenotype is confirmed by immu-

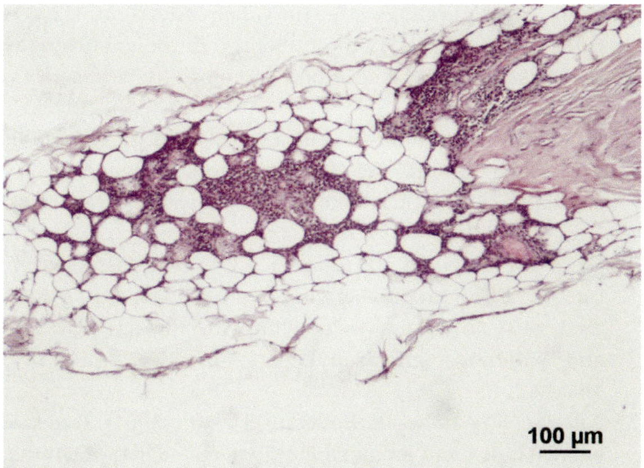

Figure 31.9 Longitudinal section, paraffin embedded sample. Waldenstrom's disease. Infiltrates of mononuclear cells in the epineurial adipose tissue; immunocytochemistry revealed that most of them specifically labeled with an anti-B cell antibody.

nohistochemistry on paraffin or deep-frozen nerve biopsy (see also Chapter 38). Cellular infiltrates may disappear on serial sections, which are required for the immunopathological studies.

In some cases, the NB may determine whether the neuropathy is due to an associated monoclonal gammopathy, to the presence of lymphoma cells or to a combination of both [65, 66]. In this context, detection of a clonal immunoglobulin or T-cell receptor gene recombination may be very useful to confirm lymphomatous infiltration. This is commonly performed by standard PCR techniques designed to assess the diversity of the junctional regions in immunoglobulin or T-cell receptor genes. PCR requires only small amounts of DNA and has a good sensitivity to detect clonality [67].

Malignant infiltrates are observed in Waldenstrom's disease, Non-Hodgkin's lymphoma, or very rarely in myeloma.

In rare cases of angiotropic lymphoma lymphomatous cells are visible in the lumen of arterioles in nerve and muscle specimens [68].

CIDP

If electrophysiological studies suggest a demyelinating polyneuropathy that appears to have no direct link with the MG, CIDP is probable. CIDP is a common and treatable immunological disorder so it is important to diagnose it [69]. The primary target antigen remains unknown. The most common association is with IgG. As for the "primitive" CIDP cases, nerve biopsy is not done in typical cases, but may be quite useful to diagnose atypical ones [70]; the pathological lesions are described in Chapter 27.

Conclusion, treatment, and future perspectives

In some patients, the precise cause of peripheral neuropathy in MG cannot be determined; it may be paraneoplastic, or lymphoma infiltration or immunoglobulin deposition may be undetected.

In these hematologic disorders it is very important to consider nerve biopsy at an early stage because, early detection of the cause of PN will determine treatment options and influence outcome. If treatment is instituted too late the outcome is poor, not unsurprisingly. The frequency of these lesions is almost certainly underestimated. Nerve biopsy may also reveal a combination of pathologies in the same case; Garces-Chancez *et al.* have shown that finding serum anti-MAG antibodies does not exclude the diagnosis of amyloidosis [53].

If therapy for the blood disorder is in progress, its possible role also requires assessment so that other strategies or drugs can be instituted.

References

1 Kelly JJ Jr, Kyle RA, O'Brien PC *et al.* (1981) Prevalence of monoclonal protein in peripheral neuropathy. *Neurology* 31, 1480–1483.

2 Kelly JJ Jr. (2008) Peripheral neuropathies associated with monoclonal gammopathies of undetermined significance. *Rev Neurol Dis* 5, 14–22.

3 Vallat JM, De Mascarel HA, Bordessoule D *et al.* (1995) Non-Hodgkin malignant lymphomas and peripheral neuropathies-13 cases. *Brain* 118, 1233–1245.

4 Silberman J, Lonial S. (2008) Review of peripheral neuropathy in plasma cell disorders. *Hematol Oncol* 26, 55–65.

5 Ramchandren S, Lewis RA. (2009) Monoclonal gammopathy and neuropathy. *Curr Opin Neurol.* 22, 480–485.

6 Gosselin S, Kyle RA, Dyck PJ. (1991) Neuropathy associated with monoclonal gammopathies of undetermined significance. *Ann Neurol* 30, 54–61.

7 Drouet A, Caudie C, Vallat JM *et al.* (2006) Polyneuropathy involving cranial nerves associated with monoclonal IgM antibodies with anti-MAG/SGPG/SGPLG/sulfatides activity. *Rev Neurol* 162, 760–766.

8 Tamhankar MA, Galetta SL, Massaro M *et al.* (2011) Pupil-involving third nerve palsy as a manifestation of anti-myelin-associated glycoprotein neuropathy. *J Neuroophthalmol* 31, 29–33.

9 Chassande B, Léger JM, Younes-Chennoufi AB *et al.* (1998) Peripheral neuropathy associated with IgM monoclonal gammopathy: correlations between M-protein antibody activity and clinical/electrophysiological features in 40 cases. *Muscle Nerve* 21, 55–62.

10 Luigetti M, Conte A, Montano N *et al.* (2012) Clinical and pathological heterogeneity in a series of 31 patients with IgM-related neuropathy. *J Neurol Sci* 319, 75–80.

11 Steck AJ, Murray N, Dellagi K *et al.* (1987) Peripheral neuropathy associated with monoclonal IgM autoantibody. *Ann Neurol* 22, 764–767.

12 Latov N, Hays AP, Sherman WH. (1988) Peripheral neuropathy and anti-MAG antibodies. *Crit Rev Neurobiol* 3, 301–332.

13 Smith IS. (1994) The natural history of chronic demyelinating neuropathy associated with benign IgM paraproteinaemia. A clinical and neurophysiological study. *Brain* 117, 949–957.

14 Ellie E, Vital A, Steck A *et al.* (1996) Neuropathy associated with "benign" anti-myelin-associated glycoprotein IgM gammopathy: clinical, immunological, neurophysiological pathological findings and response to treatment in 33 cases. *J Neurol* 243, 34–43.

15 Latov N. (1995) Pathogenesis and therapy of neuropathies associated with monoclonal gammopathies. *Ann Neurol* 37, S32–42.

16 Nobile-Orazio E, Manfredini E, Carpo M *et al.* (1994) Frequency and clinical correlates of anti-neural IgM antibodies in neuropathy associated with IgM monoclonal gammopathy. *Ann Neurol* 36, 416–424.

17 Ropper AH, Gorson KC. (1999) Neuropathies associated with paraproteinemia. *N Engl J Med* 338, 1601–1607.

18 Pestronk A, Choksi R, Logigian E *et al.* (2003) Sensory neuropathy with monoclonal IgM binding to a trisulfated heparin disaccharide. *Muscle Nerve* 27, 188–195.

19 Steck AJ, Stalder AK, Renaud S. (2006) Anti-myelin-associated glycoprotein neuropathy. *Curr Opin Neurol* 19, 458–63.

20 Kawagashira Y, Kondo N, Atsuta N *et al.* (2010) IgM MGUS anti-MAG neuropathy with predominant muscle weakness and extensive muscle atrophy. *Muscle Nerve* 42, 433–435.

21 Van den Berg L, Hays AP, Nobile-Orazio E *et al.* (1996) Anti-MAG and anti-SGPG antibodies in neuropathy. *Muscle Nerve* 19, 637–643.

22 Kuijf ML, Eurelings M, Tio-Gillen AP *et al.* (2009) Detection of anti-MAG antibodies in polyneuropathy associated with IgM monoclonal gammopathy. *Neurology* 73, 688–695.

23 Notermans NC, Franssen H, Eurelings M *et al.* (2000) Diagnostic criteria for demyelinating polyneuropathy associated with monoclonal gammopathy. *Muscle Nerve* 23, 73–79.

24 Kaku DA, England JD, Sumner AJ. (1994) Distal accentuation of conduction slowing in polyneuropathy associated with antibodies to myelin-associated glycoprotein and sulphated glucuronyl paragloboside. *Brain* 117, 941–947.

25 Attarian S, Azulay JP, Boucraut J *et al.* (2001) Terminal latency index and modified F ratio in distinction of chronic demyelinating neuropathies. *Clin Neurophysiol* 112, 457–463.

26 Capasso M, Torrieri F, Di Muzio A, *et al.* (2002) Can electrophysiology differentiate polyneuropathy with anti-MAG/SGPG antibodies from chronic inflammatory demyelinating polyneuropathy? *Clin Neurophysiol* 113, 346–353.

27 Radziwill AJ, Steck AJ, Renaud S *et al.* (2003) Distal motor latency and residual latency as sensitive markers of anti-MAG polyneuropathy. *J Neurol* 250, 962–966.

28 Vital A, Vital C, Julien J *et al.* (1989) Polyneuropathy associated with IgM monoclonal gammopathy. Immunological and pathological study in 31 patients. *Acta Neuropathol* 79, 160–167.

29 Kawagashira Y, Koike H, Tomita M *et al.* (2010) Morphological progression of myelin abnormalities in IgM-monoclonal gammopathy of undetermined significance anti-myelin-associated glycoprotein neuropathy. *J Neuropathol Exp Neurol* 69, 1143–1157.

30 Mendell JR, Sahenk Z, Whitaker JN *et al.* (1985) Polyneuropathy and IgM monoclonal gammopathy: studies on the pathogenetic role of anti-myelin-associated glycoprotein antibody. *Ann Neurol* 17, 243–254.

31 Vallat JM, Vital A, Magy L, *et al.* (2009) An update on nerve biopsy. *J Neuropathol Exp Neurol* 68, 833–844.

32 Vallat JM, Funalot B, Magy L. (2011) Nerve biopsy: requirements for diagnosis and clinical value. *Acta Neuropathol* 121, 313–326.

33 Gabriel JM, Erne B, Bernasconi L *et al.* (1998) Confocal microscopic localization of anti-myelin-associated glycoprotein autoantibodies in a patient with peripheral neuropathy initially lacking a detectable IgM gammopathy. *Acta Neuropathol* 95, 540–546.

34 Ritz MF, Erne B, Ferracin F *et al.* (1999) Anti-MAG IgM penetration into myelinated fibers correlates with the extent of myelin widening. *Muscle Nerve* 22, 1030–1037.

35 Julien J, Vital C, Vallat JM, *et al.* (1978) Polyneuropathy in Waldenström's macroglobulinemia. Deposition of M component on myelin sheaths. *Arch Neurol* 35, 423–425.

36 Tatum AH. (1993) Experimental paraprotein neuropathy, demyelination by passive transfer of human IgM anti-myelin-associated glycoprotein. *Ann Neurol* 33, 502–506.
37 Monaco S, Ferrari S, Bonetti B, *et al.* (1995) Experimental induction of myelin changes by anti-MAG antibodies and terminal complement complex. *J Neuropathol Exp Neurol* 54, 96–104.
38 Vallat JM, Jauberteau MO, Bordessoule D *et al.* (1996) Link between peripheral neuropathy and monoclonal dysglobulinemia: a study of 66 cases. *J Neurol Sci* 137, 124–130.
39 Lunn MP, Crawford TO, Hughes RA *et al.* (2002) Anti-myelin-associated glycoprotein antibodies alter neurofilament spacing. *Brain* 125, 904–911.
40 Hays AP, Latov N, Takatsu M, *et al.* (1987) Experimental demyelination of nerve induced by serum of patients with neuropathy and an anti-MAG IgM M-protein. *Neurology* 37, 242–256.
41 Nobile-Orazio E, Marmiroli P, Baldini L *et al.* (1987) Peripheral neuropathy in macroglobulinemia: incidence and antigen-specificity of M proteins. *Neurology* 37, 1506–1514.
42 Nobile-Orazio E, Francomano E, Daverio R *et al.* (1989) Anti-myelin-associated glycoprotein IgM antibody titers in neuropathy associated with macroglobulinemia. *Ann Neurol* 26, 543–550.
43 Gosselin S, Kyle RA, Dyck PJ. (1991) Neuropathy associated with monoclonal gammopathies of undetermined significance. *Ann Neurol* 30, 54–61.
44 Ilyas AA, Chou DK, Jungalwala FB *et al.* (1990) Variability in the structural requirements for binding of human monoclonal anti-myelin-associated glycoprotein immunoglobulin M antibodies and HNK-1 to sphingoglycolipid antigens. *J Neurochem* 55, 594–601.
45 Ogino M, Tatum AH, Latov N. (1994) Affinity studies of human anti-MAG antibodies in neuropathy. *J Neuroimmunol* 52, 41–46.
46 Trapp BD. (1990) Myelin-associated glycoprotein. Location and potential functions. *Ann NY Acad Sci* 605, 29–43.
47 Lach B, Rippstein P, Atack D *et al.* (1993) Immunoelectron microscopic localization of monoclonal IgM antibodies in gammopathy associated with peripheral demyelinative neuropathy. *Acta Neuropathol* 85, 298–307.
48 Vallat JM, Tabaraud F, Sindou P *et al.* (2000) Myelin widenings and MGUS-IgA: an immunoelectron microscopic study. *Ann Neurol* 47, 808–811.
49 Vallat JM, Magy L, Sindou P *et al.* (2005) IgG neuropathy: an immunoelectron microscopic study. *J Neuropathol Exp Neurol* 64, 386–390.
50 Vallat JM, Magy L, Richard L *et al.* (2008) Contribution of electron microscopy to the study of neuropathies associated with an IgG monoclonal paraproteinemia. *Micron* 39, 61–70.
51 de Waegh SM, Lee VM, Brady ST. (1992) Local modulation of neurofilament phosphorylation, axonal caliber, and slow axonal transport by myelinating Schwann cells. *Cell* 68, 451–463.
52 Yin X, Crawford TO, Griffin JW *et al.* (1998) Myelin-associated glycoprotein is a myelin signal that modulates the caliber of myelinated axons. *J Neurosci* 18, 1953–1962.
53 19.Garces-Sanchez M, Dyck PJ, Kyle RA *et al.* (2008) Antibodies to myelin-associated glycoprotein (anti-MAG) in IgM amyloidosis may influence expression of neuropathy in rare patients. *Muscle Nerve* 37, 490–495.
54 Vallat JM, Magy L, Sindou P *et al.* (2005) IgG neuropathy: An immunoelectron microscopic study. *J Neuropathol Exp Neurol* 64, 386–390.
55 Luigetti M, Frisullo G, Laurenti L, *et al.* (2010) Light chain deposition in peripheral nerve as a cause of mononeuritis multiplex in Waldenstrom's macroglobulinaemia. *J Neurol Sci* 291, 89–91.
56 Figueroa JJ, Bosch EP, Dyck PJ *et al.* (2012) Amyloid-like IgM deposition neuropathy: a distinct clinico-pathologic and proteomic profiled disorder. *J Periph Nerv Sys* 17, 182–190.
57 Vital C, Vallat JM. (1987) Ultrastructural study of the human diseased peripheral nerve. Elsevier, New York, pp 1–102.
58 Vallat JM, Magy L, Richard L, *et al.* (2008) Intranervous immunoglobulin deposits: An underestimated mechanism of neuropathy. *Muscle Nerve* 38, 904–911.
59 Kyle RA. (1999) Sequence of testing for monoclonal gammopathies. *Arch Pathol Lab Med* 123, 114–118.
60 Vital C, Vital A, Bouillot-Eimer S *et al.* (2004) Amyloid neuropathy: a retrospective study of 35 peripheral nerve biopsies. *J Periph Nerv Syst* 9, 232–241.
61 Lachmann HJ, Booth DR, Booth SE *et al.* (2002) Misdiagnosis of hereditary amyloidosis as al (primary) amyloidosis. *N Engl J Med* 346, 1786–1791.
62 Vital C, Vital A, Ferrer X *et al* (2003) Crow-Fukase (POEMS) syndrome: a study of peripheral nerve biopsy in five new cases. *J Periph Nerv Syst* 8, 136–144.
63 Mathis S, Magy L, Kaboré R *et al.* (2012) POEMS syndrome with prominent acute axonal lesions. *J Neurol Sci* 313, 185–188.
64 Kulkarni GB, Mahadevan A, Taly AB *et al.* (2011) Clinicopathological profile of polyneuropathy, organomegaly, endocrinopathy, M protein and skin changes (POEMS) syndrome. *J Clin Neurosci* 18, 356–360.
65 Kelly JJ, Karcher DS (2005) Lymphoma and peripheral neuropathy: A clinical review. *Muscle Nerve* 31, 301–313.
66 Vallat JM, De Mascarel HA, Bordessoule D, *et al.* (1995) Non-Hodgkin malignant lymphomas and peripheral neuropathies – 13 cases. *Brain* 118 (Pt 5): 1233–1245.

67 Langerak AW, Molina TJ, Lavender FL, *et al.* (2007) Polymerase chain reaction-based clonality testing in tissue samples with reactive lymphoproliferations: Usefulness and pitfalls. A report of the biomed-2 concerted action bmh4-ct98–3936. *Leukemia* 21, 222–229.

68 Vital C, Heraud A, Vital A, *et al.* (1989) Acute mononeuropathy with angiotropic lymphoma. *Acta Neuropathol* 78, 105–107.

69 Vallat JM, Sommer C, Magy L (2010) Chronic inflammatory demyelinating polyradiculoneuropathy: Diagnostic and therapeutic challenges for a treatable condition. *Lancet Neurol* 9, 402–412.

70 Vallat JM, Tabaraud F, Magy L, *et al.* (2003) Diagnostic value of nerve biopsy for atypical chronic inflammatory demyelinating polyneuropathy: Evaluation of eight cases. *Muscle Nerve* 27, 478–485.

CHAPTER 32

Paraneoplastic peripheral neuropathies

Jean-Christophe Antoine
Service de Neurologie, Hôpital Nord, CHU de Saint-Etienne, France

Introduction and definition

Clinically overt neuropathy affects up to 15% of patients with cancer and mostly results from compression or infiltration by the tumor, treatment side effects, nutritional factors, and viral infections [1]. Paraneoplastic neurological syndromes (PNS) encompass disorders that are not explained by these mechanisms and affect less than 1% of patients. Although PNS may involve any part of the central or peripheral nervous system, the neuromuscular junction or muscle in isolation or in combination, peripheral neuropathy is the most frequent manifestation representing one third of patients of the European consortium PNSEuronetwork database.

It is well established that the mechanisms by which PNS develop with carcinoma are autoimmune. Expression by the tumor of a self-antigen present in the nervous system may lead to a breakdown of immune tolerance resulting in activation of auto-aggressive B and T cells, production of auto-antibodies and development of neuropathy. These antigens and their corresponding antibodies are designated as onconeural. Two intracellular antigens are mostly associated with peripheral neuropathy, namely the HuD and CV2/CRMP5 proteins. In cases of malignant lymphoma the known mechanisms involve factors secreted by the tumor including cytokines (e.g., in POEMS syndrome) and more frequently a monoclonal immunoglobulin that can behave as an auto-antibody or acquire specific physicochemical properties. These disorders are considered elsewhere (see Chapters 31 and 38).

Criteria have been proposed for the diagnosis of PNS [2]. Definite paraneoplastic neuropathies include three categories of disorders: (1) those involving one of the aforementioned mechanisms, that is, associated with onconeural antibodies, (2) paraneoplastic neuropathy classically known to occur with a tumor but without identifiable antibodies, for example, seronegative subacute sensory neuronopathy (SSN), and (3) neuropathies that unequivocally improve with the treatment of the tumor. Other neuropathies that occur within two years of the diagnosis of cancer can be considered as a possible PNS. Many are probably coincidental.

Subacute sensory neuropathy and other peripheral nervous system disorders of the anti- Hu syndrome

SSN was first described by Denny-Brown in 1948 and results from the destruction of sensory neurons in dorsal root ganglia [3]. It is the most frequent paraneoplastic peripheral neuropathy, representing 52% of the neuropathies in the PNSEuronetwork database.

Clinical symptoms

The onset is usually subacute or rapidly progressive with paresthesia and pain. Sensory loss is mostly multifocal or asymmetrical, and the upper limbs are almost invariably involved [4]. The face, chest, or abdomen may also be affected. Pain is frequent and sensory loss, particularly of deep sensation often leads to a severe sensory ataxia in all four limbs. SSN can be very disabling, but indolent and protracted courses have been reported.

Peripheral Nerve Disorders: Pathology and Genetics, First Edition. Edited by Jean-Michel Vallat, Joachim Weis, Francoise Gray, and Katy Keohane.

CSF may show elevated protein concentration or oligoclonal bands. Pleocytosis occurs during the first months of evolution. The electrophysiological hallmark of SSN is severe and diffuse alteration of sensory nerve action potentials often with non-excitable sensory nerves. Motor conduction velocities are classically normal but are frequently mildly altered, which may lead to confusion with axonal sensory-motor neuropathy [5].

Although SSN occurs with different tumors including breast cancer and Hodgkin's disease [6], small cell lung cancer (SCLC) represents 70–80% of cases [4]. Most patients have anti-Hu antibodies, which have 99% specificity but only 82% sensitivity for the diagnosis of cancer in patients with SSN [7]. If SSN is the predominant manifestation of the anti-Hu syndrome, it is isolated in only 25% of patients; the others have some background of central nervous system involvement [4]. When the central and peripheral nervous systems are equally affected, paraneoplastic encephalomyelitis is the preferred term.

Other PNS disorders may occur with anti-Hu antibodies [4]. The commonest is dysautonomia, which is frequently associated with SSN. It affects the cardiovascular and gastrointestinal systems and may cause sudden death due to severe postural hypotension and arrhythmia or intestinal pseudo-obstruction resulting from destruction of autonomic neurons in myenteric plexuses. Lesions of the lower motor neurons induce motor deficit, muscle atrophy, and fasciculations. As most patients simultaneously have SSN, the resulting presentation is usually that of a rapidly evolving sensory-motor polyneuropathy. If the distribution is asymmetrical, it may be confused with a mononeuropathy multiplex. More symmetrical cases with fulminant progression may be misdiagnosed as Guillain–Barré syndrome. Exceptionally, there is a predominant or pure motor neuron syndrome mimicking amyotrophic lateral sclerosis.

Pathology

SSN is characterized by a loss of sensory neurons in dorsal root ganglia and a proliferation of glial cells around neurons forming Nageotte's nodules (Fig. 32.1) [3, 6]. Degeneration of the central and peripheral axonal processes results in a loss of myelinated fibers in the posterior columns of the spinal cord and in the peripheral nerves. Mononuclear cell infiltration in the ganglia is present at the initial stage. As SSN is at one end of the spectrum of paraneoplastic encephalomyelitis, patients with SSN may also have more diffuse, subclinical inflammatory lesions in their spinal cord or brain with perivascular lymphocyte cuffs, neuronal loss, and glial cell proliferation. The inflammatory lesions may also extend into the nerve roots. Motor neuron degeneration as well as neuron loss in autonomic ganglia and myenteric plexus may all occur and are well-described in autopsy cases. Positive anti-Hu antibodies in a suggestive clinical context are sufficient for the diagnosis and although feasible, biopsy of dorsal root ganglia is not recommended.

When performed, nerve biopsy shows degenerating fibers and fiber loss without clusters of regenerating axons. In some unusual cases, microvasculitis of the nerve [8] (see also Chapter 24) and demyelination [9] occur. These changes are, thus far unexplained, because Hu antigen is not expressed in the peripheral nerve.

Differential diagnosis

Paraneoplastic sensory neuronopathy represents about 15% of patients with sensory neuronopathy seen in our center. By recently published diagnostic criteria and strategies SNN can be distinguished from other sensory neuropathies and from non-paraneoplastic forms of SSN [10]. Interestingly, inflammatory changes similar to those observed in paraneoplastic SSN have been observed in the dorsal root ganglia of patients with sensory neuronopathy and Sjögren's syndrome and in some idiopathic cases that probably represent other varieties of autoimmune sensory neuron diseases for which antigens are not yet identified.

Pathogenesis and animal models

In most cases HuD is the target of the immune process in paraneoplastic SSN. This is an intracellular mRNA-binding protein expressed in both nucleus and cytoplasm of peripheral and central neurons. The blood barrier is naturally weaker in dorsal root ganglia than in the central nervous system and this probably explains why the DRG is preferentially involved. Immunoglobulin deposits containing anti-Hu antibodies have been observed around sensory neurons. The cellular infiltrate

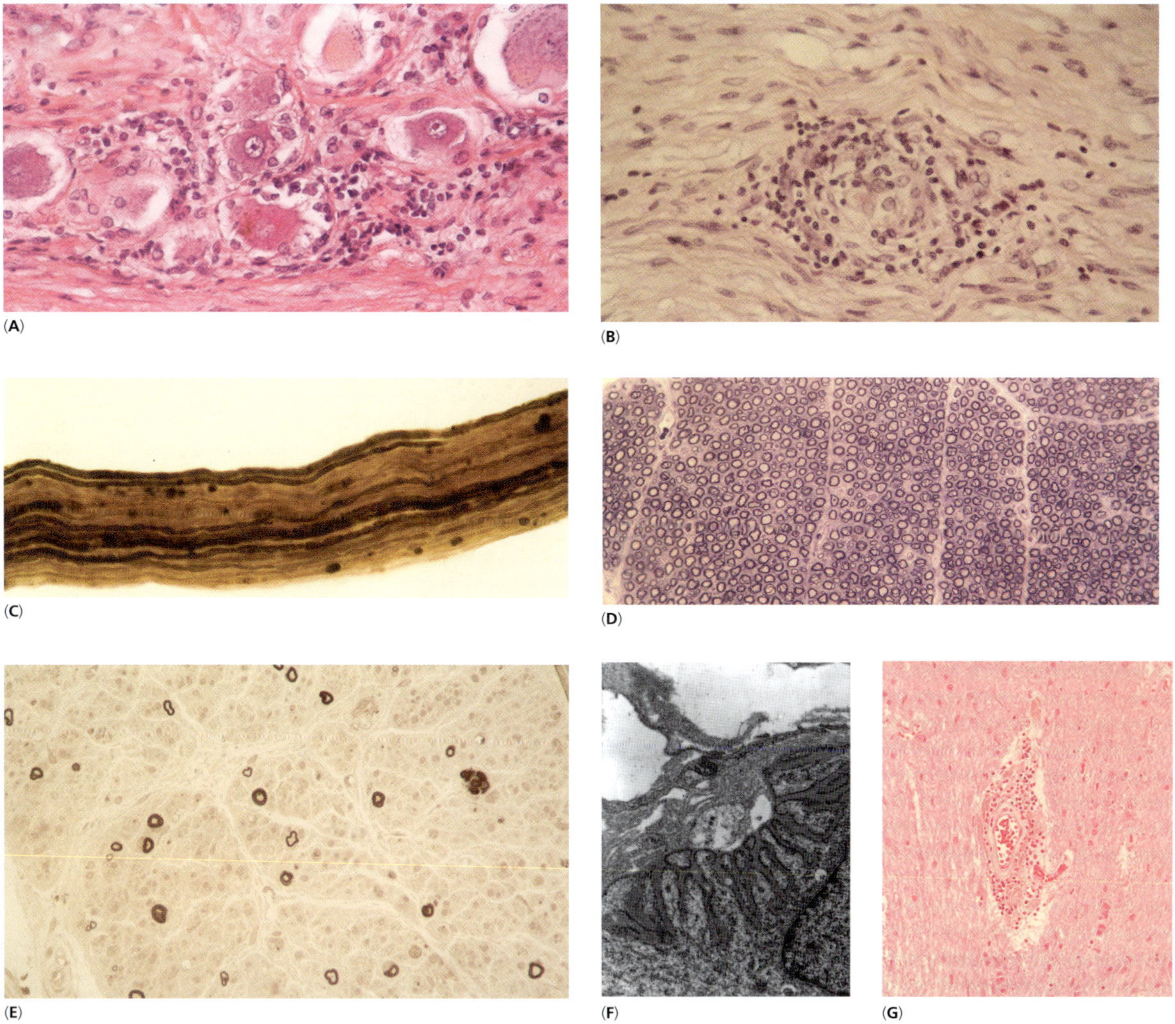

Figure 32.1 *Paraneoplastic subacute sensory neuronopathy.* (**A**) Inflammatory cell reaction around sensory neurons in a lumbar dorsal root ganglion. H&E ×20. (**B**) Perivascular mononuclear cell cuffing around an endoneurial vessel in the sensory root. H&E ×20. (**C**) Teased fiber preparation of a sensory root. Fiber loss and myelin ovoids indicating severe ongoing axonal degeneration. ×20. (**D**) Semithin section of a lumbar motor root showing a normal appearance. (**E**) Sural nerve biopsy. Semithin section. Severe fiber loss. Paraphenylendiamine, ×20. (**F**) Muscle biopsy. Electron microscopy. Motor endplate with a degenerated motor axon terminal, ×7000. (**G**) Perivascular mononuclear cell infiltrate in the spinal cord. H&E ×20.

is composed mainly of T cells. CD8-positive T cells have been shown penetrating the capsule of satellite cells surrounding the neuron cell body and secreting perforin. All of this suggests that cellular immunity plays a major role (Fig. 32.2) [11]. Immunization of animals with HuD led to the production of antibodies and immunoglobulin deposits in the nervous system, but neuronal lesions could not be reproduced. There is no clearly demonstrated genetic predisposition to paraneoplastic neurological syndromes although HLA-DQ2 and HLA-DR3 alleles have been associated with anti-Hu PNS.

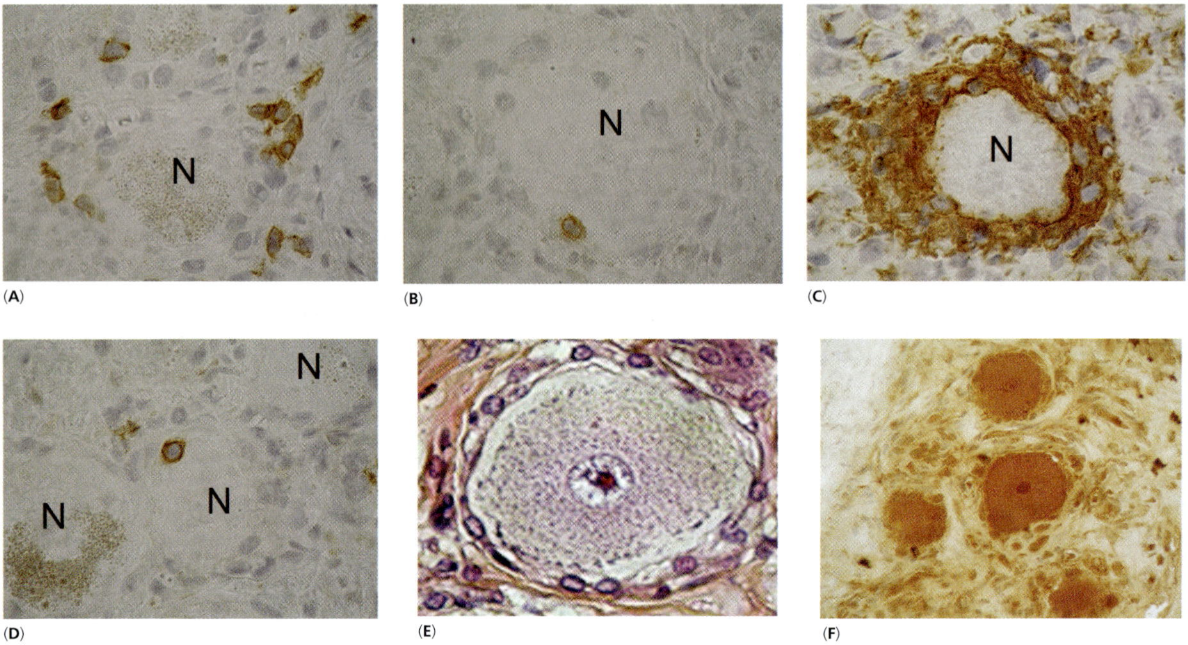

Figure 32.2 *Immunohistochemical analysis of the inflammatory cell reaction in a dorsal root ganglion of a patient with subacute sensory neuronopathy and anti-Hu antibody.* (**A**) CD4 positive helper T cells surrounding a sensory neuron. (**B**) A CD8 positive cytotoxic T cell has penetrated the satellite cell capsule of a sensory neuron and contacts the neuron cell body. (**C**) Massive expression of type I major histocompatibility complex by a sensory neuron and its capsule cells. (**D**) A perforin secreting cytotoxic T cell in contact with a neuronal cell body. (**A–D**) Immunoperoxidase method on cryocut sections counterstained with hematoxilin. × 40. N indicates the neuronal cell body. (**E**) H&S stained section showing a normal sensory neuron surrounded by its capsule of satellite cells (×40). (**F**) Immunohistochemical labeling of a normal human dorsal root ganglion with biotinylated IgGs of a patient with anti-Hu antibody. The antibody labels both cytoplasm and nuclei of sensory neurons (×20).

Peripheral neuropathy with anti-CV2/CRMP5 and other onconeural antibodies

Clinical symptoms

Peripheral neuropathy occurs in 60% of patients with anti-CV2/CRMP5 antibodies and is frequently associated with cerebellar ataxia, limbic encephalitis, or ocular involvement. This neuropathy [12] differs from that of the anti-Hu syndrome [13]. It is sensory or sensorimotor and predominates in the lower limbs. Pain is less frequent. An electroneuromyogram (ENMG) shows an axonal or mixed axonal and demyelinating pattern, but motor conduction velocities are not as slow as those in chronic inflammatory demyelinating polyneuropathies (CIDP) and conduction blocks are never seen.

It is not rare for patients to have both anti-Hu and anti-CV2/CRMP5 antibodies. These patients may develop a neuropathy blending the characteristics of the two disorders, with a mild demyelinating pattern on ENMG. Another possible association is with the Lambert–Eaton myasthenic syndrome. Any reduction of motor action potentials in a patient with anti-CV2 or anti-Hu antibodies should lead to a search for potentiation.

SCLC and thymoma are the most frequent underlying tumors with anti-CV2/CRMP5 antibodies. The prognosis of SCLC is better with anti-CV2/CRMP5 antibody than with anti-Hu antibodies [13].

Pathology

Nerve biopsy may show demyelinated fibers and onion bulbs while in other cases fiber loss predominates (Fig. 32.3) [12]. A mild inflammatory cell reaction may also occur in the endoneurial space. There are no reported autopsy cases describing the different structures of the peripheral nervous system. In two unreported cases from our series, inflammatory changes were found in the roots and in the spinal cord.

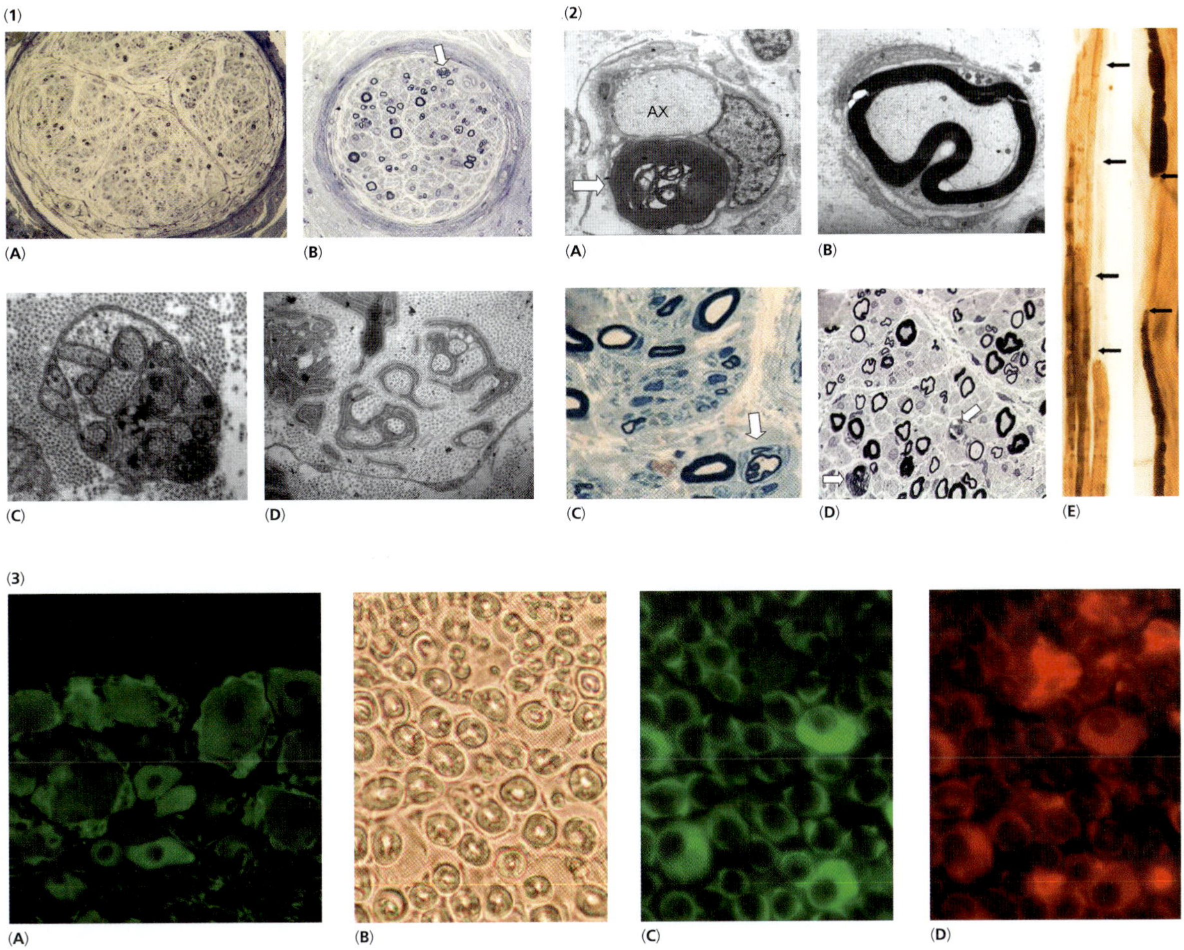

Figure 32.3 *Peripheral neuropathy in patients with anti-CV2/CRMP5 antibodies.*

(1) Predominant axonal changes in the nerve biopsy of two patients.

(**A** and **B**) Semithin sections: fiber loss and cluster of regeneration (**B**, arrow). **A** ×20. **B** ×40.

(**C** and **D**) Electron microscopy (×20.000). Collagen pockets indicating unmyelinated fiber loss.

(2) Predominant demyelinating changes in three other patients.

(**A** and **B**) Electron microscopy (×7000). (**A**) A demyelinated axon with the myelin sheath stripped in the Schwann cell cytoplasm (arrow). (**B**) An onion bulb formation.

(**C** and **D**) Semithin sections (×40). Numerous hypomyelinated fibers with onion bulbs (arrows).

(**E**) Teased fibers showing several demyelinated or hypomyelinated internodes (arrows).

(3) Expression of CRMP5 in the rat peripheral nervous system.

(**A**) Immunohistochemistry with an ani-CRMP5 antibody on a rat dorsal root ganglion (×20). The neurons and satellite cells are immunolabeled.

(B–D) Three views of the same field of rat sciatic nerve (×40). (**B**) Brightfield showing the myelinated fibers. (**C**) Immunohistochemistry with FITC labeled anti-S100 antibody staining the Schwann cell cytoplasm. (**D**) Immunohistochemistry with a TRITC labeled anti-CRMP5 antibody showing that both myelinating and non myelinating Schwann cell cytoplasm are labeled.

Pathogenesis

CRMP5 is a developmentally regulated peripheral and central nervous system protein that is down-regulated in the postnatal period. It persists in adult peripheral nerve in sensory neurons [14] and is also present in non myelinating and some myelinating Schwann cells and in unmyelinated axons. CRMP5 is massively re-expressed during nerve regeneration and down-regulated with myelination. CRMP5 expression in the peripheral nerve suggests that it is probably the target of the immune system (Fig. 32.3).

Similar to HuD, CRMP5 is also expressed by the tumor that may lead to an immunological cross reaction.

Peripheral neuropathy with other onconeural antibodies

PNS disorders occur only occasionally with anti-Yo, anti-Ma2, and anti-amphiphysin antibodies, and the clinical pattern of the neuropathy in these cases has not been well established.

Possible paraneoplastic peripheral neuropathies

Clinical symptoms

Varieties of neuropathies other than those listed above have been reported as paraneoplastic. These include cases of Gullain–Barré syndrome, CIDP, mononeuritis multiplex, lower motor neuron diseases, brachial plexopathy, autonomic, and sensory or sensorimotor axonal polyneuropathy [15]. In one study, neuropathies manifesting in parallel with the discovery of a malignancy

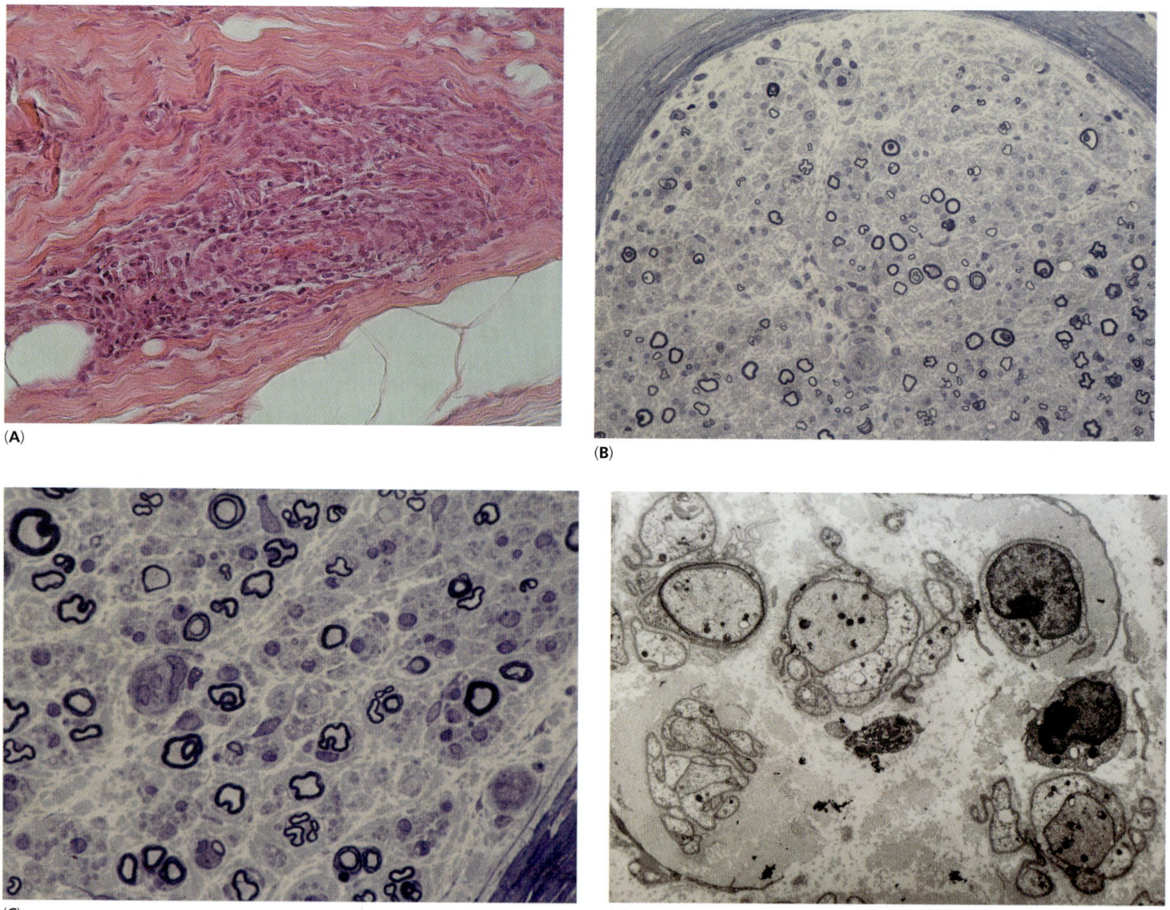

(A) (B) (C) (D)

Figure 32.4 *Different patterns of peripheral neuropathy in patients with possible paraneoplastic neuropathy.*

(A) Vasculitic lesion in the epineurium in a patient with laryngeal carcinoma and mononeuritis multiplex (H & S ×20).

(B) Fiber loss and endoneurial mononuclear cell infiltration in a patient with severe axonal sensorimotor neuropathy and kidney carcinoma (semithin section ×20).

(C) A patient with a chronic form of PIDC who recovered completely following the treatment for hepatic carcinoma. Semithin section (×40): hypomyelinated fibers and regenerating clusters.

(D) Same patient. Electron microscopy (×2000). Three demyelinated axons and a mononuclear cell.

tended to be inflammatory including Guillain–Barré syndrome, CIDP, and neuropathies with vasculitis (Fig. 32.4) [16]. In sharp contrast with neuropathies occurring with onconeural antibodies, there was no specific associated malignancy and SCLC represents a minority of cases. In lymphoma, a demyelinating neuropathy similar to CIDP is the most frequent presentation, but axonal neuropathy with microvasculitis and lower motor neuron disease have also been reported [17, 18].

Pathogenesis

All these cases have no identifiable onconeural antibodies and a direct link with the tumor is usually not demonstrated. Improvement of the neuropathy following tumor treatment is a major criterion for accepting a diagnosis of PNS, but there are only few reported cases of such a phenomenon. They include cases of lower motor neuron disease, vasculitic neuropathies, and CIDP. Rarely autoantibodies have been observed suggesting an immune mediated disorder. Ganglionic acetylcholine receptor antibodies have been reported in patients with autonomic neuropathies and tumor but these antibodies more commonly occur without cancer [19]. An antibody reacting with β-IV spectrin has been reported in a patient with breast cancer and lower motor neuron disease [20] and anti-ganglioside antibodies reacting with both the tumor and peripheral nerve have been described in patients with melanoma and CIDP [21].

Investigation for a tumor in a patient with peripheral neuropathy

In a patient with SSN or with onconeural antibodies the search for an underlying malignancy should center first on the detection of SCLC. If negative, it should be repeated every six months for four years. The primary tumor may be occult. FDG-PET scanner is the method of choice to detect tumor or lymph node metastases. As a rule, early detection and treatment of the tumor is the best way to stabilize and sometimes improve the neuropathy. With other neuropathies, the situation is difficult and there is no published recommendation. However, an underlying malignancy should be suspected and searched for in neuropathies with an unusual severe and rapid course, an absence of response to conventional treatments, symptoms of central nervous system involvement, or an inflammatory CSF reaction.

Conclusions and future perspectives

Paraneoplastic neuropathies are rare and only SSN and neuropathies associated with onconeural antibodies are definite PNS. Treatment remains disappointing and further progress is needed to improve our knowledge of the other neuropathies occurring with cancer.

References

1 Antoine JC, Camdessanché JP (2007). Peripheral nervous system involvement in patients with cancer. *Lancet Neurol* 6:75–86.

2 Graus F, Delattre JY, Antoine JC, *et al.* (2004) Recommended diagnostic criteria for paraneoplastic neurological syndromes. *J Neurol Neurosurg Psychiatry* 75:1135–1140.

3 Denny-Brown D. (1948) Primary sensory neuropathy with muscular changes associated with carcinoma. *J Neurol Neurosurg Psychiatry* 11:73–87.

4 Graus F, Keime-Guibert F, Rene R, *et al.* (2001) Anti-Hu-associated paraneoplastic encephalomyelitis: analysis of 200 patients. *Brain* 124:1138–1148.

5 Camdessanché JP, Antoine JC, Honnorat J, *et al.* (2002) Paraneoplastic peripheral neuropathy associated with anti-Hu antibodies. A clinical and electrophysiological study of 20 patients. *Brain* 125:166–175.

6 Horwich MS, Cho L, Porro RS, Posner JB. (1977) Subacute sensory neuropathy: a remote effect of carcinoma. *Ann Neurol* 2:7–19.

7 Molinuevo JL, Graus F, Serrano C, Rene R, Guerrero A, Illa I. (1998) Utility of anti-Hu antibodies in the diagnosis of paraneoplastic sensory neuropathy. *Ann Neurol* 44:976–980.

8 Younger DS, Dalmau J, Inghirami G, Sherman WH, Hays AP. (1994) Anti-Hu-associated peripheral nerve and muscle microvasculitis. *Neurology* 44:181–183.

9 Antoine JC, Mosnier JF, Honnorat J, *et al.* (1998) Paraneoplastic demyelinating neuropathy, subacute sensory neuropathy, and anti-Hu antibodies: clinicopathological study of an autopsy case. *Muscle Nerve* 21:850–857.

10 Camdessanché JP, Jousserand G, Franques J, *et al.* (2012) A clinical pattern-based etiological diagnostic strategy for sensory neuronopathies: a French collaborative study. *Journal of the peripheral nervous system: JPNS* 17:331–340.

11 Graus F, Ribalta T, Campo E, Monforte R, Urbano A, Rozman C. (1990) Immunohistochemical analysis of the immune reaction in the nervous system in paraneoplastic encephalomyelitis. *Neurology* 40:219–222.

12 Antoine JC, Honnorat J, Camdessanché JP, *et al.* (2001) Paraneoplastic anti-CV2 antibodies react with peripheral nerve and are associated with a mixed axonal and demyelinating peripheral neuropathy. *Ann Neurol* 49:214–221.

13 Honnorat J, Cartalat-Carel S, Ricard D, *et al.* (2009) Onconeural antibodies and tumour type determine survival and neurological symptoms in paraneoplastic neurological syndromes with Hu or CV2/CRMP5 antibodies. *J Neurol Neurosurg Psychiatry* 80:412–416.

14 Camdessanché JP, Ferraud K, Boutahar N, *et al.* (2012) The collapsin response mediator protein 5 onconeural protein is expressed in Schwann cells under axonal signals and regulates axon-Schwann cell interactions. *J. Neuropathol Exp Neurol* 71:298–311.

15 Rudnicki SA, Dalmau J. Paraneoplastic syndromes of the peripheral nerves. (2005) *Curr Opin Neurol* 18:598–603.

16 Antoine JC, Mosnier JF, Absi L, Convers P, Honnorat J, Michel D. (1999) Carcinoma associated paraneoplastic peripheral neuropathies in patients with and without anti-onconeural antibodies. *J Neurol Neurosurg Psychiatry* 67:7–14.

17 Briani C, Vitaliani R, Grisold W, *et al.* (2011) Spectrum of paraneoplastic disease associated with lymphoma. *Neurology* 76:705–710.

18 Viala K, Behin A, Maisonobe T, *et al.* (2008) Neuropathy in lymphoma: a relationship between the pattern of neuropathy, type of lymphoma and prognosis? *J Neurol Neurosurg Psychiatry* 79:778–782.

19 Vernino S, Low PA, Fealey RD, Stewart JD, Farrugia G, Lennon VA. (2000) Autoantibodies to ganglionic acetylcholine receptors in autoimmune autonomic neuropathies. *N Engl J Med* 343:847–855.

20 Berghs S, Ferracci F, Maksimova E, *et al.* (2001) Autoimmunity to beta IV spectrin in paraneoplastic lower motor neuron syndrome. *Proc Natl Acad Sci USA* 98:6945–6950.

21 Weiss MD, Luciano CA, Semino-Mora C, Dalakas MC, Quarles RH. (1998) Molecular mimicry in chronic inflammatory demyelinating polyneuropathy and melanoma. *Neurology* 51:1738–1741.

CHAPTER 33

Neuropathies in malnutrition and alcoholism

Martin Lammens

Department of Pathology, Antwerp University Hospital, Edegem, and University of Antwerp, Antwerp, Belgium

Introduction

Chronic alcoholism is one of the most important causes of neuropathy. Historically, alcoholism was usually accompanied by severe malnutrition. In recent years the social habits in the western world have changed and food additives may ameliorate the most severe damage. Whether the neuropathy is primarily due to the effect of alcohol, or if it is secondary to nutritional defects accompanying alcoholism has been a source of discussion for a long time [1–10]. Since some patients with chronic alcoholism and neuropathy do not have a clear nutritional deficiency, and as the neuropathy often does not respond to pure nutritional supplementation, it has become clear that there is also a direct toxic effect of alcohol.

Nutritional deficiencies should be relatively rare in the developed world, and most are secondary to poor diet. Chronic alcoholism remains an important factor, chronic illness can be a problem, but mostly responds to treatment; weight loss surgery has recently become a new challenge. Some chronic diseases, including hereditary types, lead to partial selective nutritional deficiencies, such as vitamin E or vitamin B12 deficiency. These syndromes with relative or secondary malnutrition will also be dealt with in this chapter.

Alcohol related peripheral neuropathy

Epidemiology

The term alcohol-related peripheral neuropathy (ALN) [9] is useful epidemiologically, as it combines both alcohol and neuropathy. The estimated prevalence of neuropathy in patients who suffer from alcoholism, as defined by DSM IV criteria, is between 25 and 66 % in the American population [4, 11]. The incidence of alcoholic polyneuropathy according to gender is controversial: according to Ammendola *et al.* [4] it is higher in women than in men, Zambelis *et al.* [11] found the reverse. The total lifetime amount of alcohol consumption and the duration of alcohol abuse are associated with ALN [3, 11]. ALN is more prevalent in frequent, heavy, and continuous drinkers than in episodic drinkers [3]. According to a study of Monforte *et al.* [3] consuming roughly 300 ml of 86% proof whiskey per day in a 70-kg man for several years leads to ALN. The type of beverage also plays a role, possibly due to the presence of impurities, such as lead in wine [6].

Clinical features

The usual clinical picture in patients with alcoholism is an indolent, slowly developing peripheral neuropathy with abnormalities in sensory, motor, and autonomic functions occurring over a period of months to years [1, 2, 7]. It usually starts with painful sensations with or without burning qualities in the limbs, followed by sensory loss mainly in the distal parts of the limbs in a stocking-glove distribution. Muscle weakness is present in about half of the patients, starting with foot drop and intrinsic hand muscle weakness. All patients have diminished or absent deep tendon reflexes. Autonomic changes are evident distal trophic skin changes.

Electrodiagnostic studies of the nerves reveal reduced sensory nerve action potentials, mildly reduced distal compound motor action potentials (CMAPs), and mild to moderate reduction of sensory and motor

Peripheral Nerve Disorders: Pathology and Genetics, First Edition. Edited by Jean-Michel Vallat, Joachim Weis, Francoise Gray, and Katy Keohane.

conduction velocities [7]. On electromyography distal denervation is seen. These studies are often abnormal in the presymptomatic patient [11]. In patients with chronic alcoholism combined with thiamine deficiency, CMAPs are more severely reduced [7].

Rapidly progressive motor weakness in patients with chronic alcoholism may be due to an acute myopathy, but an acute motor axonal neuropathy resembling Guillain–Barré syndrome has also been described as a complication of alcohol abuse [12, 13]. This complication is seen in patients who have thiamine deficiency with [14] or without alcoholism [15]. The entity is somewhat controversial, but the absence of typical spinal fluid changes, lack of ascending involvement of the limbs [13] and its recovery with nutritional supplementation alone strongly support its distinction from an axonal form of Guillain–Barré syndrome.

Neurarthropathy, also known as Charcot arthropathy, is a complication usually ascribed to diabetic neuropathy, but is also seen in patients with chronic alcoholism without diabetes [16]. It is a condition with marked joint instability, rocker bottom feet deformity with development of bony prominences leading to ulceration of the second and third toes, often accompanied by infections. Neurarthropathy is usually less devastating in patients with alcoholism than in diabetic patients, probably due to the higher incidence of obesity and immunocompromise in the latter population [16].

Pressure palsy (e.g., radial nerve palsy) after prolonged alcohol-induced sleep is a peculiar complication of alcohol abuse, and may occur even after a single episode of binge drinking.

The therapy of ALN consists of complete cessation of alcohol abuse and correction of nutritional deficiencies. Recovery may require many months, and can be almost complete, but liver transplantation may be required in decompensated alcoholic cirrhosis, since the aforementioned remedies alone are insufficient [17].

Pathology and pathogenesis

Although it is evident for a long time that polyneuropathy is a frequent complication of chronic alcoholism, the exact cause and mechanisms involved have been quite controversial. The concomitant nutritional deficiencies in alcoholism, especially thiamine deficiency, have often been considered as responsible for the nerve disturbances. Early studies often did not separate the direct effect of alcohol from the malnutrition, but a Danish study of Behse *et al.* [1] comparing patients with alcoholic neuropathy and postgastrectomy polyneuropathy concluded that alcohol per se plays a role in the pathogenesis of alcoholic neuropathy. In that study electron microscopy confirmed axonal degeneration of myelinated and unmyelinated fibers, with minimal evidence of primary demyelination (Fig. 33.1).

A few studies in humans have tried to differentiate the direct toxic defect of alcohol from the combined effects of alcoholism and nutritional deficiencies. A sural nerve biopsy study by Koike *et al.* [7] comparing groups of chronic alcohol patients with and without thiamine deficiency found that small-fiber-predominant axonal loss was characteristic of the pure form of alcoholic neuropathy. A clinical and electrophysiological study of non-deficient alcohol-dependent subjects found a group of exclusively large and a group of exclusively small fiber neuropathy that did not differ in any clinical or laboratory parameter [11]. Especially in the early stages of ALN the density of small myelinated and of unmyelinated fibers is more severely reduced than the density of large myelinated fibers [7].

The overall findings of the studies in "pure" alcoholism are consistent with a primary length-dependent axonal degeneration of myelinated and unmyelinated fibers (Fig. 33.1) with some secondary segmental de- and remyelination and myelin irregularity. Besides the direct neurotoxic effects of alcohol, some metabolites of alcohol play a detrimental role in alcoholic neuropathy. Accumulation of acetaldehyde may lead to dose-dependent neuronal cell death [18]. The detrimental effect of acetaldehyde is more in individuals with a mutation in acetaldehyde dehydrogenase (found in about 50% of the Asian population), who generate about 20 times higher acetaldehyde concentrations. Following ethanol intoxication, the balance between pro-oxidants and antioxidants is disturbed to such an extent that oxidative damage of biomolecules such as fats, proteins, and DNA occurs, leading to cell injury and thus alcoholic neuropathy [10]. Other molecules such as protein kinase C, the MEK/ERK pathway, and caspases play a role in the pathogenesis of alcoholic neuropathy. Glutamate receptors and the opioidergic systems are altered after chronic alcohol exposure, and play a role in pain symptoms in ALN [10]. Finally, axonal transport and cytoskeletal properties are altered by ethanol exposure as has been demonstrated in many in vitro and animal studies [10].

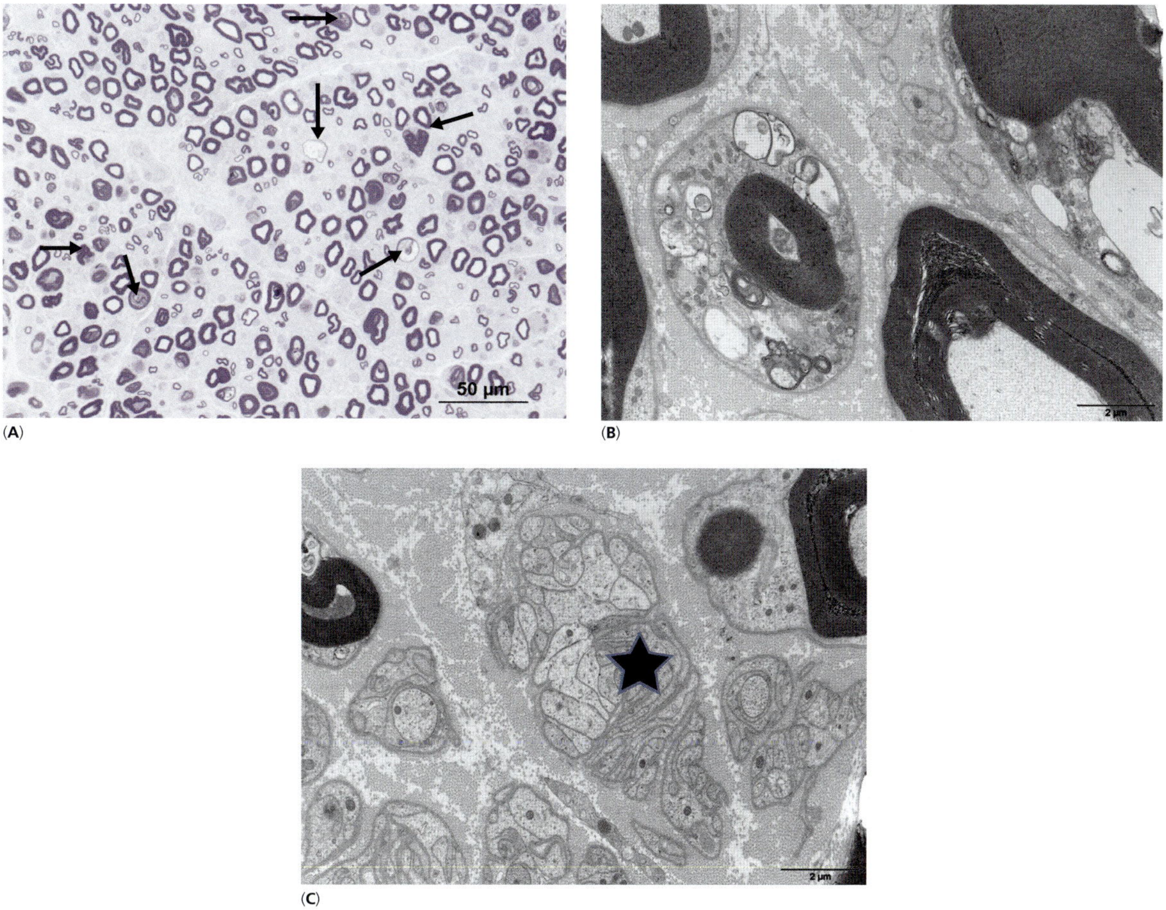

Figure 33.1 Alcoholic neuropathy (Courtesy Jean Michel Vallat) (A) Semithin transverse section. Moderate reduction of myelinated fibers, but many are destroyed: numerous "ovoids" corresponding to axonal lesions (arrows). (B) Electron micrograph, transverse section. Same case as Fig. 33.1(A). On the left, one myelinated fiber has become ovoid: note the disappearance of axons, the collapsed myelin and the accumulation of osmiophilic myelin debris in the Schwann cell cytoplasm. (**C**) Electron micrograph, transverse section. Same case as Figs 33.1(A,B). Denervated Schwann cell band from unmyelinated axons (star).

Thiamine deficiency

As already stated, thiamine deficiency is classically associated with chronic alcoholism. Recently, malnutrition is a complication following bariatric surgery in the western world [19] and often leads to thiamine deficiency, due to a combination of two important potential nutritional hazards: low food intake and persistent vomiting during the first few months, later malabsorption after surgery. Polyneuropathy has been found in up to 17% of bariatric surgery patients [20]. Other causes of thiamine (vitamin B1) deficiency are high-carbohydrate low-thiamine diets, anorexia nervosa, hyperemesis gravidarum, prolonged parenteral nutrition, and post-gastrectomy for neoplasms. It is often called "dry Beriberi neuropathy."

The characteristic neuropathy is a length-dependent dying back axonal neuropathy leading to a symmetric polyneuropathy involving the lower more than the upper limbs, with a centripetal pattern [7]. Motor weakness is a more prevalent symptom of thiamine neuropathy than pain [7]. Another clinical presentation consists of a predominant proximal weakness mimicking Guillain–Barré syndrome, often sparing the respiratory muscles, probably due to a combination of axonal neuropathy and muscle involvement [15, 21].

Thiamine replacement (50–100 mg intravenously or intramuscularly daily for 7–14 days, followed by 50–100 mg orally) is the treatment.

Vitamin B 12 deficiency

Vitamin B12 or cobalamin deficiency is well known as the cause of subacute combined degeneration, a myelopathy involving cervical and thoracic posterior and lateral columns. Cobalamin deficiency also causes a peripheral neuropathy, which is more prevalent than the myelopathy. In elderly patients, cobalamin deficiency is classically caused by pernicious anemia and food-cobalamin malabsorption [22]. Gadoth *et al.* [23] found it in 26.5% of an elderly cobalamin deficient population in Israel, Andrès *et al.* [22] found it in 28% of an elderly French population.

Neurophysiological and pathological studies reveal axonal degeneration with or without demyelination, unmyelinated fibers are also involved [24, 25]. A recent study demonstrated that low serum vitamin B12 levels (<260 pmol/L) were associated with a sensorimotor neuropathy, so it is not necessary to have actual vitamin B12 deficiency defined by an elevated methylmalonic acid level [26].

Folate deficiency

Folate deficiency is quite common despite recent folic acid fortification of food for the prevention of birth defects in some western countries. There are a few reports of apparently isolated folate deficiency [27, 28], leading to an axonal sensorineural neuropathy prevalent in the lower limbs.

Vitamin E deficiency

Alpha-tocopherol, best known as vitamin E, is a lipid-soluble vitamin absorbed in the small intestine after processing by bile acids. Vitamin E deficiency is mostly due to a fat malabsorption syndrome as seen in cystic fibrosis, chronic cholestasis, short-bowel syndrome, and other gastrointestinal disorders, or a primary or secondary defect of a specific transfer-protein. The latter is seen in several forms of hypo- or abetalipoproteinemia (see Chapter 20). In addition to central nervous system disorders such as spinocerebellar degeneration, myoclonic dystonia and seizures, polyneuropathy has been regularly reported [29–31].

The neuropathy is characterized by mostly sensory symptoms. In experimentally induced vitamin E deficiency in animals, dystrophic axonal changes are seen [32]. The few histological studies on human neuropathy

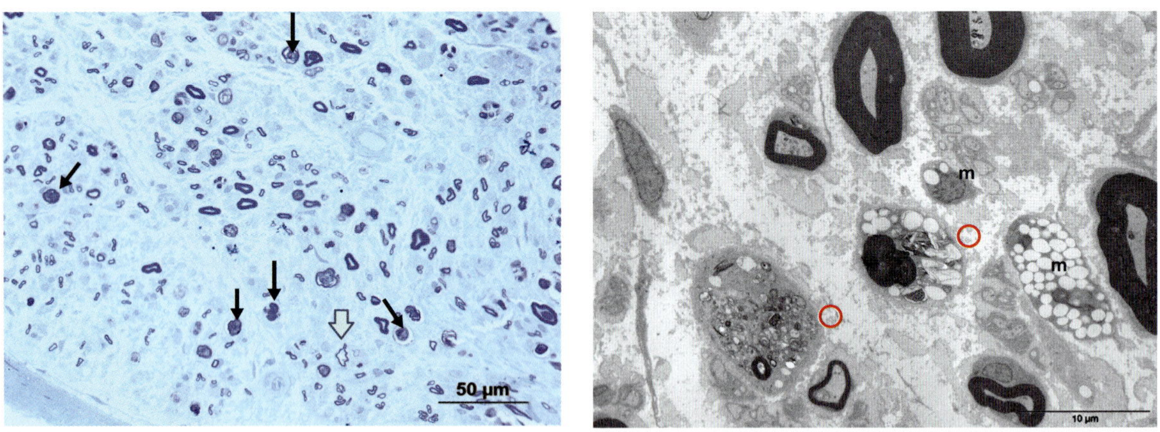

(A) (B)

Figure 33.2 Malnutrition neuropathy (Courtesy Jean Michel Vallat). (**A**) Semithin transverse section. Significant reduction of large myelinated fibers. There are many "ovoids" corresponding to axonal lesions (black arrows) and a few demyelinating fibers (open arrow). (**B**) Electron micrograph, transverse section. Same case as Fig. 33.2(A). O = "ovoids"; m = macrophages that contain lipid droplets in their cytoplasm.

revealed features that were not very specific and included axonal damage, signs of demyelination, and some inclusions in Schwann cells [29, 33].

Other deficiencies in malnutrition

Other nutrients may be absent in general malnutrition, but rarely as an isolated defect.

Niacin deficiency leads to pellagra, a disease characterized by a specific dermatitis, diarrhea, and dementia [34]. In the western world, bread is enriched by niacin, so it is rarely seen there. The deficiency leads to an axonal neuropathy resembling thiamine deficiency.

Vitamin B6 deficiency may be seen in patients treated with the antituberculosis drug isoniazid [35]. It leads to a non-specific axonal sensorimotor polyneuropathy.

In many cases, mainly in developing countries, malnutrition neuropathies cannot be related to a specific deficiency. In all these various neuropathies, the microscopic nerve abnormalities are usually severe, non-specific, mainly axonal, and rarely associated with a few demyelinating features (Fig. 33.2A,B).

References

1 Behse F, Buchthal F (1977). Alcoholic neuropathy – clinical, electrophysiological, and biopsy findings. *Ann Neurol* 2: 95–110.

2 Hawley RJ, Kurtzke JF, Armbrustmacher VW, *et al.* (1982) The course of alcoholic-nutritional peripheral neuropathy. *Acta Neurol Scan* 66: 582–589.

3 Monforte R, Estruch R, Valls-Sole J, *et al.* (1995) Autonomic and peripheral neuropathies in patients with chronic alcoholism. A dose-related toxic effect of alcohol. *Arch Neurol* 52: 45–51.

4 Ammendola A, Tata MR, Aurilio C, *et al.* (2001) Peripheral neuropathy in chronic alcoholism: a retrospective cross-sectional study in 76 subjects. *Alcohol Alcohol* 36: 271–275.

5 Koike H, Mori K, Misu K, *et al.* (2001) Painful alcoholic polyneuropathy with predominant small-fiber loss and normal thiamine status. *Neurology* 56: 1727–1732.

6 Vittadini G, Buonocore M, Colli G, *et al.* (2001) Alcoholic polyneuropathy: a clinical and epidemiological study. *Alcohol Alcohol* 36: 393–400.

7 Koike H, Iijima M, Sugiura M, *et al.* (2003) Alcoholic neuropathy is clinicopathologically distinct from thiamine-deficiency neuropathy. *Ann Neurol* 54: 19–29.

8 Koike H, Sobue G (2006) Alcoholic neuropathy. *Curr Opin Neurology* 19: 481–486.

9 Mellion M, Gilchrist JM, de la Monte S. (2011) Alcohol-related peripheral neuropathy: nutritional, toxic, or both? *Muscle Nerve* 43: 309–316.

10 Chopra K, Tiwari V (2012) Alcoholic neuropathy: possible mechanisms and future treatment possibilities. *Brit J Clin Pharm* 73: 348–362.

11 Zambelis T, Karandreas N, Tzavellas E, *et al.* (2005) Large and small fiber neuropathy in chronic alcohol-dependent subjects. *J Periph Nerv Syst* 10: 375–381.

12 Wohrle JC, Spengos K, Steinke W *et al.* (1998) Alcohol-related acute axonal polyneuropathy: a differential diagnosis of Guillain–Barre syndrome. *Arch Neurol* 55: 1329–1334.

13 Sahin S, Cinar N, Sezgin G, *et al.* (2010) Acute motor axonal neuropathy: a severe complication of alcohol abuse. *J Neuropsychiatry Clin Neurosci* 22: 451-ie16-e17.

14 Howard AJ, Kulkarni O, Lekwuwa G, *et al.* (2010) Rapidly progressive polyneuropathy due to dry beriberi in a man: a case report. *J Med Case Rep* 4: 409.

15 Koike H, Ito S, Morozumi S *et al.* (2008) Rapidly developing weakness mimicking Guillain-Barre syndrome in beriberi neuropathy: two case reports. *Nutrition* 7–8: 776–780.

16 Shibuya N, La Fontaine J, Frania SJ. (2008) Alcohol-induced neuroarthropathy in the foot: a case series and review of literature. *J Foot Ankle Surg* 47: 118–124.

17 Gane E, Bergman R, Hutchinson D (2004) Resolution of alcoholic neuropathy following liver transplantation. *Liver Transpl* 10: 1545–1548.

18 Takeuchi M, Saito T (2005) Cytotoxicity of acetaldehyde-derived advanced glycation end-products (AA-AGE) in alcoholic-induced neuronal degeneration. *Alcohol Clin Exp Res* 29 (Suppl): 220S–224S.

19 Anthone GJ, Lord RV, DeMeester TR, *et al.* (2003) The duodenal switch operation for the treatment of morbid obesity. *Ann Surg* 238: 618–627.

20 Thaisetthawatkul P, Collazo-Clavell ML, Sarr MG, *et al.* (2004) A controlled study of peripheral neuropathy after bariatric surgery. *Neurology* 63: 1462–1470.

21 Murphy C, Bangash IH, Varma A. (2009) Dry beriberi mimicking the Guillain–Barre syndrome. *Pract Neurol* 9: 221–224.

22 Andres E, Kaltenbach G, Perrin AE, *et al.* (2002) Food-cobalamin malabsorption in the elderly. *Am J Med* 113: 351–352.

23 Gadoth N, Figlin E, Chetrit A, *et al.* (2006) The neurology of cobalamin deficiency in an elderly population in Israel. *J Neurol* 253: 45–50.

24 Abarbanel JM, Frisher S, Osimani A. (1986) Vitamin-B12 deficiency neuropathy – sural nerve biopsy study. *Isr J Med Sci* 22: 909–911.

25 Schröder JM. (1999) *Pathologie des Nervensystems.* Springer, Berlin.

26 Leishear K, Boudreau RM, Studenski SA, *et al.* (2012) Relationship between vitamin B12 and sensory and motor peripheral nerve function in older adults. *J Am Ger Soc* 60: 1057–1063.

27 Botez MI, Peyronnard JM, Bachevalier J, *et al.* (1978) Polyneuropathy and folate deficiency. *Arch Neurol* 35: 581–584.
28 Koike H, Hama T, Kawagashira Y, *et al.* (2012) The significance of folate deficiency in alcoholic and nutritional neuropathies: analysis of a case. *Nutrition* 28: 821–824.
29 Landrieu P, Selva J, Alvarez F, *et al.* (1985) Peripheral nerve involvement in children with chronic cholestasis and vitamin E deficiency. A clinical, electrophysiological and morphological study. *Neuropediatrics* 16: 194–201.
30 Davidai G, Zakaria T, Goldstein R, *et al.* (1986) Hypovitaminosis E induced neuropathy in exocrine pancreatic failure. *Arch Dis Child* 61: 901–903.
31 Palmucci L, Doriguzzi C, Orsi L, *et al.* (1988) Neuropathy secondary to vitamin E deficiency in acquired intestinal malabsorption. *Ital J Neuro Sci* 9: 599–602.
32 Southam E, Thomas PK, King RH, *et al.* (1991) Experimental vitamin E deficiency in rats. Morphological and functional evidence of abnormal axonal transport secondary to free radical damage. *Brain* 114: 915–936.
33 Traber MG, Sokol RJ, Ringel SP, *et al.* (1987) Lack of tocopherol in peripheral nerves of vitamin E-deficient patients with peripheral neuropathy. *New Engl J Med* 317: 262–265.
34 Isaac S (1998) The "gauntlet" of pellagra. *Int J Dermatol* 37: 599.
35 Lubing HN. (1953) Peripheral neuropathy in tuberculosis patients treated with isoniazid. *Am Rev Tuberc Pulm* 68: 458–461.

CHAPTER 34

Critical illness polyneuropathy

Douglas C. Anthony[1] and David Lacomis[2]

[1] Department of Pathology and Laboratory Medicine, Alpert Medical School of Brown University, and Lifespan Academic Medical Center, Rhode Island, USA

[2] Department of Neurology and Pathology, University of Pittsburgh School of Medicine, Pittsburgh, USA

Definition

Critical illness polyneuropathy (CIP) is an acute onset predominantly axonal peripheral neuropathy in critically ill patients who are often on ventilator support. Typically patients are in intensive care units (ICU) and are weak; the weakness prevents weaning from ventilator support, the weaning period being 2–5 times longer in patients with CIP than in those without. Synonyms are "critical care neuropathy," "ICU neuropathy," or "ventilator-dependent neuropathy." The term critical illness polyneuropathy more accurately reflects its relationship to an acute severe illness, rather than an implied association with the care, ICU, or ventilator. It may or may not be accompanied by critical illness myopathy. The diagnostic criteria are based on the clinical setting of a critical illness, usually in intensive care and accompanied by sepsis, weakness, and sensory loss, and with electrophysiological evidence of axonal neuropathy, mainly decreased amplitudes without significant slowing on nerve conduction studies (NCS).

The commonest presenting symptom is difficulty weaning from ventilator support. Patients with CIP have profound generalized weakness that may be accentuated distally in the limbs [1, 2]. Muscle atrophy may develop rapidly, and deep tendon reflexes are usually absent or markedly reduced. Hoarseness, limb weakness, weak grip, and weak cough with abundant secretions are additional signs. The two mandatory criteria for CIP are: (1) a critically ill patient, and (2) diffuse limb weakness or difficulty weaning from a ventilator. Additional major criteria are reductions in sensory and motor nerve amplitudes, absence of conduction block or prolonged F-waves, needle EMG with reduced recruitment of normal motor unit potentials (MUP) acutely, and fibrillation potentials and reduced recruitment of long duration high-amplitude MUPs over time [1, 3]. The minor criteria include absence of decremental responses on repetitive nerve stimulation, confirmatory findings on nerve or muscle biopsy, and changes in nerve-evoked muscle action potentials.

Epidemiology

The incidence is best defined within the subset of patients with a critical illness receiving care in an intensive care unit. Within ICU patients, critical illness polyneuropathy is very common with an incidence of acute-onset weakness of 25–50% [1, 2, 4]; the prevalence is even higher if NCS are the defining criteria [2, 5]. Since myopathy and polyneuropathy often coexist in the same patient, the less specific term "critical care weakness" has also been used [6]. The incidence of CIP correlates with length of stay in ICU and severity of sepsis [2, 5]. The mortality is as high as 60% [2].

Clinical features and investigations

CIP is often first identified in patients who have profound weakness or paralysis of limbs and respiratory muscles after prolonged sedation in the ICU [6]. Onset is often during the period of sedation and ventilator support and failure to wean from ventilator support is the commonest presenting symptom. CIP includes limb and

Peripheral Nerve Disorders: Pathology and Genetics, First Edition. Edited by Jean-Michel Vallat, Joachim Weis, Francoise Gray, and Katy Keohane.

respiratory muscle weakness and may coexist with critical illness myopathy [6]. Weakness may be documented with muscle testing, handgrip testing, or maximal respiratory effort [6]. The limb weakness is usually symmetric, and facial muscles are usually spared [6]. Patients are often sedated or unable to cooperate with neurologic examination, so NCS and electroneuromyography (ENMG) are the mainstays of diagnosis, both in children and adults [1, 4, 7]. ENMG shows decreased recruitment of motor unit potentials acutely and fibrillation potentials followed by decreased recruitment of high amplitude, long duration motor unit potentials. NCS shows low amplitude sensory and motor action potentials with near-normal conduction velocity [2]. During clinical improvement, electrophysiological parameters often show recovery over the course of several weeks.

Pathology

CIP is characterized by an acute onset axonal neuropathy with widespread axonal degeneration [1, 2, 4]. The distribution of affected fibers appears to be random throughout the fascicle; axonal degeneration involves motor and sensory fibers, unmyelinated fibers, and both large and small caliber myelinated axons [8]. Distal and proximal nerve segments are affected. These lesions are diffuse rather than multifocal, affecting large proportions of nerve trunks. In the acute phase, myelinated fibers are replaced by numerous ovoids; later in the illness, biopsy may show significant axon loss. Lymphocytic inflammation is not seen. During clinical recovery from the acute illness, axonal regeneration is prominent. Muscle biopsy may show atrophy predominantly of type II fibers, selective loss of thick (myosin) filaments, acute necrotizing myopathy, and neurogenic atrophy [5, 7].

Genetics

No genetic predisposition for critical illness neuropathy is known.

Differential diagnosis

Profound weakness and failure to wean from ventilatory support after prolonged ICU sedation is common in critically-ill patients [6] and has a distinct differential diagnosis. Common causes are CNS depression (central ventilatory dependence, often due to CNS depressant therapies), stroke or other CNS neurologic problem of recent onset (cerebrovascular event, central pontine myelinolysis), weakness due to critical illness polyneuropathy, muscle weakness due to myopathy (critical illness myopathy), and endocrine or metabolic disturbance. The symmetric flaccidity of CIP helps in the distinction from stroke or other acute CNS event. Electrophysiologies (electromyography and/or NCS) are helpful in identifying recent-onset neuromuscular disease. CIP is identified by decreased amplitudes on NCS, while critical illness myopathy is characterized by myopathic findings on NCS and/or EMG. Measurement of strength by means of the MRC scale [6] or handgrip dynamometry has been used as an alternative to electrophysiological testing.

Pathogenesis, treatment, and outcome

The pathogenesis of CIP is not completely understood. There is a high incidence in patients who have sepsis and develop disseminated intravascular coagulation (DIC). Common preceding events include prolonged sedation, prolonged mechanical ventilation, sepsis, and multiple organ failure. For these reasons, a vascular etiology for CIP has been suspected. However, some patients develop CIP in the absence of DIC, and intravascular thrombi have not been demonstrated in the peripheral nerves of patients with CIP. In addition, there is a strong correlation with hyperglycemia, and changes in nerve excitability have been described [9]. The incidence of CIP may be reduced by intensive treatment of hyperglycemia, but this approach is controversial due to higher mortality.

CIP has a high morbidity and mortality, and there is no known specific treatment. Therapy is aimed at supportive care. In general, ICU care and ventilator support required in the setting of CIP is 2–5 times the duration of ICU care required in its absence [6], with high associated comorbidities and cost [10]. In the short-term, the mortality resulting from the underlying ICU illness is nearly 50% [1, 5], but increases with abnormalities on NCS [1]. The long-term outcome following CIP is worse than following CIM, and requires a longer recovery period. Many patients with CIP may have long-term residual neuropathic symptoms [1]. Severe or moderate

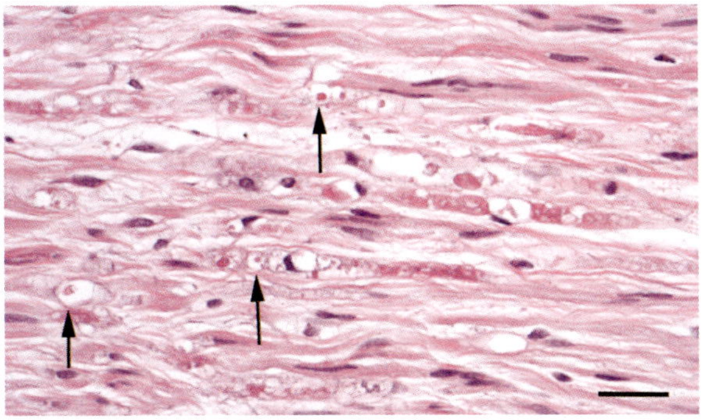

Figure 34.1 CIP nerve biopsy: acute axonal neuropathy with abundant degenerating axons visible as rows of myelin ovoids in the longitudinal plane (arrows). H&E; scale bar = 25 μm.

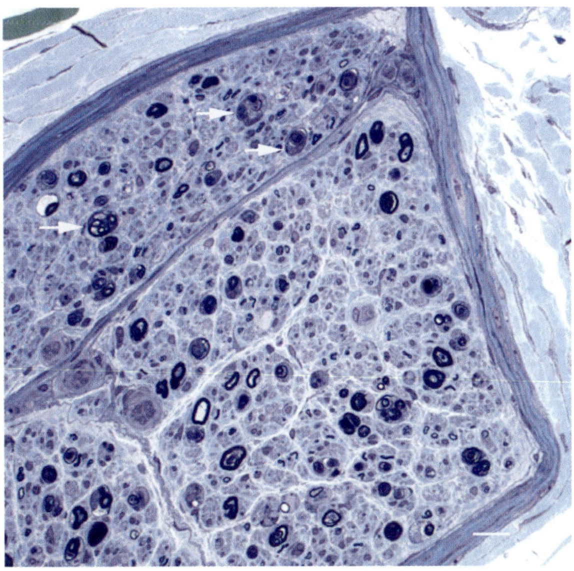

Figure 34.2 CIP nerve biopsy: acute axonal neuropathy during the acute stages, with abundant destroyed axons resembling ovoids (arrows). Semithin section, Toluidine blue. Scale bar = 20 μm.

peripheral neuropathy is common after discharge, but there is usually substantial recovery over weeks [1, 4, 11]. Up to 20% of patients have residual severe peripheral neuropathy for 1–2 years, and electrodiagnostic testing up to 5 years after critical illness still shows signs of partial denervation [1].

Animal models

Rodent models of CIP can be produced by chronic sepsis or direct injection of *Corynebacterium* and suggest that ion channels may be involved [1].

Conclusions and future perspectives

CIP is a well-defined clinical entity; however, the pathophysiology is only partially understood. Better understanding of its pathophysiology may lead to improved treatment and preventive strategies to reduce its occurrence in critically-ill patients.

References

1 Lacomis D. (2011) Neuromuscular disorders in critically ill patients: Review and update. *J Neuromusc Dis* 12, 197–218.

2 Dhand UK. (2006) Clinical approach to the weak patient in the intensive care unit. *Resp Care* 51, 1024–1040.

3 Bolton CD. (2005) Neuromuscular manifestations of critical illness. *Muscle Nerve* 32, 140–163.

4 Chawla J, Gruener G. (2010) Management of critical illness polyneuropathy and myopathy. *Neurol Clin* 28, 961–977.

5 Khan J, Harrison TB, Rich MM, Moss M. (2006) Early development of critical illness myopathy and neuropathy in patients with severe sepsis. *Neurol* 67, 1421–1425.

6 Latronico N, Rasulo FA. (2010) Presentation and management of ICU myopathy and neuropathy. *Curr Opinion Crit Care* 16, 123–127.

7 Williams S, Horrocks IA, Ouvrier RA, Gillis J, Ryan MM. (2007) Critical illness polyneuropathy and myopathy in pediatric intensive care: A review. *Pediatr Crit Care Med* 8, 18–22.

8 Ohto T, Iwasaki N, Ohkoshi N, Aoki T, *et al.* (2005) A pediatric case of critical illness polyneuropathy: clinical and pathologic findings. *Brain Dev* 27, 535–538.

9 Graggen WJ, Lin CSY, Howard RS, Beale RJ, Bostock H. (2006) Nerve excitability changes in critical illness polyneuropathy. *Brain* 129, 2461–2470.

10 Deem S. (2006) Intensive-care-unit-acquired muscle weakness. *Resp Care* 51, 1042–1052.

11 Semmler A, Okulla T, Kaiser M, Seifert B, Neneka MT. (2012) Long-term neuromuscular sequelae of critical illness. *J Neurol* 260, 151–157.

CHAPTER 35

Non-vasculitic ischemic neuropathies

Robert E. Schmidt

Department of Pathology and Immunology, Division of Neuropathology, Washington University School of Medicine, St. Louis, USA

Definition

Non vasculitic ischemic neuropathies are defined as neuropathies developing in nerves in which diminished blood flow occurs in the absence of vasculitis. Separation of vasculitis involving the vasa nervorum from non-vasculitic causes of ischemia appears relatively clear cut using the histologic presence or absence of angionecrosis, often considered the gold standard of vasculitis [1]. However, in practice, this simple distinction may be complicated. Some entities (e.g., collagen vascular diseases including rheumatoid arthritis, scleroderma, and Sjogren syndrome) may have a variety of histopathologic presentations ranging from mild epineurial perivascular lymphocytic cuffing to fibrinoid vasculitis indistinguishable from polyarteritis nodosa. One additional confounding element is the focal nature of vasculitis; fibrinoid vascular necrosis and thrombosis may be found at one level and only perivascular cuffing involving the same vessel less than a few hundred microns away.

A nerve that has suffered marked depletion of axons and, with time, Schwann cells, may show secondary decrease in blood flow as a result, that is, the presence of ischemia may not be the primary and most critical pathogenetic element. With these caveats, this chapter will focus on ischemic non-vasculitic neuropathies.

Clinical conditions, presentations, and epidemiology

Neuropathy has been described in occasional patients with chronic vascular insufficiency involving the lower limb in the absence of any other cause of neuropathy (particularly diabetes). The neuropathy is characterized by paresthesias and sensory loss, and, in other patients, with weakness, wasting, or with reduced ankle reflexes that parallel ischemia [2, 3]. Some patients with arteritis involving large vessels without accompanying involvement of the vasa nervorum may present with large vessel occlusion, claudication, and eventually gangrene. Other causes of ischemic neuropathy may follow aortic occlusion from arteriosclerotic vascular disease, abdominal aortic aneurysms or their repair, overall low cardiac output, use of an intra-aortic balloon pump or prolonged tourniquet time in surgery. Some of these conditions are age-related (e.g., aortic aneurysms) and others may have a genetic component (exaggerated atherosclerosis).

Similarly, rheumatoid arthritis or scleroderma may result in severe neuropathy in the presence of frank vasculitis of the vasa nervorum or exhibit a milder form without angionecrosis, which also may result in axon loss [4]. Patients with Sjögren syndrome may develop axonal sensorimotor neuropathy, which may have an ischemic pathogenesis [5]. Patients with chronic hypoxemia resulting from serious chronic pulmonary disease sometimes develop mild sensory complaints, particularly distally, and accompanied by diminished ankle jerks [6].

Peripheral neuropathy developing in patients with a history of vascular catheterization, particularly of the femoral artery, or those with severe aortic atherosclerosis may be the initial manifestation of cholesterol emboli syndrome (CES) [7]. Intralumenal cholesterol clefts in small epineurial arteries can sometimes be seen in peripheral nerve biopsy in CES, but are more frequently found in muscle in combined muscle and nerve biopsy (see Chapter 2). These emboli only occasionally result in

Peripheral Nerve Disorders: Pathology and Genetics, First Edition. Edited by Jean-Michel Vallat, Joachim Weis, Francoise Gray, and Katy Keohane.

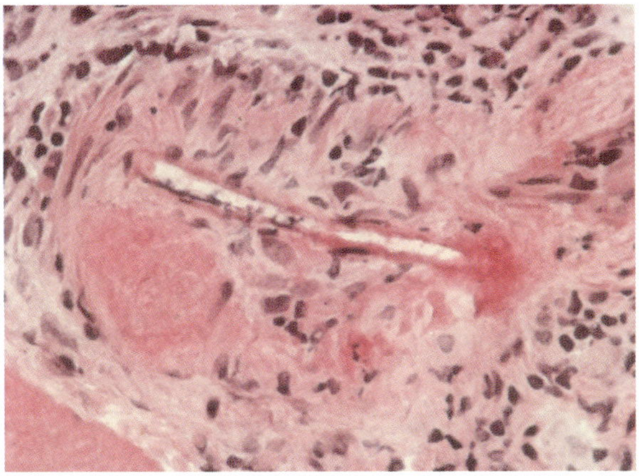

Figure 35.1 Cholesterol emboli syndrome: Cholesterol embolus in a small intramuscular artery associated with fibrinoid necrosis and inflammation of the vessel wall. H&E.

necrotizing arteritis (Fig. 35.1), but can be associated with severe degeneration of peripheral and intramuscular nerves. The underlying pathology of CES neuropathy is chronic axonal degeneration.

A variety of factors may induce ischemic neuropathy including hypercoagulable/hyperviscosity states, use of vasoconstrictors like methylsergide (for migraine) and ethanol sclerotherapy of vascular malformations prior to surgery [8, 9]. Sickle cell disease, particularly patients in crisis, represents a rare cause of neuropathy characterized by weakness, often lumbosacral and asymmetric, as well as pain and sensory loss in the leg. Amyloid compression of the epineurial vasculature may result in axon loss; however, amyloid may be simultaneously deposited in the endoneurium complicating a purely ischemic pathogenesis. Although an uncommon cause, intravascular lymphoma may be so extensive as to occlude many small vessels in the epineurium and endoneurium (Figs 35.2A–C) and produce axon loss. Arachidonic acid injection into the femoral artery may result in an ischemic insult to peripheral nerve.

Pathology

The degree of axon loss in ischemic neuropathy is quite variable ranging from minimal to near complete [2, 3]; conversely, some authors [1] suggest there is little evidence suggesting chronic large vessel ischemia causes peripheral nervous system injury. Although some studies, particularly animal studies (see next section), have described a centrofascicular predilection for axon loss in ischemic neuropathy, most experience with clinical nerve biopsies only rarely has shown a purely centrofascicular distribution. Clinical ischemic neuropathy may have diffuse, subperineurial, and centrofascicular axon loss. There is evidence of fascicle to fascicle variability in axon loss, a range of chronicity from acute axonal degeneration to chronic axon dropout. Some cases show selective involvement of large myelinated axons, or involving all populations of axons, not sparing unmyelinated axons. Additionally, ischemic neuropathy may show axonal atrophy, organelle accumulation, paranodal demyelination, perineurial thickening, and even onion-bulb formation [6, 7].

Although occasionally ischemic neuropathy has been described as demyelinative, in most cases demyelination that occurs is secondary to axonal disease (i.e., "secondary demyelination").

Vasa nervorum in chronic ischemia are thought to show increased smooth muscle, disorganized vascular layers, reduplication of basement membranes, hyperplasia, and hypertrophy of endothelial cells as well as microvascular occlusion [1, 2]. Maximal involvement preferentially occurs at mid-arm and mid-thigh levels that are vascular watershed regions of nerve [10].

Animal models

Animal models of ischemic neuropathy have been produced by ligating multiple large vessels (abdominal aorta and both iliac arteries) in experimental rodents or by the use of intra-arterial injection of large numbers of polystyrene microspheres [11]. Fourteen micron diameter microspheres plug capillaries and pre-capillaries to decrease hindlimb intraneural blood flow [11]. Nukuda and Dyck [11] demonstrated that occlusion of many microvessels results in central fascicular axonal degeneration, thought to represent a watershed region of poor perfusion. The clinical and pathologic effect of microsphere injection was dose-related as measured by the degree of hind limb paresis, reduction in nerve blood flow, degree of fiber pathology, and ischemic conduction failure in the tibial nerve. These authors described increased capillary density in subperineurial areas of sciatic nerve, which accompanied the preferential loss of central fascicular axons, especially in large proximal nerve fascicles. Sites of increased vulnerability also

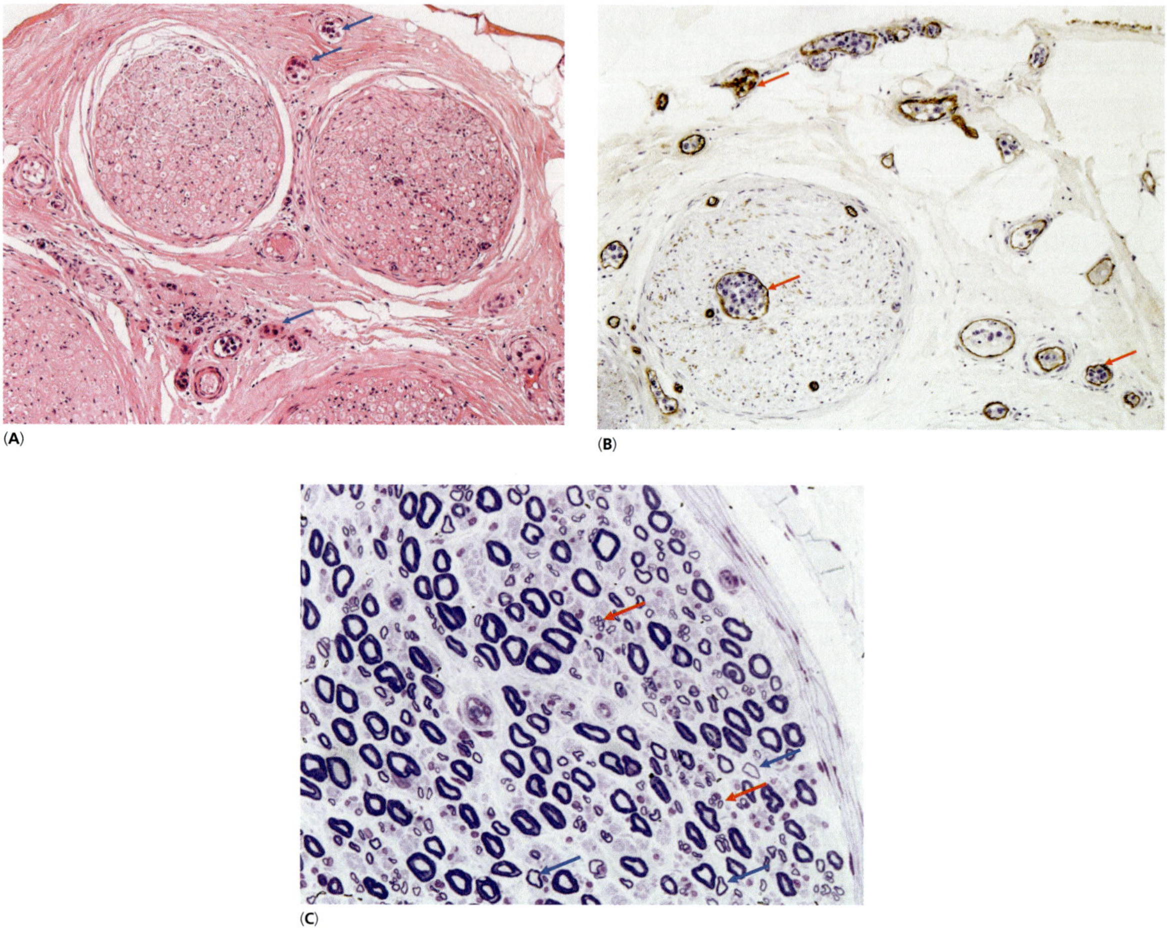

Figure 35.2 Intravascular lymphoma, a rare cause of ischemic neuropathy. (**A, B**) Intravascular lymphoma (arrows) diffusely involving epineurial and endoneurial vasculature. (**A**): H&E, (**B**) Ulex europaeus stain. (**C**) Surprisingly, semithin sections (Toluidine blue) show only mild loss of axons as well as axon clusters (red arrows) and axons with myelin too-thin-for-axon-caliber (blue arrows). Original magnification: 1: ×2000; 2 A, B: ×200; C: ×1000.

included lower sciatic and upper tibial/peroneal regions. Nerve edema and ischemic fiber degeneration consistently became more severe with reperfusion, which results in an increase in nerve lipid hydroperoxides and oxidative stress, impairing the blood-nerve barrier and causing ischemic axonal degeneration.

References

1 Midroni G, Bilbao JM. (1995) Vasculitic neuropathy, Chapter 13 In: *Biopsy Diagnosis of Peripheral Neuropathy*, Midroni G and Bilbao JM (eds), pp. 341–262. Butterworth-Heinemann, Boston.

2 Eames RA, Lange LS. (1967) Clinical and pathologic study of ischemic neuropathy. *J Neurol Neurosurg Psychiatry* 30, 215–226.

3 Farinon AM, Marbini A, Gemignani F, *et al.* (1984) Skeletal muscle and peripheral nerve changes caused by chronic arterial insufficiency: significance and clinical correlations, histological, histochemical and ultrastructural study. *Clin Neuropathol* 3, 240–252.

4 Olney RK. (1992) Neuropathies in connective tissue disease. *Muscle Nerve* 15, 531–542.

5 Gemignami F, Marbini A, Pavesi G, *et al.* (1994) Peripheral neuropathy associated with primary Sjogren's syndrome. *J Neurol Neurosurg Psychiatry* 57, 983–986.

6 Malik RA, Masson EA, Sharma AK, *et al.* (1990) Hypoxic neuropathy: relevance to human diabetic neuropathy. *Diabetologia* 33, 311–318.

7 Bendixen BH, Younger DS, Hair LS, *et al.* (1992) Cholesterol emboli neuropathy. *Neurology* 42, 428–430.

8 Ney JP, Shih W, Landau ME. (2006) Sciatic neuropathy following endovascular treatment of a limb vascular malformation. *J Brach Plex Perip Nerve Injury* 1, 8.

9 Laghi Pasini F, Pastorelli M, Beermann U, *et al.* (1996) Peripheral neuropathy associated with ischemic vascular disease of the lower limbs. *Angiology* 47, 569–577.

10 Dyck PJ, Conn DL, Okazaki H. (1972) Necrotizing angiopathic neuropathy: three-dimensional morphology of fiber degeneration related to sites of occluded vessels. *Mayo Clin Proc* 47, 461–475

11 Nukada H, Dyck PJ. Microsphere embolization of nerve capillaries and fiber degeneration. *Am J Pathol* 115, 275–287.

CHAPTER 36

Traumatic and compressive lesions of peripheral nerves

Carlos Ortiz-Hidalgo[1] and Roy O. Weller[2]

[1] *Department of Tissue and Cell Biology, Universidad Panamericana, and Department of Surgical and Molecular Pathology, The American British Cowdray (ABC) Medical Centre, Mexico*

[2] *Department of Neuropathology, Clinical and Experimental Sciences, Faculty of Medicine, University of Southampton, Southampton, UK*

Definition

Trauma to peripheral nerves results in injury of varying type and severity [1, 2]. *Compression injury* is the monophasic application of force compressing a nerve against a rigid structure such as bone. An example is compression from a tourniquet. *Entrapment injury* to a nerve occurs when it passes through an opening that is too small for a nerve of that size. The opening may be bounded by muscle, ligament, or bone and injury may be due to compression, stretching, and ischemia. In both compression and entrapment injuries, the connective tissue elements of the nerve remain intact and, in many cases, nerve fibers regenerate and return to almost normal. *Transection injuries* are the most severe form of nerve trauma in which the nerve trunk, blood supply, perineurium, and epineurium are completely severed. Regeneration is much less successful as fewer nerve fibers grow across the gap between the severed ends of the nerve [3].

Epidemiology

Nerve trauma may occur at any age. Compression injuries may be caused by a tourniquet or tumor, whereas entrapment injuries occur around joints and in ligamentous channels such as the carpal tunnel at the wrist and are more common in the elderly [2]. Transection injuries of peripheral nerves occur mainly in younger people and are associated with penetrating injuries or bone fractures in industrial and road traffic accidents. Ulnar nerves are most frequently injured in this way, followed by radial and median nerves in the upper limb, and the sciatic and common peroneal nerve in the lower limb. In one survey, the mean age was 31.8 years (range 2–81 years) and the male:female ratio was 2.4:1 [4].

Clinical features and investigations

The major clinical signs associated with peripheral nerve injury are disturbed sensation, weakness or paralysis of muscle, vasomotor and sudomotor paralysis in the distribution of the affected nerve [1]. The severity of clinical signs depends on the degree of nerve injury; signs are less severe in mild compression and entrapment syndromes and most severe following transection in penetrating injuries or in damage associated with a bone fracture. Complete division of a nerve is often painless whereas an incomplete division may be painful [1]. Abnormal sensitivity at the point of injury is probably due to regenerating nerve fibers. Sympathetic paralysis, leaving the skin warm and dry, is an important sign evident 24 hours after injury [1]. The Hoffman–Tinel sign, used in the diagnosis of entrapment neuropathies such as carpal and cubital tunnel syndromes, is positive when a tingling sensation occurs in a specific anatomical distribution if the nerve is lightly percussed. Persistent continuous or episodic neuropathic pain with dysesthesia and allodynia occurs as a consequence of several peripheral nerve lesions, including entrapment syndromes. Direct injuries to nerves in the limbs including the brachial plexus, radial, ulnar, and peroneal nerves result in neuropathic pain in some 50% of affected patients [5].

Peripheral Nerve Disorders: Pathology and Genetics, First Edition. Edited by Jean-Michel Vallat, Joachim Weis, Francoise Gray, and Katy Keohane.

Electrophysiology is used to determine the site and extent of nerve trauma and to assess whether the damage is demyelinating or axonal [3]. MRI is used to assess damage to deep structures, such as the brachial plexus or to detect tumors compressing peripheral nerves.

Pathology

The most commonly adopted schemes to classify traumatic injuries of peripheral nerves were developed by Seddon and by Sunderland [3, 6] and are summarized in Table 36.1. The Seddon scheme is used more frequently and injuries are classified with increasing severity as neurapraxia, axonotmesis, and neurotmesis [6].

Schemes to classify traumatic injuries of peripheral nerves

Neurapraxia

Neurapraxia is the mildest form of peripheral nerve injury. There is motor and sensory loss and no evidence of axonal degeneration. The nerve distal to the injury conducts normally, although there is conduction block at the site of injury, which is usually the result of focal demyelination as discussed next. Complete recovery of function may require weeks or a few months. Such injuries occur during acute compression. Examples are lying awkwardly in an armchair resulting in acute wrist drop ("Saturday night palsy"), entrapment syndromes including carpal tunnel syndrome from median nerve compression at the wrist and cubital tunnel syndrome from ulnar nerve compression at the elbow. Nerves associated with joints such as the elbow and wrist glide through the tissue during flexion and extension; the median nerve glides as much as 14.5 mm at the wrist [2]. Nerve entrapment results in a mixture of stretching, compression and damage to the blood supply. Applying a tourniquet in experimental studies produced graded severity of peripheral nerve damage [7]. The least severe was a reversible physiological conduction block, or more accurately a conduction failure in the nerve segment distal to the site of ischemia that recovered quickly if the tourniquet was released within 40 minutes. A common clinical example of such transient ischemia is when a leg "goes to sleep" on crossing the legs and symptoms recover once the limb posture is changed. This type of lesion has no recognizable microscopic or ultrastructural pathology. More severe damage from the tourniquet led to compression and displacement of myelin resulting in paranodal or internodal demyelination. The most severe cases had frank axonal degeneration. This work suggests that, following nerve compression, fluid is expressed from the endoneurial compartments, with subsequent damage to myelin and ultimately to axons.

Table 36.1 Classification of nerve injuries.

Seddon Classification (By Name)	Sunderland Classification (By Grade)	Pathology	Prognosis
Neurapraxia	I First Degree	Mild demyelination of nerve sheath.	Recovery of nerve conduction deficit is full, and requires days to months.
Axonotmesis	II Second Degree	Loss of continuity of axon. Endoneurial tubes intact. Perineurium and epineurium intact.	Recovery can occur by axonal regrowth along endoneurial tubes (months).
	III Third Degree	Loss of axons and endoneurial tubes. Perineurium/epineurium intact.	Recovery depends on axons finding endoneurial tubes. Mild to moderate loss of function.
	IV Fourth Degree	Axon loss with disruption of endoneurial tubes and perineurium. Epineurium intact.	Prognosis poor without surgical intervention.
Neurotmesis	V Fifth Degree	Axon loss. Endoneurial tubes/perineurium/ epineurium severed.	Recovery not possible without appropriate surgical treatment.

Adapted from Robinson, 2000 [3].

Changes to myelin occur immediately on nerve compression, suggesting they are due to direct compression of myelin and axons rather than to ischemia that would take longer to develop [7]. Post-mortem examination of human ulnar nerves at the elbow and median nerves under the flexor retinaculum in an unselected population revealed increased fibrosis and increased Renaut bodies, suggesting some degree of compressive or entrapment damage even in unaffected individuals [8]. Renaut bodies are frequently found at sites of nerve entrapment, but can also occasionally be present in a sural nerve biopsy (see Fig. 7.20).

Axonotmesis

Axonotmesis is commonly seen in entrapment and stretching injuries such as birth-related brachial plexus injuries, or with fractures, as in radial nerve injury secondary to fracture of the humerus. Axons and myelin are damaged but endoneurial, perineurial, and epineurial structures are partially or entirely preserved [3, 6]. The degree of recovery depends on the severity of the injury but, since connective tissue elements are preserved, axons may regrow along Schwann cell bands, guided by an intact perineurium.

Neurotmesis

Neurotmesis is the most severe type of nerve injury in which axons, myelin, perineurium, and epineurium are damaged. The nerve may be completely severed. Regrowth of axons is distorted by lack of perineurial sheaths and blocked by the development of scar tissue at the site of injury. This type of injury occurs with major trauma and surgical intervention may be necessary to avoid severe paralysis and sensory loss [1].

Focal lesions associated with trauma and compression

Traumatic (amputation) neuromas

Traumatic neuroma (TN) or amputation neuroma is an exuberant reparative nerve process secondary to amputation or trauma resulting in disorganized tangles of regenerating axons that may occur in numerous sites. Following nerve damage, regenerating axons grow along columns of Schwann cells (the bands of Büngner) to reinnervate the affected area [9]. If regeneration fails due to separation of the proximal and distal portions of the nerve, regeneration to the distal stump is blocked by scar tissue and axons may grow outside the original course sometimes creating free-nerve endings (terminals of Perroncito). These small bundles of regenerating neurites, often surrounded by perineurial cells, form a swelling – a TN (Fig. 36.1). Immunohistochemistry for neurofilament proteins (axons), EMA, GLUT-1 and claudin-1 (perineurial cells), and S-100 protein (Schwann cells) identify the components of a TN. Numerous α-smooth muscle actin-positive myofibroblasts are present surrounding and within the neuroma. Macrophages migrate into the neuroma within the first two weeks after injury and ingest cell and myelin debris. Macrophages may also contribute to chronic pain by releasing substances influencing axon regeneration or by direct action on the denuded remodeling membranes [10]. Immunohistochemistry and radioimmunoassay have shown focal accumulation of sodium channels within the tips of injured axons that may be partly responsible for ectopic axonal excitability and the resulting abnormal pain and paresthesia [10]. Myofibroblasts in TN participate in the scar contracture, and the neuroma may crush regenerating nerve fibers leading to persistent neuroma-associated pain [11].

All elements of the nerve fascicle are present in TN, so neurofibromas enter into the differential diagnosis. The similarities may be striking; sometimes identifying the characteristic collagen bundles of a neurofibroma enables a final diagnosis. Solitary circumscribed neuroma (SCN) is another differential diagnosis. SCN is of unknown etiology, is regarded as benign, and can be conceptualized as a hyperplastic expansion of cutaneous peripheral nerve Schwann cells and axons [12].

Morton's neuroma

Morton's neuroma (MN) (Fig. 36.2), also known as Morton's metatarsalgia, or localized interdigital neuritis, is an entrapment neuropathy with fibrosis mainly involving the perineurium. MN is usually located in the third web space between the third and fourth metatarsal heads; similar lesions occur in the hand, some have been related to chronic work-related or recreational injuries [13] The exact cause of this condition is unknown. Several hypotheses have been put forward including chronic repetitive trauma of the plantar nerve against the transverse intermetatarsal ligament combined with local ischemia. Nerve compression due to excessive weight bearing on the forefoot related to the use of high-heeled shoes has been implicated and may explain the higher prevalence of MN in middle-aged

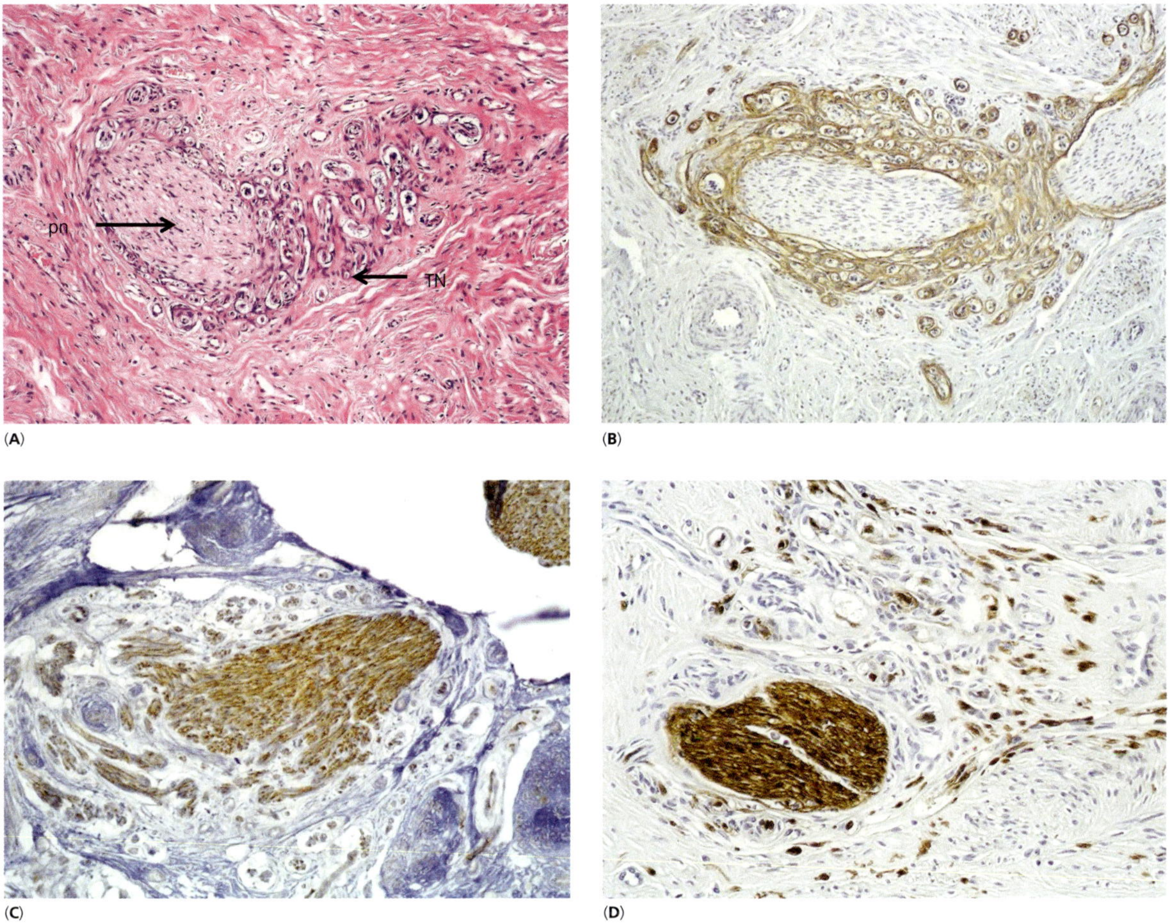

Figure 36.1 Traumatic neuroma. Histological and immunocytochemical stains show the elements in a traumatic neuroma. (**A**) A peripheral nerve (pn) stained by H&E is associated with numerous small nerve fascicles that represent the traumatic neuroma (TN). Immunocytochemistry for epithelial membrane antigen (**B**) shows that each of the small fascicles is surrounded by perineurial cells and (**C**) contain small numbers of axons stained with an antibody against neurofilament protein. (**D**) S-100 positive Schwann cells are present in the main nerve fascicle and in the small fascicles of the traumatic neuroma. Magnifications: (**A**): ×100; (**B**): ×100; (**C**): ×200; (**D**): ×100.

women. MNs in feet with *cavus* or forefoot deformity further support a mechanical pathogenesis.

Symptoms of MN include pain, a burning sensation, numbness, and paresthesia, primarily occurring during weight bearing on the bottom of the foot in the region of the intermetatarsal spaces; symptoms are relieved by rest and removing the shoe. Ultrasound can differentiate a bursa (which is compressible) from a neuroma (which is not compressible). MRI has detected MN in asymptomatic patients [13]. On physical examination, a mass may be palpated in 33% of patients with radiating pain into the affected toes. Mulder's sign is a "click" produced by direct pressure between the two metatarsal heads, while simultaneously putting pressure on the interdigital space with the other hand [13].

Histologically, there is perineurial fibrosis around the intermetatarsal nerves associated with vascular hyalinization, edema, and neural degeneration. Elastic fibers are increased at the periphery, focally resembling an elastofibroma. Thrombosed blood vessels are sometimes present. Immunohistochemistry for neurofilament and S-100 proteins demonstrates a reduction of axons and Schwann cells reflecting nerve damage (Fig. 36.2). Variable numbers of CD163/CD68-positive macrophages

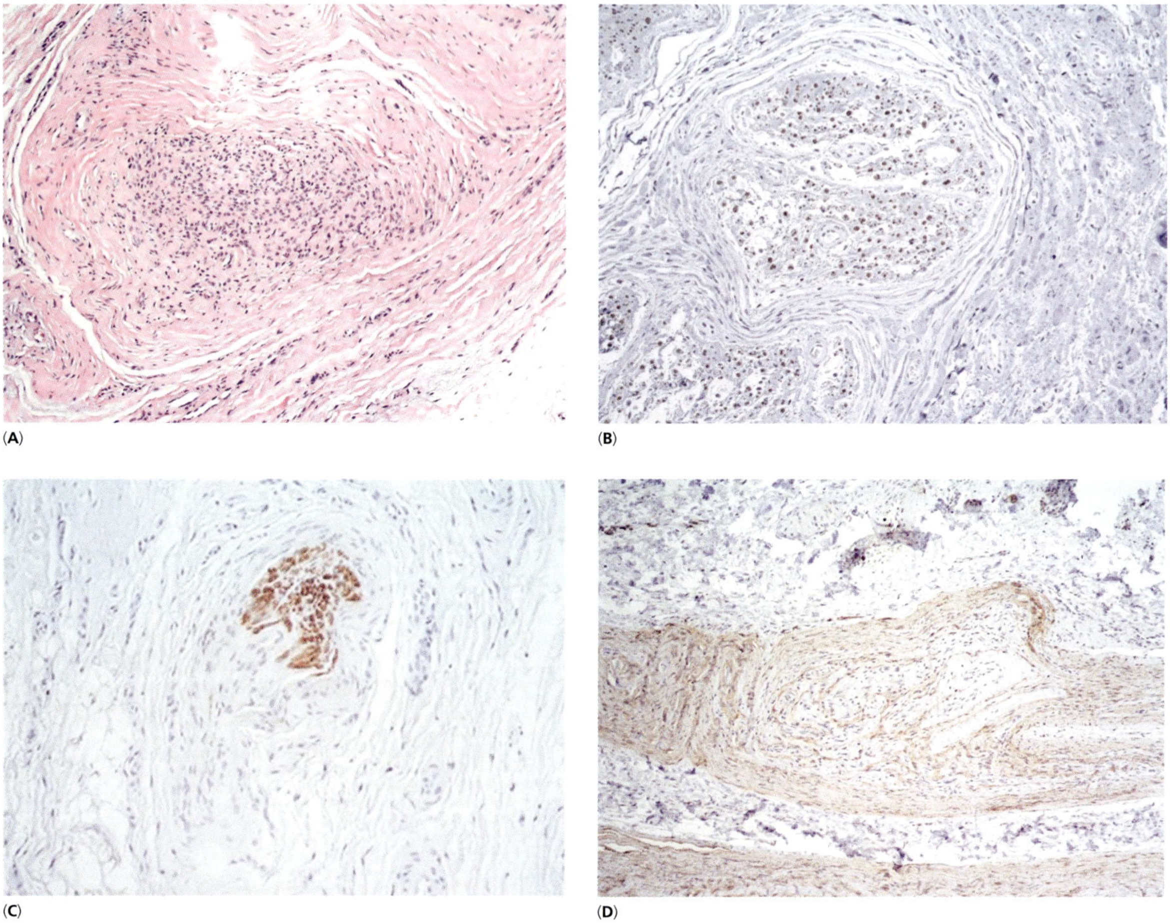

Figure 36.2 Morton's neuroma. An H&E stain (**A**) shows a nerve fascicle surrounded by dense fibrous tissue, but neural elements are preserved as seen in (**B**) where axons are stained with an antibody to neurofilament protein and (**C**) Schwann cells are identified by the S-100 stain; (**D**) shows the distorted nature of the damaged perineurium in the EMA stain. Magnifications: (**A**): ×200; (**B**): ×200; (**C**): ×200; (**D**): ×100.

are present throughout the lesion and a lymphocyte infiltrate may also be seen. Similar changes in plantar digital nerves from asymptomatic patients suggest the changes in MN may not be responsible for the symptoms of interdigital metatarsalgia [14].

The differential diagnosis of MN includes metatarsal stress fracture, intermetatarsal bursitis, true neuroma, inflammatory arthritis, pigmented villonodular synovitis, osteomyelitis, foreign body granuloma, stress fracture, osteochondritis of the metatarsal head (Freiberg's disease), and metatarsophalangeal joint dislocation. In these instances, MRI has a proven value in establishing the underlying cause of the intermetatarsal pain.

Reparative perineurial hyperplasia (RPH)

Beer found hyperplastic proliferation of perineurial cells associated with fine nerves in the mid or deep dermis of re-excision skin specimens [15]. This resulted from concentric proliferation of perineurial cells around nerves intimately associated with fibrosis. Awareness of RPH in healing surgical wounds or in some traumatic conditions is important to avoid its misdiagnosis as malignant perineurial invasion [15].

Traumatic localized hypertrophic neuropathy (LHN)

Focal enlargement of peripheral nerves has been reported involving the median nerve above the elbow [16] and at sites of nerve compression or entrapment involving the posterior interosseous branch of the radial nerve in the forearm and the common peroneal nerve at the head of the fibula [17]. Histology of the lesions varies; lesions at sites of compression or entrapment may result from local perineurial damage with formation of micro-fascicles encompassing small numbers of nerve fibers similar to traumatic neuromas (see Figs. 36.1A,B) [17, 18]. These lesions possibly result from recurrent demyelination due to compression or entrapment of the nerve. LHN should be distinguished from neoplastic perineuriomas [19] and other forms of neoplastic or hereditary localized hypertrophic neuropathy (see Chapter 37), which may contain onion bulbs formed by Schwann cells [16] and more closely resemble generalized hypertrophic neuropathy.

Genetics

Hereditary neuropathy with liability to pressure palsy (HNPP), also known as "tomaculous neuropathy" (*tomaculum*=Latin for sausage), is about the only genetic disorder associated with nerve trauma (see also Chapter 15). Tomaculous neuropathy can mimic an entrapment neuropathy [20].

Differential diagnosis

Nerve entrapment syndromes should be distinguished from peripheral nerve diseases such as multifocal motor neuropathy and neuralgic amyotrophy that can mimic entrapment neuropathies [21] The differential diagnosis in nerve trauma includes diverse entities such as amyotrophic lateral sclerosis, diabetic neuropathy, HIV polyneuropathy, multiple sclerosis, various peripheral neuropathies, polyarteritis nodosa, and syringomyelia [21].

Pathogenesis

In acute compression lesions of peripheral nerves, there is distortion of myelin with nodal and internodal demyelination; more severe compression results in axonal degeneration [7]. In more chronic compressive and entrapment lesions, ischemia appears important in inducing nerve damage as nerves are stretched and compressed due to restriction of gliding movement [2]. Blood vessels associated with nerves are damaged in transection injuries and the resulting ischemia may interfere with regeneration of damaged axons.

Animal models

Animal models have been used to study the pathology of acute and chronic peripheral nerve compression and nerve transection [7, 20]. In one study, rats were trained to reach for a food pellet several times per day for 3–12 weeks. At 5–6 weeks there were numerous macrophages in the nerves and at week 12, collagen type I immunoreactivity was detected in the epineurium at the wrist, similar to that seen in humans [22].

Conclusions and future perspectives

Molecular therapy for treatment of nerve injuries is currently under development [23] but only animal models have been studied. Neurotrophic factors such as nerve growth factor (NGF), brain-derived neurotrophic factor (BDNF), neurotrophin-3 (NT-3), neurotrophin-4/5 (NT-4/5), and neurotrophin-6 (NT-6) have well-documented potential to support neuron survival and stimulate neurite outgrowth, making them excellent candidates for stimulating repair of injured nerves [24]. Nerve repair is enhanced by the controlled release of a combination of neurotrophins, at higher concentrations [25] but such therapy has yet to be successfully used in the treatment of peripheral nerve injuries [25].

References

1 Birch R. (2005) Operating on peripheral nerves. In: Dyck PJ, Thomas PK, (eds). *Peripheral Neuropathy*. 4th edn, pp. 1511–1532. Elsevier, Philadelphia.

2 Rempel D, Dahlin L, Lundborg G. (1999) Pathophysiology of nerve compression syndromes: response of peripheral nerves to loading. *J Bone Joint Surg Am* 81,1600–1610.

3 Robinson LR. (2000) Traumatic injury to peripheral nerves. *Muscle Nerve* 23,863–873.

4 Eser F, Aktekin LA, Bodur H, Atan C. (2009) Etiological factors of traumatic peripheral nerve injuries. *Neurol India* 57,434–437.

5 Ciaramitaro P, Mondelli M, Logullo F, *et al.* (2010) Traumatic peripheral nerve injuries: epidemiological findings, neuropathic pain and quality of life in 158 patients. *J Peripher Nerv Syst* 15,120–127.

6 Burnett MG, Zager EL. (2004) Pathophysiology of peripheral nerve injury: a brief review. *Neurosurg Focus* 16,1–7.
7 Ochoa J, Fowler TJ, Gilliatt RW. (1972) Anatomical changes in peripheral nerves compressed by a pneumatic tourniquet. *J Anat* 113,433–455.
8 Neary D, Ochoa J, Gilliatt RW. (1975) Sub-clinical entrapment neuropathy in man. *J Neurol Sci* 24,283–298.
9 Zochodne DW. (2012) The challenges and beauty of peripheral nerve regrowth. *J Peripher Nerv Syst* 17,1–18.
10 Zochodne DW. (2000) The microenvironment of injured and regenerating peripheral nerves. *Muscle Nerve* Suppl 9,S33–38.
11 Yan H, Gao W, Pan Z, Zhang F, Fan C. (2012) The expression of alpha-SMA in the painful traumatic neuroma: potential role in the pathobiology of neuropathic pain. *J Neurotrauma* 29,2791–2797.
12 Jokinen CH, Ragsdale BD, Argenyi ZB. (2010) Expanding the clinicopathologic spectrum of palisaded encapsulated neuroma. *J Cutan Pathol* 37,43–48.
13 Bencardino J, Rosenberg ZS, Beltran J, Liu X, Marty-Delfaut E. (2000) Morton's neuroma: is it always symptomatic? *AJR Am J Roentgenol* 175,649–653.
14 Bourke G, Owen J, Machet D. (1994) Histological comparison of the third interdigital nerve in patients with Morton's metatarsalgia and control patients. *Aust N Z J Surg* 64,421–424.
15 Beer TW. (2009) Reparative perineural hyperplasia: a series of 10 cases. *Am J Dermatopathol* 31,50–52.
16 Koszyca B, Jones N, Kneebone C, Blumbergs P. (2009) Localized hypertrophic neuropathy: a case report and review of the literature. *Clin Neuropathol* 28,54–58.
17 Weller RO. (1974) Letter: "Localised hypertrophic neuropathy" and hypertrophic polyneuropathy. *Lancet* 2,592–593.
18 Neary D, Ochoa J. (1975) Letter: Localized hypertrophic neuropathy, intraneural tumour, or chronic nerve entrapment? *Lancet* 1,632–633.
19 Koutlas IG, Scheithauer BW, Folpe AL. (2010) Intraoral perineurioma, soft tissue type: report of five cases, including 3 intraosseous examples, and review of the literature. *Head Neck Pathol* 4,113–120.
20 Goebbels S, Oltrogge JH, Wolfer S, Wieser GL, Nientiedt T, Pieper A, Ruhwedel T, Groszer M, Sereda MW, Nave KA. (2012) Genetic disruption of Pten in a novel mouse model of tomaculous neuropathy. *EMBO Mol Med* 4,486–499.
21 England JD. (1999) Entrapment neuropathies. *Curr Opin Neurol* 12,597–602.
22 Keir PJ, Rempel DM. (2005) Pathomechanics of peripheral nerve loading. Evidence in carpal tunnel syndrome. *J Hand Ther* 18,259–269.
23 Jaggi AS, Singh N. (2011) Therapeutic targets for the management of peripheral nerve injury-induced neuropathic pain. *CNS Neurol Disord Drug Targets* 10,589–609.
24 Alsina FC, Ledda F, Paratcha G. (2012) New insights into the control of neurotrophic growth factor receptor signaling: implications for nervous system development and repair. *J Neurochem* 123,652–661.
25 Deister C, Schmidt CE. (2006) Optimizing neurotrophic factor combinations for neurite outgrowth. *J Neural Eng* 3,172–179.

CHAPTER 37

Localized hypertrophic neuropathy, intraneural perineurioma, polyneuropathy with perineurial cell hyperplasia, and minifascicular neuropathy

Joachim Weis

Institute of Neuropathology, RWTH Aachen University Hospital and JARA Brain Translational Medicine, Aachen, Germany

Introduction

In the past, the term "localized hypertrophic neuropathy" has been used to describe lesions characterized by numerous onion bulb formations and increased extracellular matrix, leading to diffuse focal enlargement of individual nerves and their branches. Most cases did not show evidence of hereditary or inflammatory hypertrophic neuropathy, or of a nerve sheath tumor or neurofibromatosis. In recent years it became clear that, even if all these differential diagnoses are excluded, at least two forms of focal hypertrophic neuropathy have to be distinguished. In the "classical" form of localized hypertrophic neuropathy the onion bulbs are formed by Schwann cells. The second entity is characterized by onion bulbs that are mostly composed of cells that show perineurial differentiation. Two further entities included in this chapter, polyneuropathy with perineurial cell hyperplasia and minifascicular neuropathy, are not focal in nature, but are also characterized by prominent alterations of the perineurium and of perineurial cells, and are therefore discussed here.

Localized hypertrophic neuropathy

Definition, clinical presentation, and genetics

This entity is defined as a rare, non-hereditary, localized Schwann cell proliferation involving isolated nerves and characterized by onion bulb formation [1, 2]. The clinical presentation is that of a localized neuropathy. Among the few cases published so far, the trigeminal nerve is predominantly affected [2].

Histopathology, differential diagnosis, and pathogenesis

Macroscopically, the nerve shows a diffuse, fusiform enlargement.

Light microscopically, the lesion is characterized by numerous, often multilayered, S100-immunoreactive Schwann cell onion bulb formations encircling variably myelinated axons [1]. Collagen content of the extracellular matrix is increased, and alcian-blue-positive mucoid substance may accumulate in the extracellular space. Inflammatory infiltrates are absent. The histological picture is similar to that seen in generalized hypertrophic neuropathies [1, 2].

Ultrastructurally, the cells are covered by a continuous basal lamina and lack the pinocytotic vesicles and numerous cell-cell contacts of perineurial cells [1].

The differential diagnosis also includes localized hypertrophic neuritis and CIDP, which feature onion bulb formation combined with mononuclear inflammatory infiltration (see Chapter 27). Localized hypertrophic neuropathy must be distinguished from perineurioma, a macroscopically similar process leading to diffuse nerve enlargement. The multilayered onion bulbs in perineuriomas, however, are formed by proliferating cells showing perineurial features

Peripheral Nerve Disorders: Pathology and Genetics, First Edition. Edited by Jean-Michel Vallat, Joachim Weis, Francoise Gray, and Katy Keohane.

("pseudo-onion bulbs," see next). The pathogenesis of localized hypertrophic neuropathy is unclear [2]. Some authors consider a reactive, traumatic cause, others favor a neoplastic process [2].

Intraneural perineurioma

Definition, genetics, and epidemiology

Perineurioma has been defined as a tumor composed entirely of cells showing perineurial differentiation [3]. Intraneural perineuriomas infiltrate the perineurium and the endoneurium. Extraneural soft tissue perineuriomas are often located in the subcutaneous tissue. They grow without obvious connection to a larger nerve, but may show residual entrapped Schwann cells and axons [4]. Sclerosing and reticular (retiform) variants of extraneural soft tissue perineurioma exist [4]. In two case of intraneural perineurioma, cytogenetic analysis revealed a homozygous deficiency of chromosomal material 22q11.2qter [5]. In a second case of the same series, 53% of interphase nuclei showed three FISH signals with a chromosome 14/22 probe, suggesting either monosomy for the centromere of chromosome 14 or that of chromosome 22 [5]. These findings were interpreted as evidence of a clonal and thus neoplastic nature of perineuriomas [5]. Chromosomal alterations in this region have been reported more frequently in soft tissue perineuriomas [6]. Whether this is true for all perineuriomas remains an open question [7]. No clear association with neurofibromatosis has been found for either form of perineurioma [4, 7] with the exception of one case [6]. Intraneural perineurioma usually affects children and young adults [7].

Clinical presentation

Large nerve trunks, in particular the sciatic nerve and its branches, are the most frequent sites of intraneural perineurioma [7]. However, plexus or smaller nerves including the sural nerve may also be affected [7, 8]. The nerve segments infiltrated by perineuriomas show a fusiform enlargement; the lesions range from a few cm to more than 30 cm in length. Motor symptoms are more frequent than sensory symptoms [7, 9]. A characteristic MRI pattern with isointensity on T1 and hyperintensity on T2 imaging and prominent contrast enhancement has been reported [7]. Most lesions run a benign course with little, if any progression or spread over time [7].

Histopathology

Perineuriomas consist of spindle-shaped cells with long processes and isomorphic nuclei that infiltrate the perineurium and the endoneurium, forming so-called "pseudo-onion bulbs" around single or small groups of myelinated or unmyelinated nerve fibers (Fig. 37.1A).

Perineurioma cells are EMA, and often claudin and human erythrocyte glucose transporter-1 (GLUT-1) immunoreactive, but are negative for S100 [4, 5].

Ultrastructurally, they display elongated cytoplasmic processes with pinocytotic vesicles, frequent cell-cell contacts including poorly developed tight junctions and an incomplete basal lamina [4, 6].

Rarely, aberrant differentiations including ossification, granular or adipocytic transformation, or plexiform spread have been reported [4]. Malignant perineuriomas/malignant peripheral nerve sheath tumors with perineurial differentiation are rare [10].

Polyneuropathy with perineurial cell hyperplasia

Cases of polyneuropathy associated with prominent, focally accentuated perineurial cell hyperplasia have been described repeatedly. In these cases, endoneurial "pseudo-onion blubs" consisting of abnormal perineurial cells and/or abnormal compartmentalization of the endoneurium by dysplastic perineurial cells or subperineurial perineurial cell hyperplasia were observed (Fig. 37.1B). Interestingly, this peculiar neuropathy could be part of a variable syndromic picture that includes cataracts, mental retardation and/or optic nerve atrophy [11–15].

Minifascicular neuropathy (MIM 607080)

Minifascicular neuropathy (MFNP) was first described in a patient with 46XY mixed gonadal dysgenesis and symptoms of distal, predominantly sensory neuropathy and slowing of motor and sensory nerve conduction [16]. Sural nerve biopsy revealed about 50 fascicles that contained many smaller subfascicles (minifascicles), each surrounded by cells with perineurial differentiation. These cells extended processes into the endoneurium, indicating ongoing minifascicle formation. The

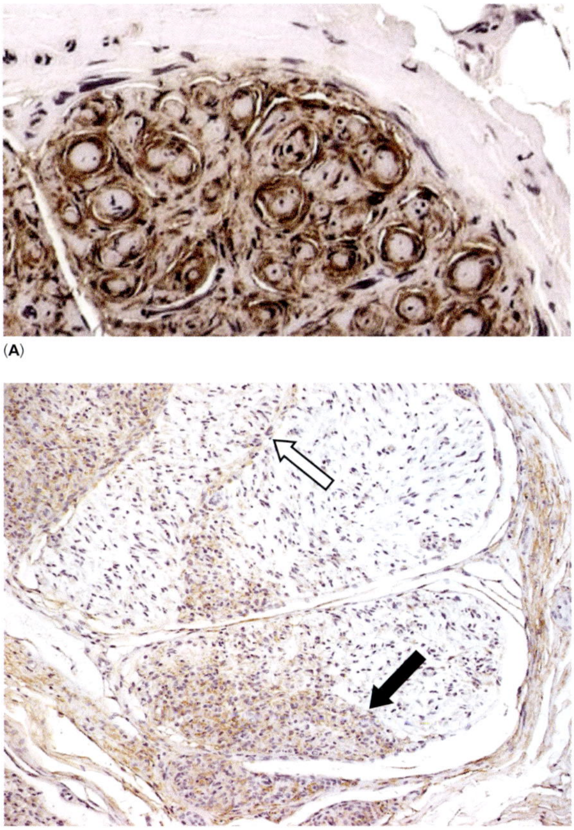

(**A**)

(**B**)

Figure 37.1 (**A**) Perineurioma: Endoneurial whorls of EMA-immunoreactive tumor cells ("pseudo-oninon bulb formations"). (**B**) Polyneuropathy with perineurial cell hyperplasia: Patchy, often subperineurial (black arrow) proliferations of EMA-immunoreactive perineurial cells. White arrow: Abnormal septum formed by EMA-immunoreactive cells.

density of myelinated fibers was decreased; there were no onion bulb formations. Similar cases were reported subsequently, and a desert hedgehog homolog (DHH) gene mutation was found in one patient and the patient´s father, indicating that the DHH protein might be involved in the formation and maintenance of the perineurium [17]. Cases of hereditary motor and sensory neuropathy with minifascicle formation in a patient with 46XY pure gonadal dysgenesis [18], of MFNP in a patient with 46XY gonadal dysgenesis and normal DHH gene [19], of MFNP in a patient with normal karyotype [20], and of motor-sensory neuropathy without minifascicles in 46XY gonadal dysgenesis have also been reported [21].

References

1 Scheithauer BW, Woodruff JM, Erlandson RA (1999) *Tumors of the Peripheral Nervous System*: Armed Forces Institute of Pathology, Washington D.C.

2 Koszyca B, Jones N, Kneebone C, Blumbergs P (2009) Localized hypertrophic neuropathy: a case report and review of the literature. *Clin Neuropathol;*28:54–58.

3 Scheithauer BW, Woodruff JM, Antonescu CR (2007) Perineurioma. *In:* Louis DN, Ohgaki H, Wiestler OD, Cavenee WK (eds). WHO *Classification of Tumours of the Central Nervous System*, pp. 158–159. International Agency for Research on Cancer, Lyon.

4 Macarenco RS, Ellinger F, Oliveira AM (2007) Perineurioma: a distinctive and underrecognized peripheral nerve sheath neoplasm. *Arch Pathol Lab Med;*131:625–636.

5 Emory TS, Scheithauer BW, Hirose T *et al.* (1995) Intraneural perineurioma. A clonal neoplasm associated with abnormalities of chromosome 22. *Am J Clin Pathol;*103: 696–704.

6 Boyanton BL, Jr., Jones JK, Shenaq SM *et al.* (2007) Intraneural perineurioma: a systematic review with illustrative cases. *Arch Pathol Lab Med;*131:1382–1392.

7 Mauermann ML, Amrami KK, Kuntz NL *et al.* (2009) Longitudinal study of intraneural perineurioma – a benign, focal hypertrophic neuropathy of youth. *Brain;*132: 2265–2276.

8 Sciacco M, Scarpini E, Baron PL *et al.* (1992) Sural nerve immunoreactivity for nerve growth factor receptor in a case of localized hypertrophic neuropathy. *Acta Neuropathol;*83: 547–553.

9 Scheller C, Richter HP, Scheuerle A *et al.* (2008) Intraneural perineuriomas; a rare entity. Clinical, surgical and neuropathological details in the management of these lesions. *Zentralbl Neurochir;*69:134–138.

10 Mitchell A, Scheithauer BW, Doyon J *et al.* (2012) Malignant perineurioma (malignant peripheral nerve sheath tumor with perineural differentiation). *Clin Neuropathol;*31:424–429.

11 Wolfe GI, Brower RD, Burns DK (2000) Perineurial cell hyperplasia in early-onset polyneuropathy with multiple cranial neuropathies. *Neuromuscul Disord;*10:503–506.

12 Jay V, Vajsar J, Haslam R (1996) Axonal neuropathy with perineurial hyperplasia: report of a case with multifocal involvement. *J Child Neurol;*11:400–403.

13 Thomas PK, King RH, Workman JM, Schroder JM (2000) Hypertrophic perineurial dysplasia in multifocal and generalized peripheral neuropathies. *Neuropathol Appl Neurobiol;* 26:536–543.

14 Schroder JM, Rollnik JD, Schubert M, Dengler R (1999) Demyelinating sensorimotor neuropathy with congenital cataract, mental retardation, and unique, dysplastic perineurial cells within the endoneurium. *Acta Neuropathol;*98:421–426.

15 Nakamura N, Oka N, Nakamura S *et al.* (1995) [A case with hereditary motor and sensory neuropathy with

multiple cranial nerves involvement]. *Rinsho Shinkeigaku;* 35:516–520.

16 Umehara F, Yamaguchi N, Kodama D *et al.* (1999) Polyneuropathy with minifascicle formation in a patient with 46XY mixed gonadal dysgenesis. *Acta Neuropathol;*98:309–312.

17 Umehara F, Tate G, Itoh K, Yamaguchi N *et al.* (2000) A novel mutation of desert hedgehog in a patient with 46,XY partial gonadal dysgenesis accompanied by minifascicular neuropathy. *Am J Hum Genet;*67:1302–1305.

18 Sugie K, Futamura N, Suzumura A *et al.* (2002) Hereditary motor and sensory neuropathy with minifascicle formation in a patient with 46XY pure gonadal dysgenesis: a new clinical entity. *Ann Neurol;*51:385–388.

19 Baets J, Dierick I, Groote CC *et al.* (2009) Peripheral neuropathy and 46XY gonadal dysgenesis: a heterogeneous entity. *Neuromuscul Disord;*19:172–175.

20 Malandrini A, Gambelli S, Muglia M *et al.* (2005) Motor-sensory neuropathy with minifascicle formation in a woman with normal karyotype. *Neurology;*65:776.

21 Malandrini A, Gambelli S, Muglia M *et al.* (2008) Motor-sensory neuropathy without minifascicles in a patient with 46XY gonadal dysgenesis. *Brain Dev;*30:291–294.

CHAPTER 38

Neurolymphomatosis and rare focal or multifocal lesions

Joachim Weis
Institute of Neuropathology, RWTH Aachen University Hospital and JARA Brain Translational Medicine, Aachen, Germany

Introduction

In most cases, a nerve biopsy is performed to obtain diagnostic information when a disease process affects large parts of the peripheral nervous system in a more or less disseminated, diffuse manner. In some cases, however, a nerve selected for biopsy demonstrates a focal lesion confined to the biopsied nerve segment, or a systemic disease causing multiple focal lesions. This chapter provides an overview on such neoplastic and non-neoplastic, often space-occupying processes that can be found in sural and other diagnostic nerve biopsies. These lesions present clinically with symptoms of focal or generalized neuropathy such as sensory deficits, dysesthesias, pain, and pareses. They include malignant lymphoma of the peripheral nerve, nerve ganglion cysts, and other rare disorders. The differential diagnoses include inflammatory and neurofibromatous neuropathies.

Neurolymphomatosis (lymphomatous neuropathy)

Definition and epidemiology

Non-Hodgkin's lymphoma may invade cranial or peripheral nerve roots, plexus or nerves (neurolymphomatous neuropathy or neurolymphomatosis) [1, 2]. The meninges might be affected simultaneously. Spread of a lymphoma from the CNS or elsewhere to the PNS is more common than a primary PNS manifestation. It is estimated that neurolymphomatosis has a relative incidence of around 3% of newly diagnosed intermediate- or high-grade Non-Hodgkin's lymphomas [1, 2]. In some cases, symptoms of neuropathy precede the diagnosis of neurolymphomatosis for many months; this has been interpreted as evidence suggesting that lymphoma may arise by malignant degeneration of an autoreactive B cell clone targeting peripheral neural structures [1]. Neurolymphomatosis may be combined with vasculitis, monoclonal gammopathy or cryoglobulinemia. Hodgkin's lymphoma less frequently infiltrates peripheral nerves than Non-Hodgkin's lymphoma, but both can be associated with autoimmune disorders that affect the PNS [2].

Clinical presentation

Neurolymphomatosis may manifest as cranial neuropathy, painful or painless polyneuropathy or polyradiculopathy, or peripheral mononeuropathy [1, 2]. At the later stages of disease, lymphomas primarily manifesting in the PNS may spread to the CNS [1]. Median survival has been reported to be in the range of 10 months after diagnosis [1]. Differential diagnoses include GBS, vasculitic neuropathy, carcinomatous meningitis, and neuropathies caused by infectious agents such as HIV or *Borrelia Burgdorferi* [3]. Imaging, especially MRI or PET-CT, may demonstrate diffuse or focally accentuated infiltration and thickening of peripheral nerves [2].

Histopathology

Nerve biopsies in neurolymphomatosis show tumor cell infiltration of the epineurium with a predilection for the perivascular space, indicating hematogenous spread [2]. Vessel wall destruction is usually absent,

Peripheral Nerve Disorders: Pathology and Genetics, First Edition. Edited by Jean-Michel Vallat, Joachim Weis, Francoise Gray, and Katy Keohane.

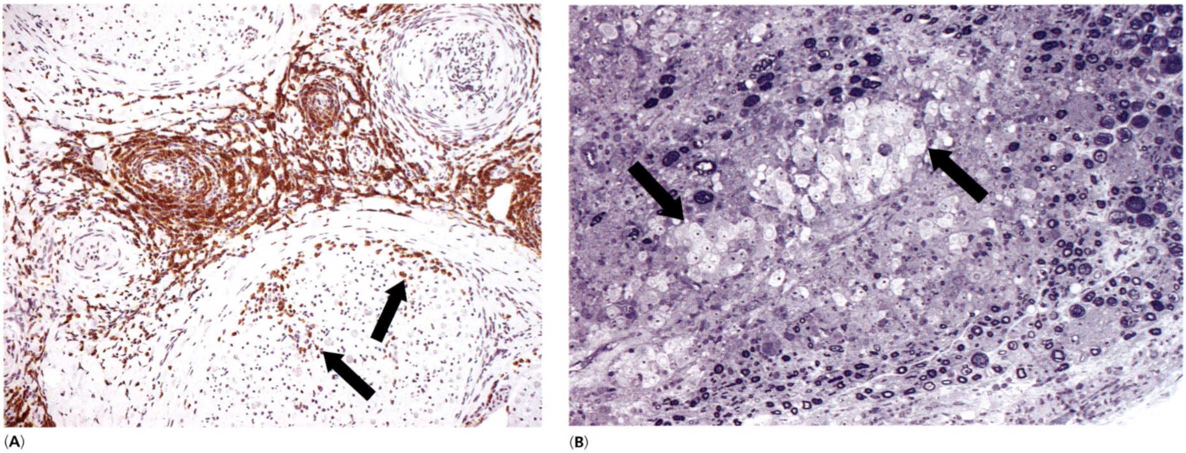

Figure 38.1 (**A**) Sural nerve in a case of neurolymphomatosis due to B cell lymphoma [3]. The neoplastic cells are CD79a-immunoreactive (brown) and show predominantly epineurial spread. Arrows: minor subperineurial and endoneurial infiltration. (**B**) Endoneurial infiltration of a peripheral nerve by adenocarcinoma cells (arrows). Semithin section, Toluidine blue.

unlike in vasculitis. Perineurium and endoneurium may be infiltrated by neoplastic cells to a variable extent. Most lymphomas that spread to peripheral nerves are B cell lymphomas and thus display B cell-associated antigens such as CD20 [1, 2] and CD79a [3] (Fig. 38.1A). The Ki67 index is high in most cases. The neoplastic cell infiltration leads to focally accentuated nerve fiber loss. Angiotropic lymphoma may also manifest in the PNS and can be found in nerve and muscle biopsies [4, 5].

Animal models

Marek's disease in chickens is a T cell lymphoma, which selectively affects peripheral nerves and is caused by avian cytomegalovirus infection [6].

Other malignant neoplastic lesions

Chronic lymphocytic leukemia and Waldenström´s macroglobulinemia may cause nerve damage indirectly by inducing autoimmunity or – in the case of Waldenström´s disease – by inducing amyloidosis. They also may infiltrate the nerve diffusely in a pattern similar to neurolymphomatosis [2] (see the previous section and Chapter 31). Peripheral neuropathy involving multiple nerves due to infiltration of nerve fascicles by carcinoma cells has rarely been reported, but may appear in sural [7] and other peripheral nerve biopsies (Fig. 38.1B).

Non-malignant neoplastic lesions

Schwannomas and other nerve sheath tumors rarely affect nerves used for diagnostic biopsy in an isolated manner [8]. In contrast, involvement of such nerves by so-called schwannoid tumorlets is common in neuropathies in the context of neurofibromatosis-2 (see Chapter 23). A granular cell tumor may arise from the sural nerve [9].

Non-neoplastic focal lesions

In a series of 36 cases with isolated sural neuropathy, Stickler and colleagues reported 16 patients with ankle trauma, three with vasculitis, and one patient each with schwannoma and ganglionic cyst [8]. Ganglionic cysts of the sural nerve have also been described by other authors [10–12]. Neuritis ossificans is another non-neoplastic focal lesion regarded as a reactive process, similar to myositis ossificans, in which zonally arranged fibrovascular tissue, osteoid, and bone formation occurs in the nerve. It may be of importance to pathologists examining sural nerve biopsies [13, 14].

References

1 Baehring JM, Batchelor TT (2012) Diagnosis and management of neurolymphomatosis. *Cancer J*;18:463–468.

2 Kelly JJ, Karcher DS (2005) Lymphoma and peripheral neuropathy: a clinical review. *Muscle Nerve*;31:301–313.

3 Urban PP, Kaczmarek E, Wellach I, *et al.* (2008) Neurolymphomatosis. Subacute sensorimotor polyneuropathy as a first sign of non-Hodgkin's B cell lymphoma. *Nervenarzt;* 79:699–702.

4 Levin KH, Lutz G (1996) Angiotropic large-cell lymphoma with peripheral nerve and skeletal muscle involvement: early diagnosis and treatment. *Neurology;*47:1009–1011.

5 Prayson RA (1996) Angiotropic large cell lymphoma: simultaneous peripheral nerve and skeletal muscle involvement. *Pathology;*28:25–27.

6 Lee LF, Roizman B, Spear PG, *et al.* (1969) Marek's disease herpes virus: a cytomegalovirus. *Proc Natl Acad Sci U S A;*64: 952–956.

7 Saikumar J, Li G, Chaudhary RT (2011) Reversible neuropathy after chemotherapy for metastatic adenocarcinoma from an unknown primary tumor to the sural nerve. *Am J Ther;* 18:e264–268.

8 Stickler DE, Morley KN, Massey EW (2006) Sural neuropathy: etiologies and predisposing factors. *Muscle Nerve;*34:482–484.

9 Daentzer D, Schmidinger A, Boker DK (2003) Atypical granular cell tumour of the sural nerve mimicking a Schwannoma. *Acta Neurochir (Wien);*145:1019–1020

10 Spinner RJ, Amrami KK, Ibrahim Elshiekh MA, Blitz NM (2012) Sural intraneural ganglion cysts are joint-related. *Arch Plast Surg;*39:77–79.

11 Blitz NM, Prestridge J, Amrami KK, Spinner RJ (2008) A posttraumatic, joint-connected sural intraneural ganglion cyst-with a new mechanism of intraneural recurrence: a case report. *J Foot Ankle Surg;*47:199–205.

12 Acciarri N, Giuliani G, Poppi M, *et al.* (1990) Sural neuropathy produced by intraneural ganglion. *J Foot Surg;*29: 231–232.

13 Katz LD, Lindskog D, Eisen R (2011) Neuritis ossificans of the tibial, common peroneal and lateral sural cutaneous nerves. *J Bone Joint Surg Br;*93:992–994.

14 George DH, Scheithauer BW, Spinner RJ, *et al.* (2002) Heterotopic ossification of peripheral nerve ("neuritis ossificans"): report of two cases. *Neurosurgery;*51:244–246.

Index

Note: Page references in *italics* refer to Figures; those in **bold** refer to Tables

Peripheral Nerve Disorders: Pathology and Genetics, First Edition. Edited by Jean-Michel Vallat, Joachim Weis, Francoise Gray, and Katy Keohane.